Guide to Advanced Medical Billing: A Reimbursement Approach

THIRD EDITION

Sharon Brown, Esq.

Lori Tyler, MS
President/Owner Lori Tyler & Associates

Boston   Columbus   Indianapolis   New York   San Francisco   Upper Saddle River
Amsterdam   Cape Town   Dubai   London   Madrid   Milan   Munich   Paris   Montreal   Toronto
Delhi   Mexico City   São Paulo   Sydney   Hong Kong   Seoul   Singapore   Taipei   Tokyo

Publisher: Julie Levin Alexander	**Production Editor:** Peggy Kellar
Publisher's Assistant: Regina Bruno	**Senior Media Editor:** Matt Norris
Editor-in-Chief: Marlene McHugh Pratt	**Media Project Manager:** Lorena Cerisano
Executive Editor: Joan Gill	**Manufacturing Manager:** Lisa McDowell
Associate Editor: Bronwen Glowacki	**Creative Director:** Andrea Nix
Editorial Assistant: Stephanie Kiel	**Senior Art Director:** Maria Guglielmo
Director of Marketing: David Gesell	**Interior Designer:** Ilze Lemesis
Marketing Manager: Katrin Beacom	**Cover Designer:** Ilze Lemesis
Senior Marketing Coordinator: Alicia Wozniak	**Cover Image:** Shutterstock/RoJo Images
Marketing Specialist: Michael Sirinides	**Composition:** Aptara®, Inc.
Marketing Assistant: Crystal Gonzalez	**Printing and Binding:** R.R. Donnelley/Harrisonburg
Managing Production Editor: Patrick Walsh	**Cover Printer:** R.R. Donnelley/Harrisonburg
Production Liaison: Julie Boddorf	

Credits and acknowledgments borrowed from other sources and reproduced, with permission, in this textbook appear on appropriate page within text.

Every effort has been made to provide accurate and current Internet information in this book. However, the Internet and information posted on it are constantly changing, so it is inevitable that some of the Internet addresses listed in this textbook will change.

Library of Congress Cataloging-in-Publication Data

Brown, Sharon E.
   Guide to advanced medical billing: a reimbursement approach / by Sharon Brown and Lori Tyler.—3rd ed.
     p. ; cm.
   Rev. ed. of: Guide to health claims examining. 2nd ed. c2007.
   Includes bibliographical references and index.
   ISBN-13: 978-0-13-504305-9
   ISBN-10: 0-13-504305-0
   I. Tyler, Lori.   II. Guide to health claims examining.   III. Title.
   [DNLM: 1. Practice Management, Medical—economics.   2. Forms and Records Control—methods.   3. Patient Credit and Collection.   4. Reimbursement Mechanisms. W 80]
   LC Classification not assigned
   368.38'2—dc23

2012046784

10 9 8 7 6 5 4 3 2

PEARSON

ISBN 13: 978-0-13-504305-9
ISBN 10:   0-13-504305-0

Disclaimer

This text is a guide for learning advanced concepts related to the billing, coding, examination, and processing of a healthcare claim. Decisions for coding and processing of claims should not be based solely on information within this guide. Decisions that affect the practice of processing health claims must be based on individual circumstances, including legal and ethical considerations, local conditions, and payer policies.

The information contained in this text is based on experience and research. However, in the complex, rapidly changing insurance environment, this information may not always prove correct. Data used are widely variable and can change at any time. Readers should follow current coding regulations as outlined by official coding organizations.

Any *Current Procedural Terminology* (*CPT*®) codes, services, descriptions, instructions, and/or guidelines are copyright 2012 (or other date of publication of *CPT* as defined in the federal copyright laws), American Medical Association, All Rights Reserved.

The *CPT* manual is a listing of descriptive terms and five-digit numeric identifying codes and modifiers for reporting medical services that are performed by physicians and other healthcare practitioners. This text includes only *CPT* descriptive terms, numeric identifying codes, and modifiers for reporting medical services and procedures that were selected for use in this publication. The most current version of the *CPT* is available from the American Medical Association. No fee schedules, basic unit values, relative value guides, conversion factors, or components thereof are included in the *CPT*.

The American Medical Association assumes no responsibility for the consequences attributable to, or related to, any use or interpretation of any information or views contained in or not contained in this publication.

Claims and forms contained in this text are examples only. The publisher and author do not accept responsibility for any adverse outcome from undetected errors, opinion, and analysis contained in this manual that may prove inaccurate or incorrect, or any outcome that results from the reader's misunderstanding of an extremely complex topic. All names used in this text are completely fictitious. Any resemblance to persons or companies, current or no longer existing, is purely coincidental.

Brief Contents

Preface xi

SECTION 1: Introduction to Issues Related to Health Claims Processing 1

1 Introduction to Technical and Legal Issues 2

2 Resource Manuals and Billing Forms 24

SECTION 2: Contract Interpretation and Administration 61

3 Medical Plan Provisions 62

4 Medical Benefit 94

SECTION 3: Medical Claims Examining Guidelines and Procedures 123

5 Medical Claims Administration 124

6 Physician's, Clinical, and Hospital Services Claims 157

7 Surgery and Anesthesia Claims 184

8 Medicare and Medicaid 214

9 Workers' Compensation 232

10 Managed Care Claims 246

SECTION 4: Management of Claims Examining 265

11 Claims Auditing 266

12 Processing Non-Medicare Claims 275

13 Processing Medicare Claims 286

14 Processing Workers' Compensation Claims 306

Appendix A: Contracts 315

Appendix B: Forms 322

Appendix C: Tables 331

Glossary 352

Index 363

Contents

Preface   xi

SECTION 1
Introduction to Issues Related to Health Claims Processing   1

1   Introduction to Technical and Legal Issues   2
The Rising Cost of Healthcare   4
Types of Insurance   5
Employee Benefits   6
Types of Health Benefit Plans   6
Medical Billing and Claims Examiner   7
The Regulatory Departments of Insurance   9
Legal Issues Pertaining to Disclaimers   10
Legal Issues Pertaining to Privacy Guidelines   11
Legal Issues Pertaining to Fraud   14
Healthcare Fraud and Abuse   17
Investigation   18
Embezzlement   19
Legal Damages   19
Maintenance of Records   20
Subpoenas Duces Tecum   21
Chapter Review   22

2   Resource Manuals and Billing Forms   24
ICD-CM (PCS)   25
CPT®/RVS   26
Health Care Common Procedure Coding System   27
Physicians' Desk Reference   28
Medical Dictionary   29
Merck Manual   29
Red Book and Blue Book   30
CMS-1500 Form   30
Version 5010: CMS-1500 and UB-04   37
Chapter Review   57

SECTION 2
Contract Interpretation and Administration   61

3   Medical Plan Provisions   62
Contract Validity   63
Group Contracts   64
Contract Provisions   65
Contract Benefits   66
Eligibility   69
Open Enrollment   73
Termination of Coverage   73
Continuation of Coverage   73
General Plan Provisions   78

Acts of Third Parties   78
Subrogation   84
Preexisting Conditions   85
Health Insurance Portability and Accountability Act   87
STATE Mandates   90
Prompt-Pay Laws   91
External or Independent Grievance Systems   91
Chapter Review   92

4   Medical Benefit   94
Benefit Definitions   95
Benefit Calculations   96
Calculating the Deductible   97
Common Accident Provision   98
Basic Benefits   100
Common Basic Benefits   101
Major Medical Benefits   104
Comprehensive Major Medical Benefits   105
Computing Stop-loss   105
Usual, Customary, and Reasonable   106
Resource-Based Relative Value Studies   107
Geographical Practice Cost Index   112
Formulas for Determining Physician Fees   114
Cost Containment Programs   115
Managed Care   118
Medical Case Management   119
Chapter Review   120

SECTION 3
Medical Claims Examining Guidelines and Procedures   123

5   Medical Claims Administration   124
Maintenance of Claim Files   125
Documentation to Substantiate a Claim   126
Claims Investigations   128
Referrals   128
Pending Claims   128
Claim Processing   129
Good Claim Practices for the Insurance Claims Examiner   132
Unbundling of Services   133
Separate Procedures   134
Payment Worksheet   134
The Examiner Processing of a Claim   134
Quick Reference Formulas   142
Billing or Claims Management Office Administration   142
Prescription Drug Claims   142
Claims Examiner Handling of Prescription Drug Claims   145
Coordination of Benefits   145

Definitions   146
Order of Benefit Determination Rules   148
Right to Receive and Release Information   148
Right of Recovery   148
Health Maintenance Organizations   149
Preferred Provider Organizations   149
TRICARE   149
Recognizing the Presence of Dual Coverage   150
Adjustments   152
Chapter Review   154

6   Physician's, Clinical, and Hospital Services Claims   157
Coding Evaluation and Management   159
CPT Coding Medicine   162
Modifiers for Evaluation and Management and Medicine Codes   167
X-Ray and Laboratory Services   168
Radiology (X-Ray)   168
Modifiers for Radiology (X-Ray) Codes   169
Pathology and Laboratory (80047–89398)   169
Component Charges   171
Modifiers for Pathology (Lab) Codes   172
Hospital Services   172
UB-04 Billing Form   172
Ambulance Services   177
Durable Medical Equipment Billing Procedures   178
DME for Patient's Home Use   179
Types of Durable Medical Equipment   180
Chapter Review   181

7   Surgery and Anesthesia Claims   184
Surgical Procedures   186
Surgery and the CPT   187
General Guidelines   189
Maternity Expenses   192
Cosmetic Surgery   194
Obesity Surgery   198
Cosurgeons   199
Assistant Surgeons   199
Podiatry   200
Surgical Coding for Podiatry   200
Conditions of the Foot and Treatment Procedures   201
Surgery Modifiers   205
Anesthesia   205
Anesthesia CPT Coding   206
Anesthesia Handling Procedures   206
Calculating Anesthesia   208
Modifiers   208
Monitored Anesthesia Care   209
Medical Direction of Anesthesiology   210

Pain Control   210
Miscellaneous   211
Chapter Review   211

8   Medicare and Medicaid   214
TEFRA/DEFRA   216
Medicare Eligibility   216
Providers of Service   216
The Parts of Medicare   217
Approved or Reasonable Charges   219
Medicare Assignment of Benefits   219
Coordination of Benefits with Medicare   220
Estimating Medicare Coverage   226
Diagnosis-Related Group Billing   226
Medicaid   227
Chapter Review   228

9   Workers' Compensation   232
Employee Activities   234
Types of Claims   235
Privacy in Processing Workers' Compensation Claims   236
Fraud and Abuse   239
Liens   240
Reversals   243
Chapter Review   244

10   Managed Care Claims   246
Health Maintenance Organizations   247
HMO Coverage   249
Preferred Provider Organizations   250
Groups/Independent Physician Associations   250
Capitation Payments   252
Billing for Services   253
Authorizations, Referrals, and Second Opinions   253
Miscellaneous Services   257
Claim Payments   258
Processing the Claim   259
Denial of a Claim or Service   261
Appeals   262
Reinsurance/Stop-loss   262
Chapter Review   262

SECTION 4
Management of Claims Examining   265

11   Claims Auditing   266
Office of Inspector General   267
Auditing   269
Audit Findings   269
Certificate of Compliance Agreement   270
Self-Disclosure Protocol   273
Chapter Review   273

12 Processing Non-Medicare Claims 275

Billing for Services Rendered 276

Committee Review of Claims 277

Examining Claims 281

Chapter Review 285

13 Processing Medicare Claims 286

Evaluation and Management Coding for Medicare Claims 287

Use of Encounter Forms 288

Final Claim Audit 294

Postaudit Review 299

Electronic Billing Systems 303

Requests for Supplemental Information 304

Chapter Review 304

14 Processing Workers' Compensation Claims 306

Workers' Compensation—The Billing Perspective 307

Doctor's First Report 307

Progress Reports and Termination of Treatment 309

Investigating Workers' Compensation Claims 310

Workers' Compensation Clean Claims Criteria 311

Chapter Review 312

Appendix A: Contracts 315

Appendix B: Forms 322

Appendix C: Tables 331

Glossary 352

Index 363

Introduction

Health claims examining and medical billing and coding are two of the fastest-growing employment opportunities in the United States today. Health claims examining is the study of health claims from the coding and billing perspective, including the examining procedures of claims processing. Insurance companies, intermediaries, carriers, medical offices, hospitals, and other healthcare providers are in great need of trained personnel to code and process claims.

The most important ingredient for success for an aspiring medical biller or claims examiner is the desire to learn, without which the learning process is ineffective. The desire to learn can lead to a rewarding career in the health claims examining field.

Writing Style

The straightforward easy-to-understand writing style of this text presents information clearly and concisely. Designed with professional real-life applicability, the information presented here allows students to fully grasp the knowledge they need to perform the tasks involved in processing medical claims.

Text Features

Special features of the text include learning objectives, key terms and definitions, end-of-chapter exercises, and multiple activities to enhance readers' understanding and retention of the material.

Learning Objectives: Each chapter begins with a bulleted list of learning objectives to help focus the student on the most pertinent topics, key skills, and concepts covered in that chapter.

Key Terms and Definitions: Key terms are listed at the beginning of the chapter and defined within the text. Key terms are bolded and defined when they are introduced, allowing readers to quickly identify them. This structural element allows the student to read the term in context with the related material. In addition, the student can remain focused on reading the material without having to stop and refer to the glossary for a definition.

Practice Pitfalls: This special feature provides the student with a professional insider's point of view. These practice pitfalls provide guidance for professional success and ideas, shortcuts, and good habits to follow in the office, as well as warnings about bad work habits, the outcomes of sloppy work, and common mistakes that the student can avoid.

Critical Thinking Questions: As a challenge to the student thought process, critical thinking questions apply the information covered to real-life decisions in workplace situations.

Activities: Each chapter has practice activities throughout the chapter as well as supplemental activities after the end-of-chapter review questions. These varied activities are designed to give the reader practice in applying the information presented in that chapter. The activities provide real-life work practice completing tasks from coding to examining. The information that was used to build these activities complies with the latest updates in HIPAA laws, HITECH, the Patient Protection and Affordable Care Act, the Administration Simplification Rule, and the *ICD-10-CM/PCS*.

Summaries: Each chapter ends with a bulleted list of key concepts. These summaries are useful study tools that enable students to assess their level of knowledge and also are useful as a quick study reference.

End-of-Chapter Exercises: Questions for Review located at the end of the chapter helps to reinforce key concepts. Answering questions without looking back at the chapter will help students determine whether they have grasped the principles within the chapter or whether they need to study further. The questions also prepare students for examinations, giving the opportunity to put their knowledge into practice, and help to ensure competence in health claims examining. Answers are contained in the Instructor Resource Guide for this text.

Online Features: Throughout the chapters, online resources are indicated for students to access up-to-date information online.

Pedagogy: *Guide to Advanced Medical Billing: A Reimbursement Approach* will aid the student in learning the skills necessary to become a successful health claims examiner. The material is designed to be comprehensive, yet user friendly. The text follows a logical learning format by beginning with a broad base of information and then, step by step, following the course for learning the specifics of medical billing and coding and health claims examiner job duties.

New to the Edition

In addition to updating the content to include new legislative actions and changes in the industry, *Guide to Advanced Medical Billing: A Reimbursement Approach* focuses on the reimbursement process.

New Chapters
- Chapter 11: Claims Auditing
- Chapter 12: Processing Non-Medicare Claims
- Chapter 13: Processing Medicare Claims
- Chapter 14: Processing Workers' Compensation Claims

New Features
- Activities throughout the chapter have been enhanced to meet new coding, processing, and auditing protocols.
- Forms have been added to provide the student with improved tools for ensuring the reimbursement process goes smoothly.
- Online resources have been noted in each chapter to extend student resources.

- Critical thinking questions have been added to spark students' thought process around applicability of the content to the workplace.

Content Additions and Enhancements
- Information about legal and technical issues has been updated to include new healthcare legislation and requirements for electronic reimbursement procedures.
- Billing forms have been changed to the CMS-1500 and UB-04 with step-by-step instructions for accurate completion.
- Contract interpretation now includes the mandated changes from HIPAA and HITECH.
- Medical benefits have been updated to show the impact of the new legislation on insurance companies.
- Medical claims information now includes updated *CPT* codes and prepares the student for the *ICD-10-CM* conversion.
- Content about Medicare and Medicaid has been updated with new audits and qualification standards from the Office of the Inspector General.
- Workers' compensation now includes the entire process, from the incident report to the investigation and appeal process.
- All case studies, physician notes, encounter forms, history and physicals, and other data for the activities are new.

Organization of the Text

Guide to Advanced Medical Billing: A Reimbursement Approach provides students with all the theoretical knowledge and practical skills they need to achieve success as a medical biller or coder and/or a health claims examiner. The text reviews billing/coding and health claims examining before proceeding to cover the more in-depth procedures and practices of sending, receiving, reviewing, and processing claims. The text covers all aspects of health claims examining procedures. Content provides updated information from the following legislative actions: the Healthcare Insurance Portability and Accountability Act (HIPAA), Health Information Technology for Economic and Clinical Health Act (HITECH), Patient Protection and Affordable Care Act, and the OIG Corporate Compliance Act. Current (as of 2012) versions of Medicare billing forms, examples of newer electronic notices to beneficiaries, information about RAC and ZPAC auditing strategies, and transition recommendations for *ICD-10-CM/PCS* are included. As of the publication of this text, the *CPT, ICD-9-CM,* and Healthcare Common Procedure Coding System (HCPCS) codes are up-to-date as indicated.

Ancillary and Program Material

The *Guide to Advanced Medical Billing Instructor Resource Guide* are designed to reinforce the concepts learned in *Guide to Advanced Medical Billing: A Reimbursement Approach*

and provide students with an opportunity to practice and sharpen their skills.

- **Instructor Resource Guide** provides detailed lesson plans and answers to in-text exercises.
- **PowerPoint Presentation** slides are included, presenting an outline of book content that students may use for in-class presentations.
- **MyTest**—The questions and exams are developed from chapter objectives.

Additional Resources

The following additional resources are available to accompany this text:

- CPT (Current Procedural Terminology) **Manual**
- ICD-9-CM (International Classification of Diseases) **Manuals**
- ICD-10-CM/PCS **Manual**
- HCPCS (Healthcare Common Procedure Coding System) **Manual**
- Taber's Medical Dictionary
- PDR (Physicians' Desk Reference)
- Merck Manual

Before You Start

Claims: The claims should be processed on the basis of the information noted.

Dates: Please note that when YY is used in reference to a date, YY indicates the current year (12/01/YY). When PY is used in reference to a date, PY indicates the prior year or last year (12/01/PY). When NY is used in reference to a date, NY indicates the next year (12/01/NY).

Birth Dates: Birth dates will be referenced using MM/DD/CCYY.

Forms: The forms needed for processing claims in this text are located in Appendix C. These forms should be copied and used as needed.

Relative Value Study, Contracts, and UCR Conversion Factor Report: A Relative Value Study, Contracts, and a UCR Conversion Factor Report are included in Appendices A and B. These materials are to be used for processing the claims in this text.

About the Author

For 20 years, Lori Tyler was a faculty member, program director, and dean at two- and four-year colleges. She taught a number of courses, including medical billing, medical coding, law and ethics, medical office management, medical terminology, and medical office computer software. Prior to working in education, Lori worked in healthcare for 10 years. Her passion for education and her desire to help both faculty and students led her to the publishing industry. In addition to providing consulting and workshops to education facilities, Lori has developed her own company and has been successful at authoring various educational materials, including six textbooks. She also has handled the job of Developmental Editor for materials published through Pearson Education.

Acknowledgments

Many people have contributed to the development and success of the *Guide to Advanced Medical Billing: A Reimbursement Approach*. We extend our thanks and deep appreciation to the many students and classroom instructors who have provided us with helpful suggestions for this edition of the text.

We would also like to extend our appreciation to the following reviewers for providing valuable feedback throughout the review process:

Mollie Banks, MPS, RHIT, CPC, CMRS
Daymar College of Bowling Green
Bowling Green, KY
Dana Garrett
Brookline College
Albuquerque, NM

Terra L. Hunt, RHIT
Daymar College
Louisville, Kentucky
Michelle Lenzi, M.Ed., CPC, CPC-H, CPC-I
Hesser College
Manchester, NH
Wendy Schmerse, CMRS, CPI
Charter College
Oxnard, CA
Sandra A. Silvestro, MEd, CPC
Hesser College
Manchester, NH
Teresa Tarkington, CPC, CMRS
Daymar Institute
Murfreesboro, TN
Simone F. Thomas, MHSc, MHL, CCS
Miami Dade College
Miami, FL

Learning Objectives—Each chapter begins with a list of the skills that students will have after completing the chapter.

Keywords and concepts you will learn in this chapter:

Accident
Active Work
Actively-at-Work
Acts of Third Parties (ATP)
Affordable Care Act of 2010
Aggregate
Alternative Medicine Treatments
Basic Benefit
Beneficiary
Carryover Deductible
Coinsurance
Coinsurance Limit
Consideration
Consolidated Omnibus Budget Reconciliation
Act of 1985 (COBRA)
Contract
Contributory Plan
Conversion
Copayment
Deductible
Effective Date
Eligibility
Eligible

After completing this chapter, you will be able to:

- List the items that are necessary for a contract to be valid and enforceable.
- Describe the elements of a group contract.
- Define the provisions for coverage (i.e., eligibility, effective date, termination of coverage).
- Describe various benefits that a contract can offer.
- Define eligibility.
- Explain open enrollment.
- Discuss provisions for terminating an individual's coverage.
- Identify the main situations in which benefits can be extended beyond normal eligibility.
- Explain how the Affordable Care Act of 2010 has affected insurance coverage.
- Identify possible third-party liability.
- Define subrogation.

Key Words and Concepts—A list of the important concepts that students need to know or need to have reinforced appears at the beginning of each chapter. These terms appear in boldface type and are defined upon first appearance in the chapter; they also appear in the Glossary at the end of the book.

Basic Benefit
Beneficiary
Carryover Deductible
Coinsurance

- Describe various benefits that a contract can offer.
- Define eligibility.

Written **contracts** are present in every aspect of society. Essentially, any agreement between two or more persons that is enforceable by law is considered a contract. Written contracts have several advantages

Introduction—An introduction to the main topic of the chapter is presented at the beginning of each chapter to provide students with a flavor of what is going to be covered.

Every healthcare plan is required by law to have a written description of the benefits available to the members of that plan. This plan document must indicate, in detail, and in layman's terms, the provisions of the coverage.

Three major types of indemnity coverage are currently available:

- Basic only
- Basic–Major Medical
- Comprehensive Major Medical

Within these types, there may be numerous variations. In addition, under managed care provisions there can be PPO and HMO contracts.

As the benefit payments calculated under each type of coverage can be identical, focus on the concept of the benefit being offered. Medical billers and health claims examiners should understand the type of benefit payments before submitting or processing claims. Accurate benefit payment calculation is essential to being a good biller or claims examiner. Inaccurate payments can cost providers or insurance carriers money.

▶ CRITICAL THINKING QUESTION: What is the purpose of making sure that all healthcare plans have a written description of the benefits available to the members of that plan?

Practice Pitfalls—This special feature provides students with a professional insider's point of view. Practice pitfalls provide additional information to increase professional success, including ideas, shortcuts, and good habits to follow in the office, as well as the bad work habits, the outcomes of sloppy work, and common mistakes that students can avoid.

PRACTICE PITFALLS

A claimant is injured while on the premises of a grocery store. He submits the claims for his injuries to his benefit plan for payment. Subsequently, he also seeks recovery from the store. When recovery is successful, the claimant is required to reimburse the benefit plan for its losses.

Critical Thinking Questions—These questions challenge the students' thought processes and ask him or her to apply the information learned to real-life decisions at work.

▶ CRITICAL THINKING QUESTION: What will lifting lifetime limits do to insurance companies' bottom line?

Activities—Each chapter has practice activities throughout the chapter and supplemental activities after the end-of-chapter review questions.

These varied activities are designed to give the student practice applying the topic of the chapter. In addition, the activities provide real-life work practice completing tasks from coding to examining. The information that was used to build these activities complies with the latest updates in HIPAA laws, HITECH, The Patient Protection and Affordable Care Act, The Administration Simplification Rule, and the ICD-10-CM/PCS.

ACTIVITY #1

Jonny Lang Breaks a Leg

Directions: Complete CMS-1500 claim forms for the listed events and supplemental bills for the patient on the example patient bill form. Find the CMS-1500 and Patient Bill forms in Appendix B.

1. On March 3, CCYY, eight-year-old Jonny Lang fell out of a tree and broke his tibia. His parents brought him to the office, where he received the following services:
   a. Complex office visit of an established patient ($50.00)
   b. X-ray of the affected tibia ($120.00)
   c. Closed conscious sedation for setting of the tibia bone ($320.00)
   d. Casting of the leg ($120.00)
   e. Second X-ray of leg to assure proper casting ($120.00)
   f. Administration of a tetanus shot ($25.00)
2. On April 15, CCYY, Jonny returned to have his cast removed, incurring the following charges:
   a. Office visit of established patient, 40 minutes ($65.00)
   b. Cast removal ($100.00)

Examples—Examples are provided throughout the chapters to demonstrate how to complete forms and figure computations.

The following information will explain how to complete the sections of the payment worksheet.

Step 1. Complete the information regarding the patient and insured first. This information is contained in the box in the upper left-hand corner of the payment worksheet.

Payment Worksheet Field	CMS-1500	CMS-1500 Block Number	UB-04	UB-04 Form Locator
Eligible Employee	Nancy Normal	Block 4	Betty B. Bossy	FL 58
Company	XYZ Corporation	Block 11b	Ninja Enterprises	FL 65
Insured's Identification Number	777-77-WXYZ	Block 1a	999-99 NIN	FL 60
Patient	Nancy Normal	Block 2	Betty B. Bossy	FL 12
Relationship	Self	Block 6	18 (self)	FL 59
Provider's ZIP Code	89578	Block 33	12890	FL 1

Step 2. Next, each CPT code should be listed in the "Procedure Type of Service" column. Only codes that are the same should be combined together. Otherwise, list one code per line, even if this means using more than one payment worksheet.

Procedure Type of Service	1. 99201 2. 85025 3. 87040	Field 24D	111 (inpatient hospital claim)	FL 4

Step 3. List the date(s) of service in the "Dates of Service" column.

Dates of Service	1. 02/05/CCYY 2. 02/05/CCYY 3. 02/05/CCYY	Field 24A	02/06/CCYY through 02/14/CCYY	FL 6

Figures—The figures within each chapter represent a variety of supplemental information and/or illustrations.

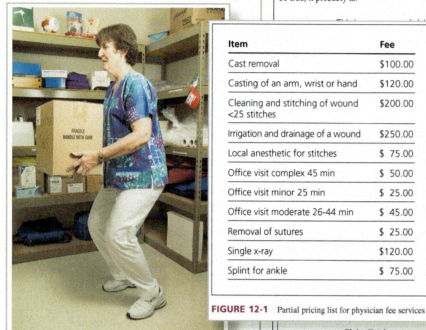

Medicare Summary Notice

July 1, 2012

BENEFICIARY NAME
STREET ADDRESS
CITY, STATE ZIP CODE

CUSTOMER SERVICE INFORMATION

Your Medicare Number: 111-11-1111A

If you have questions, write or call:
Medicare (#12345)
555 Medicare Blvd., Suite 200
Medicare Building
Medicare, US XXXXX-XXXX

BE INFORMED: Beware of "free" medical services or products. If it sounds too good to be true, it probably is.

Call: 1-800-MEDICARE (1-800-633-4227)
Ask for Hospital Services
TTY for Hearing Impaired: 1-877-486-2048

This _____ of claims processed from 05/10/2012 through 08/10/2012.

___TIENT CLAIMS

	Benefit Days Used	Non-Covered Charges	Deductible and Coinsurance	You May Be Billed	See Notes Section
	0	$0.00	$0.00	$0.00	
	0	$0.00	$0.00	$0.00	

___ATIENT FACILITY CLAIMS

	Amount Charged	Non-Covered Charges	Deductible and Coinsurance	You May Be Billed	See Notes Section
	293.00	0.00	58.60	58.60	
Claim Total	**$293.00**	**$0.00**	**$58.60**	**$58.60**	

(continued)

FIGURE 13-10 Medicare Summary Notice

Item	Fee
Cast removal	$100.00
Casting of an arm, wrist or hand	$120.00
Cleaning and stitching of wound <25 stitches	$200.00
Irrigation and drainage of a wound	$250.00
Local anesthetic for stitches	$ 75.00
Office visit complex 45 min	$ 50.00
Office visit minor 25 min	$ 25.00
Office visit moderate 26-44 min	$ 45.00
Removal of sutures	$ 25.00
Single x-ray	$120.00
Splint for ankle	$ 75.00

FIGURE 12-1 Partial pricing list for physician fee services

FIGURE 9-1 Lifting injuries are common Workers' Compensation claims
Source: Michal Heron/Pearson Education/PH College

Tables—Tables throughout the text provide information that students require to complete the activities or show examples of national indexes that are used to make billing computations.

TABLE 4-1 2012 CMS RVUs for Physician Fee Schedules

DATA RECORD			
HCPCS Code	1-5	X(5)	CPT or Level 2 HCPCS number for the service. NOTE: See copyright statement on cover sheet.
Modifier	6-7	X(2)	For diagnostic tests, a blank in this field denotes the global service and the following modifiers identify the components:
			—26 = Professional component
			—TC = Technical component
			—For services other than those with a professional and/or technical component, a blank will appear in this field with one exception: the presence of CPT modifier -53 indicates that separate RVUs and a fee schedule amount have been established for procedures which the physician terminated before completion. This modifier is used only with colonoscopy CPT code 45378, or with G0105 and G0121. Any other codes billed with modifier -53 are subject to carrier medical review and priced by individual consideration.
			—53 = Discontinued Procedure - Under certain circumstances, the physician may elect to terminate a surgical or diagnostic procedure. Due to extenuating circumstances, or those that threaten the well being of the patient, it may be necessary to indicate that a surgical or diagnostic procedure was started but discontinued.
Description	8-57	X(50)	
Status Code	58-58	X(1)	Indicates whether the code is in the fee schedule and whether it is separately payable if the service is covered. See Attachment A for description of values. Only RVUs associated with status codes of "A", "R", or "T", are used for Medicare payment.
Work RVU	60-65	999.99	Relative Value Unit (RVU) for the physician work in the service as published in the Federal Register Fee Schedule for Physicians Services for CY 2012.
Transitioned Non-Facility Practice Expense RVU	67-72	999.99	Relative Value Unit (RVU) for the transitioned resource-based practice expense for the non-facility setting, as published in the Federal Register Fee Schedule for Physicians Services for CY 2012.

Online Features—Throughout the chapters, online resources indicate where students can access up-to-date information online.

● **ONLINE INFORMATION:** Several automobile insurance companies have websites that help a medical biller determine whether to bill the automobile insurance or the patient's healthcare insurance policy. Conduct a search on the differences and add it to your resource file.

Summary—Each chapter ends with a brief restatement of key points in the chapter.

CHAPTER REVIEW

Summary

- Determining the appropriate E/M procedural codes is essential to filing an accurate Medicare claim. Review the extent of history taken at the encounter, the examination time and technicality, and the level of medical decision making that was necessary to verify that the E/M code is correct.
- To identify why a Medicare audit downcoded a service, review the diagnosis and the procedure to ensure that they match. The most frequent audit reason for downcoding is lack of substantiation for the E/M code used.

- To prevent downcoding during an audit, choose key information from the medical record to complete a claim (rather than just using the codes indicated by the practitioner). Reviewing the Medicare claim for accuracy and medical necessity will also prevent declarations of overpayment due to an audit.
- When further information is requested from Medicare, produce the information from the medical record in a timely and thorough manner. This is the opportunity to justify the claim coding and avoid a reduction in payment.

End-of-Chapter Material—A review section at the end of each chapter reinforces key concepts, provides students with an additional opportunity to practice skills, and offers resources for additional learning.

Chapter Review Questions—The review questions located at the end of the chapter help to reinforce key concepts. Answering questions without looking back at the chapter material will help students determine whether they have grasped the principles within the chapter or whether they need to do further study. The questions also prepare students for examinations and give students the opportunity to put their knowledge into practice. Answers are contained in the Instructor Resource Guide for this textbook.

CHAPTER REVIEW

Summary

- The term "contract," in general, is an agreement among two or more persons that is enforceable by law. In order for a contract to be valid, the parties must agree on its terms. There must also be some form of offer and acceptance.
- When an offer has been properly communicated and accepted, a binding contract is formed.
- A group contract allows an insurance company to meet the financial security needs of a group of persons.
- It is vital that medical billers and health claims examiners understand how to interpret contracts. It will take practice to accurately understand the coverages provided under contracts and to pay benefits properly.
- Basic and major medical plans are generally classified as indemnity contracts.
- These plans indemnify or reimburse the insured for medical expenses incurred and typically require the insured to complete and file claims.
- These plans often also contain deductible and coinsurance provisions and may restrict coverage for certain types of medical care expenditures.
- The three contracts found in Appendix A will be used throughout the course to calculate benefits on sample claims and to clarify examples to demonstrate the application of plan provisions.
- These sample contracts are based on actual plans and should be used as examples of what is possible within the industry. There is no such thing as a definitive plan.

As you will discover, there are a multitude of possible contract provisions. Therefore, use these samples as learning tools only.
- Eligibility and effective dates of coverage are probably the most important factors to consider when you process a claim.
- Thus, the first things you should check when you receive a claim for payment are eligibility and effective date. If the patient is not eligible, no further action need be taken on the claim.
- Acts of Third Parties and subrogation can drastically alter the way a claim is paid and who is responsible for the claim payment.
- Preexisting conditions and lifetime limit benefits will be prohibited in 2014.
- Some preventative care services are now mandated to be covered at 100% by insurance.
- The health claims examiner and medical biller must understand these concepts and must know when they come into play.

Review Questions

Directions: Answer the following questions after reviewing the material just covered. Write your answers in the space provided.

1. True or False? Every health benefit plan, whether it is insured or not, is required by law to have a written document describing the plan benefits. _____

SECTION 1

INTRODUCTION TO ISSUES RELATED TO HEALTH CLAIMS PROCESSING

CHAPTER 1
Introduction to Technical and Legal Issues

CHAPTER 2
Resource Manuals and Billing Forms

Introduction to Technical and Legal Issues

Keywords and concepts you will learn in this chapter:

Actuarial Statistics
Benefit
Claim
Compensatory Damages
Disclaimer
Effective Date of Coverage
Electronic Data Interchange
Electronic Health Records (EHR)
Eligibility Requirements
Embezzlement
Fraud
Group Insurance
Individual Insurance
Insurance
Insurance Policy
Insurance Speculation
Investigation
Lapse in Coverage
Legal Damages
Malice
Oppression
Pended
Premium

After completing this chapter, you will be able to:

- Explain what insurance is and how it works.

- Explain the reasons for the rising cost of healthcare.

- Identify and explain the various types of insurance available.

- Identify and explain various types of health benefit plans.

- Identify and explain the duties of a health claims examiner.

- Identify the responsibilities of the state insurance regulatory departments.

- Explain what disclaimers are and how to use them appropriately.

- List HIPAA guidelines regarding privacy issues.

- Identify advantages to the national use of EHR.

- Describe the updates to HIPAA fraud statutes.

- List the steps that should be taken to build evidence of fraud in a claim.

Privacy Guidelines
Punitive Damages
Reinstated
Reinsurance
Renewal
Self-Funded Plan
State Insurance Regulatory Department
Stop-Loss Insurance
Subpoena Duces Tecum
Termination Date
Third-Party Administrator (TPA)
Waiting Period

List items that may indicate fraud or embezzlement in various situations (e.g., provider fraud).

Discuss how to determine whether a plan has met the obligation of good faith and fair dealing.

Explain the process used to correct information in a medical record.

List the appropriate procedures to be followed for a subpoena of records.

Because healthcare costs are rising, it is virtually impossible for each person to have the necessary funds available to cover his or her expenses in a disaster, whether it is a large-scale disaster or a personal one. For this reason, purchasing **insurance** has become a necessary part of life in American society.

Essentially, insurance is an agreement between insurance companies, who collect fees or **premiums,** and individuals, who pay the premiums in return for specific **benefits.** These benefits are outlined in the **insurance policy** and may include payment of healthcare expenses, the replacement or repair of personal property, or the payment of expenses for others who have been injured by you or on your property.

A person does not have insurance until he or she completes an insurance application, pays the premium, and has the application accepted by the insurance company. If the insurance is a provision from an employer, there may be a **waiting period** before coverage begins (e.g., 30 days after date of hire). All policies have an **effective date of coverage** and most have a **termination date.** To continue the coverage, the person must pay a premium and maintain **eligibility requirements,** such as sustained employment. Also, the insured person must renew the insurance before the coverage expires in order to remain insured. A **renewal** allows the individual to pay a premium in order to continue coverage after the initial or subsequent policy periods have expired. If the insured does not renew the insurance, he or she may have a **lapse in coverage** and in some cases will not be able to get the insurance back, even by paying the premium. In most cases, if the insurance has lapsed, the individual must pay the premium and then the insurance is **reinstated.**

It is best to pay premiums as agreed to avoid complications, which range from having no coverage at all to experiencing a large increase in premiums. After a person enrolls in an insurance plan, the insurance company will send the individual an insurance identification card and/or policy. The individual is now considered a *member* of that insurance. Possession of the insurance card itself does not constitute insurance coverage. The provider must always verify insurance coverage because the policy only remains valid as long as the member continues to pay the insurance premiums Figure 1-1 ● gives an example of an insurance identification card.

The member (or provider on the member's behalf) is reimbursed for any benefits available under his or her insurance policy. In order to be reimbursed, the person must file a health insurance

URHealthInsurance

Account **12344567**
Issuer (80844)

ID: **555678899 01**

Name: **Jane Smith**
Coverage Effective Date: 01/01/2012

PCP: **James Smith**

PCP Phone: 555-214-3400

Network
Copays:
PCP Visit **$15**
Specialist **$15**
Hospital ER**$50**
Urgent Care**$50**

FIGURE 1-1 Valid date of insurance is indicated on the front of this insurance identification card

claim with the insurance company (this is done electronically by the provider). By filing a claim, the insured individual (via the provider) is notifying the insurance company of the member's loss or entitlement to reimbursement for any losses incurred. Failure to notify the insurance carrier of a claim in a timely manner could result in denial or a reduction of benefits. Therefore, it is wise to file claims as soon as possible.

Insurance companies operate on the principle that most of those who pay premiums will not need services, or that the services they need will cost less than the premiums they have paid. This means that insurance companies place restrictions on the amount and type of benefits that they will pay. These restrictions can include eligibility requirements, deductibles, maximum benefits, exclusions to a policy, and other policy provisions. The medical biller and health claims examiner are responsible for ensuring that each claim falls within the guidelines set by the company or the policy.

The Rising Cost of Healthcare

The inflation that affects so many areas of the American economy has had a severe impact on the cost of healthcare. National health expenditures are expected to continue to rise steadily in the next decade. This trend has prompted the federal government to introduce major changes in the healthcare system in an effort to control costs and to help insure a higher percentage of Americans.

There are a number of reasons for the enormous increase in the cost of healthcare. Significant factors include:

1. More people are seeking healthcare now than 20 years ago.
2. Medical treatments are more extensive and sophisticated than ever before. In addition, the equipment required for many treatments is extremely expensive. For example, one magnetic resonance imaging (MRI) unit, shown in Figure 1-2 ●, can easily cost $1 million dollars or more.
3. The cost of training healthcare professionals, such as physicians, nurses, and laboratory technicians is much greater than ever before.
4. The price that healthcare professionals pay for malpractice insurance has increased dramatically because of the increase in lawsuits.
5. When a significant part of a person's medical expenses are paid for by a health plan, neither the patient nor the healthcare provider has much incentive to control costs or limit the utilization of services.
6. There is little competition among healthcare providers and insurance providers within each state. Consequently, the marketplace does not place restraints on costs.
7. As people live longer, they require more healthcare services, thus prolonging the need for care and increasing costs.
8. Fraud by both providers and members (insured persons) is increasing.

For these reasons, the cost of healthcare has been rising steadily for the past few decades. Unless major steps are taken to curb this increase, many Americans will find themselves unable to afford healthcare, and many companies will no longer be able to afford to insure their employees.

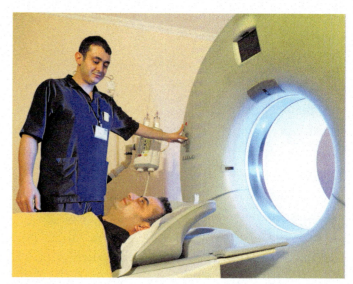

FIGURE 1-2 Patient undergoing an MRI
Source: Levent Konuk/Shutterstock

ACTIVITY #1

Rise in Healthcare Costs

Directions: Review the information covered previously, and list five reasons for the rising cost of healthcare in the United States. Write your answers in the space provided.

1. _____

   _____

   _____

2. _____

   _____

   _____

3. _____

   _____

   _____

4. _____

   _____

   _____

5. _____

   _____

Types of Insurance

There are various types of insurance coverage. Employers often offer multiple supplemental benefits in addition to healthcare insurance. The following types of insurance coverage are the most common types available:

- **Accidental Death and Dismemberment Insurance** pays a benefit to the beneficiary in the event of the insured person's death by accidental means. It also pays a benefit to the insured when an accident causes the loss of a limb.
- **Disability Insurance** covers an employee's salary, or a percentage of it, while the employee is on disability leave. Short-term disability insurance usually covers the insured for up to 12 weeks, and long-term disability insurance covers the insured for the length of the disability.
- **Health Insurance** covers medical and hospital services. Such policies are sold as individual or group policies.
- **Life Insurance** is coverage on a person's life. In the event of the insured person's death, a benefit is paid to the named beneficiary.
- **Workers' Compensation** is a medical and disability reimbursement program that provides full medical coverage and a scheduled weekly disability benefit for job-related injuries, illnesses, or conditions arising out of or in the course of employment.

Here are some other non-employer-sponsored insurance programs:

- **Medicaid** is a federal program established under Title XIX of the Social Security Act of 1965. Its purpose is to provide the needy with access to medical care.

- **Medicare** is the Federal Health Insurance Benefit Plan for the Aged and Disabled under Title XVIII of Public Law 89-97 of the Social Security Act. This program is for people 65 years of age and older and certain individuals who are disabled.
- **TRICARE** is a health insurance benefit provided to active and retired military personnel and their beneficiaries.

Numerous other types of coverage may be purchased from insurance companies. It is possible to be insured against almost any loss if you are willing to pay the premium. In addition, the term *insurance* is often incorrectly used to refer to all types of health coverage. In reality, medical insurance is only one way people are covered for healthcare expenses.

Individual vs. Group Insurance

Insurance coverage is categorized as either individual or group. **Individual insurance** is issued to insure the life or health of a named person or persons, rather than the life or health of the members of a group. That means premiums are usually higher because of the higher risks associated with insuring individuals on a case-by-case basis. With *individual insurance*, there is nowhere to spread risks, and the chance that losses may exceed the premiums collected is greater than in group insurance. The number of participants in a plan does not determine whether or not the plan is individual or group. The difference is defined by the type of contract, not the number of participants.

Group insurance provides coverage for several people under one contract, called a *master contract*. It is available to all people who qualify on a class basis, regardless of individual considerations. A group consists of any number of people who have a common purpose other than obtaining insurance coverage. Under this definition, members of unions, trade associations, and other organizations are able to purchase insurance as a group.

EXAMPLES:

Group Insurance: A company purchases insurance for all its employees, or a club or organization offers insurance to its members through a specified insurance company. All members of the group or organization may buy the policy that the organization has chosen.

Individual Insurance: A person purchases an insurance policy from an insurance carrier that is customized according to the person's specifications (e.g., auto insurance where the insured may choose the amount of coverage, deductible, and other factors).

Often individuals only purchase insurance when they feel that they have a reasonable chance of needing the benefits. Therefore, individual insurance poses a greater risk to the insurance carrier because healthy people tend not to purchase coverage. However, there is less risk for the insurance carrier in a group coverage situation because an employer will purchase coverage for all the employees, not just those who are likely to be ill. Thus, the premiums for the healthy employees help cover the costs of those employees who need benefits.

Conventional Insurance

In a conventional insurance arrangement, an employer or individual purchases an insurance plan and agrees to pay premiums to the insurance company. In return, the insurance company agrees to pay specific benefits. The premium cost is based on the "experience" of the plan, which includes the actuarial statistics, inflation, and administrative expenses of the company. **Actuarial statistics** are studies that an insurance company uses. For a carrier which covers health insurance, these can include statistics covering average lifespan, number of days in hospital per year for each age group, number of doctor visits, costs of all medical services, and so on.

In the past few years, the rise in healthcare costs has affected the increase in premiums. As a result, it has become almost prohibitively expensive for small employers and individuals to purchase coverage. For many larger employers, benefits have decreased, the portion paid by the employee has increased, or the plan has become self-funded.

Self-Funded Plans

In a **self-funded plan**, the total and ultimate responsibility for providing all plan benefit payments rests solely with the employer, group, or association. For example, a state healthcare association may offer self-funded insurance for healthcare providers. In self-funding the risk of loss is assumed by the funding entity. Because of this economic risk, it is not uncommon for portions of the benefits to be self-funded (i.e., employer, group, or association pays for benefits) and other portions to be insured (i.e., insurance company pays for benefits). For example, the medical benefits may be self-funded and the dental benefits may be insured. This potential risk may be decreased by the employer purchasing **reinsurance** or **stop-loss insurance**. Reinsurance is a program that reimburses the employer when losses exceed a specific amount agreed on by the employer and the reinsurance carrier.

In this text, the term "plan benefits" refers to coverage—medical or dental—without distinguishing whether those benefits are insured or self-funded. Such a distinction is irrelevant for our purposes, because handling and processing of claims within both arrangements are nearly identical.

EXAMPLE:

Self-funded Plan: The Giant-Mega Corporation has 10,000 employees. The company determines that the yearly insurance premiums for all its employees would be approximately $10 million. However, the company does not expect the employees to receive $10 million in benefits during the year. Thus, the company chooses to become self-funded. The $10 million is placed in an account, and the company pays the benefits to the employees directly.

Third-Party Administrators

A **Third-Party Administrator (TPA)** is a professional firm that is under contract by the insurance company to deal solely with administering the eligibility and claim payment services, including all of the paperwork (and various other administrative services), for self-funded benefit plans. The administrator provides all of the equipment and personnel required to meet the plan's needs. In turn, the plan supplies the funds or monies needed for payment of the administrator's services and for amounts paid out for claims. The insurance company handles all plan administration, provides all of the equipment and personnel required, and supplies the funds for claim payments.

In response to the increase in the number of self-funded plans, many insurance companies now offer what are known as Administrative Services Only (ASO) contracts. These contracts basically work the same way as a TPA insofar as all of the funding is provided by the client, and the expertise, equipment, and personnel are provided by the insurance company. As with all areas of the benefit industry, a multitude of variations are possible on both of these concepts.

EXAMPLE:

The Giant-Mega Corporation has decided that it takes too much time and effort for their claims department to process the claims submitted by its employees. The corporation hires a TPA to process the claims and pay the benefits out of the account that the corporation has set up.

Employee Benefits

Auto, home, and most other personal property insurance are purchased by individuals. However, healthcare insurance is often supplied (partly or fully) by a person's employer. The supplying of healthcare insurance comes under the heading of an employee benefit. Healthcare benefits are an extremely important part of almost everyone's economic security. Today, many employees consider them to be a major consideration for job seekers.

Types of Health Benefit Plans

There are many different types of insurance health plans that provide medical benefits. Some insurance types for people in the United States are discussed in this section.

Indemnity Plan

Traditional indemnity plans are almost nonexistent today, but they used to be the most common type of benefit plan. Under an indemnity insurance plan, the member pays an insurance premium and the insurance pays a fixed percentage of covered expenses. The member pays deductibles and copayments (a portion of the payment); however, the member can choose his or her own physician and other healthcare providers and specialists, and can otherwise make independent decisions about what type of care to seek.

Preferred Provider Organization

A preferred provider organization (PPO) operates much like an indemnity plan, except the plan provides incentives for insured individuals to seek care from providers who are on a list provided by the insurance company. A PPO plan is one type of managed care plan. Under a PPO plan, the insurance company generally covers a higher percentage of the cost, and sometimes allows the member to pay a lower deductible, if he or she chooses a preferred provider. However, a PPO lets the member seek services from providers outside the network if the member is willing to pay a larger portion of the cost.

Health Maintenance Organization, Open Access

A Health Maintenance Organization (HMO) with open access provides coverage for many services but requires that the member seek care first from either a Gatekeeper or a Primary Care Provider (PCP) before he or she goes to any other physicians or health facilities. The HMO provides a list of physicians from which a member may select a PCP. The insurance will cover visits to the PCP and most services that the PCP recommends.

Services that the individual seeks independently (without consulting the PCP) are generally not covered. If the member needs to see a specialist, be hospitalized, or have lab or X-ray work, the member's PCP must refer him or her to a provider or facility. The member's PCP must authorize these services to be covered by the HMO. In all cases, the member is responsible for paying the indicated copayment with this type of plan.

Health Maintenance Organization, Closed Panel

An HMO with closed panel is one in which the physicians and other practitioners work directly for the HMO. All services must be provided directly by the HMO and its staff. Services which the member seeks outside the HMO are generally not covered.

Point-of-Service

Point-of-service (POS) plans combine characteristics of HMOs and PPOs. The member chooses a PCP who controls all aspects of care, including referrals to specialists. All care received under that physician's guidance (including referrals) is fully covered. Care received by out-of-network providers is reimbursed, but the member must pay a significant copayment or deductible. So basically, the member decides each time he or she needs medical care whether to use the plan as an HMO or a PPO.

Dental Insurance

Dental insurance covers preventive and restorative services of the teeth and gums. Dental plans come in almost as many forms as health coverage. This coverage can be included as a benefit under an indemnity, PPO, or dental maintenance organization (DMO) plan, or it can be an entirely separate plan. Some DMOs are associated with dental practices. Other companies provide the same kind of in-network low-pay and out-of-network/higher-pay options for dental services as they do with their healthcare. Still others opt for a traditional indemnity approach, allowing members to go to the dentist of their choice, pay up front, and wait for reimbursement. Basic dental coverage in managed care plans usually includes 100% payment for annual checkups and makes the member responsible for a percentage of other necessary treatments (e.g., X-rays, surgeries).

Vision Insurance

Vision insurance coverage can be included as a benefit under an indemnity, PPO, or HMO plan, or it can be an entirely separate plan. Some plans offer coverage for annual eye exams and a percentage of the frame and prescription lens or contact lens costs every 24 months. HMOs usually have eye-care professionals on site; other types of plans may have in-network and out-of-network restrictions.

Prescription Drug Insurance

Prescription drug coverage can be included as a benefit under an indemnity, PPO, or HMO plan, or it can be an entirely separate plan. One of the highest costs of healthcare today is prescription drugs. Some health plans do not cover prescription drugs at all. HMOs generally have pharmacies on site that fill prescriptions from doctors in the network. Other plans cover a specific list of approved medications called a "formulary" for a small copayment, and still others reimburse the member for a percentage of the costs after the member has purchased the prescription drug.

Medical Billing and Claims Examiner

The medical billing and claims examiner positions have similar duties as they work with claims. The medical biller is usually responsible for coding a claim and responding to requests for more information from insurance companies. The claims examiner can either work for a provider to review claims for accuracy prior to sending them to the insurance company or work for an insurance company to evaluate the validity of submitted claims and/or process said claims.

Claims Examiner

The conduct of all claims personnel is extremely important. Claims personnel are more visible because most of the public

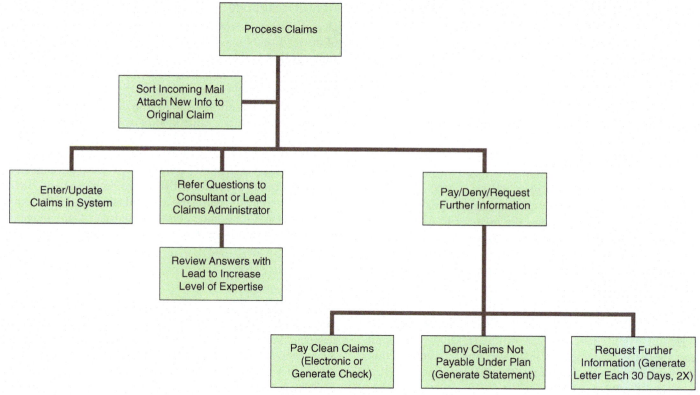

FIGURE 1-3 Sample Workflow Model

interfaces either with the customer service representative or directly with claims processing personnel. The public's opinion of the insurance payer is based primarily on contacts with claims personnel. Therefore, it is important for claims examining personnel to establish and adhere to basic principles. The claims examiner's guiding philosophy should be to provide timely, competent, fair, and friendly claims service to all members. A proposed workflow model is illustrated in Figure 1-3 ●. If you review this model periodically, it will ensure that you have taken the basic steps toward proper claims processing. Keep in mind that this is a basic outline, and the specifics may vary from company to company.

The start of the day for claims examiners begins with receipt of **Electronic Data Interchange (EDI)** information. The computer software being used will define the tasks involved in this retrieval of information. In any case, the examiner will likely have new claims to review, supplemental information that was previously requested to process, and appeals of denied claims to review.

If the claim is appropriate to be processed, it is either paid or denied according to the terms of the insurance policy. The claims examiner then generates an electronic check or statement. If additional information is needed, the examiner puts the claim on hold and a letter is generated by the system or the claims examiner manually fills out a form letter identifying the additional information needed. When a claim is on hold it is considered **pended**. If the insured

has not responded within 30 days, a follow-up letter is sent. A maximum of two follow-up letters should be sent. If no reply has been received within 30 days of the last follow-up letter, the pended claim should be denied for lack of information.

If the claims examiner is unable to make a decision based on his or her expertise, the claim is referred for supervisory or consultant review. Many insurance companies have a listing of certain types of claims that are always referred for review. These claims are reviewed for appropriateness by a supervisor or consultant who is hired for his or her credentialing and experience. The consultant will inform the claims examiner of the action to be taken, and the claim is processed accordingly. It can be a learning experience for the claims examiner to review the consultant's decision and ask questions for clarification. This work does not negate the need for the consultant to examine some identified claim issues.

Medical Biller

In contrast, medical billers spend their time using the EDI to send and receive information. The standard healthcare claim form is the CMS-1500. Most computer software systems since January 2012 utilize this form and are equipped with coding and database information for the medical biller to use. Specific coding skill is discussed later in this text.

PRACTICE **PITFALLS**

The following list of nine guiding principles will assist the biller or examiner in adopting a professional philosophy:

1. Know the plan provisions of the contracts you are responsible for handling/billing.
2. Be sure you understand the application of the provisions. If you are not sure, ask before you process claims.
3. Conduct claim reviews that reflect a prompt and diligent search for accuracy.
4. If additional information or clarification is required, review the claim and ask for all the information that is needed at one time. For example, if you are billing for a patient and the date of the injury is not in the medical record, you should send a letter to the patient requesting said information. Before this action is taken, you should review the entire claim and make sure there is no other information needed from the patient. Similarly, if a claims examiner requires more information from a provider, he or she should make one request for everything needed to complete the claim.
5. Conclude each claim, large or small, on the basis of its own merits, in light of the facts, the law, and the coverage afforded.
6. Claims examiners should give a prompt, courteous, and forthright explanation to each provider or insured party about the company's position with respect to the claim.
7. Medical billers should respond promptly, when a response is indicated, to all communications from policyholders, claimants, attorneys, and other involved persons. (Or they should refer the communication promptly to the designated person responsible for responding in those situations.)
8. Seek and support new methods designed to improve billing and claims service.
9. Suggest or help establish procedures and practices to
   a. Prevent misrepresentation of the pertinent facts or policy provisions.
   b. Avoid unfair advantage by reason of superior knowledge.
   c. Maintain accurate claim records as privileged and confidential.

ACTIVITY #2

Biller and Claims Examiner Guiding Principles

Directions: List four guiding principles to assist the biller/examiner in adopting a professional philosophy.

1. _____
2. _____
3. _____
4. _____

The Regulatory Departments of Insurance

The insurance industry is overseen in each state by a **state insurance regulatory department**. This department in each state holds the primary legal authority over the operations of all insurance companies within that state. Therefore, it has influence over insured benefit plans but generally does not have authority over self-funded plans. The many responsibilities of these regulatory departments include

- Issuing certificates and licenses authorizing insurance companies to operate and insured products to be sold in the state.
- Licensing agents to sell insurance and revoking licenses when warranted.
- Reviewing the annual statements of insurance companies to verify solvency.
- Ensuring that policy forms include the required provisions and are printed in the proper format.
- Performing on-site inspections of insurance companies.
- Maintaining an office for receiving and acting on consumer complaints.
- Ensuring that insurance companies observe the rules affecting policy reserve maintenance and investment activities.

▶ **CRITICAL THINKING QUESTION:** How can a medical biller and/or health claims examiner stay abreast of new insurance and/or coding changes related to each insurance program?

ACTIVITY #3

State Insurance Regulatory Departments

Directions: Review the information covered previously, and list five responsibilities of the state regulatory departments over insurance. Write your answers in the space provided.

1. _____
   _____
   _____
2. _____
   _____

(Continued)

3. _____
   _____

4. _____
   _____

5. _____
   _____

Legal Issues Pertaining to Disclaimers

There are several legal issues that affect the health claims examiner on a daily basis. One of the most common is disclaimers. Insurance companies are in the business of providing healthcare benefits to their members. There are times when a health claims examiner may quote benefits to a provider or member, but due to changes in circumstances the benefits quoted may not be available when the claim is received (e.g., it is found that the member's coverage has terminated since the benefits were quoted, the group has not paid their premiums, or there is some other extenuating circumstance). Because of this possibility, it is highly advisable for the health claims examiner to use a disclaimer when giving benefit information.

A **disclaimer** is a denial or renunciation of responsibility. In the health claims examiner's world, it means to use words and phrases that refuse to promise an outcome.

Disclaimers are one of the best ways to protect oneself from possible legal action. Disclaimers use phrases such as "it appears that" or "this may be." These words allow the examiner to provide a general answer to a question without making any type of promise. If the examiner makes a statement that is later found to be in error, it can cause numerous problems in customer satisfaction and may raise legal issues. To combat this, insurance companies often have conversations recorded for their own protection.

EXAMPLE:

Ms. Smith called the claims examiner in charge of her claim and was told, "Yes, you are covered for a hysterectomy." It was later discovered that there was no medical reason to perform the hysterectomy; Ms. Smith wanted it as a form of foolproof contraception. Because contraceptive devices and procedures were not covered by the contract, the insurance carrier later denied the claim. Ms. Smith insisted that she had been told that the procedure would be covered, and therefore the insurance carrier must pay, regardless of what it said in the contract. She insisted she had a verbal agreement from the insurance carrier that it would pay for the procedure.

All claims examiners should practice using disclaimers in their conversations. When confirming a member's eligibility and benefits, they should always include disclaimers.

The following disclaimers may be used in your verbal and written responses:

Eligibility—We show that _____ is currently effective on group _____. To receive benefits, he or she must be eligible at the time services are rendered.

Benefits—These are the benefits now in effect for this contract. To receive benefits, your membership must be in good standing on the dates that services are rendered.

Remember that the main purpose when using disclaimers is to clarify an issue or answer a customer's question without making a promise that the company may be held to later. The intent is not to mislead the customer in any way or neglect to answer their questions. Rather, disclaimers should be used to ensure that the claims examiner is not making any promises that might not be accurate in the future.

ACTIVITY #4

Disclaimer Statements

Directions: Reword the statements that follow to include the use of a disclaimer in the sentence.

1. _____ Yes, your plan does include that coverage.
   _____
   _____

2. Yes, you are a member of that plan. _____
   _____

3. Yes, that is a covered service and we will be paying for it. _____
   _____

4. Your check will arrive in five days. _____
   _____

5. Your deductible and stop-loss have been met so you will not have to put out any more money on this bill.
   _____
   _____

6. You have worked for over 90 days so your company's insurance should cover the services. _____
   _____

7. Do not worry; your insurance will cover the bill. ____
   _____

8. All hospitalization expenses are covered under your plan. _____
   _____

9. We pay 80% of the billed amount. _____
   _____

10. All preventive care is covered under your contract. ___

_____

11. Your insurance will cover the cost of these services. __

_____

12. Your policy includes coverage for those services, so we will pay a portion of the cost. _____

_____

13. We process all claims upon receipt, so you should have your payment within 10 working days. _____

_____

14. Yes, your child is an eligible dependent. _____

_____

15. If your claim reaches us by the 15th, it should be paid by the end of the month. _____

_____

Legal Issues Pertaining to Privacy Guidelines

In addition to disclaimers, **privacy guidelines** are another common legal issue that affects the health claims examiner on a daily basis. The very nature of health benefits administration requires a great deal of personal information to be gathered and maintained about many individuals. Therefore, the needs of the company must be carefully weighed against individuals' right to privacy to avoid unwarranted invasions of that right.

In particular, claims information is considered to be privileged and confidential in the context of the administrator–member relationship. Unauthorized disclosure of information may represent a violation of that confidentiality and may be prosecuted under the Health Information Portability and Accountability Act (HIPAA). The confidentiality of claims records has assumed a new importance for several reasons:

1. People are becoming more litigation-minded.
2. Health plans are reimbursing for more sensitive services that were excluded in the past (for example, alcohol detoxification, mental health treatment, and AIDS-related illnesses).
3. More employers are self-administering or self-funding their health plans, which could mean that an employee's highly personal medical information is in some instances routinely handled by fellow employees.
4. New HIPAA regulations require that all personnel involved in the healthcare process respect the patient's right to privacy and confidentiality.

HIPAA

In 1996, President William Clinton signed into law the Health Insurance Portability and Accountability Act (HIPAA). The portability issues of this law will be addressed in another chapter. Here we will discuss the patient privacy and fraud and abuse issues.

The Act encompasses two main issues:

1. Portability, the ability to change insurance companies and still be covered for pre-existing conditions (which will be discussed in more depth in a later chapter)
2. Accountability, which generally deals with the patient's right to privacy from the medical provider, health insurer, and any other parties in the healthcare process (e.g., billers, clearinghouses).

Regarding the Privacy section of HIPAA, the Department of Health and Human Services states

The privacy requirements limit the release of patient Protected Health Information (PHI) without the patient's knowledge and consent beyond that required for patient care. Patient's personal information must be more securely guarded and more carefully handled when conducting the business of health care.

> ● **ONLINE INFORMATION:** To learn more about HIPAA and privacy, visit the following website: www.hhs.gov/ocr/privacy/

Health Information Technology for Economic and Clinical Health Act

Electronic Health Records (EHR) are flourishing. In EHR, all the information on a patient is kept in an electronic record rather than in a traditional medical chart or record. To address the confidentiality issues created as EHR becomes the standard, the American Recovery and Reinvestment Act of 2009 (ARRA) included the Health Information Technology for Economic and Clinical Health Act (HITECH). HITECH is intended to increase the use of electronic health records in the United States. There are many advantages to national use of the EHR system:

1. Improved patient care
2. Increased patient safety
3. Simplified compliance with privacy standards
4. Lower costs in the long term
5. Minimized errors
6. Increased productivity in administrative efficiency

There is a progression within the HITECH portion of the ARRA to allow creation of national privacy certification standards for EHR system implementation. Financial incentives are built into HITECH to encourage physicians and hospitals to have electronic health information systems in place by 2015.

> ● **ONLINE INFORMATION:** To learn more about the impact of the HITECH Act, visit www.hipaa.com/2009/02/what-does-the-hitech-act-mean-to-you/.

PRACTICE PITFALLS

The following general rules can help ensure that privacy guidelines are met:

1. Always obtain an authorization to release information *before* releasing any information. Most releases routinely signed in a medical practice only authorize the physician to release information necessary to process a patient's claim. Additional authorization should be obtained to release any information to other parties. These releases should include exactly what information is to be released, the dates of any services provided which fall within the release, the person to whom the information may be released, the signature of the patient, the date of the signature, and the date the release expires. An example is given in Figure 1-4 ●.

2. Make sure that a *release* was signed by the member before you process a claim for reimbursement. If possible, ask the provider for a copy of the patient's signature on the release form. This will ensure that you have the right to look at the information contained on the claim.

3. Gather only the information that is necessary and relevant to the billing or processing of the claim.

MEDICAL RECORD RELEASE FORM (SAMPLE)

I, _____ ACTING ON
BEHALF OF: (Print Name of Patient or Legally Authorized Representative)

_____ HEREBY AUTHORIZE THE RELEASE
(Print Name of Patient)
OF INFORMATION AS INDICATED:

My Healthcare Information

_____ I authorize disclosure of healthcare information (related to my medical history, diagnosis, treatment, or prognosis) to all inquiries or only to the following people or entities (for example, family friends, employer, insurance companies, clergy):

<u>List Names</u>:

_____

_____

Limited Healthcare Information

_____ I wish to limit disclosure of only certain kinds of healthcare information (related to my medical history, diagnosis, treatment, or prognosis) to the following people or entities:

<u>List Names</u>   <u>List information that may be released</u>

_____   _____

_____   _____

No Information

_____ I do not authorize release of any information regarding my admission or treatment. I wish to be a "no information" patient, and I realize that flowers, telephone calls, and visitors will be refused on my behalf.

_____   _____

(Signature of Patient or Legally Authorized Representative)   **(Date)**

FIGURE 1-4 • Sample of Medical Record Release Form

4. Use only legal and ethical means to collect the information required. Whenever permission is necessary, obtain written authorization from the insured or claimant (guardian or parent if the claimant is a minor) before disclosing information.

5. At the request of the insured or claimant, and not subject to any applicable legal or ethical prohibition or privilege, provide the insured with the nature of the information and its general uses.

6. Make every reasonable effort to ensure that the information on which an action is based is accurate, relevant, timely, and complete.

7. Upon request from the provider's office or claims examiner, the claimant or insured should be given the opportunity to correct or clarify the information given by or about him or her, and the file should be amended to the extent that it is fair to both the insurer and the member or claimant. Requests for review or clarification of medical information will be accepted only from the healthcare provider from whom the information was obtained.

8. In general, disclosures of information to a third party (other than those described to the insured or claimant) should be made only with the written authorization of the member or claimant. This includes disclosure to employers, family members, or former spouses.

9. All practical precautions should be taken to ensure that claim files are physically secure and that access to such files is limited to authorized personnel. Precautions include not leaving files out, locking all files, and even turning your computer screen away from where it might be seen by other persons. You may also need to use security passwords and other security measures, depending on your office situation.

10. All personnel involved in the processing of claims should be advised of the need to protect insured persons' Right of Privacy in obtaining required information and should treat all individually identifiable information as confidential. Willful abuse of the privacy of any insured or claimant by the employee may be cause for dismissal.

11. The disclosure of a diagnosis should never be made to a member or his or her family. If the member requests this information, refer the member to the physician. There may be a reason the patient does not know his or her diagnosis.

12. Never release any information to an ex-spouse. This includes the member's address, phone number, when a claim was paid, to whom it was paid, and other information. The ex-spouse should be instructed to contact the member directly.

13. When you are working with hard-copy files, do not leave files or members' records open on your desk or in an area where they may be seen by others. Instead, be sure that all files are closed or are turned over on your desk. When you are working with EHR, be careful when using member files or information that may be displayed on a computer screen. Computer screens must be placed in such a way that they cannot be seen by anyone passing by. If necessary, use a screen saver or be ready to click on another document (an unrestricted one) to replace the EHR instantaneously.

14. If a minor patient has the legal right to authorize treatment for services, then to disclose that treatment or service to the minor's parents or legal guardians or to other persons may be a violation of HIPAA or the confidentiality of the Medical Information Privacy and Security Act (MIPSA).

15. Be cautious about releasing information to a patient's employer, even if the patient has provided an authorization to release information.

These guidelines cover some of the basic aspects of HIPAA privacy regulations. For detailed information regarding HIPAA guidelines, you may review the complete rules and regulations regarding HIPAA, which are printed in the Federal Register and on the Centers for Medicare and Medicaid Services (CMS) (www.cms.org) or Office for Civil Rights (OCR) (www.hhs.gov/ocr/privacy/) websites.

ACTIVITY #5

Privacy Guidelines

Directions: After reviewing the information covered previously, list at least 10 privacy guidelines that should be followed. Write your answers in the space provided.

1. _____

2. _____

3. _____

4. _____

5. _____

6. _____

7. _____

8. _____

9. _____

10. _____

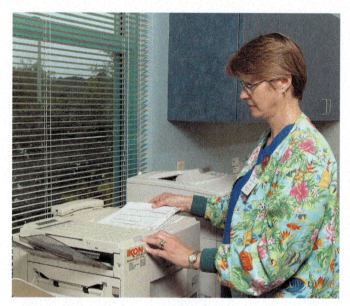

FIGURE 1-5 When sending a fax be sure and use a cover sheet
Source: Michal Heron/Pearson Education/PH College

Electronic Transmission of Personal Health Information

Electronic transmission of Personal Health Information (PHI) is a common practice. Some of the methods include faxing and email. Transmission is the term used when information is sent through electronic methods.

FAXING. When faxing items, be aware of sensitive information on a fax document. All faxes should contain a cover sheet that announces the intended recipient of the fax, the sender, and a confidentiality statement asserting that the enclosed information is personal and confidential, as seen in Figure 1-5 ●. The following paragraph is sample wording for a fax confidentiality statement:

> The enclosed information is intended exclusively for the individual or entity to which it is addressed and contains information which is privileged, confidential, or exempt from disclosure under federal or state laws. If the reader of this message is not the recipient or the agent or employee responsible for delivering this facsimile transmission to the intended recipient,

you are hereby notified that any dissemination, distribution, or copying of the information contained in this facsimile is strictly prohibited. If you have received this facsimile in error, please notify our office immediately by telephone and return the original facsimile to us at the above address.

Best practices to help in maintaining confidentiality include calling ahead to ensure that the recipient is near the fax machine (in case the fax is located in a public area), making sure faxes are retrieved immediately, verifying the fax number prior to sending a fax, and removing the fax you sent from the fax machine as soon as it is sent.

EMAIL/ELECTRONIC DATA INTERCHANGE. Data sent through email and other electronic transmissions are encrypted to protect the confidentiality of patients. Developing the standards for encryption and creating safe electronic data interchange are goals of the U.S. Department of Health and Human Services. The Office for Civil Rights is responsible for enforcing the regulations related to HIPAA and other privacy-related acts. The National Institute of Standards and Technology has issued several special publications to assist entities in complying with HIPAA and HITECH electronic data interchange standards.

Legal Issues Pertaining to Fraud

Legal issues pertaining to fraud commonly affect the health claims examiner on a daily basis. **Fraud** is the use of deception to cause a person to give up property or something to which they have a lawful right. Fraud is synonymous with deceit, trickery, and being an imposter. Schemes for gain involve almost every conceivable form of deception, from a subtle omission of fact to the most flagrant lie.

Fraud can be perpetrated by anyone and can involve every type of claim. Doctors, lawyers, hospitals, claimants, beneficiaries, and claims handlers working for an insurance company are capable of committing fraud. It is estimated that millions of dollars annually are paid out by the health benefits industry on fraudulent claims. HIPAA and HITECH were passed to assist in identifying and preventing fraud. Regardless of who submitted the expenses for payment or how they were submitted, the overall impact of fraud on claim payments, premiums, administrative costs, and other expenses is devastating.

PRACTICE **PITFALLS**

The following scenarios may be helpful in identifying fraudulent situations:

1. A member is covered under two policies for group hospital benefits. The member conceals this fact to avoid receiving reduced payments by one or both of the insurers.

2. A prospective insured has been receiving medical treatment for hypertension. The person denies receiving such treatment on an application for life insurance in an effort to obtain coverage that is not otherwise available or to receive a better rate.

3. A member has a medical condition that requires prescription medication. The member alters dates on the bills and files photocopies plus the originals in order to receive multiple payments for the same charges.

4. An employee copies another claimant's bills, replacing the actual claim data with his own. The bills are marked "paid," and the fake claims are submitted as his own.

5. The insured's attending physician signs a return-to-work release. Discarding this release, the insured shops for another doctor who will extend her disability status.

6. The insured stages an intentional injury to appear accidental.
7. A worker strains his back lifting a TV set at home. The next day, coworkers find the insured lying at the bottom of a flight of stairs complaining of back pain. The insured files a workers' compensation claim for loss of wages and medical expenses.

8. The member's spouse sustains a stroke and requires constant custodial care at home. Instead of paying for home help, the member claims that her formerly stable, chronic condition has suddenly become acute, rendering her unable to continue working and enabling her to remain at home and care for her spouse.

Forms of Fraud

Fortunately, most claims are legitimate and forthright. Therefore, a claims examiner should not automatically assume fraud. However, it is important to remain aware of the possibility in order to properly recognize and detect those instances of fraud. The two major areas of fraud concern are

1. Internal fraud, which involves the employees of the company against which the fraud is perpetrated. The employee may act alone or with other employees.
2. External fraud, which involves people outside the company against which the fraud is directed. Claims personnel are often the innocent parties who discover fraud during routine claim-paying activities.

Some forms of fraud are more obvious than others. With training and experience, a competent examiner develops a sense about claims that just do not appear right. In such cases, the examiner needs to listen to that intuition and take steps to explore the possibility of fraud.

Although the list of potential fraud situations is endless, maintaining an attitude of alertness and making thorough, conscientious efforts can curb the success of the various scenarios.

Establishing a Fraud Case

The following procedures can assist in establishing a case of fraud and successfully prosecuting it.

QUESTION DISCREPANCIES. If the file is out of the ordinary in any way or contains discrepancies, be inquisitive. Try to determine why file statements or circumstances conflict with expected conclusions. Notice whether the claim was filed in a timely manner. Information about other insurance; the how, when, and where of the accident; and the names and addresses of all attending physicians and witnesses should be freely available from the claimant. Appearance of undue anxiety or anger on the part of the claimant or beneficiary related to the promptness of payment could be a fraud indicator. You should question any alteration of a claim form or bill.

Sometimes routine, in-depth reviews of original claim files disclose questionable elements or trends. You should pursue and develop suspicious elements, rather than ignoring them.

A questionable element in one area of a claim file often points to further discrepancies in other areas until you discover an entire series of payments that were paid in error. Follow up on all leads and clues. Be sure claims are handled promptly. Use tact in pursuing possible fraud indicators.

Attempts to recognize and deal with fraud are a basic part of an overall philosophy of good claim practices. There is not only a contractual obligation to properly handle possible fraudulent situations, but a social obligation as well. Like any other crime, insurance fraud is detrimental to society in many ways, including the influence it may have in increasing the overall price of benefit coverage.

THOROUGH INVESTIGATION. Although investigation of fraudulent claims may be thorough and complete and the documentation may seem irrefutable, it is often difficult to prove fraud in court. In some cases, depending on the nature of the fraud, the insurance company or administrator may be hesitant to prosecute because of the possibility of a countersuit on the charge of libel. This does not mean that efforts to resolve fraudulent claims should be restricted. Rather, this possibility emphasizes the need for in-depth investigation and development of a complete, accurate claim file so that any fraud case that is prosecuted will be as solid as possible. Thorough investigation increases the chances that the case will be prosecuted in the courts, that prosecution will be successful, and that the occurrence of countercharges for libel will be reduced.

COMMUNICATION. Although each examiner must recognize and investigate each case of potential fraud, management should retain actual and overall control. In the process of prosecuting fraud, the responsibility is spread among many persons. Cooperation among and between several different departments is essential. For example, the investigator must keep the management informed about the investigation. The records department must cooperate and provide information requested in a timely manner. Communication plays a critical role in the investigation process.

Indicators of Fraud

Some indicators may help to isolate situations of possible fraud. No single indicator is necessarily suspicious, nor is it evidence that fraud has occurred. The claims examiner must assume the identity of an investigator and put all of the facts and indicators together to see whether fraud is actually present. The following indicators have been put into categories for easier reference.

Here are indicators associated with the claimant or insured (employee):

1. Claimant is overly pushy and demanding a quick claim settlement.
2. Claimant is unusually familiar with insurance terminology or claims procedures.
3. Claimant handles business in person or by phone, apparently avoiding use of the mail. (Using the mail for such purposes is a federal offense.)
4. Attorney or claimant is willing to accept less than the actual claim estimate just to help out and resolve the matter quickly.

5. Insured/claimant contacts the insurance agent to verify coverage or extent of coverage just before loss.
6. Attorney representation is coincident with or shortly after injury date, and the attorney threatens a bad-faith lawsuit unless the carrier or administrator agrees to settle quickly.
7. No police report was made or only an over-the-counter report occurred when police would usually investigate the actual scene.
8. Claimants or witnesses use a post office box or a hotel address.
9. Claimant has multiple policies covering the same loss.
10. Claimant is requesting reimbursement for an accident with no witnesses, a one-car accident, or a hit-and-run accident.
11. The injured party declines medical treatment at the time of the accident, but is later hospitalized for extensive injuries.
12. Claimant has a history of previous loss with similar treatment, or the same doctor or attorney repeatedly handles medical or lost earnings claims following minor accidents.
13. Claimant has a history of numerous past questionable claims.
14. Billing statements show trends or treatments by providers appear to show excessive charges. These charges may include the same fees and treatment regardless of condition, and differences between amounts billed to the patient and amounts on claim forms.

CLAIM PROCESSING AND CLAIM INFLATION INDICATORS.
Frequently, discrepancies found in a claim are red flags that warn the claims examiner to go over the claim papers more thoroughly or to check past history at length. Rather than being obvious, these indicators often are seen only after a number of payments have occurred. Things to look for include

1. A minor accident produces major accident costs, lost wages, and so on.
2. Medical bills indicate routine treatment being provided on Sundays, holidays, or a doctor's day off.
3. Summary medical bills are submitted without itemizing office visits or treatments.
4. Claimant submits photocopies of medical, prescription, or dental bills; third or fourth generation bills are especially suspect. Photocopies of claim forms contain alterations or corrections.
5. Receipts or bills are submitted without provider's letterhead.
6. Several different typefaces, handwritings, or colors of ink are on claim forms or bills.
7. Claimant receives an unusually high number of treatments for a relatively minor condition. Such ailments persist for weeks or months.
8. Insurance became effective or employment commenced just a short time before the claim.
9. Condition is diagnosed subjectively as nausea, fatigue, inability to sleep, headaches, low-back pain, sprain, whiplash, and so on.
10. Patient states that services were not received as shown on the billing.
11. Provider accepts claim payment as payment in full for services rendered, regardless of the billed amount.

12. Unassigned benefits are seen on large medical claim amounts with questionable evidence to support payment in full and with a claim form as the only information submitted. Supporting bills are seldom, if ever, included.
13. Incorrect or incomplete forms are submitted. For example, there are questionable signatures from providers (e.g., doctor's name is signed Doctor J. Jones instead of J. Jones, MD).
14. Claim includes unusual or unfamiliar medical terms, misspelled medical words, or a nonexistent diagnosis.
15. The claim file indicates that the insured does not have other coverage, but photocopies of unassigned medium or large dollar-amount claims are frequently submitted.
16. Claim lists improbable, impossible treatment or unlikely surgery (e.g., second appendectomy, hysterectomy on a male, two gallbladder removals).
17. Doctor's specialty is not related to the patient's diagnosis (e.g., male treated by an obstetrician, severe heart problem treated by a chiropractor).

INSURANCE SPECULATION INDICATORS. Insurance Speculation occurs when someone buys insurance coverage for the purpose of making a profit. The insured may stage a fake death or accident to file claims under more than one policy. Collusion with others may occur. The following indicators may suggest that insurance speculation has occurred:

1. An attorney makes a demand or threatens a lawsuit even before a claimant files a claim.
2. Claims are reported late.
3. There is instant pressure from the claimant or provider to pay quickly.
4. The claimant holds multiple hospital indemnity coverage policies or combined hospital, medical, accident, and hospital indemnity policies.
5. The claimant denies or omits information about other insurance coverage.

OTHER INDICATORS OF FRAUD. Indicators pointing to employee embezzlement usually apply to employees within or even outside the claim operation. Access to a claim file is usually involved. Look for the following indicators of fraud:

1. Payee name and address does not match claim form, bills, or other pertinent material.
2. Change in lifestyle is inconsistent with expected income level.
3. There are undocumented claim file actions, such as voids, reversals, or reissued payments by employee.
4. Provider bills and claim forms do not match explanation of benefits; there is an unusual payee or questionable assignments/nonassignments.
5. Claim payments are split by examiner to keep payment within dollar-authorized levels.
6. There is no documentation for many payments on a claimant's file. System production records and manual counts of work do not match, and claim papers are missing from daily correspondence files.

7. The claimant is overutilizing certain benefits, such as claims for hospitalization or extensive treatment indicating total disability even though the claimant was not observed to have been absent or ill from work.
8. There is a pattern of accident claims by an individual or family.
9. The patient name is altered to that of another family member (for example, to allow payment under another member's history and avoid paying a deductible).

ACTIVITY #6

Fraud Indicators

Directions: After reviewing the information covered previously, list 10 items or situations that may indicate fraud (either internal or external). Write your answers in the space provided.

1. _____
   _____
2. _____
   _____
3. _____
   _____
4. _____
   _____
5. _____
   _____
6. _____
   _____
7. _____
   _____
8. _____
   _____
9. _____
   _____
10. _____
   _____

> ▶ **CRITICAL THINKING QUESTION:** How can you protect yourself if you know that fraud and/or abuse are occurring in your workplace?

Healthcare Fraud and Abuse

The HIPAA fraud statutes have greatly broadened the scope of the federal government for prosecuting fraud and abuse in the healthcare industry. There are frequent updates to these statutes. Here is a summary of recent updates:

False Claims Act

The False Claims Act was amended in 2009 by the Fraud Enforcement and Recovery Act of 2009 (FERA). Basically anyone involved in the healthcare industry who knowingly and willfully falsifies or conceals a scheme that causes failure of payment for a government obligation is guilty of fraud. In addition, if anyone involved in the healthcare industry knowingly makes any fictitious or fraudulent statements (including written) that cause failure to pay an obligation owing to the government, such statements also constitute a false claim. The updates also make it fraudulent to fail to report an overpayment from a government insurance plan. These false claims are punishable by fines and/or imprisonment.

The Anti-Kickback Statute

The Anti-Kickback Statute prohibits the "knowing and willful" offer, payment, solicitation, or receipt of remuneration to induce or reward the improper referral of items or services reimbursable by a federal healthcare program, regardless of any alternative explanation for remuneration. (*Note:* "Knowing" does not mean one has to have first-hand knowledge of the anti-kickback statute nor intent to violate the statute.) If a marketer makes a deal with a provider to refer patients to the provider in exchange for money, this is a violation of the anti-kickback statute.

Administrative Sanctions—Civil Monetary Penalties

Healthcare providers engaging in fraudulent or abusive activities are subject to a number of administrative sanctions. In addition to being excluded from participation in Medicare and Medicaid, providers can be assessed civil monetary penalties for each claim that is deemed improper. An "improper" claim is any claim that is false or fraudulent or is in violation of the anti-assignment rule. An improper transaction might involve the transfer of funds to a Medicare or state health plan beneficiary to entice the beneficiary to improperly order or receive services from a particular institution or healthcare provider. An example of an improper claim is when a sister gives her insurance card to her sister to use as if she, the member, were being treated.

The Office of the Inspector General

The updated standards extend the basis under which the Office of the Inspector General (OIG) is authorized to impose civil monetary penalties (CMPs) and/or exclude healthcare entities from participation in federal healthcare programs. CMPs are imposed in the following cases:

- Knowingly making, using, or causing to be made or used a false record or statement material to a false claim for payment under federal healthcare programs ($50,000 per false record or statement).
- Failing to grant timely access to the Inspector General (IG) after the IG makes a reasonable request to conduct

audits, investigations, evaluations, or other statutory functions of the OIG ($15,000 per day).

- Ordering or prescribing a medical or other item or service during a period in which the person was excluded, knowing that the claim for such service or item will be made to a federal healthcare program ($10,000 plus three times the amount of the potential claim).

Investigation

Investigation is an organized effort to discover the facts or truth of a matter. Legitimate claims should be paid promptly and in accordance with scheduled allowances. The handling of such claims should reflect a positive service attitude. The same amount of effort and determination should go into the denial of every illegitimate claim. The claims examiner cannot accomplish this purpose without exercising investigative efforts whenever claim discrepancies occur.

During the review of every claim, the examiner must be alert to items that do not look right. Because most claims are payable without further questions, it is only necessary to investigate claims that raise questions.

Although investigation of facts takes time, it is absolutely necessary to properly document the claim file. Even if the claimant or an attorney threatens to contact the state insurance regulatory department or to file a lawsuit, these threats should not deter continued investigation as long as the examiner and his or her supervisor are relatively sure that the claim investigation is justified. The claimant or the provider should be kept well informed of the claim's status regarding what has been requested and what items are necessary or outstanding in order to complete the processing of the claim. Be aware that there are legal standards regarding timely responses to claimants and regular communication during investigation.

Be candid with persons who are inquiring about the claim, to a point. Do not hesitate to let an inquirer know that the claim needs further research to determine the validity of the facts presented. Avoid words that can be damaging to a case, such as "crook" and "thief," and never make accusations (see Table 1-1 ●).

Prompt, cautious contact with information sources is essential in every investigation. When possible fraud indicators are present, you must exercise a greater degree of caution and take into account the source of suspected fraud when you make various contacts.

TABLE 1-1 Investigation Terminology

Words to Avoid	Words to Use
Investigation	Clarification of charges, services, etc.
Fraud	Incomplete/omitted information
Lied	Inconsistency in information reported
Any other derogatory remark/term	It appears that . . .

Remember that all insurance plans have the right to investigate and confirm the validity of the submitted information.

Inside Sources of Fraud

Whenever a company's employees within or outside the claim processing area appear to be involved in questionable activity, the claims examiner should contact his or her supervisor, personnel director, or others in management. Under no circumstances should the matter be discussed with anyone other than management personnel in a secluded area. It is then up to management to decide how the matter will be handled.

Outside Sources of Fraud

Whenever insureds, members, claimants, or other persons (not including the provider of service) appear to be involved in fraud, you should be careful about your contact with providers of services. These contacts involve the verification of dates, type of service rendered, and amounts charged to the patient. Verification of disability and accident-related information should also be investigated. The use of an outside investigator may be required to expedite the investigation. All contacts should be documented in writing. If possible, the information should be requested in writing, and the reply should also be given in writing with the name and the title of the person supplying the information.

When providers of services appear to be involved in fraud, you should be careful about your contact with the member/claimant. Limit verification to dates, types of treatment, and amounts of charges for those services. Avoid discussions regarding diagnoses. As previously indicated, all information requested and received should be documented in writing whenever possible.

Building the Claim File

Use the following five steps to build evidence in a claim file:

1. Carefully document all discrepancies, conflicting facts, and omissions. Do not write on any of the original submitted claim documents. Make notes on a notepad or separate pieces of paper.
2. Make a written record of pertinent points of phone conversations. Summarize conflicting facts that were obtained by phone, and note any new information carefully. Include dates of conversations, names, and phone numbers of contacts.
3. Place all documents in the order in which the events they describe occurred or the order in which they were received. Keep a log that clearly shows the dates of all communications and the parties that were communicating.
4. Retain the envelopes for all documents mailed to the office. Attach the envelope to the back of the documentation received.
5. Coordinate the investigation with the insurance company's or administrator's legal department or counsel.

PRACTICE **PITFALLS**

Every claims examiner should be aware of the possibility of fraud and check each claim for fraudulent indicators. The following checklist should alert you to the need for further investigation, although the existence of one or more of these factors does not prove that fraud exists. Look carefully for the following situations:

- The insured lists no insurance coverage on hospital admissions forms.
- The insured does not assign benefits on inpatient hospital bills.
- Proof of accident or illness includes photocopies of documents, forms, or bills with altered dates or receipts with serialized numbers.
- Prescription bills submitted for payment are consecutively numbered.
- Claimants say that the insurance company is being billed for services that were not received or treatment that was not provided.
- Claims are submitted for injuries that were not reported or witnessed.
- The doctor's portion of the bill or claim form has erasures or strikeouts.

ACTIVITY #7

Investigation

Directions: Review the information covered previously, and list three examples of items that should be investigated in reviewing a claim.

1. _____

2. _____

3. _____

Embezzlement

When an employee illegally takes funds from his or her company, it is **embezzlement**. Embezzlement can be committed by anyone in a firm.

To protect against embezzlement, keep accurate records of all transactions. Be sure to follow these procedures when issuing claim payment checks:

1. Clearly notate any amounts paid out, including the payee, the amount, the date, the check number, and the reason for payment.
2. Immediately report any discrepancies to a supervisor.
3. If you suspect embezzlement, notify the proper person. If you suspect your coworker, notify his or her supervisor. If you know of embezzlement by a coworker and say nothing, you are guilty of being an accomplice to the crime.

4. Obtain a bond (insurance against embezzlement) for each member of the company who deals directly with the company's receipts or processes payments.
5. If you notice poor bookkeeping or inaccurate records that were kept by a previous employee or a current coworker, bring it to the attention of your supervisor or employer.
6. You should then document the problems in writing, and ask the supervisor or employer to initial a copy for you to keep. This record may provide minimal protection in case the problems with the records are found to conceal embezzlement or mismanagement of funds.

Insurance carriers are responsible for the acts of their employees. If embezzlement is found, the insurance carrier may be considered guilty and may be responsible for monies embezzled by their employees.

Legal Damages

Legal damages are monetary awards above and beyond the benefits provided by the group plan that a plan member may attempt to recover.

In the legal climate today, it is not uncommon for plan members to seek legal channels to obtain benefits or to obtain greater benefits than are generally provided by a plan. Usually, such cases are based on what is known as "bad faith."

An **insurance policy** is a written contract defining the insurance plan, its coverage, its exclusions, its eligibility requirements, and all benefits and conditions that apply to individuals insured under the plan. It is considered a legal contract. Under contract law, the claimant can only recover benefits up to the policy or plan limits.

However, with the development of consumerism, the courts have become more liberal. In some states, a body of law has developed that says there is an implied obligation of good faith and fair dealings in every contract. A breach of this obligation is termed bad faith. Generally, the law of bad faith allows an insured to attempt to recover various types of damages above and beyond the benefits provided by the plan. The courts will consider two questions to determine whether a plan has met the obligation of good faith and fair dealing:

1. Did the plan give the claimant's interest and the company's interest equal consideration?
2. Was the claim handled or denied in accordance with the plan provisions and in a timely manner?

The following examples show how courts often view policy interpretations:

1. The meaning of a plan of benefits is determined by the member's reasonable expectations of coverage.
2. Uncertain wording that could be subject to more than one interpretation will usually be resolved against the plan and in favor of the member.
3. When there are two equally believable interpretations, the one that gives the greatest amount of protection to the member will prevail.

There are two types of damages that a court may award: compensatory damages and punitive damages.

Compensatory damages are designed to compensate an insured for all of the actual losses or damages to make that person whole again. For example, if a person has not been able to pay his home mortgage or car payment because he did not receive a monthly disability check and, therefore, his home was foreclosed and his car was repossessed, he may be able to recover equity for the home and car, attorney fees, and damages for emotional stress.

Punitive damages are often the larger of the two awards and are intended primarily to punish wrongdoing by the defendant and make an example of the defendant to help deter such actions in the future. Unlike compensatory damages, punitive damages are not automatically recoverable if bad faith is found. In some states, such as California, for example, a plan member must prove the insurance plan not only to have acted in bad faith but to be the cause of fraud, oppression, or malice. **Malice** is intentional conduct to cause injury or conduct that is carried on with the conscious disregard of the rights of others. **Oppression** is putting a person through cruel and unjust hardships with conscious disregard of rights. For example, if the insured is denied coverage and as a result experiences cruel and unjust hardships, a case can be made for oppression of the insurance member.

Bad Faith Awards

The dollar amount of a bad faith award is based on two concepts, the degree of wrongfulness and the wealth of the defendant.

All lawsuits are expensive not only in the dollar cost of the damages, but in other costs as well. These costs remain even if the case is settled out of court. If the case is settled out of court, the plaintiff's attorney costs, miscellaneous costs, the attorney costs for the plan, and the benefit not originally paid must be paid. In addition, the payments may include substantial pain and suffering costs. The value of the claim usually has no relation to the amount of restitution (award) sought.

Part of the reason for the continuing escalation of premium costs is the necessity of being prepared for lawsuits, because whether the case is settled in court or out of court, the monetary damage to the plan is usually significant and often preventable.

In light of the foregoing information, it is important that every claim be handled quickly, correctly, and fairly. This responsibility falls on each and every claims examiner. To fulfill this responsibility, you should adhere to the following four guidelines during the routine handling and processing of claims.

PROMPT COMMUNICATION. Every customer and claimant is entitled to courteous, fair, and just treatment. Send claimants a reasonably prompt acknowledgment of all communications with respect to a claim or bill.

EQUAL TREATMENT. Treat customers and claimants equally and without outside considerations other than those dictated by the office policy or plan provisions.

EQUITABLE SETTLEMENT. Promptly investigate all pertinent facts and objectively evaluate every claim in order to ensure a fair and equitable settlement.

PROMPT PAYMENT. Pay all just claims promptly.

ACTIVITY #8

Bad Faith

Directions: Answer the following questions after reviewing the information covered previously. Write your answers in the space provided.

1. What are the two types of damages that may be awarded in bad faith actions?

   a. _____

   b. _____

2. What are the two questions that the court will consider when deciding the dollar amount of a bad faith award?

   a. _____

   _____

   b. _____

   _____

Maintenance of Records

Records should be accurate and contain details of the claims processing history. If information must be changed on a record, a single line should be drawn through the old information, and the correct data should be placed above or beside it. The date of the change should be notated and initialed by the person responsible for the change (see Figure 1-6 ●).

All records should be kept as long as they are needed. Most insurance carriers put their medical records on microfiche and keep them indefinitely.

Date	Time	Order	Doctor	Administered by
9/9/05	3 pm	Erythromycin ~~500 mg~~ 250 mg BT 9/9	Williams	B. Fremgen RN.

FIGURE 1-6 A corrected chart notation

Local and state laws govern how long claims records should be preserved, usually from 7 to 10 years.

Subpoenas Duces Tecum

Occasionally, the records of a member may be needed in a court action. In such a case, the court issues a subpoena requesting the records. A **subpoena duces tecum** is a demand for a witness or a document to appear. Sometimes a witness will need to turn the records over to the court personally. Other times the documents may be mailed.

One person in the office should be designated to handle subpoenas. This person should be the only person to accept a subpoena of claims records. If you are the designated person, the subpoena must be served (given to you) in person. It cannot be laid on a desk or sent through the mail. No one else should accept the subpoena in your absence.

A witness fee or mileage amount may be given to a witness. You should request any payable fees at the time the subpoena is served.

Usually, you are given a specified amount of time to produce the records. Occasionally the records will need to be turned over at the time of the subpoena. In all cases, consult with your supervisor before you turn over the records. If your supervisor is unavailable, let the server know that you are unable to turn over the records without proper authorization, and tell the server when they can come back and serve the subpoena directly on your supervisor. This will give you time to be sure that the record is complete, accurate, and in good order. Also be sure all signatures are identifiable, and make copies.

In most cases you must send the original record. Always keep a copy of all the records you send. This practice allows you to check for changes in the records and protects against loss of information if the records are lost. Number the pages before you make copies so you can determine if any pages are missing.

If you are unable to accept the subpoena and no one is present who is authorized to accept it, explain the situation to the person serving the subpoena. Suggest a time when he or she can come back or ask the person to contact the insurance carrier's legal department. Then inform the legal department of the situation.

After a subpoena has been served, check over the records to be sure they are accurate and complete, number the pages, and make the copy. You should then send the original file immediately (if delivery by certified mail is allowed), or place it under lock and key to avoid tampering. Find out the day of the trial and comply with all orders given by the court. Be sure not to allow anyone to see the records or tamper with them. The records should only be turned over to the judge and should only be left in the care of the judge or jury, never in the care of an attorney. Be sure to obtain a receipt for the records if you are leaving them.

Subpoena Notification

If a subpoena is served to request claims records, many insurance carriers will notify the member in writing that the records have been requested. This practice allows the member's attorney to file papers with the court to block the subpoena.

If there is very little time between the date the subpoena was served and the date the records have been requested, the member

---

MEMBER NOTIFICATION OF SUBPOENA

Date:

To:
Address:

Dear Member and your Attorney of Record:

Please note that records pertaining to you are being sought by _____; as shown in the subpoena attached to this Notice.

If you object to us furnishing any part of the records described in this action, you must file papers with the court prior to our release of these records. This subpoena requires that we furnish the records on or by (date).

You or your attorney of record may contact the attorney for the party seeking to examine such records and determine whether they are willing to agree to cancel or limit this subpoena. If no such agreement is reached and you are not already represented by an attorney in this action, **you should consult an attorney to advise you of your rights in this matter.**

If we do not have notification in writing regarding the cancellation or limitation of this subpoena at least 24 hours prior to the above date, we will assume you have no objection to us releasing this information.

Signed: _____ Date: _____

FIGURE 1-7   Subpoena Notification

---

notification letter may be faxed or the member may be contacted by phone. In either case, be sure to let the member know that he or she does not have the authority to stop you from releasing the records. The member must have his or her attorney file a petition with the court in order to have the subpoena rescinded. For a sample of a subpoena notification, see Figure 1-7 ●.

ACTIVITY #9

Subpoena

Directions: Answer the following questions after reviewing the information that was covered previously. Write your answers in the space provided.

1. True or False: When someone enters the office with a subpoena you should immediately turn over all records that are requested. _____

2. What should you do if the person who handles subpoenas is not in the office and someone attempts to serve a subpoena? _____

CHAPTER REVIEW

Summary

- There are several types of insurance companies, and each provides benefits in exchange for receiving premium payments from its members.
- Insurance companies are overseen by the state insurance regulatory agency, which holds the primary legal authority over the operations of insurance companies within that state.
- As a health claims examiner, you need to understand the principles that underlie the Claims Department's primary objective, which is to deliver timely, competent, fair, and friendly claim service. When these principles are conscientiously and consistently applied, they enable a company to build and maintain a respectable image with its customers and the general public.
- The maintenance of strong customer goodwill and the creation of a favorable public position are vital to the progress of a company, as well as to each individual employee.
- Always use disclaimers when you are speaking to patients or providers. This practice can help prevent the insurance carrier from being held liable for a promise made by a claims examiner.
- Submission of fraudulent claims has hit epidemic levels. Payments for fraudulent claims cost administrators millions of dollars annually.
- One of the qualities of a good claims examiner is the ability to use good judgment in making claim decisions.
- Fraud is a very sensitive issue, and the guidelines we have covered should be practiced at the provider and insurance company levels to ensure that claims decisions are accurate and fair.
- Records should be maintained properly and requests for subpoenas should be answered promptly and correctly.

Review Questions

Directions: Answer the following questions without looking back at the material just covered. Write your answers in the space provided.

1. What is insurance? _____
_____

2. What are the two categories of insurance plans, and how do they differ?

   a. _____

   b. _____

3. What does TPA stand for, and what do these companies do? _____
_____

4. What are employee benefits? _____
_____

5. What does the word "disclaimer" mean? _____
_____

6. What is insurance speculation? _____
_____

7. Define *fraud*. _____
_____

8. Define *embezzlement*. _____
_____

9. What are the two main areas of fraud concern?

   a. _____

   b. _____

10. What is an investigation? _____
_____

If you were unable to answer any of these questions, refer back to that section and then fill in the answers.

ACTIVITY #10

Definitions

Directions: Complete this activity by filling in the word for each definition.

1. Deception to cause a person to give up property or something to which the person has a lawful right.
_____

2. A denial or renunciation of responsibility. _____

3. An item covered by an insurance policy, or something paid to or on behalf of a recipient. _____

4. A written request by the insured individual for payment by the insurance company of expenses that are covered under the insurance policy. _____

5. Items or services offered for sale by a company. Within the insurance industry, this term refers to various benefit plans. _____

6. Intentional conduct to cause injury, or conduct that is carried on with the conscious disregard of the rights of others. _____

7. A demand for a witness or a document to appear in court. _____

ACTIVITY #11

Matching

Directions: Match the following terms with the proper definition by writing the letter of the correct definition in the space next to the term.

1. _____ Actuarial Statistics
2. _____ Compensatory Damages
3. _____ State Regulatory Department of Insurance
4. _____ Individual Insurance
5. _____ Insurance Policy
6. _____ Insurance Speculation
7. _____ Lapse in Coverage
8. _____ Reinsurance
9. _____ Renewal
10. _____ Self-Funded Plan
11. _____ Third-Party Administrator

a. A person or entity buying insurance or maintaining coverage for the purpose of making a profit.

b. A plan administration firm that deals solely with administering the eligibility and claim payment services, including all of the paperwork (along with various other administrative services) for self-funded benefit plans.

c. A break in continuous insurance coverage, usually resulting from nonpayment of premium.

d. When the total and ultimate responsibility for providing all plan benefit payments rests solely with the employer, group, or association.

e. An insurance that would reimburse the employer when losses exceed a specific amount agreed on by the employer and the insurance carrier.

f. Paying a premium in order to continue coverage after the initial policy period has expired.

g. An insurance policy issued to insure the life or health of a named person or persons, rather than the life or health of the members of a group.

h. Damages designed to compensate an insured for all of the actual losses or damages to make that person whole again.

i. Studies that an insurance company uses. For a carrier that covers health insurance, these studies can include statistics covering average lifespan, number of days in hospital per year for each age group, number of doctor visits, costs of all medical services, and so on.

j. A written contract defining the insurance plan, including its coverage, exclusions, and eligibility requirements, and all benefits and conditions that apply to individuals insured under the plan.

k. The legal entity that oversees the operations of all insurance companies within the state.

Resource Manuals and Billing Forms

Keywords and concepts you will learn in this chapter:

Centers for Medicare and Medicaid Services (CMS)

CMS-1500

Current Dental Terminology (CDT)

Current Procedural Terminology (CPT)

Healthcare Common Procedure Coding System (HCPCS)

International Classification of Diseases – 9th Revision Clinical Modification (ICD-9-CM)

International Classification of Diseases – 10th Revision Clinical Modification Manual (ICD-9-CM)

International Classification of Diseases – 10th Revision Procedure Coding System (ICD-10-PCS)

Medical Dictionary

Merck Manual

Modifier Codes

Physicians' Desk Reference (PDR)

Procedure Code

Red Book and Blue Book

Relative Value Scale (RVS)

Uniform Bill-2004 (UB-04)

Version 4010/4010A

Version 5010

After completing this chapter, you will be able to:

- Describe the layout of the ICD-9-CM manual.

- State the purpose of the CPT.

- Discuss how HCPCS codes are used.

- Explain the contents of the *Physician's Desk Reference*.

- Explain how to use a medical dictionary properly

- Describe the contents of the *Merck Manual*.

- Compare and contrast the red book and the blue book.

- Identify information required for an accurately completed CMS-1500 health insurance claim form.

- Explain the elements that comprise an accurately completed UB-04 billing form.

In health claims billing, coding, and examining, a number of books are utilized as reference materials:

- The *International Classification of Diseases—9th Revision Clinical Modification (ICD-9-CM)*—Will be used until September 30, 2013, for coding healthcare claims with diagnostic information. *International Classification of Diseases—10th Revision Clinical Modification and Procedure Coding System (ICD-10-CM/PCS)*—Will be used after October 1, 2014, for coding healthcare claims with diagnostic and procedural information.
- *Current Procedural Terminology (CPT®)*—Used for coding healthcare claims with procedural items.
- *Relative Value Scale (RVS)*—Provides information on fees that can be used for the area in which the service was provided.
- *Current Dental Terminology (CDT)*—Provides language for dental healthcare claims.
- *Health Care Common Procedure Coding System (HCPCS)*—Used for coding hospital or inpatient procedures on healthcare claims.
- *Physicians' Desk Reference (PDR)*—Provides pictures, descriptions, and other useful information on drugs.
- *Merck Manual*—A medical dictionary with pictures and descriptions to aid the healthcare worker to find appropriate terms.
- *Red Book*—Used to understand drugs and compare wholesale prices.
- *Blue Book*—A resource for patients to compare common healthcare pricing in their geographical area.

ICD-CM (PCS)

The *International Classification of Diseases (ICD)* is an indexing system of conditions that serves a dual purpose for health benefits personnel. (See Figure 2-1 ●.) It enables medical billers and claims examiners to convert verbal descriptions of illnesses, injuries, and other conditions into numerical or alphanumeric codes. Secondly, it allows diseases to be classified for statistical purposes. This reference identifies symptoms, diseases, injuries, and procedure services, assigning each an entirely numerical code or a combination of letters and numbers. The *ICD-10-CM* has updated codes that allow the use of up to seven alphanumeric digits, whereas the *ICD-9-CM* only used up to five digits. There are significant changes to the procedural coding in the *ICD-10-PCS*.

ICD-9-CM

The *ICD-9-CM* consists of three volumes:

- Volume I—A tabular listing of diseases.
- Volume II—An alphabetical listing of diseases by English language description.
- Volume III—A numerical and alphabetical listing of surgical or nonsurgical procedures that may be performed by a physician in a hospital or inpatient setting.

The order and degree of use varies for each volume.

VOLUME I. Volume I is structured numerically according to body system.

001–139	Infectious and parasitic diseases
140–239	Neoplasms
240–279	Endocrine, nutritional, and metabolic disease and immunity disorders

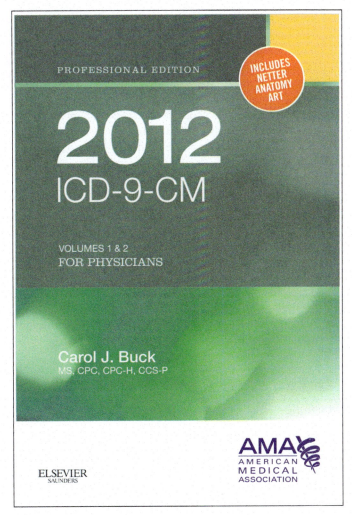

FIGURE 2-1   The ICD-9-CM code book
Source: Michal Heron/Merrill

280–289	Diseases of the blood and blood-forming organs
290–319	Mental, behavior, and neurodevelopmental disorders
320–389	Diseases of the nervous system and sense organs
390–459	Diseases of the circulatory system
460–519	Diseases of the respiratory system
520–579	Diseases of the digestive system
580–629	Diseases of the genitourinary system
630–679	Complications of pregnancy, childbirth, and the puerperium
680–709	Diseases of the skin and subcutaneous tissue
710–739	Diseases of the musculoskeletal system and connective tissue
740–759	Congenital anomalies
760–779	Certain conditions originating in the perinatal period
780–799	Symptoms, signs, and ill-defined conditions
800–999	Injury and poisoning

The *ICD-9-CM* is used when

1. An *ICD-9-CM* code is provided, but there is no language description of the diagnosis.
2. A language diagnosis is included, but an *ICD-9-CM* is not indicated and the terms used by the provider cannot be found in Volume II. If you can identify the body system, you may be able to locate an appropriate *ICD-9-CM* code. (See Table 2-1 ● for the categories found in the Tabular List of Volume I.) V codes and E codes are supplementary classifications found in Volume I. V codes deal with classification of factors influencing health status and contact with health services. E codes are used for classification of external causes of injury and poisoning.

VOLUME II. Volume II is the alphabetical listing of diagnoses. This section is most commonly used first. It is divided into four sections:

1. An alphabetical index of diseases and injuries.
2. A table of drugs and chemicals, hypertension, and neoplasms.
3. An alphabetical index of external causes of injuries and poisonings (accidents, known as E codes).
4. A listing of factors affecting the health status of an individual (V codes).

TABLE 2-1 Tabular List Volume I

Sections	Code Ranges
Evaluation and Management	99201-99499
Anesthesia	00100-01999
Surgery	10040-68899
Radiology	70010-79999
Pathology and Laboratory	80047-89398
Medicine	90281-99607

VOLUME III. Volume III of the *ICD-9-CM* is used for coding diagnoses and procedures performed in a hospital. Volume III contains both a tabular listing and index. In the tabular listing, procedures are arranged according to body sections. The body sections are arranged as follows:

1. Operations on the Nervous System
2. Operations on the Endocrine System
3. Operations on the Eye
4. Operations on the Ear
5. Operations on the Nose, Mouth, and Pharynx
6. Operations on the Respiratory System
7. Operations on the Cardiovascular System
8. Operations on the Hemic and Lymphatic System
9. Operations on the Digestive System
10. Operations on the Urinary System
11. Operations on the Male Genital Organs
12. Operations on the Female Genital Organs
13. Obstetrical Procedures
14. Operations on the Musculoskeletal System
15. Operations on the Integumentary System
16. Miscellaneous Diagnostic and Therapeutic Procedures

The index lists procedures in alphabetical order. Thus, it is the easiest way to look up a procedure. The medical biller or health claims examiner should confirm that the correct code has been selected by looking in the tabular listing and checking all referrals, exclusions, and notes included.

ICD-10-CM/PCS

The *ICD-10-CM/PCS* codes became available for dual use starting on October 1, 2012. The *ICD-10-CM/PCS* has two manuals:

1. **Clinical Manual**
   The *ICD-10-CM* is similar to the *ICD-9-CM* except that the codes are more specific and have been expanded to allow the addition of more codes in the future. Volumes I and II remain in this manual. All healthcare settings will utilize this portion.
2. **Procedural Service Codes**
   This *ICD-10-PCS* manual has been drastically upgraded for inpatient hospital settings to code procedures. This manual contains Volume III. It is tentatively set to release in summer 2012 for use in fall 2012. Full implementation is expected in 2014. The *ICD-11* is in the works and will be implemented between 2014 and 2020.

> ● **ONLINE INFORMATION:** To find the latest updates on the *ICD-10* conversion, visit the website of the *Centers for Medicare and Medicaid Services (CMS)* (www.cms.gov/icd10).

CPT/RVS

The **Current Procedural Terminology (CPT)** is a systematic listing for coding the procedures or services performed by a physician. (See Figure 2-2 ●.) Within this text, the word "physician" is used generically to apply to any provider of services other than a hospital or other facility. A **procedure code** is a five-digit numerical code that is used to designate medical

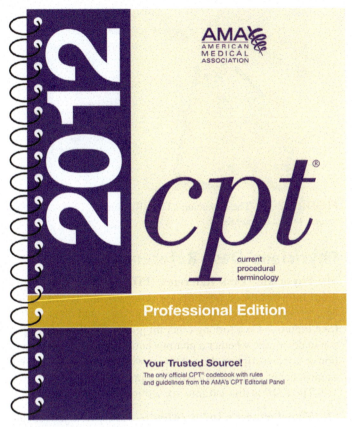

FIGURE 2-2 The CPT manual
Source: Michal Heron/Merrill

services according to standardized, industry-accepted methods, usually reflected in the *CPT* manual. The purpose of the *CPT* is to provide a uniform method of accurately describing medical, surgical, and diagnostic services, which facilitates effective communication among physicians, patients, and claim administrators. **Modifier codes** are two-digit numerical codes or alphanumeric codes attached to a *CPT* code to indicate special circumstances that affect reimbursement for that particular service.

The ***Relative Value Scale (RVS)*** is payment methodology devised by Harvard University and adapted by HCFA now known as CMS to be used in the American Medicare system. It assigns a value to procedures performed by a physician. The relative value differs by geographic region and is adjusted annually. So, a procedure performed in Miami, Florida, is worth more than the same procedure performed in Topeka, Kansas. The following year, the value of the procedure in each location could increase, decrease, or remain the same. The value is multiplied by a conversion factor to determine the amount of payment for that particular procedure. The *RVS* bases prices on three factors: physician work, practice expense, and malpractice expense.

The *CPT* has six major sections:

1. Evaluation and Management 99201–99499
2. Anesthesiology 00100–01999, 99100–99150
3. Surgery 10021–69990
4. Radiology 70010–7999
5. Pathology & Laboratory 80047–89398
6. Medicine 90281–99189; 99500–99607

To properly code using the *CPT*, choose the number code associated with the English-language description of the procedure performed. Sometimes the procedure is described using different terminology (e.g., *testectomy* is found under *orchiectomy*, even though both are legitimate medical terms). Therefore, it is important to check all related codes and alternate terminology for a procedure. It may also be necessary to consult a medical dictionary for alternate terminology for a specified procedure.

In each section of the *CPT*, prior to the first codes there are specific instructions relating to that section. It is important to read each of these instructions in order to properly code the procedures contained in that section or review the appropriateness of the codes (in the case of the claims examiner). Within each section, there are instructions related to each body system as well. For example, in the surgery section there are instructions for the musculoskeletal system, then instructions for organs, and so on.

Some descriptions in the *CPT* are subprocedures of other descriptions. These subheading descriptions will be indented under the main procedure. To properly read an indented procedure, read the description of the main procedure (the one not indented) up to the semicolon. Then add the remaining description found in the indented wording.

For example, codes 21208 and 21209 read as follows:

21208   Osteoplasty, facial bones; augmentation (autograft, allograft, or prosthetic implant)

21209   reduction

Therefore, the correct description for 21209 is Osteoplasty, facial bones; reduction. It is important to carefully read the full description of all related procedures before you choose the one that best describes the procedure performed. A slight change in the main description can significantly alter the meaning of the indented procedure.

Using the CPT Index

The *CPT* index lists all main procedures, often with a choice of several codes. Once again, some procedures are indented, indicating that in each case, the unindented procedure listed directly above is part of the description.

Listings in the *CPT* are arranged by the procedure done, then by the site of the procedure. For example, the heading Transplantation lists numerous portions of the body that can be transplanted and their related codes. Some portions of the body also have a heading. Thus, you may locate the code for transplantation of the liver by looking under either Transplantation and Liver or Liver and Allotransplantation. In most cases, it is best to check both descriptions, as there may be additional codes located under one of the descriptions.

Health Care Common Procedure Coding System

The **Health Care Common Procedure Coding System (HCPCS)** (commonly referred to as "hicpics" in the medical community) was created because there were limitations in the

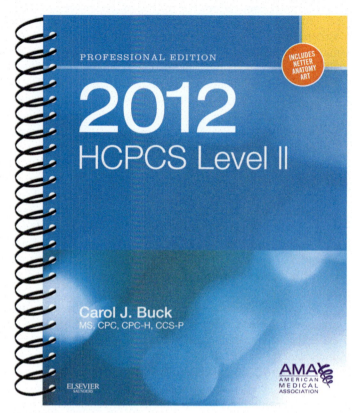

FIGURE 2-3   The HCPCS manual
Source: Michal Heron/Merrill

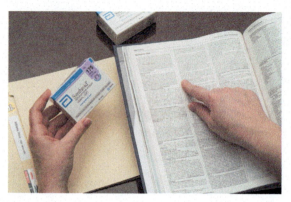

FIGURE 2-4   The Physician's Desk Reference
Source: Michal Heron/Merrill

Physicians' Desk Reference

The **Physicians' Desk Reference (PDR)** is a manual that provides information on prescription drugs, including usage, dosage, appearance, prescription status, makeup, and other factors. (See Figure 2-4 ●.) Among other things, the *PDR* enables a person to determine whether a pharmaceutical product is a prescription or nonprescription drug. This is a very important distinction, as most health plans do not cover nonprescription drugs.

The *PDR* is divided into six sections:

1. **Manufacturer's Index (white)**—Arranged alphabetically by manufacturer, then by drug name. The name and address of the manufacturer are included. This section includes prescription and nonprescription drugs. The related information has been provided by the manufacturer.
2. **Product Name Index (pink)**—Arranged alphabetically by brand name or generic name (if provided). Prescription and nonprescription drugs are included. This section is usually used first to locate the manufacturer's name and the page number to obtain further information.
3. **Product Category Index (blue)**—Arranged alphabetically by drug action category, that is, according to the most common use of the drug. If the drug is an antidepressant, it is listed under the antidepressant category. If it is an antacid, it is listed under the antacid category.
4. **Product Identification Section (gray)**—Arranged alphabetically by manufacturer, then by brand name. This section contains the actual size and full-color reproductions. Only the reproductions submitted by the manufacturer are included.
5. **Product Information Section (white)**—Arranged alphabetically by manufacturer, then brand name. Most pharmaceuticals are described by indications and usage, dosage, administration, description, clinical pharmacology, supply warnings, contraindications, adverse reactions, overdosage precautions, and other information.
6. **Diagnostic Product Information (green)**—Arranged alphabetically by manufacturer, then by product. This section provides a description of diagnostic products only.

CPT and *RVS* for billing services such as injections, medication, supplies, durable medical equipment, and chiropractic and dental services. (See Figure 2-3 ●.) These codes are most often used for billing Medicare claims, but they may also be used for Medicaid claims and for some private insurance carriers (with the exception of J codes, which are used for all drugs within all insurance companies). The HCPCS system actually includes three levels of coding:

• Level I utilizes the current *CPT* codes for most procedures.
• Level II utilizes the HCPCS codes listed in the HCPCS manual.
• Level III utilizes codes that were specific to the local Medicare/Medicaid carrier. Level III codes were discontinued on December 31, 2003.

One way to code using the HCPCS system is to check Level II codes first and then go to the *CPT* manual. Another way is to go to the *CPT* codes first and then check the HCPCS. It depends on the type of coding being done.

To use the HCPCS manual, follow these instructions:

1. If you have a code number, but you need the English language equivalent, look in the front section of the HCPCS. HCPCS codes are a letter followed by several numbers. The codes are listed by the letter, then the numbers following that letter (e.g., V2100, V2101, V2102). In addition, codes are assigned within groups. Therefore, the items within a group will be found near each other (e.g., medications, orthopedic devices).
2. If you have an English language equivalent and you need to look up a HCPCS code, look up the item in the index.

> ● **ONLINE INFORMATION:** Search online to find a medication that you or a family member take. Can you find the generic name, side effects, and a picture of the medication? Report the ease and/or difficulty you encounter in researching this information.

Claims examiners use the Product Information Section (white) the most. However, because generic drugs are cheaper than brand-name medications, many plans encourage their members to purchase generic versions and offer increased payment incentives. Therefore, use of the Product Name Index (which includes both brand names and generic names) is increasing. For instance, instead of paying for generic drugs at the plan's regular coinsurance rate of 80%, members may find that generics are covered at 100%. As with all benefits, this incentive varies widely by plan.

Medical Dictionary

Medical dictionaries list medical terms and their definitions, synonyms, illustrations, and supplemental information. There are numerous medical dictionaries on the market. These dictionaries can be very helpful in assisting the examiner to identify diagnoses, symptoms, prognoses, and common treatment protocols. A dictionary also can assist the medical biller in interpreting the physician's notes, coding the claim, and determining whether the diagnosis or services are allowed under a plan.

As a rule, the medical dictionary should be used mainly to verify a diagnosis or affected body area or to check definitions and the spelling of terms. If you need greater detail on symptomatology and treatment protocols, the *Merck Manual* is more definitive. As with most dictionaries, entries are arranged alphabetically.

When you are using the medical dictionary, it is important to first read through the foreword and any instructions or general guidelines contained in the front of the book. As each publisher uses different symbols and information, you must read these instructions to understand the symbols and terms and their meanings.

Merck Manual

Even the most experienced medical biller will occasionally have questions regarding the appropriateness of services for a reported diagnosis. Medical professionals rely on the **Merck Manual** to assist in identifying the symptomatology, prognosis, treatment protocols, etiology, and other miscellaneous information regarding diagnoses.

When an examiner receives a claim with services that are unusual for that diagnosis, he or she may use the *Merck Manual* to identify whether the treatment is appropriate for the reported diagnosis or symptoms.

The *Merck Manual* has two main sections: a listing of diseases and an index. The index is arranged alphabetically by disease. To look something up, simply turn to the index to find the page containing the disease information.

The information provided includes the diagnosis, symptoms, prognosis, and treatment. If the treatment provided is not consistent with the diagnosis, the claim may be forwarded to a medical review board or a consultant, causing a delay in its processing.

PRACTICE **PITFALLS**

Many medical dictionaries include the following information regarding the word or term, in addition to the basic definition:

1. The etymology of the word (i.e., the original language and meaning).
2. The pronunciation of the word.
3. Biographical information on diseases, symptoms, conditions, procedures, or cures that have been given an eponym (named after a person).
4. Synonyms. Often diseases or conditions are known by more than one name. In these instances, they are listed as synonyms in the dictionary
5. Abbreviations. The standard abbreviation, if there is one in the medical community.
6. Etiology. The causes of the disease.
7. Treatment. Common medical treatments are stated for some diagnoses or conditions. It is understood that these may not be the only effective medical treatments and that specifics of the treatment are not given.
8. Cross-reference. Cross-referencing treatments allows the user to locate possible drugs or treatments that may prove to be effective.
9. Prognosis. A generalized prognosis for the disease is given. At times it will include a prognosis for patients who are not treated and for those who are.

10. Nursing implications. The implications of care of the patient. These may include the need for monitoring of certain conditions or vital signs.
11. Nursing diagnosis cross-reference. Some dictionaries list an appendix of nursing diagnoses and implications. Certain diseases or conditions will be cross-referenced to this section.
12. Subentries. Contain more specific information regarding a term or condition and list some of the different types of conditions that can occur. For example, the subentries under the term "acid" can include acetic a., boric a., citric a., fatty a., and sulfuric a., as well as many others. It is understood that a small letter followed by a period refers to a repetition of the original term or condition. In the preceding example, the "a." stands for the word "acid."
13. Illustration cross-reference. An illustration placed either near the word or under another heading depicts either the term or a portion of the definition. The user is directed to the correct page on which or term under which the illustration can be found.
14. Cautions or warnings. Certain terms or conditions have a warning placed within the definition. Warnings appear most often with drugs and treatments and can include any side effects, adverse reactions, or conditions that can result from use of the drug or treatment. Often this caution or warning is in boldface or marked off within a section to help call attention to it.

(Continued)

When you are using the medical dictionary, it is imperative to read through the entire entry. If the definition uses terms that you do not understand, you should also look up the unknown word, either in the medical dictionary (if it is a medical term) or in a standard dictionary (if it is not).

There are numerous diseases, conditions, or terms that are very similar to each other in spelling or pronunciation but vastly different in meaning. It is important to use the proper term and its proper spelling when you are billing, coding, and examining a claim.

▶ **CRITICAL THINKING QUESTION:** How can the medical dictionary assist the medical biller in properly coding healthcare claims? Provide two examples.

Red Book and Blue Book

The *Red Book* and the *Blue Book* list wholesale prices of drugs. The **Red Book** is primarily used by pharmacists to obtain drug information and wholesale pricing, and the **Blue Book** is used normally by providers and patients to compare pricing within their geographical area.

Some plans have a separate coverage for prescriptions. Drugs on these plans are often paid according to a set price schedule, regardless of the amount charged by the pharmacy or dispensing physician. These schedules are often based on the *Red Book* or the *Blue Book*. Often the plan provisions will specify payment at 150% or 175% of the *Red Book* or *Blue Book* price.

ACTIVITY #1

Resource Manuals

Directions: Determine the correct resource manual needed to answer the question, and then use that reference to find the answer. Do not be concerned if you do not understand all the words in the description or answer.

1. _____ What is the English-language description for diagnosis codes 460 and 487.1?

2. Describe diagnosis 1 (code 460) from question 1. ___

3. Define catarrhal. _____

4. Is fever most commonly a symptom of diagnosis 1 (460) or diagnosis 2 (487.1)? _____

5. What is a synonym for the common cold? _____

6. How long is a person contagious with this disease? ___

7. Name two symptoms or signs of diagnosis 1 (460). ___

8. What causes the condition from diagnosis 1 (460)? ___

9. What is the incubation period for this disease?_____

10. What does the procedure code 87070 indicate, and is it appropriate for diagnosis code 460?_____

ACTIVITY #2

Coding Practice

Directions: Determine the correct resource manual needed to answer the question, and then use that reference to find the answer. Do not be concerned if you do not understand all the words in the description or answer.

1. What is the English-language description for diagnosis code 696.1? _____

2. Describe the disease from question 1. _____

3. What are erythematous papules? _____

4. What is the cause of the disease in question 1? _____

5. Name two symptoms or signs of this disease. _____

6. Name two possible treatments for this disease. _____

7. What is the English-language description for procedure code 97028? _____

8. Is procedure code 97028 a valid treatment for diagnosis code 696.1? _____

9. Should a patient with this disease expose himself to sunlight? _____

10. Does smoking affect this condition? If so, in what way?

CMS-1500 Form

There are two types of forms commonly used for billing claims, the CMS-1500 and the UB-04. We will discuss the CMS-1500 here and the UB-04 later in this chapter. The

CMS-1500 claim form is a standardized form, approved by the American Medical Association for use as a "universal" form for billing outpatient professional services (see Figure 2-5 ●). All healthcare providers who use the CMS-1500 form are required to be covered under HIPAA. These forms are updated to accommodate the *ICD-10-CM/PCS*. These forms in electronic version have been required since January 1, 2012.

CMS-1500 CLAIM FORM

```
1500

HEALTH INSURANCE CLAIM FORM
APPROVED BY NATIONAL UNIFORM CLAIM COMMITTEE 08/05

PICA                                                                            PICA

1. MEDICARE   MEDICAID   TRICARE      CHAMPVA   GROUP        FECA    OTHER   1a. INSURED'S I.D. NUMBER          (For Program in Item 1)
                         CHAMPUS                HEALTH PLAN  BLK LUNG
   (Medicare #) (Medicaid #) (Sponsor's SSN) (Member ID#) (SSN or ID) (SSN) (ID)

2. PATIENT'S NAME (Last Name, First Name, Middle Initial)   3. PATIENT'S BIRTH DATE    SEX   4. INSURED'S NAME (Last Name, First Name, Middle Initial)
                                                               MM   DD   YY
                                                                            M    F

5. PATIENT'S ADDRESS (No, Street)                           6. PATIENT RELATIONSHIP TO INSURED   7. INSURED'S ADDRESS (No, Street)
                                                               Self  Spouse  Child  Other

CITY                                       STATE            8. PATIENT STATUS                    CITY                                STATE
                                                               Single  Married  Other

ZIP CODE        TELEPHONE (Include Area Code)                       Full-Time  Part-Time         ZIP CODE        TELEPHONE (Include Area Code)
                (      )                                   Employed  Student  Student                           (      )

9. OTHER INSURED'S NAME (Last Name, First Name, Middle Initial)  10. IS PATIENT'S CONDITION RELATED TO:   11. INSURED'S POLICY GROUP OR FECA NUMBER

a. OTHER INSURED'S POLICY OR GROUP NUMBER                   a. EMPLOYMENT? (Current or Previous)   a. INSURED'S DATE OF BIRTH         SEX
                                                               YES  NO                                 MM   DD   YY              M    F

b. OTHER INSURED'S DATE OF BIRTH       SEX                  b. AUTO ACCIDENT?    PLACE (State)   b. EMPLOYER'S NAME OR SCHOOL NAME
   MM   DD   YY                  M    F                         YES  NO

c. EMPLOYER'S NAME OR SCHOOL NAME                           c. OTHER ACCIDENT?                    c. INSURANCE PLAN NAME OR PROGRAM NAME
                                                               YES  NO

d. INSURANCE PLAN NAME OR PROGRAM NAME                      10d. RESERVED FOR LOCAL USE          d. IS THERE ANOTHER HEALTH BENEFIT PLAN?
                                                                                                     YES  NO  If yes, return to and complete item 9 a-d

READ BACK OF FORM BEFORE COMPLETING & SIGNING THIS FORM.
12. PATIENT'S OR AUTHORIZED PERSON'S SIGNATURE I authorize the release of any medical or other information    13. INSURED'S OR AUTHORIZED PERSON'S SIGNATURE I authorize payment of medical
    necessary to process this claim. I also request payment of government benefits either to myself or to the party who   benefits to the undersigned physician or supplier for services described below.
    accepts assignment below.

    SIGNED _____   DATE _____         SIGNED _____

14. DATE OF CURRENT    ILLNESS (First symptom) OR   15. IF PATIENT HAS HAD SAME OR SIMILAR ILLNESS.   16. DATES PATIENT UNABLE TO WORK IN CURRENT OCCUPATION
    MM   DD   YY        INJURY (Accident) OR              GIVE FIRST DATE   MM   DD   YY                   MM   DD   YY              MM   DD   YY
                        PREGNANCY (LMP)                                                              FROM                    TO

17. NAME OF REFERRING PHYSICIAN OR OTHER SOURCE    17a.                                         18. HOSPITALIZATION DATES RELATED TO CURRENT SERVICES
                                                   17b.  NPI                                         MM   DD   YY              MM   DD   YY
                                                                                                FROM                    TO

19. RESERVED FOR LOCAL USE                                                                     20. OUTSIDE LAB?              $ CHARGES
                                                                                                   YES  NO

21. DIAGNOSIS OR NATURE OF ILLNESS OR INJURY (Relate Items 1,2,3 or 4 to Item 24E by Line)     22. MEDICAID RESUBMISSION
    1. _____        3. _____                                                   CODE            ORIGINAL REF. NO.
    2. _____        4. _____                                               23. PRIOR AUTHORIZATION NUMBER

24. A. DATE(S) OF SERVICE       B.        C.   D. PROCEDURES, SERVICES, OR SUPPLIES   E.          F.          G.      H.      I.        J.
    From        To           PLACE OF         (Explain Unusual Circumstances)      DIAGNOSIS   $ CHARGES   DAYS   EPSDT   ID.      RENDERING
    MM  DD  YY  MM  DD  YY    SERVICE  EMG    CPT/HCPCS    MODIFIER                 POINTER                 OR    Family  QUAL.   PROVIDER ID. #
                                                                                                          UNITS  Plan

1                                                                                                                          NPI
2                                                                                                                          NPI
3                                                                                                                          NPI
4                                                                                                                          NPI
5                                                                                                                          NPI
6                                                                                                                          NPI

25. FEDERAL TAX ID NUMBER   SSN EIN   26. PATIENT'S ACCOUNT NO.   27. ACCEPT ASSIGNMENT?   28. TOTAL CHARGE   29. AMOUNT PAID   30. BALANCE DUE
                                                                    (For govt. claims, see back)
                                                                    YES  NO               $                $                $

31. SIGNATURE OF PHYSICIAN OR SUPPLIER   32. SERVICE FACILITY LOCATION INFORMATION   33. BILLING PROVIDER INFO & PH. # (      )
    INCLUDING DEGREES OR CREDENTIALS
    (I certify that the statements on the reverse
    apply to this bill and are made a part thereof)

    SIGNED _____ DATE _____   a.            b.                                   a.            b.

NUCC Instruction Manual available at: www.nucc.org                                  APPROVED OMB 0938-0999 FORM CMS-1500 (08/05)
WCMS-1500CS
```

FIGURE 2-5   CMS 1500 form

As you use the CMS-1500, you will become familiar with the various blocks and know where to obtain the information required for completing and processing claim forms. The listing that follows will explain the uses of the various blocks. It contains the block number, the name of the block, and a brief description of the information needed. The word "same" means that the description is the same as the title of the block. Explanations that are too lengthy to be included here have been recorded after this brief listing.

As it is easier to remember information that has been grouped together, we have broken the CMS-1500 into sections for understanding. These sections include information about the patient, the insured, the secondary insurance, third-party liability, the authorization signature, the illness, the procedures performed, and the provider of services.

Block Number and Block Name/Description

Following are the numbers, titles, and descriptions of the blocks found on the CMS-1500 form, along with a description of the information that the coder needs in order to fill in that block.

INFORMATION ABOUT THE PATIENT. These blocks contain information about the patient.

1. Medicare, Medicaid, TRICARE, CHAMPVA, Group Health Plan, FECA Black Lung or Other. Check the box of the organization to which you are submitting this claim for payment.

2. Patient's Name. Enter patient name.

3. Patient's Birth Date and Sex. All dates should be recorded as Month/Day/Year (e.g., 01/13/2012). Check the box for the appropriate sex.

5. Patient's Address, City, State, ZIP code, and Phone Number. Enter address.

6. Patient's Relationship to Insured. Spouse, self, etc.

8. Patient's Status. Check applicable boxes.

INFORMATION ABOUT THE INSURED. These blocks contain information on the insured, their insurance, and their employment.

1a. Insured's ID Number. Social security number, ID number, or policy number of insured.

4. Insured's Name. Subscriber's name (or Same, as title suggests).

7. Insured's Address, City, State, ZIP code, and Phone Number. Same, as title suggests.

11. Insured's Policy Group or FECA (Federal Employees Compensation Act) Number. Subscriber's Group Number. This number refers to the primary insured listed in 1a.

11a. Insured's Date of Birth and Sex. Same, as title suggests.

11b. Employer's Name or School Name. Name of insured party's employer or school.

11c. Insurance Plan Name or Program Name. Name of insurance company or group plan.

11d. Is There Another Health Benefit Plan? Check appropriate box. If "YES" is checked, then items 9a–9d must be completed.

INFORMATION ABOUT THE SECONDARY INSURANCE. These blocks contain information about a secondary insurance policy (if any), which may provide coverage on this patient.

9. Other Insured's Name. Other insured whose coverage may be responsible, in whole or in part, for the payment of this claim.

9a. Other Insured's Policy or Group Number. Same, as title suggests.

9b. Other Insured's Date of Birth and Sex. Same, as title suggests.

9c. Employer's Name or School Name. Name of other insured party's employer or school.

9d. Insurance Plan Name or Program Name. Name of insurance company or group plan for other insured.

INFORMATION ABOUT THIRD-PARTY LIABILITY. These blocks contain information on whether a third party may be liable for payment on this claim.

10a. Is Patient's Condition Related to: Employment? If "YES" is marked, then Workers' Compensation Insurance is involved. If "NO" is marked, then Workers' Compensation is not involved. Circle whether employment is current or previous.

10b. Is Condition Related to: Auto Accident? If "YES" is marked, then check for an injury date (Block 14) and an injury diagnosis (Block 21). Also indicate the state in which the accident occurred. If "NO" is marked, then the claim may not be for an auto accident injury. Also use this block for workers' compensation.

10c. Is Condition Related to: Other Accident? If "YES" is marked, then check for an injury date (Block 14) and an injury diagnosis (Block 21). If "NO" is marked, then the claim may not be for an accident injury.

10d. Reserved for Local Use. Used for Medicaid crossover claims.

AUTHORIZATION SIGNATURES. These blocks should be signed by the insured, or a signed permanent release of information and assignment of benefits form should be kept on file. If there is a permanent release of information or assignment of benefits on file, the words SIGNATURE ON FILE should be placed in these boxes.

12. Patient's or Authorized Person's Signature and Date Signed. Acknowledging patient's release of medical information form is on file.

13. Assignment of Benefits. Acknowledging patient's assignment of benefits form is on file.

INFORMATION ABOUT THE ILLNESS. These blocks contain information about the current illness.

14. Date of Illness, Injury, Accident or Pregnancy. All injury claims (i.e., injury diagnosis) must have an injury, accident, or workers' compensation date. If the patient's condition is a pregnancy, the date of the last menstrual period (LMP) should be indicated.

15. If Patient Has Had Same or Similar Illness, Give First Date. Same.

16. Dates Patient Unable To Work in Current Occupation. Enter dates.

17. Name of Referring Physician or Other Source. If this patient was referred to the current physician by another physician, hospital, or clinic, the referring party should be listed here.

17a. ID Number of Referring Physician. National Practitioner Identifier (NPI) number of referring physician (if there is one).

17b. Provider's NPI Number. NPI number of provider.

18. Hospitalization Dates Relating to Current Services. Enter dates.

19. Reserved for Local Use. Leave blank.

20. Outside Lab. Was laboratory work performed outside your office and your office is billing for it? If so, check the yes box, and indicate the total of the charges.

21. Diagnosis or Nature of Illness or Injury. The diagnosis states why the patient went to see the provider. You can list up to four diagnostic codes.

22. Medicaid Resubmission Code. Leave blank, unless the claim is a Medicaid resubmission, in which case you add the claim number here.

INFORMATION ABOUT THE PROCEDURES PERFORMED.

These blocks contain information about the procedures that were performed.

23. Prior Authorization Number. Authorization number for services that were approved prior to being rendered.

24a. Date(s) of Service. The date(s) when the provider rendered service. A complete date must be given, unless it is the same date of service, in which case you only have to enter the date once.

24b. Place of Service. The location where the services were performed (located at the front of the *CPT* manual).

24c. EMG (Emergency). If service was rendered in the hospital emergency room, this should match the service code in block 24b.

24d. Procedures, Services, or Supplies. The five-digit procedure code as found in the *CPT* and HCPCS manuals. These are codes that have been assigned to each procedure the provider can perform. By selecting the proper code, billers can describe the type of service performed with a few numbers. This practice eliminates the confusion that used to arise from various abbreviations and descriptions of a procedure. It also allows for easy computer tabulation of the different procedures performed. You can list up to six codes on the form.

24d. Modifier Code. The two-digit modifier from the *CPT/RVS* further describing the procedure code. You can list up to four modifiers.

24e. Diagnosis Pointer. This block is used in conjunction with block 21. The number placed in block 24e (e.g., 1, 2,

3, 4) refers to diagnosis 1, 2, 3, or 4 in block 21. In other words, the doctor can perform different services for different illnesses or injuries on different dates and submit them all on one claim form as long as the dates are consecutive.

24f. Charges. The charge per line of service.

24g. Days or Units. The number of times a service was performed.

24h. EPSDT (Early Periodic Screening, Diagnosis, and Treatment) Family Plan. Leave blank.

24i. ID Qualifier. Enter the ID qualifier 1C (meaning Medicare Provider ID Number) in the shaded portion.

24j. Rendering Provider ID #. Enter the provider's NPI number.

28. Total Charge. The total charge of the claim.

29. Amount Paid. The amount paid by the patient or subscriber.

30. Balance Due. The difference between the total charge and the amount paid by the patient or subscriber (if any).

INFORMATION ABOUT THE PROVIDER OF SERVICES. These blocks contain information about the provider of services.

25. Federal Tax ID Number. This may be the TIN (Tax Identification Number) if the provider is an independent practitioner. If the provider of service is a facility, an Employer Identification Number (EIN) should be used. Check the appropriate box, indicating whether the TIN or EIN was used.

26. Patient's Account Number. Indicate the account number.

27. Accept Assignment for Government Claims. For all insurance carriers, if you have signed a contract as a provider, then you should check Yes. Both 13 and 27 need to be complete. However, some carriers don't care about 13 if the provider is contracted, and they automatically send payment to the provider due to the contract provisions. This block is always used if they are a participating provider.

31. Signature of Physician or Supplier of Service. Must be electronically signed by the provider, indicating that the said services have indeed been rendered. Degrees or credentials (e.g., M.D., D.O.) should follow the name.

32. Service Facility Location Information. Enter facility address here.

33. Physician's/Supplier's Billing Name, Address, ZIP Code, and Phone #. The name, address, and phone number of the physician or supplier of service. This is the address to which payments will be addressed if assignment of benefits has been indicated in block 13 and 27.

33a. NPI of the Billing Provider or Group. This is a required field.

33b. Effective May 23, 2008, Item 33b is not to be reported.

Block 24b, Place of Service

This item needed further description for which space was not available in the preceding text. This is a numerical code to indicate the place where the service was rendered (see Table 2-2 ●).

TABLE 2-2 **Place of Service Codes**

Place of Service Code	Place of Service Name	Place of Service Description
01	Pharmacy	A facility or location where drugs and other medically related items and services are sold, dispensed, or otherwise provided directly to patients. (effective 10/1/05)
02	Unassigned	N/A
03	School	A facility whose primary purpose is education.
04	Homeless shelter	A facility or location whose primary purpose is to provide temporary housing to homeless individuals (e.g., emergency shelters, individual or family shelters).
05	Indian health service freestanding facility	A facility or location, owned and operated by the Indian Health Service, which provides diagnostic, therapeutic (surgical and nonsurgical), and rehabilitation services to American Indians and Alaska Natives who do not require hospitalization.
06	Indian health service provider-based facility	A facility or location, owned and operated by the Indian Health Service, which provides diagnostic, therapeutic (surgical and nonsurgical), and rehabilitation services rendered by, or under the supervision of, physicians to American Indians and Alaska Natives admitted as inpatients or outpatients.
07	Tribal 638 freestanding facility	A facility or location, owned and operated by a federally recognized American Indian or Alaska Native tribe or tribal organization under a 638 agreement which provides diagnostic, therapeutic (surgical and nonsurgical), and rehabilitation services to tribal members who do not require hospitalization.
08	Tribal 638 provider-based facility	A facility or location, owned and operated by a federally recognized American Indian or Alaska Native tribe or tribal organization under a 638 agreement which provides diagnostic, therapeutic (surgical and nonsurgical), and rehabilitation services to tribal members admitted as inpatients or outpatients.
09	Prison-correctional facility	A prison, jail, reformatory, work farm, detention center, or any other similar facility maintained by either Federal, State, or local authorities for the purpose of confinement or rehabilitation of adult or juvenile criminal offenders.
10	Unassigned	N/A
11	Office	Location, other than a hospital, skilled nursing facility (SNF), military treatment facility, community health center, State or local public health clinic, or intermediate care facility (ICF), where the health professional routinely provides health examinations, diagnosis, and treatment of illness or injury on an ambulatory basis.
12	Home	Location, other than a hospital or other facility, where the patient receives care in a private residence
13	Assisted living facility	Congregate residential facility with self-contained living units providing assessment of each resident's needs and on-site support 24 hours a day, seven days a week, with the capacity to deliver or arrange for services, including some health care and other services.
14	Group home	A residence, with shared living areas, where clients receive supervision and other services such as social and/or behavioral services, custodial service, and minimal services (eg. medication administration) (effective 4/1/04).
15	Mobile unit	A facility or unit that moves from place to place and is equipped to provide preventive, screening, diagnostic, and/or treatment services.
16	Temporary lodging	A short term accommodation such as a hotel, camp ground, hostel, cruise ship, or resort where the patient receivers care, and which is not identified by any other POS code
17	Walk-in retail health clinic	A walk-in health clinic, other than an office, urgent care facility, pharmacy, or independent clinic, and which is not described by any other Place of Service code, that is located within a retail operation and provides on an ambulatory basis, preventive and primary care services. (This code is available for use immediately with a final effective date of May 1, 2010.)
18-19	Unassigned	N/A
20	Urgent care facility	Location, distinct from a hospital emergency department, an office, or a clinic, whose purpose is to diagnose and treat illness or injury for unscheduled, ambulatory patients seeking immediate medical attention.
21	Inpatient hospital	A facility, other than psychiatric, which primarily provides diagnostic, therapeutic (both surgical and nonsurgical), and rehabilitation services by, or under, the supervision of physicians to patients admitted for a variety of medical conditions.
22	Outpatient hospital	A portion of a hospital that provides diagnostic, therapeutic (both surgical and nonsurgical), and rehabilitation services to sick or injured persons who do not require hospitalization or institutionalization.
23	Emergency room–hospital	A portion of a hospital where emergency diagnosis and treatment of illness or injury is provided.
24	Ambulatory surgical center	A freestanding facility, other than a physician's office, where surgical and diagnostic services are provided on an ambulatory basis.

TABLE 2-2 (*Continued*)

Place of Service Code	Place of Service Name	Place of Service Description
25	Birthing center	A facility, other than a hospital's maternity facilities or a physician's office, which provides a setting for labor, delivery, and immediate postpartum care as well as immediate care of newborn infants.
26	Military treatment facility	A medical facility operated by one or more of the Uniformed Services. Military Treatment Facility (MTF) also refers to certain former U. S. Public Health Service (USPHS) facilities now designated as Uniformed Service Treatment Facilities (USTF).
27-30	Unassigned	N/A
31	Skilled nursing facility	A facility that primarily provides inpatient skilled nursing care and related services to patients who require medical, nursing, or rehabilitative services but does not provide the level of care or treatment available in a hospital.
32	Nursing facility	A facility that primarily provides to residents skilled nursing care and related services for the rehabilitation of injured, disabled, or sick persons, or, on a regular basis, health-related care services above the level of custodial care to other than mentally retarded individuals.
33	Custodial care facility	A facility that provides room, board and other personal assistance services, generally on a long-term basis, and that does not include a medical component.
34	Hospice	A facility, other than a patient's home, in which palliative and supportive care for terminally ill patients and their families are provided.
35-40	Unassigned	N/A
41	Ambulance—land	A land vehicle specifically designed, equipped, and staffed for lifesaving and transporting the sick or injured.
42	Ambulance—air or water	An air or water vehicle specifically designed, equipped, and staffed for lifesaving and transporting the sick or injured.
43-48	Unassigned	N/A
49	Independent clinic	A location, not part of a hospital and not described by any other Place of Service code, that is organized and operated to provide preventive, diagnostic, therapeutic, rehabilitative, or palliative services to outpatients only. (effective 10/1/03)
50	Federally qualified health center	A facility located in a medically underserved area that provides Medicare beneficiaries preventive primary medical care under the general direction of a physician.
51	Inpatient psychiatric facility	A facility that provides inpatient psychiatric services for the diagnosis and treatment of mental illness on a 24-hour basis, by or under the supervision of a physician.
52	Psychiatric facility-partial hospitalization	A facility for the diagnosis and treatment of mental illness that provides a planned therapeutic program for patients who do not require full time hospitalizations, but who need broader programs than are possible from outpatient visits to a hospital-based or hospital-affiliated facility.
53	Community mental health center	A facility that provides the following services: outpatient services, including specialized outpatient services for children, the elderly, individuals who are chronically ill, and residents of the CMHC's mental health community area who have been discharged from inpatient treatment at a mental health facility; 24 hour a day emergency care services; day treatment, other partial hospitalization services, or psychosocial rehabilitation services; screening for patients being considered for admission to State mental health facilities to determine the appropriateness of such admission; and consultation and education services.
54	Intermediate care facility/mentally retarded	A facility that primarily provides health-related care and services above the level of custodial care to mentally retarded individuals but does not provide the level of care or treatment available in a hospital or SNF.
55	Residential substance abuse treatment facility	A facility which provides treatment for substance (alcohol and drug) abuse to live-in residents who do not require acute medical care. Services include individual and group therapy and counseling, family counseling, laboratory tests, drugs and supplies, psychological testing, and room and board.
56	Psychiatric residential treatment center	A facility or distinct part of a facility for psychiatric care which provides a total 24-hour therapeutically planned and professionally staffed group living and learning environment.
57	Non-residential substance abuse treatment facility	A location that provides treatment for substance (alcohol and drug) abuse on an ambulatory basis. Services include individual and group therapy and counseling, family counseling, laboratory tests, drugs and supplies, and psychological testing.
58-59	Unassigned	N/A

(*Continued*)

TABLE 2-2 *(Continued)*

Place of Service Code	Place of Service Name	Place of Service Description
60	Mass immunization center	A location where providers administer pneumococcal pneumonia and influenza virus vaccinations and submit these claims as electronic medical claims, paper claims, or using the roster billing method. This generally takes place in a mass immunization setting, such as a public health center, pharmacy, or mall but may include a physician office setting.
61	Comprehensive inpatient rehabilitation facility	A facility that provides comprehensive rehabilitation services under the supervision of a physician to inpatients with physical disabilities. Services include physical therapy, occupational therapy, speech pathology, social or psychological services, and orthotics and prosthetics services.
62	Comprehensive outpatient rehabilitation facility	A facility that provides comprehensive rehabilitation services under the supervision of a physician to outpatients with physical disabilities. Services include physical therapy, occupational therapy, and speech pathology.
63-64	Unassigned	N/A
65	End-stage renal disease treatment facility	A facility other than a hospital that provides dialysis treatment, maintenance, and/or training to patients or caregivers on an ambulatory or home-care basis.
66-70	Unassigned	N/A
71	Public health clinic	A facility maintained by either State or local health departments that provides ambulatory primary medical care under the general direction of a physician.
72	Rural health clinic	A certified facility that is located in a rural medically underserved area that provides ambulatory primary medical care under the general direction of a physician.
73-80	Unassigned	N/A
81	Independent laboratory	A laboratory certified to perform diagnostic and/or clinical tests independent of an institution or a physician's office.
82-98	Unassigned	N/A
99	Other place of service	Other place of service not identified above.

▶ **CRITICAL THINKING QUESTION:** Where might coders, billers, and health claims administrators find continued updates to the CMS-1500 form?

PRACTICE **PITFALLS**

Tips on Understanding the CMS-1500

Properly using the CMS-1500 is vital to receiving the proper reimbursement on claims. The following tips will help to minimize errors and speed processing of a claim.

1. Be sure that the patient information contained on the claim matches that in your records.
2. Be sure that all necessary blocks are filled in.
3. Be sure that all diagnoses have related procedures, and all procedures have a related diagnosis.
4. Do not write additional comments on the form. Instead, attach a separate paper for comments.
5. Do not sign or write in red ink. Many scanners used by insurance carriers are programmed to pass over everything in red on the form and just pick up the data. Therefore, anything in red will not be picked up by the scanner.
6. Do not use a highlighter on the form. Some scanners will pick up the highlighter and turn it into a black mark, thus obliterating the information in that field.

ACTIVITY #3

CMS-1500

Directions: Look at the CMS-1500 form in Figure 2-5, and then indicate the box that provides the information given. Write your answer in the space provided.

1. What is the patient's name? _____
_____

2. What is the name of the insured person on this claim?
_____

3. What is the procedure code for the procedure performed?
_____

4. What is the diagnosis code given? _____
_____

5. What is the patient's marital status? _____
_____

6. Under what insurance plan is the patient covered?
_____

7. Has the authorization to release information been signed? _____

8. Is this patient covered under more than one insurance policy? _____

9. Have benefits been assigned on this claim? _____
   _____

10. What is the name of the provider on this claim? ____
    _____

Version 5010: CMS-1500 and UB-04

The CMS-1500 for outpatient services and the UB-04 for hospital or inpatient services are universally accepted health insurance claim forms. The previous version was **Version 4010/4010A**. Although the forms were originally designed for use to bill Medicare and Medicaid consistently, they are now required for those health facilities covered by HIPAA and billing insurance agencies.

CMS-1500

The Modifications to the HIPAA Electronic Transaction Standards Final Rule, published on January 16, 2009, replaced the current versions of the standards (4010/4010A) with **Version 5010** and Version D.0, respectively. The National Council for Prescription Drug Program (NCPDP) also adopted a new standard for Medicaid subrogation for pharmacy claims known as 3.0.

Version 5010 includes the following changes to accommodate the *ICD-10* codes:

- Increased field size for *ICD* codes from five spaces to seven spaces
- Added one-digit version indicator to the *ICD* code to indicate Version 9 versus Version 10
- Increased number of diagnosis codes allowed on a claim

There are several added data modifications for the HIPAA Standards in Version 5010:

- Standardized business information related to the transaction
- Utilization of TR3 (Technical Reports Type 3 (TR3)—guidelines that represent data consistently and are less confusing
- Specification of what data need to be collected and transmitted
- Accommodation of reporting of clinical data (i.e., *ICD-10-CM* diagnosis codes and *ICD-10-PCS* procedure codes)
- Distinction between principal diagnosis, admitting diagnosis, external cause of injury, and patient reason for visit codes
- Support of monitoring of certain illness mortality rates, outcomes for specific treatment options, some hospital length of stays, and clinical reasons for care
- Address of currently unmet business needs, such as an indicator on institutional claims with a diagnosis that is "present upon admission"

CMS system improvements include the following changes:

- Implementation of standard acknowledgment and rejection transactions across all jurisdictions
- Improved claims receipt, control, and balancing procedures
- Increased consistency of claims editing and error handling
- Return of claims that need correction earlier in the process
- Assignation of claim numbers closer to the time of receipt

The CMS website contains several resources for obtaining these new forms and provides crossover and training information for healthcare providers to effectively implement these changes.

> ▶ **CRITICAL THINKING QUESTION:** If the 5010 format does not accommodate the information you need to document to bill appropriately, what action should you take?

UB-04

The National Uniform Billing Committee (NUBC) is responsible for updating the **Uniform Billing Form 2004 (UB-04)**. The UB-04 is intended to be used by hospitals or other hospital-type facilities for inpatient and outpatient billing (see Figure 2-6 ●). This form was designed to provide the basic data needed by most payers to adjudicate a large majority of their claims. The objective was to accommodate a wide range of needs while eliminating the need for attachments.

As you use this form, you will become familiar with the various boxes and know where to obtain the information required for completing and processing claim forms. The following list will assist in explaining the uses of the various fields. It contains the field number, the name of the field, and a brief description of the information needed. The word "same" refers to a description that is the same as the title of the box. Explanations that are too lengthy to be included here have been recorded after this brief listing. Be sure to always be looking at the most updated manual.

FORM LOCATOR #, NAME, AND DESCRIPTION. The form locator number helps the coder find the block in which to put the indicated information.

1. Provider Name and Address (required). Name and address of hospital or clinic where services were rendered.

2. Pay-to Name and Secondary Identification Fields (situational). When this information is different from the provider name and address, use this field.

3a. Patient Control Number (required). Patient's account number.

3b. Medical/Health Record Number (situational). If patient's medical record number is different from the account number, use this field.

4. Type of Bill (required). This four-digit alphanumeric code gives three specific pieces of information after a leading zero. CMS will ignore the leading zero. CMS will continue to process three specific pieces of information. The second digit identifies the type of facility. The third classifies the type of care. The fourth indicates the sequence of this bill in this particular episode of care. It is referred to as a "frequency" code. (See Table 2-3 ● for further information.)

5. Federal Tax Number (required). Provider's identification number or social security number.

6. Statement Covers Period (required). The dates of service that this billing statement represents. Dates should match

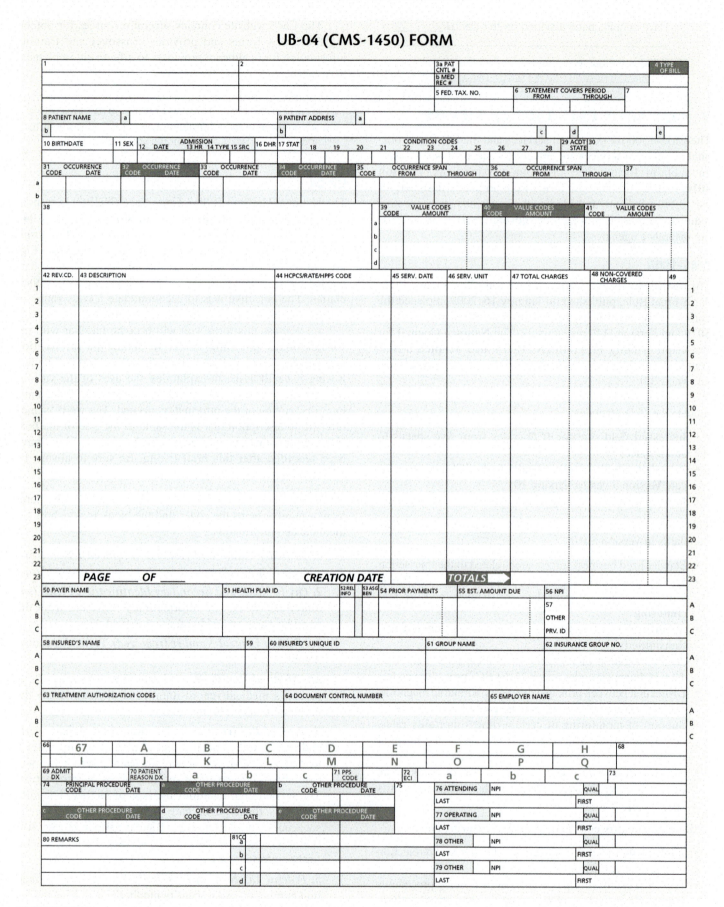

FIGURE 2-6 UB-04 form

TABLE 2-3 Hospital Revenue Codes

Major Category	Subcategory (Standard Abbreviation)
001	**Total Charges.** To reflect the total of all charges on this bill.
01X	**Reserved for internal payer use.** Leave blank.
02X-06X	**Reserved for National Assignment.** Leave blank.
07X-09X	**Reserved for State Assignment.** Leave blank.
10X	**All-inclusive Rate.** Flat fee charge incurred on either a daily basis or total stay basis for services rendered. Charge may cover room and board plus ancillary services or room and board only.
	0 All-inclusive room and board plus ancillary (ALL-INCL R&B/ANC)
	1 All-inclusive room and board (ALL-INCL R&B)
11X	**Room and Board—Private (Medical or General).** Routine service charges for single-bed rooms.
	0 General Classification (R&B/PVT)
	1 Medical/Surgical/Gyn (MED-SER-GYN/PVT)
	2 OB (OB/PVT)
	3 Pediatric (PEDS/PVT)
	4 Psychiatric (PSYCH/PVT)
	5 Hospice (HOSPICE/PVT)
	6 Detoxification (DETOX/PVT)
	7 Oncology (ONCOLOGY/PVT)
	8 Rehabilitation (REHAB/PVT)
	9 Other (OTHER/PVT)
12X	**Room and Board--Semiprivate Two-Bed (Medical or General).** Routine service charges incurred for accommodations with two beds.
	0 General Classification (R&B/SEMI)
	1 Medical/Surgical/Gyn (MED-SUR-GYN/2 Bed)
	2 OB (OB/2 Bed)
	3 Pediatric (PED/ 2 Bed)
	4 Psychiatric (PSYCH/2 Bed)
	5 Hospice (HOSPICE/2 Bed)
	6 Detoxification (DETOX/2 Bed)
	7 Oncology (ONCOLOGY/2 Bed)
	8 Rehabilitation (REHAB/2 Bed)
	9 Other (OTHER/2 Bed)
13X	**Semiprivate—Three and Four Beds.** Routine service charges incurred for accommodations with three and four beds.
	0 General Classification (R&B/3&4 Bed)
	1 Medical/Surgical/Gyn (MED-SUR-GYN/3&4 Bed)
	2 OB (OB/3&4 Bed)
	3 Pediatric (PED/3&4 Bed)
	4 Psychiatric (PSYCH/3&4 Bed)
	5 Hospice (HOSPICE/3&4 Bed)
	6 Detoxification (DETOX/3&4 Bed)
	7 Oncology (ONCOLOGY/3&4 Bed)
	8 Rehabilitation (REHAB/3&4 Bed)
	9 Other (OTHER/3&4 Bed)
14X	**Private (Deluxe).** Deluxe rooms are accommodations with amenities substantially in excess of those provided to other patients.
	0 General Classification (R&B/PVT/DLX)
	1 Medical/Surgical/Gyn (MED-SUR-GYN/DLX)
	2 OB (OB/DLX)
	3 Pediatric (PED/DLX)
	4 Psychiatric (PSYCH/DLX)
	5 Hospice (HOSPICE/DLX)
	6 Detoxification (DETOX/DLX)
	7 Oncology (ONCOLOGY/DLX)
	8 Rehabilitation (REHAB/DLX)
	9 Other (OTHER/DLX)

(Continued)

TABLE 2-3 *(Continued)*

Major Category	Subcategory (Standard Abbreviation)
15X	**Room and Board—Ward (Medical or General).** Routine service charge for accommodations with five or more beds.
	0 General Classification (R&B/WARD)
	1 Medical/Surgical/Gyn (MED-SUR-GYN/WARD)
	2 OB (OB/WARD)
	3 Pediatric (PED/WARD)
	4 Psychiatric (PSYCH/WARD)
	5 Hospice (HOSPICE/WARD)
	6 Detoxification (DETOX/WARD)
	7 Oncology (ONCOLOGY/WARD)
	8 Rehabilitation (REHAB/WARD)
	9 Other (OTHER/WARD)
16X	**Other Room and Board.** Any routine service charges for accommodations that cannot be included in the more specific revenue center codes.
	0 General Classification (R&B)
	4 Sterile Environment (R&B/STRL)
	7 Self-Care (R&B/SELF)
	9 Other (R&B/Other)
17X	**Nursery.** Charges for nursing care to newborn and premature infants in nurseries.
	0 General Classification (NURSERY)
	1 Newborn (NURSERY/NEWBORN)
	2 Premature (NURSERY/PREMIE)
	5 Neonatal ICU (NURSERY/ICU)
	9 Other (NURSERY/OTHER)
18X	**Leave of Absence.** Charges for holding a room while the patient is temporarily away from the provider.
	0 General Classification (LOA)
	1 Reserved (RESERVED)
	2 Patient Convenience (LOA/PT CONV)
	3 Therapeutic Leave (LOA THER)
	4 ICF/MR--any reason (LOA/ICF/ MR)
	5 Nursing Home (for hospitalization) (LOA/NURS HOME)
	6 Other Leave of Absence (LOA/OTHER)
19X	**Not Assigned.**
20X	**Intensive Care.** Routine service charge for medical or surgical care provided to patients who require a more intensive level of care than is rendered in the general medical or surgical unit.
	0 General Classification (ICU)
	1 Surgical (ICU/SURGICAL)
	2 Medical (ICU/MEDICAL)
	3 Pediatric (ICUPEDS)
	4 Psychiatric (ICU/PSYCH)
	6 Post-ICU (POST ICU)
	7 Burn Care (ICU/BURN CARE)
	8 Trauma (ICU/TRAUMA)
	9 Other Intensive Care (ICU/OTHER)
21X	**Coronary Care.** Routine service charge for medical or surgical care provided to patients with coronary illness who require a more intensive level of care than is rendered in the general medical care unit.
	0 General Classification (CCU)
	1 Myocardial Infarction (CCU/MYO INFARC)
	2 Pulmonary Care (CCU/PULMON)
	3 Heart Transplant (CCU/TRANS-PLANT)
	4 Post-CCU (POST CCU)
	9 Other Coronary Care (CCU/OTHR)

TABLE 2-3 (*Continued*)

Major Category	Subcategory (Standard Abbreviation)
22X	**Special Charges.** Charges incurred during an inpatient stay or on a daily basis for certain services.
	0 General Classification (SPCL CHGS)
	1 Admission Charge (ADMIT CHG)
	2 Technical Support Charge (TECH SUPPT CHG)
	3 UR Service Charge (UR CHG)
	4 Late Discharge, Medically Necessary (LATE DISCH/MED NEC)
	9 Other Special Charges (OTHER SPEC CHG)
23X	**Incremental Nursing Charge Rate.** Charge for nursing service assessed in addition to room and board.
	0 General Classification (NURSING INCREM)
	1 Nursery (NUR INCR/NURSERY)
	2 OB (NUR INCR/OB)
	3 ICU (NUR INCR/ICU)
	4 CCU (NUR INCR/CCU)
	5 Hospice (NUR INCR/HOSPICE)
	9 Other (NUR INCR/OTHER)
24X	**All-Inclusive Ancillary.** A flat rate incurred on either a daily basis or total stay basis for ancillary services only.
	0 General Classification (ALL INCL ANCIL)
	9 Other Inclusive Ancillary (ALL INCL ANCIL/OTHER)
25X	**Pharmacy.** Charges for medication produced, manufactured, packaged, controlled, assayed, dispensed, and distributed under the direction of a licensed pharmacist. This category includes blood plasma, other components of blood, and IV solutions.
	0 General Classification (PHAR)
	1 Generic Drugs (DRUGS/GENRC)
	2 Nongeneric Drugs (DRUGS/ NONGENRC)
	3 Take Home Drugs (DRUGS/ TAKEHOME)
	4 Drugs Incident to Other Diagnostic Services (DRUGS/INCIDENT OTHER DX)
	5 Drugs Incident to Radiology (DRUGS/INCIDENT RAD)
	6 Experimental Drugs (DRUGS/ EXPERIMT)
	7 Nonprescription (DRUGS/ NONPSCRPT)
	8 IV Solutions (IV SOLUTIONS)
	9 Other Pharmacy (DRUGS/OTHER)
26X	**IV Therapy.** Administration of intravenous solution by specially trained personnel to individuals requiring such treatment.
	0 General Classification (IV THER)
	2 Infusion Pump (IV THER/INFSN PUMP)
	3 IV Therapy--Pharmacy Services (IV THER/PHARM/ SVC)
	4 IV Therapy/Drug/Supply Delivery (IV THER/DRUG/ SUPPLY DELV)
	9 Other IV Therapy (IV THERP/ OTHER)
	NOTE: Providers billing for home IV therapy should use the HCPCS code that describes the pump in Item 44.
27X	**Medical/Surgical Supplies and Devices.** Charges for supply items required for patient care.
	0 General Classification (MED-SUR SUPPLIES)
	1 Nonsterile Supply (NON-STER SUPPLY)
	2 Sterile Supply (STERILE SUPPLY)
	3 Take Home Supplies (TAKE HOME SUPPLY)
	4 Prosthetic/Orthotic Devices (PROSTH/ORTH DEV)
	5 Pacemaker (PACE MAKER)
	6 Intraocular Lens (INTRA OC LENS)
	7 Oxygen-Take Home (O2/ TAKEHOME)
	8 Other Implants (SUPPLY/ IMPLANTS)
	9 Other Supplies/Devices (SUPPLY/ OTHER)
28X	**Oncology.** Charges for the treatment of tumors and related diseases.
	0 General Classification ONCOLOGY
	9 Other Oncology (ONCOLOGY/ OTHER)

(*Continued*)

TABLE 2-3 (*Continued*)

Major Category	Subcategory (Standard Abbreviation)
29X	**Durable Medical Equipment (Other Than Renal).** Charges for medical equipment that can withstand repeated use (excluding renal equipment).
	0 General Classification (DME)
	1 Rental (MED EQUIP/RENT)
	2 Purchase of new DME (MED EQUIP/NEW)
	3 Purchase of used DME (MED EQUIP/USED)
	4 Supplies/Drugs for DME Effectiveness (Home Health Agency Only) (MED EQUIP/SUPPLIES/ DRUGS)
	9 Other Equipment (MED EQUIP/ OTHER)
30X	**Laboratory.** Charges for the performance of diagnostic and routine clinical laboratory tests.
	0 General Classification (LAB)
	1 Chemistry (LAB/CHEMISTRY)
	2 Immunology (LAB/IMMUNLGY)
	3 Renal Patient (Home) (LAB/RENAL HOME)
	4 Nonroutine Dialysis (LAB/NR DIALYSIS)
	5 Hematology (LAB/HEMAT)
	6 Bacteriology & Microbiology (LAB/BACT-MICRO)
	7 Urology (LAB/UROLOGY)
	9 Other Laboratory (LAB/OTHER)
31X	**Laboratory Pathological.** Charges for diagnostic and routine lab tests on tissues and culture.
	0 General Classification (PATH LAB)
	1 Cytology (PATHOL/CYTOLOGY)
	2 Histology (PATHOL/HYSTOL)
	4 Biopsy (PATHOL/BIOPSY)
	9 Other (PATHOL/OTHER)
32X	**Radiology--Diagnostic.** Charges for diagnostic radiology services provided for the examination and care of patients. Includes taking, processing, examining, and interpreting radiographs and fluorographs.
	0 General Classification (DX X-RAY)
	1 Angiocardiography (DX X-RAY/ ANGIO)
	2 Arthrography (DX X-RAY/ARTH)
	3 Arteriography (DX X-RAY/ ARTER)
	4 Chest X-Ray (DX X-RAY/CHEST)
	9 Other (DX X-RAY/OTHER)
33X	**Radiology--Therapeutic.** Charges for therapeutic radiology services and chemotherapy that are required for care and treatment of patients. Included therapy by injection or ingestion of radioactive substances.
	0 General Classification (RX X-RAY)
	1 Chemotherapy--Injected (CHEMOTHER/INJ)
	2 Chemotherapy--Oral (CHEMOTHER/ORAL)
	3 Radiation Therapy (RADIATION RX)
	5 Chemotherapy--IV (CHEMOTHERP-IV)
	9 Other (RX X-RAY/OTHER)
34X	**Nuclear Medicine.** Charges for procedures and tests performed by a radioisotope laboratory utilizing radioactive materials as required for diagnosis and treatment of patients.
	0 General Classification (NUC MED)
	1 Diagnostic (NUC MED/DX)
	2 Therapeutic (NUC MED/RX)
	9 Other (NUC MED/OTHER)
35X	**CT Scan.** Charges for computed tomographic scans of the head and other parts of the body.
	0 General Classification (CT SCAN)
	1 Head Scan (CT SCAN/HEAD)
	2 Body Scan (CT SCAN/BODY)
	9 Other CT Scans (CT SCAN/OTHR)

TABLE 2-3 (*Continued*)

Major Category	Subcategory (Standard Abbreviation)
36X	**Operating Room Services.** Charges for services provided to patients in the performance of surgical and related procedures during and immediately following surgery.
	0 General Classification (OR SERVICES)
	1 Minor Surgery (OR/MINOR)
	2 Organ Transplant--Other than kidney (OR/ORGAN TRANS)
	7 Kidney Transplant (OR/KIDNEY TRANS)
	9 Other Operating Room Services (OR/OTHER)
37X	**Anesthesia.** Charges for anesthesia services in the hospital.
	0 General Classification (ANESTHE)
	1 Anesthesia Incident to Radiology (ANESTHE/INCIDENT RAD)
	2 Anesthesia Incident to Other Diagnostic Services (ANESTHE/ INCDNT OTHER DX)
	4 Acupuncture (ANESTHE/ ACUPUNC)
	9 Other Anesthesia (ANESTHE/ OTHER)
38X	**Blood.**
	0 General Classification (BLOOD)
	1 Packed Red Cells (BLOOD/PKD RED)
	2 Whole Blood (BLOOD/WHOLE)
	3 Plasma (BLOOD/PLASMA)
	4 Platelets (BLOOD PLATELETS)
	5 Leucocytes (BLOOD/ LEUCOCYTES)
	6 Other Components (BLOOD/ COMPONENTS)
	7 Other Derivatives (Cryoprecipitates) (BLOOD/DERIVATIVES)
	9 Other Blood (BLOOD/OTHER)
39X	**Blood Storage and Processing.** Charges for storage and processing of whole blood.
	0 General Classification (BLOOD/ STOR-PROC)
	1 Blood Administration (BLOOD/ ADMIN)
	9 Other Blood Storage and Processing (BLOOD/OTHER STOR)
40X	**Other Imaging Services.**
	0 General Classification (IMAGE SVS)
	1 Diagnostic Mammography (DIAG MAMMOGRAPHY)
	2 Ultrasound (ULTRASOUND)
	3 Screening Mammography (SCRN MAMMOGRAPHY)
	4 Positron Emission Tomography (PET SCAN)
	9 Other Imaging Services (OTHER IMAGE SVS)
	NOTE: High-risk beneficiaries should be noted by the inclusion of one of the following ICD-9CM diagnosis codes:
	V10.3 Personal History--Malignant neoplasm breast cancer
	V16.3 Family History--Malignant neoplasm breast cancer (mother, sister or daughter with breast cancer)
	V15.89 Other specified personal history representing hazards to health (not given birth prior to 30, a personal history of biopsy proven breast disease). Must be coded to the appropriate 4th or 5th digit.
41X	**Respiratory Services.** Charges for administration of oxygen and certain potent drugs through inhalation or positive pressure and other forms of rehabilitative therapy through measurement of inhaled and exhaled gases and analysis of blood and evaluation of the patient's ability to exchange oxygen and other gases.
	0 General Classification (RESPIR SVC)
	2 Inhalation Services (INHALATION SVC)
	3 Hyperbaric Oxygen Therapy (HYPERBARIC O2)
	9 Other Respiratory Services (OTHER RESPIR SVS)
42X	**Physical Therapy.** Charges for therapeutic exercises, massage, and utilization of light, heat, cold, water, electricity, and assistive devices for diagnosis and rehabilitation of patients who have neuromuscular, orthopedic, and other disabilities.
	0 General Classification (PHYS THERP)
	1 Visit Charge (PHYS THERP/ VISIT)
	2 Hourly Charge (PHYS THERP/ HOUR)
	3 Group Rate (PHYS THERP/ GROUP)
	4 Evaluation or Reevaluation (PHYS THEREVAL)
	9 Other Physical Therapy (OTHER PHYS THERP)

(Continued)

TABLE 2-3 (*Continued*)

Major Category	Subcategory (Standard Abbreviation)
43X	**Occupational Therapy.** Charges for teaching manual skills and independent personal care to stimulate mental and emotional activity on the part of patients.
	0 General Classification (OCCUP THERP)
	1 Visit Charge (OCCUP THERP/ VISIT)
	2 Hourly Charge (OCCUP THERP/ HOUR)
	3 Group Rate (OCCUP THERP/ GROUP)
	4 Evaluation or Reevaluation (OCCUP THER/EVAL)
	9 Other Occupational Therapy (OTHER OCCUP THERP)
44X	**Speech-Language Pathology.** Charges for services provided to persons with impaired functional communications skills.
	0 General Classification (SPEECH PATHOL)
	1 Visit Charge (SPEECH PATH/ VISIT)
	2 Hourly Charge (SPEECH PATH/ HOUR)
	3 Group Rate (SPEECH PATH/ GROUP)
	4 Evaluation or Reevaluation (SPEECH PATHEVAL)
	9 Other Speech-Language Pathology (OTHER SPEECH PAT)
45X	**Emergency Room.** Charges for emergency treatment to those ill and injured persons who require immediate unscheduled medical or surgical care.
	0 General Classification (EMERG ROOM)
	9 Other Emergency Room (OTHER EMER ROOM)
46X	**Pulmonary Function.** Charges for tests that measure inhaled and exhaled gases and analysis of blood and for tests that evaluate the patient's ability to exchange oxygen and other gases.
	0 General Classification (PULMON FUNC)
	9 Other Pulmonary Function (OTHER PULMON FUNC)
47X	**Audiology.** Charges for the detection and management of communication handicaps centering in whole or in part on the hearing function.
	0 General Classification (AUDIOL)
	1 Diagnostic (AUDIOLOGY/DX)
	2 Treatment (AUDIOLOGY/RX)
	9 Other Audiology (OTHER AUDIOL)
48X	**Cardiology.** Charges for cardiac procedures rendered in a separate unit within the hospital. Such procedures include but are not limited to heart catheterization, coronary angiography, Swan-Ganz catheterization, and exercise stress test.
	0 General Classification (CARDIOL)
	1 Cardiac Cath Lab (CARDIAC CATH LAB)
	2 Stress Test (STRESS TEST)
	9 Other Cardiology (OTHER CARDIOL)
49X	**Ambulatory Surgical Care.**
	0 General Classification (AMBUL SURG)
	9 Other Ambulatory Surgical Care (OTHER AMBL SURG)
50X	**Outpatient Services.** Outpatient charges for services rendered to an outpatient who is admitted as an inpatient before midnight of the day following the date of service. These charges are incorporated on the inpatient bill of Medicare patients.
	0 General Classification (OUTPATIENT SVS)
	9 Other Outpatient Services (OUTPATIENT/OTHER)
51X	**Clinic.** Clinic (nonemergency/scheduled outpatient visit) charges for providing diagnostic, preventive, curative, rehabilitative, and education services on a scheduled basis to ambulatory patients.
	0 General Classification (CLINIC)
	1 Chronic Pain Center (CHRONIC PAIN CL)
	2 Dental Clinic (DENTAL CLINIC)
	3 Psychiatric Clinic (PSYCH CLINIC)
	4 OB-GYN Clinic (OB-GYN CLINIC)
	5 Pediatric Clinic (PEDS CLINIC)
	9 Other Clinic (OTHER CLINIC)

TABLE 2-3 (*Continued*)

Major Category	Subcategory (Standard Abbreviation)
52X	**Free-Standing Clinic.**
	0 General Classification (FR/STD CLINIC)
	1 Rural Health--Clinic (RURAL/ CLINIC)
	2 Rural Health--Home (RURAL/ HOME)
	3 Family Practice (FAMILY PRAC)
	9 Other Freestanding Clinic (OTHER FR/STD CLINIC)
53X	**Osteopathic Services.** Charges for a structural evaluation of the cranium, entire cervical, dorsal, and lumbar spine by a doctor of osteopathy.
	0 General Classification (OSTEOPATH SVS)
	1 Osteopathic Therapy (OSTEOPATH RX)
	9 Other Osteopathic Services (OTHER OSTEOPATH)
54X	**Ambulance.** Charges for ambulance service, usually unscheduled, to the ill/ injured who require immediate medical attention.
	0 General Classification (AMBUL)
	1 Supplies (AMBUL/SUPPLY)
	2 Medical Transport (AMBUL/MED TRANS)
	3 Heart Mobile (AMBUL/ HEARTMOBL)
	4 Oxygen (AMBUL/OXY)
	5 Air Ambulance (AIR AMBUL)
	6 Neonatal Ambulance Services (AMBUL/NEONAT)
	7 Pharmacy (AMBUL/PHARMACY)
	8 Telephone Transmission EKG (AMBUL/TELEPHONIC EKG)
	9 Other Ambulance (OTHER AMBULANCE)
	NOTE: Units may be either miles or trips.
	NOTE: On items 55-58, charges should be reported to the nearest hour.
55X	**Skilled Nursing.** Charges for nursing services that must be provided under the direct supervision of a licensed nurse to ensure the safety of the patient and to achieve the medically desired result. This code may be used for nursing home services or a service charge for home health billing.
	0 General Classification (SKILLED NURS)
	1 Visit Charge (SKILLED NURS/ VISIT)
	2 Hourly Charge (SKILLED NURS/ HOUR)
	9 Other Skilled Nursing (SKILLED NURS/OTHER)
56X	**Medical Social Services.** Charges for services such as counseling patients, interviewing patients, and interpreting problems of social situation rendered to patients on any basis.
	0 General Classification (MED SOCIAL SVS)
	1 Visit Charge (MED SOC SERVS/ VISIT)
	2 Hourly Charge (MED SOC SERVS/HOUR)
	9 Other Medical Social Services (MED SOCIAL SERVS/OTHER)
57X	**Home Health Aide (Home Health).** Charges made by a home health agency for personnel that are primarily responsible for the personal care of the patient.
	0 General Classification (AIDE/ HOME HEALTH)
	1 Visit Charge (AIDE/HOME HLTH/ VISIT)
	2 Hourly Charge (AIDE/HOME HLTH/HOUR)
	9 Other Home Health Aide (AIDE/ HOME HLTH/OTHER)
58X	**Other Visits (Home Health).** Charges by a home health agency for visits other than physical therapy, occupational therapy or speech therapy, which must be specifically identified.
	0 General Classification (VISIT/ HOME HEALTH)
	1 Visit Charge (VISIT/HOME HLTH/ VISIT)
	2 Hourly Charge (VISIT/HOME HLTH/HOUR)
	9 Other Home Health (VISIT/HOME HLTH/OTHER)
59X	**Units of Service (Home Health).** Revenue code used by a home health agency that bills on the basis of units of service.
	0 General Classification (UNIT/ HOME HEALTH)
	9 Home Health Other Units (UNIT/ HOME HLTH/OTHER)

(Continued)

TABLE 2-3 *(Continued)*

Major Category	Subcategory (Standard Abbreviation)
60X	**Oxygen Home Health.** Charges by a home health agency for oxygen equipment, supplies, or contents, excluding purchased items. If a beneficiary has purchased a stationary oxygen system, and oxygen concentrator or portable equipment, revenue codes 292 or 293 apply. DME other than oxygen systems is billed under codes 291, 292, or 293. 0 General Classification (O2/HOME HEALTH) 1 Oxygen--Stationary Equipment, Supplies or Contents (O2/STAT EQUIP/SUPPL/CONT) 2 Oxygen--Stationary Equipment or Supplies Under 1 LPM (O2/STAT EQUIP/UNDER 1 LPM) 3 Oxygen--Stationary Equipment or Supplies Over 4 LPM (O2/STAT EQUIP/OVER 4 LPM) 4 Oxygen--Portable Add-on (O2/ PORTABLE ADD-ON)
61X	**MRI.** Charges for Magnetic Resonance Imaging of the brain and other parts of the body. 0 General Classification (MRI) 1 Brain (including brain stem) (MRI-BRAIN) 2 Spinal Cord (including spine) (MRI-SPINE) 9 Other MRI (MRI-OTHER)
62X	**Medical/Surgical Supplies.** Charges for supplies required for patient care. This code is an extension of code 27X and allows for the reporting of additional breakdown, if needed. Subcategory 1 is for providers who are not able to bill supplies used for radiology procedures under radiology. Subcategory 2 is for providers who are not able to bill supplies used for other diagnostic procedures under diagnostic procedures. 1 Supplies Incident to Radiology (MED-SUR SUPP/INCDNT RAD) 2 Supplies Incident to Other Diagnostic Services (MED-SUR UPP/INCDNT ODX)
63X	**Drugs Requiring Specific identification.** Charges for drugs and biologicals requiring specific identification required by the payer. If you are using HCPCS to identify the drug, the HCPCS code should be entered in Item 44. 0 General Classification (DRUGS) 1 Single Source Drug (DRUG/ SNGLE) 2 Multiple Source Drug (DRUG/ MULT) 3 Restrictive Prescription (DRUG/ RSTR) 4 Erythropoietin (EPO) less than 10,000 units (DRUG/EPO10,000 Units) 5 Erythropoietin (EPO) more than 10,000 units (DRUG/EPO10,000 Units) 6 Drugs requiring detailed coding (DRUGS/DETAIL CODE) NOTE: Revenue Code 636 relates to a HCPCS code. Therefore, the appropriate HCPCS code should be entered in Item 44. The specific units of services to be reported should be in hundreds (100s) rounded to the nearest hundred.
64X	**Home IV Therapy Services.** Charge for IV drug therapy services that are done in the patient's home. For home IV providers, the appropriate HCPCS code must be entered for all equipment and covered therapy. 0 General Classification (IV THER SVC) 1 Nonroutine Nursing, Central Line (NON RT NURSING/CENTRAL) 2 IV Site Care, Central Line, HCPCS related(IV SITE CARE/CENTRAL) 3 IV Start/Change Peripheral Line (IV STRT/CHNG/PERIPHRL) 4 Nonroutine Nursing Peripheral Line (NON RT NURSING/PERIPHRL) 5 Training Patient/Caregiver, Central Line (TRNG PT/CAREGVR/ CENTRAL) 6 Training Disabled Patient, Central Line (TRNG DSBLPT/CENTRAL) 7 Training Patient/Caregiver, Peripheral Line (TRNG PT/ CAREGVR/PERIPHRL) 8 Training Disabled Patient, Peripheral Line (TRNG DSBLPT/ PERIPHRL) 9 Other IV Therapy Services (OTHER IV THERAPY SVC) NOTE: Units need to be reported in 1-hour increments.
65X	**Hospice Service.** Charges for hospice care services for a terminally ill patient. The patient would need to elect these services in lieu of other services for a terminal condition. 0 General Classification (HOSPICE) 1 Routine Home Care (HOSPICE/RTN HOME) 2 Continuous Home Care (HOSPICE/ CTNS HOME) 3 RESERVED 4 RESERVED 5 Inpatient Respite Care (HOSPICE/ IP RESPITE) 6 General Inpatient Care (Nonrespite) (HOSPICE/IP NONRESPITE)

TABLE 2-3 (*Continued*)

Major Category	Subcategory (Standard Abbreviation)
	7 Physician Services (HOSPICE/ PHYSICIAN)
	9 Other Hospice (HOSPICE/OTHER)
	NOTE: There must be a minimum of 8 hours of care (not necessarily continuous) during a 24-hour period to receive the Continuous Home Care rate from Medicare under code 652. If less than 8 hours of care are provided, code 651 should be used. Any portion of an hour counts as an hour. When billing Medicare under code 657, a physician procedure code must be entered in Item 44. Code 657 is used by the hospice to bill for physician's services furnished to hospice patients when the physician is employed by the hospice or receives payment from the hospice for services rendered.
66X	**Respite Care.** Charges for hours of service under the Respite Care Benefit for homemaker or home health aide, personal care services, and nursing care provided by a licensed professional nurse.
	0 General Classification (RESPITE CARE)
	1 Hourly Charge/Skilled Nursing (RESPITE/SKILLED NURSE)
	2 Hourly Charge/Home Health Aide/ Homemaker (RESPITE/HMEAID/ HMEMKR
67X	**Not Assigned.**
68X	**Not Assigned.**
69X	**Not Assigned.**
70X	**Cast Room.** Charges for services related to the application, maintenance, and removal of casts.
	0 General Classification (CAST ROOM)
	9 Other Cast Room (OTHER CAST ROOM)
71X	**Recovery Room.**
	0 General Classification (RECOV RM)
	9 Other Recovery Room (OTHER RECOV RM)
72X	**Labor Room/Delivery.** Charges for labor and delivery room services provided by specially trained nursing personnel to patients, including prenatal care during labor, assistance during delivery, postnatal care in the recovery room, and minor gynecological procedures if they are performed in the delivery suite.
	0 General Classification (DELIVROOM/LABOR)
	1 Labor (LABOR)
	2 Delivery (DELIVERY ROOM)
	3 Circumcision (CIRCUMCISION)
	4 Birthing Center (BIRTHING CENTER)
	9 Other Labor Room/Delivery (OTHER/DELIV-LABOR)
73X	**EKG/ECG (Electrocardiogram).** Charges for operation of specialized equipment to record electromotive variations in actions of the heart muscle on an electrocardiograph for diagnosis of heart ailments.
	0 General Classification (EKG/ECG)
	1 Holter Monitor (HOLTER MON)
	2 Telemetry (TELEMETRY)
	9 Other EKG/ECG (OTHER EKG/ECG)
74X	**EEG (Electroencephalogram).** Charges for operation of specialized equipment to measure impulse frequencies and differences in electrical potential in various areas of the brain to obtain data for use in diagnosing brain disorders.
	0 General Classification (EEG)
	9 Other EEG (OTHER EEG)
75X	**Gastrointestinal Services.**
	0 General Classification (GASTR-INTS SVS)
	9 Other Gastrointestinal (OTHER GASTROINTS)
	NOTE: Use 759 with the procedure code for endoscopic procedure
76X	**Treatment/Observation Room.** Charges for the use of a treatment room, or observation room charges for outpatient observation services.
	0 General Classification (TREATMT/OBSERVATION RM)
	1 Treatment Room (TREATMT RM)
	2 Observation Room (OBSERV RM)
	9 Other Treatment/Observation Room (OTHER TREAT/OBSERV RM)
77X	**Not Assigned.**
78X	**Not Assigned.**

(*Continued*)

TABLE 2-3 (*Continued*)

Major Category	Subcategory (Standard Abbreviation)
79X	**Lithotripsy.** Charges for using lithotripsy in the treatment of kidney stones.
	0 General Classification (LITHOTRIPSY)
	9 Other Lithotripsy (LITHOTRIPSY/ OTHER)
80X	**Inpatient Renal Dialysis.** A waste removal process that uses an artificial kidney when the body's own kidneys have failed. The waste may be removed directly from the blood (hemodialysis) or indirectly from the blood by flushing a special solution between the abdominal covering and the tissue (peritoneal dialysis). In-unit lab nonroutine tests are medically necessary tests in addition to or at greater frequency than routine tests that are performed in the dialysis unit.
	0 General Classification (RENAL DIALY)
	1 Inpatient Hemodialysis (DIALY/ INPT)
	2 Inpatient Peritoneal (Non-CAPD) (DIALY/INPT/PER)
	3 Inpatient Continuous Ambulatory Peritoneal Dialysis (DIALY/ INPT/CAPD)
	4 Inpatient Continuous Cycling Peritoneal Dialysis (DIALY/ INPT/CCPD)
	9 Other Inpatient Dialysis (DIALY/ INPT/OTHER)
81X	**Organ Acquisition.** The acquisition of a kidney, liver, or heart for use in transplantation. Organs other than these are included in category 89X. Living donor is a living person from whom kidney is obtained for transplantation. Cadaver is an individual who has been pronounced dead according to medical and legal criteria from whom organs have been obtained for transplantation.
	0 General Classification (ORGAN ACQUISIT)
	1 Living Donor--Kidney (KIDNEY/ LIVE)
	2 Cadaver Donor--Kidney (KIDNEY/ CADAVER)
	3 Unknown Donor--Kidney (KIDNEY/UNKNOWN)
	4 Other Kidney Acquisition (KIDNEY/OTHER)
	5 Cadaver Donor--Heart (HEART/ CADAVER)
	6 Other Heart Acquisition (HEART/ OTHER)
	7 Donor--Liver (LIVER ACQUISIT)
	9 Other Organ Acquisition (ORGAN/ OTHER)
82X	**Hemodialysis--Outpatient or Home.** A program under which a patient performs hemodialysis away from the facility using his or her own equipment and supplies. Hemodialysis is the removal of waste directly from the blood.
	0 General Classification (HEMO/OP OR HOME)
	1 Hemodialysis/Composite or Other Rate (HEMO/COMPOSITE)
	2 Home Supplies (HEMO/HOME/ SUPPL)
	3 Home Equipment (HEMO/HOME/ EQUIP)
	4 Maintenance 100% (HEMO/HOME/ 100%)
	5 Support Services (HEMO/HOME/ SUPSERV)
	9 Other Outpatient Hemodialysis (HEMO/HOME/OTHER)
83X	**Peritoneal Dialysis--Outpatient or Home.** A program under which a patient performs peritoneal dialysis away from the facility using his or her own equipment and supplies. Waste is removed by flushing a special solution between the tissue and the abdominal covering.
	0 General Classification (PERTNL/ OP OR HOME)
	1 Peritoneal/Composite or Other Rate (PERTNL/COMPOSITE)
	2 Home Supplies (PERTNL/HOME/ SUPPL)
	3 Home Equipment (PERTNL/ HOME/EQUIP)
	4 Maintenance 100% (PERTNL/ HOME/100%)
	5 Support Services (PERTNL/HOME/ SUPSERV)
	9 Other Outpatient Peritoneal (PERTNL/HOME/OTHER)
84X	**Continuous Ambulatory Peritoneal Dialysis (CAPD)--Outpatient or Home.** A program under which a patient performs continual dialysis away from the facility using his or her own equipment and supplies. The patient's peritoneal membrane is used as a dialyzer.
	0 General Classification (CAPD/OP OR HOME)
	1 CAPD/Composite or Other Rate (CAPD/COMPOSITE)
	2 Home Supplies (CAPD/HOME/ SUPPL)
	3 Home Equipment (CAPD/HOME/ EQUIP)
	4 Maintenance 100% (CAPD/HOME/ 100%)
	5 Support Services (CAPD/HOME/ SUPSERV)
	9 Other Outpatient CAPD (CAPD/ HOME/OTHER)

TABLE 2-3 (*Continued*)

Major Category	Subcategory (Standard Abbreviation)
85X	**Continuous Cycling Peritoneal Dialysis (CCPD)--Outpatient or Home.** A program under which a patient performs continual dialysis away from the facility using his or her own equipment and supplies. A machine is used to make automatic exchanges at night. 0　General Classification (CCPD/OP OR HOME) 1　CCPD/Composite or Other Rate (CCPD/COMPOSITE) 2　Home Supplies (CCPD/HOME/ SUPPL) 3　Home Equipment (CCPD/HOME/ EQUIP) 4　Maintenance 100% (CCPD/HOME/ 100%) 5　Support Services (CCPD/HOME/ SUPSERV) 9　Other Outpatient CCPD (CCPD/ HOME/OTHER)
86X	**Reserved for Dialysis (National Assignment).**
87X	**Reserved for Dialysis (National Assignment).**
88X	**Miscellaneous Dialysis.** Charges for dialysis services not identified elsewhere. *Rationale:* Ultrafiltration is the process of removing excess fluid from the blood of dialysis patients by using a dialysis machine but without the dialysis solution. The designation is only used when the procedure is not performed as a part of a normal dialysis session. 0　General Classification (DIALY/ MISC) 1　Ultrafiltration (DIALY/ ULTRAFILT) 2　Home Dialysis Aid Visit (HOME DIALY AID VISIT) 9　Miscellaneous Dialysis Other (DIALY/MISC/OTHER)
89X	**Other Donor Bank.** Charges for the acquisition, storage, and preservation of all human organs (excluding kidneys). 0　General Classification (DONOR BANK) 1　Bone (DONOR BANK/BONE) 2　Organ (other than Kidney) (DONOR BANK/ORGN) 3　Skin (DONOR BANK/SKIN) 9　Other Donor Bank (OTHER DONOR BANK)
90X	**Psychiatric/Psychological Treatments.** Charges for providing treatment for emotionally disturbed patients, including patients admitted for diagnosis and for treatment. 0　General Classification (PSYCH TREATMENT) 1　Electroshock Treatment (ELECTRO SHOCK) 2　Milieu Therapy (MILIEU THER) 3　Play Therapy (PLAY THERAPY) 9　Other (OTHER PSYCH RX)
91X	**Psychiatric/Psychological Services.** Charges for providing nursing care and professional services for emotionally disturbed patients, including patients admitted for diagnosis and those admitted for treatment. 0　General Classification (PSYCH SVS) 1　Rehabilitation (PSYCH/REHAB) 2　Day Care (PSYCH/DAYCARE) 3　Night Care (PSYCH/NIGHTCARE) 4　Individual Therapy (PSYCH/INDIV RX) 5　Group Therapy (PSYCH/GROUP RX) 6　Family Therapy (PSYCH/FAMILY RX) 7　Biofeedback (PSYCH/BIOFEED) 8　Testing (PSYCH/TESTING) 9　Other (PSYCH/OTHER)
92X	**Other Diagnostic Services.** Charges for other diagnostic services not otherwise categorized. 0　General Classification (OTHER DX SVS) 1　Peripheral Vascular Lab (PERI-VASCUL LAB) 2　Electromyogram (EMG) 3　Pap Smear (PAP SMEAR) 4　Allergy Test (ALLERGY TEST) 5　Pregnancy Test (PREG TEST) 9　Other Diagnostic Service (ADDL DX SVS)
93X	**Not Assigned.**

(Continued)

TABLE 2-3 (*Continued*)

Major Category	Subcategory (Standard Abbreviation)
94X	**Other Therapeutic Services.** Charges for other therapeutic services not otherwise categorized.
	0 General Classification (OTHER RX SVS)
	1 Recreational Therapy (RECREA-TION RX)
	2 Education/Training (EDUC/TRNG)
	3 Cardiac Rehabilitation (CARDIAC REHAB)
	4 Drug Rehabilitation (DRUG REHAB)
	5 Alcohol Rehabilitation (ALCOHOL REHAB)
	6 Complex Medical Equipment--Routine (CMPLX MED EQUIP-ROUT)
	7 Complex Medical Equipment--Ancillary (CMPLX MED EQUIP-ANC)
	9 Other Therapeutic Services (ADDITIONAL RX SVS)
	NOTE: Use 930 with a procedure code for plasmapheresis. Use 932 for dietary therapy and diabetes-related services, education, and training.
95X	**Not Assigned.**
96X	**Professional Fees.** Charges for medical professionals that the hospitals or third party payers require to be separately identified.
	0 General Classification (PRO FEE)
	1 Psychiatric (PRO FEE/PSYCH)
	2 Ophthalmology (PRO FEE/EYE)
	3 Anesthesiologist (MD) (PRO FEE/ ANES MD)
	4 Anesthetist (CRNA) (PRO FEE/ ANES CRNA)
	9 Other Professional Fees (OTHER PRO FEE)
97X	**Professional Fees (continued).**
	1 Laboratory (PRO FEE/LAB)
	2 Radiology--Diagnostic (PRO FEE/RAD/DX)
	3 Radiology--Therapeutic (PRO FEE/RAD/RX)
	4 Radiology--Nuclear Medicine (PRO FEE/NUC MED)
	5 Operating Room (PRO FEE/OR)
	6 Respiratory Therapy (PRO FEE/ RESPIR)
	7 Physical Therapy (PRO FEE/ PHYSI)
	8 Occupational Therapy (PRO FEE/ OCUPA)
	9 Speech Pathology (PRO FEE/ SPEECH)
98X	**Professional Fees (continued).**
	1 Emergency Room (PRO FEE/ER)
	2 Outpatient Services (PRO FEE/ OUTPT)
	3 Clinic (PRO FEE/CLINIC)
	4 Medical Social Services (PRO FEE/ SOC SVC)
	5 EKG (PRO FEE/EKG)
	6 EEG (PRO FEE/EEG)
	7 Hospital Visit (PRO FEE/HOS VIS)
	8 Consultation (PRO FEE/CONSULT)
	9 Private Duty Nurse (FEE/PVT NURSE)
99X	**Patient Convenience Items.** Charges for items that are generally considered by the third party payors to be strictly convenience items and, as such, are not covered.
	0 General Classification (PT CONV)
	1 Cafeteria/Guest Tray (CAFETERIA)
	2 Private Linen Service (LINEN)
	3 Telephone/Telegraph (TELEPHN)
	4 TV/Radio (TV/RADIO)
	5 Nonpatient Room Rentals (NONPT ROOM RENT)
	6 Late Discharge Charge (LATE DISCH)
	7 Admission Kits (ADMIT KITS)
	8 Beauty Shop/Barber (BARBER/BEAUTY)
	9 Other Patient Convenience Items (PT CONVENCE/OTH)

those on the itemized billing statement. If services were rendered on the same day, both dates should be the same.

7. Future Use. Leave blank.

8. Patient Name (required). Patient name.

9. Patient Address (required). Patient address.

10. Patient Birthdate (required). Patient date of birth.

11. Patient Sex (required). Same (see Table 2-4 • for further information).

12. Admission Date (required for Inpatient and Home Health). Date patient was admitted to hospital.

TABLE 2-4 Hospital Form Locator Codes

Type of Bill Codes (Form Locator 4)	
Code	**1st Digit: Type of Facility**
1	Hospital
2	Skilled nursing facility
3	Home health
4	Christian science (hospital)
5	Christian science (extended care)
6	Intermediate care
7	Clinic
8	Special Facility
Code	**2nd Digit: Bill Classifications (Clinics only)**
1	Rural Health
2	Clinic - Hospital Based or Independent Renal dialysis center
3	Free-standing
4	Other rehabilitation facility
5	Clinic - CORF
6	Clinic - CMHC
9	Other
Code	**2nd Digit - Bill Classifications (Except Clinics & Special Facilities)**
1	Inpatient (including Medicare Part A)
2	Inpatient (Medicare Part B only)
3	Outpatient
4	Other
5	Intermediate Care, Level I
6	Intermediate Care, Level II
7	SubAcute Inpatient
8	Swing Beds
Code	2nd Digit - Bill Classifications (Special Facilities only)
1	Hospice (Non Hospital Based)
2	Hospice (Hospital Based)
3	Ambulatory Surgical Center
4	Free Standing Birth Center
5	Critical Access Hospital
6	Residential Facility
9	Other
Code	3rd Digit: Frequency
0	Non-Payment/Zero
1	Admit through discharge claim
2	Interim: first claim

(Continued)

TABLE 2-4 (*Continued*)

Type of Bill Codes
(Form Locator 4)

Code	1st Digit: Type of Facility
3	Interim: continuing claims
4	Interim: last claim
5	Late charge only
6	Reserved
7	Replacement of prior claim
8	Void/cancel of prior claim
9	Final Claim for a Home Health PPS Episode

Sex Codes
(Form Locator 15)

Code	Definitions
M	Male
F	Female
U	Unknown

Marital Status Codes
(Form Locator 16)

Code	Definition
S	Single
M	Married
X	Legally separated
D	Divorced
W	Widowed
U	Unknown
P	Life partner

Type of Admission Codes
(Form Locator 19)

Code	Definition
1	Emergency
2	Urgent
3	Elective
4	Newborn
5	Trauma Center
9	Information not available

Source of Admission Codes Except Newborns
(Form Locator 20)

Code	Definition
1	Physician referral
2	Clinical referral
3	HMO referral

TABLE 2-4 (*Continued*)

Source of Admission Codes Except Newborns
(Form Locator 20)

Code	Definition
4	Transfer from a hospital
5	Transfer from a skilled nursing facility
6	Transfer from another health facility
7	Emergency room
8	Court/law enforcement
9	Information not available
A	Transfer from a critical access hospital
B	Transfer from another HHA
C	Readmission to same HHA

Additional Source of Admission Codes for Newborns
(Form Locator 20)

Code	Definition
1	Normal delivery
2	Premature delivery
3	Sick baby
4	Extramural birth
5	Information not available

Patient Status
(Form Locator 22)

Code	Definition
01	Discharged to home or self-care (routine discharge)
02	Discharged/transferred to another short-term general hospital
03	Discharged/transferred to a skilled nursing facility
04	Discharged/transferred to an intermediate care facility
05	Discharged/transferred to another type of institution (including distinct parts) or referred for outpatient services to another institution
06	Discharged/transferred to home under care of organized home health service organization
07	Left against medical advice or discontinued care
08	Discharged/transferred to home under care of home IV therapy provider
09	Admitted as an inpatient to this hospital
20	Expired (or did not recover - Christian Science patient)
30	Still a patient or expected to return for outpatient services
31-39	Reserved for National Assignment
40	Expired at home (for hospice care only)
41	Expired in a medical facility such as a hospital, SNF, ICF, or free-standing hospice (for hospice care only)
42	Expired, place unknown (for hospice care only)
43	Discharged/transferred to a Federal Hospital
50	Discharged to a hospice, Home
51	Discharged to hospice, Medical Facility

(*Continued*)

TABLE 2-4 (*Continued*)

Condition Codes
(Form Locator 24-30)

Code	Definition
02	Enter this code if the patient alleges that the medical condition causing this episode of care is due to environment/event from his/her employment.
03	Indicates that patient/patient representative has stated that coverage may exist beyond that reflected on this bill.
04	Indicates bill is submitted for informational purposes only. Examples would include a bill submitted as a utilization report, or a bill for a beneficiary who is enrolled in a risk-based managed care plan (such as Medicare+Choice) and the hospital expects to receive payment from the plan.
05	Enter this code if you have filed a legal claim for recovery of funds potentially due to a patient or on behalf of a patient.

Release of Information Indicator
Codes (Form Locator 52)

Code	Definitions
Y	Yes
R	Restricted or modified release
N	No release

Member's Relationship to the Insured Codes
(Form Locator 59)
(Date of Service is before October 16, 2003)

Code	Definition
01	Patient is the insured
02	Spouse
03	Natural child/insured has financial responsibility
04	Natural child/insured does not have financial responsibility
05	Stepchild
06	Foster child
07	Ward of the court
08	Employee
09	Unknown
10	Handicapped dependent
11	Organ donor
12	Cadaver donor
13	Grandchild
14	Niece/nephew
15	Injured plaintiff
16	Sponsored dependent
17	Minor dependent of a minor dependent
18	Parent
19	Grandparent
20	Life partner

TABLE 2-4 *(Continued)*

Member's Relationship to the Insured Codes
(Form Locator 59)
(Date of Service is after October 16, 2003)

Code	Definitions
01	Spouse
04	Grandfather or Grandmother
05	Grandson or Granddaughter
07	Niece/nephew
10	Foster Child
15	Ward
17	Stepson or Stepdaughter
18	Self
19	Child
20	Employee
21	Unknown
22	Handicapped dependent
23	Sponsored dependent
24	Dependent of minor dependent
29	Significant other
32	Mother
33	Father
36	Emancipated minor
39	Organ donor
40	Cadaver donor
41	Injured plaintiff
43	Child where insured has no financial responsibility
53	Life partner
G8	Other relationship

Valid Employment Status Codes
(Form Locator 64)

Code	Definition
1	Employed full-time
2	Employed part-time
3	Not employed
4	Self-employed
5	Retired
6	On active military duty
9	Unknown

13. Admission Hour (not required). Leave blank. If submitted, the data will be ignored.

14. Type of Admission/Visit (required on inpatient bills only). Numerical code denoting the priority of this admission (see Table 2-4 for further information).

15. Source of Admission (required). (See Table 2-4 for further information).

16. Discharge Hour (not required). Leave blank. Data entered will be ignored.

17. Patient Status (required). (See Table 2-4 for further information).

18.–28. Condition Codes (situational). Same.

29. Accident State (not used). Leave blank. Data entered will be ignored.

30. *Future Use.* Leave blank.

31.–34. *Occurrence Codes and Dates (situational).* (See Table 2-4 for further information).

35.–36. *Occurrence Span Codes and Dates (required for inpatient).* (See Table 2-4 for further information).

37. *Future Use.* Leave blank.

38. *Responsible Party Name and Address (not required).* For claims that involve payers of higher priority than Medicare. Name and address of person ultimately responsible for ensuring payment of the bill. This is usually the patient, or the parent or legal guardian if the patient is a minor.

39.–41. *Value Codes and Amounts (required).* Codes and the related dollar amount that identify data of a monetary nature that are necessary for the processing of this claim.

42. *Revenue Code (required).* Revenue code referencing the type of services provided (see Table 2-3 for more information).

43. *Revenue Description (not required).* A description of the services provided. Abbreviations may be used. Accommodation (room) descriptions must be entered first on the bill and must be in chronologic order of appearance (e.g., 03/01/YY ICU, 03/02/YY semi-private room).

44. *HCPCS/Rates (required).* The accommodation rate for inpatient bills, or the *CPT* or HCPCS code for ancillary or outpatient services. Outpatient Workers' Compensation and Medicaid require HCPCS coding in this space.

45. *Service Date (required outpatient).* The date the service was provided if this is a series bill in which the date of service differs from the from/through date on the bill.

46. *Units of Service (required).* Quantitative measure of services: days, miles, pints of blood, units, or treatments (e.g., if a patient was hospitalized for three days, place a 3 here).

47. *Total Charges (by Revenue Code) (required).* Total charges for that line of services. Not applicable for electronic billers.

48. *Noncovered Charges (required).* The amount per line of service that is not covered by the primary payer.

49. *Future Use.* Leave blank.

50. *A, B, and C Payer Name (required).* Name of insurer(s) covered by the patient who may be responsible for payment on this bill. Insurers should be listed in order of Primary Payer, Secondary Payer, and Tertiary Payer(s). If required, numbers identifying each payer organization should be listed.

51. *Health Plan ID.* A—Required (must put a number here); B—Situational (only if required by the insurance company or other agency; C—Situational.

52. *A, B, and C Release of Information Certification (required).* A "Y" (yes) or "N" (no) designation stating whether or not patient's signature is on file authorizing the release of information. An "R" indicates that a hospital has restricted authorization to release information, and the authorization should be attached. If no Authorization to Release Information is on file, you must obtain one before you send in the claim (see Table 2-4 for further information).

53. *Assignment of Benefit Certification.* Leave blank. Data entered will be ignored.

54. *Prior Payments (situational).* The amount that has been paid toward this bill prior to the current billing date. These payments can include payments by the patient, other payers, and so on.

55. *Estimated Amount Due (not required).* The amount estimated by the provider to be due from the indicated payer. This is usually the total amount due minus any previous payments.

56. *National Provider Identifier (required).* The NPI assigned to the provider.

57. *Other Provider IDs (situational).* NPI of any other provider involved in service.

58. *Insured's Name (required).* Name of the person listed on the insurance forms (subscriber's name).

59. *Patient's Relationship to Insured (required).* Numerical code designation indicating the relationship between the patient and the insured. The insured may be a spouse or parent of the patient (see Table 2-4 for further information).

60. *Insured's Unique ID (required).* The policy number under which the insured is covered if it is an individual policy. If the insured is covered under a group policy (such as one offered by his/her employer), often the insured's social security number is used as the subscriber number.

61. *Insured Group Name (situational, required if known).* The name of the group or company that holds the insured's policy. Often this is the employer of the insured. This information is required by Medicare when Medicare is not the primary payer.

62. *Insurance Group Number (situational, required if known).* The group number denoting the group policy or plan under which the insured is covered.

63. *Treatment Authorization Code (situational).* A number indicating that the treatment described by this bill has been authorized by the payer.

64. *Document Control Number (situational).* A number might be used here for various purposes.

65. *Employer Name (situational).* Name of the employer of the insured person as needed for insurance or workers' compensation information.

66. Diagnosis and Procedure Code Qualifier (required). Enter code qualifiers.

67. Principal Diagnosis Code (required). *ICD* code for the diagnosis of the patient's condition. E codes cannot be listed as first diagnosis.

67A.–67Q. Other Diagnoses Codes (inpatient/ outpatient required). *ICD* codes for up to eight additional diagnoses.

68. Future Use. Leave blank.

69. Admitting Diagnosis (required). The *ICD* code provided at the time of admission.

70. Patient's Reason for Visit Code (situational). (See Table 2-4 for further information).

71. PPS/DRG Code (not used). Leave blank. Data entered will be ignored.

72. External Cause of Injury Code (not used). Leave blank. Data entered will be ignored.

73. Future Use. Leave blank.

74. Principal Procedure Code and Date (situational). *CPT* code for procedure if appropriate.

75. Future Use. Leave blank.

76. Attending Name/ID (situational, including NPI). NPI number.

77. Operating Provider Name and Identifiers (including NPI). NPI number.

78.–79. Other Provider Name and Identifiers (situational, including NPI). NPI number.

80. Remarks (situational). Pertinent data for which there is no other specific place on the form. Often this space is used to record the nature of an accident (e.g., fell and hit head on concrete, 06/09/PY). Also, multiple visits to the ER on the same day should be recorded here.

81. Code–Code Field (situational). (See Table 2-4 for further information).

ACTIVITY #4

UB-04

Directions: Look at the UB-04 form in Figure 2-6, and indicate which box contains the following information. Write your answer in the space provided.

1. What is the patient's name? _____

2. What is the name of the insured person on this claim? _____

3. What is the procedure code for the procedure performed? _____

4. What is the diagnosis code given? _____

5. What is the patient's marital status? _____

6. Under what insurance plan is the patient covered? _____ _____

7. Has the authorization to release information been signed? _____

8. Is this patient covered under more than one insurance policy? _____

9. Have benefits been assigned on this claim? _____

10. What is the name of the provider on this claim? _____ _____

CHAPTER REVIEW

Summary

- Health claims examiners should familiarize themselves with the use of the reference books in this chapter. If you do not utilize them properly, the claims you submit to payers may be subject to delays and denials.
- The International Classification system (*ICD-9-CM* and *ICD-10-CM*) are used to code diagnoses, conditions, and hospital procedures.

- The *CPT, ICD-10-PCS,* and HCPCS are used to code procedures and services rendered by providers.
- The *PDR* assists in determining whether a drug is prescription or nonprescription and lists some of the properties (e.g., manufacturer, chemical makeup, side effects, appearance) of a specific drug.
- Medical dictionaries list medical terms and their meanings, and the *Merck Manual* can assist in determining whether a service or procedure is appropriate for a given diagnosis or condition.

- The CMS-1500 is the only accepted form for billing professional services if the healthcare provider is covered under HIPAA.
- The UB-04 is the claim form used when billing for hospital services.
- The information in each field of these forms allows the claim to be processed quickly and accurately.
- While understanding the forms may seem simple, it takes practice to be able to accurately process these claims.
- You should familiarize yourself with these forms and know where to find the necessary information for claims processing.

Review Questions

Directions: After reviewing the material just covered, answer the following questions. Write your answers in the space provided.

1. For what is the CMS-1500 billing form used? _____

_____

2. If the provider of service is an individual, what is shown in the block titled Federal Tax ID Number? _____

_____

3. Which CMS-1500 block denotes that Workers' Compensation is involved in the claim? _____

_____

4. For what is the block at the top of the CMS-1500 form, labeled "Medicare, Medicaid, TRICARE, FECA, Black Lung, and Other"? _____

_____

5. What does the term "Assignment of Benefits" mean? _____

_____

6. On the CMS-1500, what information is placed in block 24G "Days or Units"? _____

_____

7. True or false: When a physician or provider of service signs a medical billing form, he/she is legally stating that the service(s) for which he or she is seeking payment has actually been performed. _____

_____

8. What is a "Unit of Service?" _____

_____

9. For what is the UB-04 billing form used? _____

_____

10. What does form locator 17 on the UB-04 indicate? _____

_____

11. True or false: Occurrence codes and occurrence span codes are the same thing. _____

_____

12. What would code 20 indicate in form locator 21 on the UB-04? _____

_____

13. What would the code 03 indicate in form locator 22 on the UB-04? _____

_____

14. On the UB-04, for what is a value code used? _____

_____

15. What do the following revenue codes indicate on a UB-04?

  a. 722 _____
  b. 351 _____
  c. 559 _____
  d. 207 _____
  e. 450 _____
  f. 622 _____
  g. 815 _____
  h. 657 _____
  i. 490 _____
  j. 341 _____

16. Which manual is used for coding diagnoses? _____

_____

17. Name the two manuals that serve the same purpose and may be referred to interchangeably.

  1. _____
  2. _____

18. The full name of the *PDR* is _____

_____

19. If you needed to verify a diagnosis, affected body area, or the spelling of terms and definitions, you would probably refer to the _____

_____

20. The _____ is useful in determining the appropriateness of services for a reported diagnosis.

_____ If there were any questions that you could not answer, refer back to that section and then fill in the answers.

ACTIVITY #5

Matching

Directions: Match the following terms with the proper definition by writing the letter of the correct definition in the space next to the term.

1. _____ CMS-1500

2. _____ Health Care Common Procedure Coding System

3. _____ International Classification of Disease—9th Revision Clinical Modification

4. _____ Current Procedural Terminology

5. _____ UB-04

a. An indexing of conditions.

b. A systematic listing for coding the procedures or services performed by a physician.

c. The claim form most commonly used to bill for hospital services.

d. The claim form most commonly used to bill for provider's services.

e. A coding book that was developed to overcome the limitations in the *CPT* and *RVS* for billing injections, medication, supplies, and durable medical equipment.

SECTION 2

CONTRACT INTERPRETATION AND ADMINISTRATION

CHAPTER 3
Medical Plan Provisions

CHAPTER 4
Medical Benefit

Medical Plan Provisions

Keywords and concepts you will learn in this chapter:

Accident

Active Work

Actively-at-Work

Acts of Third Parties (ATP)

Affordable Care Act of 2010

Aggregate

Alternative Medicine Treatments

Basic Benefit

Beneficiary

Carryover Deductible

Coinsurance

Coinsurance Limit

Consideration

Consolidated Omnibus Budget Reconciliation Act of 1985 (COBRA)

Contract

Contributory Plan

Conversion

Copayment

Deductible

Effective Date

Eligibility

Eligible

After completing this chapter, you will be able to:

- List the items that are necessary for a contract to be valid and enforceable.

- Describe the elements of a group contract.

- Define the provisions for coverage (i.e., eligibility, effective date, termination of coverage).

- Describe various benefits that a contract can offer.

- Define eligibility.

- Explain open enrollment.

- Discuss provisions for terminating an individual's coverage.

- Identify the main situations in which benefits can be extended beyond normal eligibility.

- Explain how the Affordable Care Act of 2010 has affected insurance coverage.

- Identify possible third-party liability.

- Define subrogation.

Evidence of Insurability
Exclusions
Group Contract
Individual Deductible
Insurance Carrier
Insurance Company
Insurance Premium
Insured or Member
Major Medical Benefits
Mandates
Mental Health and Substance Abuse
Treatment Expenses
Nonaggregate
Noncontributory Plan
Offer
Open Enrollment
Out-of-Pocket
Policy
Preadmission Testing
Preexisting Condition
Qualified Beneficiary
Qualifying Event
Second Surgical Opinion
Subrogation
Termination of Coverage
Third-Party Liability (TPL)
Usual, Customary and Reasonable (UCR)

- Discuss preexisting conditions.

- Explain the impact HIPAA has had on health insurance.

- Identify the mandates that affect payment.

- Describe the requirements of prompt-pay laws.

- Discuss external and independent grievance systems.

Written **contracts** are present in every aspect of society. Essentially, any agreement between two or more persons that is enforceable by law is considered a contract. Written contracts have several advantages over nonwritten (oral) contracts: The existence of a written contract cannot be denied, and the terms of a written contract can be enforced more easily in the event of the death or incapacity (e.g., insanity, coma) of one of the parties of the contract.

In health insurance, a contract is used to determine eligibility requirements and covered services and to determine how those covered services are to be paid. The contract also indicates services that are excluded and services that have limitations. Therefore, the medical biller and the health claims examiner must read and interpret the contract in order to pay the proper benefits.

Contract Validity

In order for a contract to be valid, the persons signing the contract must agree on the terms. For the parties to agree there must be some form of offer and acceptance. The party who is **offering** is proposing to undertake, to do, or to give something to the other party, in exchange for a return promise from that person. An offer must be communicated in one form or another before it can be accepted (see Figure 3-1 ●). However, acceptance need not always be communicated to create a contract.

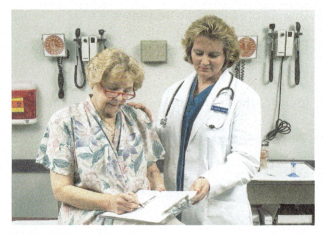

FIGURE 3-1 Patient signing a contract agreeing to receiving care
Source: Michal Heron/Merrill

For example, banks often send a letter to their patrons informing them of a change in interest rates or other terms regarding their accounts. These letters often state that if the patron does not contact the bank within a specified period of time, it will be assumed that the patron has agreed to and accepted the new terms or rates.

In order for a contract to be valid and enforceable, it must adhere to the following principles:

1. The contract must be based on a mutual agreement by the parties to do or not to do a specific thing or things.
2. The contract must be made by parties who are able and competent to enter into the contract and to enforce the terms of the contract. In some states, minors may not enter into certain types of contracts.
3. The contract must include consideration to pay money, deliver services, or promise to do or refrain from doing some lawful act that has not yet occurred (i.e., a contract cannot be made to enforce an event that has already occurred).
4. The purpose of the contract must be lawful. Contracts for unlawful acts are unenforceable.
5. If the contract falls into a class of contracts that are required by law to be in a special form, the format of the contract must meet those laws or requirements.

> ● **ONLINE INFORMATION:** Learn about what invalidates a healthcare contract by researching healthcare contracts on the Internet (see web.finweb.com/insurance/characteristics-of-insurance-contracts.html)

Group Contracts

Every health benefit plan, whether it is insured or not, is required by law to have a written document describing the plan benefits. This written legal document is used both by the plan members and by the administrator in determining how claims are to be paid. If any settlement disputes develop, the document provides evidence of what is and is not covered, what allowances are provided towards specific services, what books are used for reference in calculating benefits, and what the appeal procedures are.

Insured plans call this written document a contract or **policy**. Noninsured plans usually refer to it as a summary plan description. For our purposes, we will refer to the documents generically as contracts without implying whether a plan is insured.

The **group contract** offers an instrument through which an insurance company can meet the financial security needs of a group of persons. In essence, it is an agreement between the insurance company and the policyholder to insure the lives and/or health of the members of a defined group of persons and to pay the insurance benefits to the insured person or their beneficiaries. An **insured** person (also called a **member**, employee, subscriber, guarantor, or simply an insured) obtains or is otherwise covered by insurance on his or her health, life, or property. The specific terms and conditions of the contract are determined by negotiation between the insurance company and the policyholder. With the exception of benefit provisions, the terms are largely determined by standard provisions that are generally accepted throughout the industry.

The group contract must consist of the following three parts:

1. The group master policy.
2. The application of the group policyholder.
3. The individual applications, if any, of the persons insured.

The term **insurance company** is often used to refer to companies that sell policies offered by insurance carriers. The parties to a group contract are the insurance company and the group policyholder. In most cases, this is an employer. However, the policyholder may be a union or the trustee of a fund established by employers, unions, or both. In order for a group contract to be valid, a written application must be made. In order for it to remain valid, premiums must continue to be paid.

A basic principle of the law of contracts is consideration. Consideration can be a very broad term. For our purposes, **consideration** is anything that is given, done, promised, forbidden, or suffered by one party as an inducement for the agreement. The most common form of consideration is the payment of money in exchange for a promise. In the case of insurance, consideration is the premium paid by the group policyholder. The individual insured may contribute toward these premiums or provide the entire amount. In most cases, the premium is paid by the policyholder to the insurer, even though the individual insured may contribute part or all of the monies.

Interpreting and understanding contracts is one of the most important aspects of working in a healthcare billing or claims examining function. The healthcare contract document is used to determine the benefits which the insurance carrier will pay for services rendered. The **insurance carrier**, the corporation or association whose business is to make contracts of insurance, offers the health insurance policy.

The wording and terminology of health insurance contracts can often be confusing to someone who is not well versed in the insurance field. For this reason, medical billers or health claims examiners are often called on to interpret the provisions of a contract for billing purposes or to explain benefits to a patient.

Contract Provisions

In the following sections, we will briefly look at each of the items in a contract. These items, and how to calculate them, will be discussed in more detail in subsequent chapters. For now, just familiarize yourself with where to find items in a contract.

Eligibility

The first item that is considered on the contract is **eligibility**, or the qualifications which make the person eligible for coverage. Usually, these qualifications include items such as working full-time for a company and the description of what is considered full time. For example, in the Winter contract (see Appendix A), an employee must work a minimum of 30 hours per week to be eligible for coverage. The contract also discloses who is considered a dependent of the employee.

If subscribers have purchased individual coverage are not covered by their place of work, they have no minimum work requirements. However, they must still meet qualifications in order to have coverage under the plan.

Dependent eligibility is usually defined by the relationship of the dependent to the employee and the age (if the dependent is a child). For example, in the Winter contract, a child is covered until he or she reaches age 26. Children include unmarried natural children, legally adopted children, foster children, and those for whom the employee is considered the legal guardian.

In some contracts, there are provisions which state that if a husband and wife (or parent and child) work for the same employer and are covered under the same contract, the spouse or child cannot be covered as a dependent on the employee's policy. Also, some contracts state that if both spouses are working at the same company and are covered under the same contract, the children may be covered by one parent or the other, but not both. These rules prevent the insurance carrier from having to pay twice for the same patient and services rendered.

Effective Date

The next item we will consider is whether the contract was in force at the time the services were rendered. Often, an employee must work a minimum length of time for a company in order for the contract to be in force. The **effective date** is when the contract begins to be in force.

Many contracts include an **actively-at-work** stipulation. This clause states that a person must be at work (or actively engaged in his or her normal activities if he or she is a dependent) on the date that coverage becomes effective. If the person is not at work or actively engaged in his or her normal activities, the contract does not become effective until the employee or dependent returns to work or to normal activities.

It should be noted that the employee does not have to be actively-at-work if the effective date of coverage falls on a date when the employee would not normally be scheduled to work (e.g., an employee works Monday through Friday, but his effective date falls on Saturday). In this instance, the employee's coverage would become effective on Saturday. For an eligible dependent, if the dependent is confined to a hospital on the date that coverage was to become effective, the coverage will not become effective until after the dependent is released from the hospital.

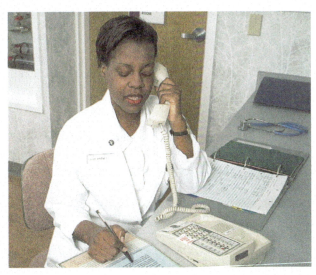

FIGURE 3-2 Contacting the insurance company to ensure coverage is important
Source: Michal Heron/Merrill

As a medical biller or health claims examiner, it is important that you ensure that a patient is eligible and is covered under an insurance policy in order to receive benefits. Many providers contact the insurance company prior to performing a procedure to be sure that the patient is covered (see Figure 3-2 ●). It is especially important to check eligibility when a patient is covered under an individual policy and pays a monthly premium for coverage.

Termination of Coverage

This section provides information regarding when coverage ends if an employee is terminated. It is important to note when coverage ceases, as the insurance carrier will not pay benefits after this date. **Termination of coverage** is a cessation of eligibility under the plan. However, coverage will often continue until the end of the month in which an employee terminates.

ACTIVITY #1

Contracts

Directions: Answer the following questions after reviewing the material just covered. Write your answers in the space provided.

1. For a contract to be valid and enforceable, what five principles must be met?

   a. _____

   b. _____

   c. _____

   d. _____

   e. _____

2. What are the three parts of a group contract?

a. _____ *pg. 64*

b. _____

c. _____ *all 3*

Contract Benefits

The contract benefits section of a contract details the benefits that the policy covers. These benefits can include basic and major medical benefits. Premiums are based on the number and amount of benefits which a contract covers. The greater the coverage, the higher the cost of the premiums. For example, a contract that covers charges at 90% of the allowed amount and that has a $100 deductible will usually cost more than a similar contract that covers charges at 70% of the allowed amount and that has a $250 deductible.

Basic Benefits

A **basic benefit** provides a specified allowance for a certain type of service (e.g., preventative tests), is usually paid at 100% of covered expenses, and is paid before major medical benefits are paid. Therefore, it is possible for the insurance plan to pay basic benefits even when the patient has not yet met his or her deductible. Since the implementation of the Affordable Care Act from 2009 to 2014, basic benefits are mandated to include certain preventative care services at no additional cost to the insured. This topic will be covered in further detail later. Basic benefit plans are often called managed care plans.

> ● ONLINE INFORMATION: How are mandatory preventative services determined? Research this subject online. Hint: Check out www.cms.gov.

In some contracts, the basic benefit is the unit value (a number based on the difficulty of a procedure and the overhead needed) multiplied by a basic conversion factor (see the Ball contract in Appendix A). This way, a small portion of most services is paid at 100% and the remaining portion is paid at the normal coinsurance percentage. Often, these types of basic benefits do not cover all procedures.

ACCIDENT BENEFITS. One of the most common basic benefits is an **accident** benefit, an unintentional injury which has a specific time, date, and place. For example, if an insurance company's policy has an accident benefit, it likely covers an amount (such as the first $300 of services that are due to the accident) at 100%. The remaining charges are then paid at 90%. This benefit is usually for a set amount of charges that are incurred within 120 days of the date of an accident.

On the CMS-1500 form, blocks 10b and 10c indicate services due to an accident, and the date of the accident is indicated in block 14.

PREADMISSION TESTING. In the past, a patient would enter the hospital the day before surgery for routine tests such as a chest X-ray and blood tests. The hospital would then admit the patient and watch over him or her to ensure that the patient did

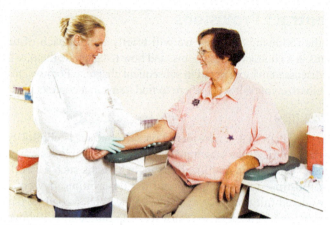

FIGURE 3-3 Patient having blood drawn for preadmission testing
Source: Michal Heron/Pearson Education/PH College

not eat or drink in the 24 hours prior to surgery. Insurance carriers realized there would be a great cost savings if the patient could visit the hospital for the tests, return home, and return the next day for the surgery. This practice eliminated the charges for an overnight hospital stay.

To encourage this practice, some insurance carriers offer an extra incentive for **preadmission testing**. Preadmission testing consists of routine laboratory and X-ray tests performed on an outpatient basis before a scheduled inpatient admission. Some insurance carriers now cover these charges at 100% rather than at their normal coinsurance percentage. Usually, only tests done at the facility where the patient will be admitted and done within 24 hours of admittance are allowed under this benefit (see Figure 3-3 ●).

SECOND SURGICAL OPINIONS. A **second surgical opinion** allows the insurance company to verify that another physician also recommends surgery for the patient. This provision is designed to ensure that the diagnosis of a disease and recommendations of treatment are accurate or to investigate alternative and less invasive treatment.

Some insurance carriers pay 100% of allowable charges for a second surgical opinion. This practice originally started as a cost containment measure. The hope was that only those surgeries that were necessary would be confirmed, and that some patients would receive alternative, less expensive treatments or no treatments.

Second surgical opinions have become less popular among insurance carriers because the cost savings seems to be minimal, if any. Many doctors are reluctant to go against the word or prescribed treatments of another physician. They do not want to contradict their peers and also do not want to open themselves up to a lawsuit by suggesting a less radical treatment which may eventually prove less effective. Therefore, they often simply confirm the diagnosis and prescribed treatment of the original physician.

OUTPATIENT FACILITY CHARGES. Some surgeries are simple or routine enough to be performed on an outpatient basis. This means the patient enters the facility in the morning, has surgery, and, after a brief recovery period, returns home the same day. There are no overnight or room and board charges. To encourage outpatient surgery when and where possible, some insurance carriers will cover such charges at 100%. Common examples are cholecystectomy, oral surgery, and invasive biopsy.

Major Medical Benefits

Major medical benefits are the benefits that are paid after basic benefits. They are usually subject to a deductible and/or coinsurance. Major medical plans usually cover a broad list of medical expenditures. This section of the contract lists the particular benefits and stipulations which a major medical contract provides. For example, cancer treatment, dialysis, inpatient surgeries, and heart disease procedures are included in major medical benefits.

INDIVIDUAL DEDUCTIBLE. The first item of contracts is the amount of the **deductible**. This is the amount that the member must pay toward medical costs before the insurance will pay benefits. If an **individual deductible** is assigned, the individual family member must pay the deductible before benefits become payable by the plan. Deductibles are usually accumulated according to a calendar year. Thus, each January 1st, the amount that a patient has paid toward his or her deductible returns to zero and the patient must start paying again.

The exception to this rule is in contracts that have a carryover deductible provision. A **carryover deductible** means that any amounts that the patient pays toward his or her deductible in the last three months of the year will carry over and will be applied toward the next year's deductible. Remember, the member pays his or her deductible before the insurance is required to pay any benefits. Therefore, if the patient is still paying a deductible in the last three months of the year, the insurance carrier has not had to pay any major medical benefits on this patient up to that time.

FAMILY DEDUCTIBLE. Family deductibles work the same way that individual deductibles do, in that once the family pays up to a certain limit, they are not responsible for paying any more. There are two ways to accumulate family deductible amounts: aggregate and nonaggregate. **Aggregate** means that any amounts paid toward the deductible by any member of the family will be added up to reach the deductible. **Nonaggregate** means a specified number of individual deductibles must be satisfied before the family limit is met.

OUT-OF-POCKET LIMIT. A member's **out-of-pocket** costs include the deductible, cost-sharing arising from the operation of the coinsurance clause, and medical expenditures that are deemed by the plan to be in excess of **usual, customary, and reasonable (UCR)** charges.

COPAYMENT. **Copayments** allow the insured party to share in the cost of the service. They vary depending on the service but are a set amount each time the insured obtains that service. Copayment provisions are frequently found in PPO and HMO plans.

COINSURANCE. **Coinsurance** is similar to a copayment, but it is a percentage, and the out-of-pocket expense for the insured

usually has a limit. The percentage listed is what the insurance company will pay (e.g., the insurance covers 80% of the approved amount of a bill, and the member covers 20%).

COINSURANCE LIMIT. Many insurance companies are aware that the costs of a catastrophic illness can ruin a family financially. Because insurance carriers want to keep people on the member rolls, they must leave them with enough resources to consistently pay premiums. For this reason, many insurance carriers have a **coinsurance limit**. This limit stipulates that if the coinsurance portion of a patient's bills reaches a certain amount, the insurance carrier will pay all subsequent claims at 100% of the allowed amount.

MENTAL HEALTH/SUBSTANCE ABUSE TREATMENT EXPENSES. **Mental Health and Substance Abuse Treatment Expenses** include claims submitted for psychiatric services, marriage and family counseling services, and drug and alcohol treatment. A lower coinsurance percentage (e.g., 50%) and/or a higher copayment may apply. Also, the coverage may depend on whether treatment is provided on an inpatient or outpatient basis. Many contracts have a calendar year maximum or a maximum number of visits for these types of services.

ALTERNATIVE MEDICINE TREATMENT EXPENSES. **Alternative Medicine Treatment Expenses** include claims for chiropractic care, acupuncture, massage therapy, and other nontraditional medical expenses. Each insurance company has different coverage amounts for these types of expense or may not cover them at all. As in the case of mental health benefits, the copay may be higher than for other procedures and services, or there may be a limit on the number of covered treatments per year.

PRACTICE **PITFALLS**

The Ball Insurance Carriers contract has a coinsurance limit of $400. Because the coinsurance amount is based on 20% of the allowed amount (with the insurance covering 80% of the allowed amount), the patient must have bills with approved amounts totaling over $2,125 in a calendar year before the coinsurance limit is reached ($125 is applied toward the deductible, and $2,000 multiplied by 20% equals the $400 limit).

LIFETIME LIMIT. Until 2014, when the Affordable Care Act of 2010 removes the lifetime limit cap, most insurance contracts have a lifetime limit payment amount. After the patient reaches the **lifetime limit** amount, the insurance carrier will not cover any additional expenses. Essentially this amount is the total dollar payments that the insurance carrier will make toward the care of this member. However, this amount is so high that it is seldom reached, except in extreme cases.

▶ CRITICAL THINKING QUESTION: What will lifting lifetime limits do to insurance companies' bottom line?

PREEXISTING CONDITION. A **preexisting condition** is a medical condition that a member had before he or she purchased an insurance policy. Depending on the policy, a preexisting condition may be defined according to when it originated, when symptoms first appeared, or when the patient first sought treatment. Depending on the insurance company's policies, the company may or may not be able to withhold payment for conditions that existed before a patient became covered under a contract. This rule prevents a patient who has not been paying for insurance coverage suddenly discovering that he or she has a serious illness and seeking insurance to cover that illness.

According to the Affordable Care Act of 2010 law, preexisting limitations must be included in the contract (new legislation may affect whether this law continues to be allowable). The term *preexisting* is different for each contract. Most often it is defined as a condition for which the patient has sought treatment within a given time period before insurance coverage has begun. If the patient has sought treatment for such a condition within this time period, benefits for treatment may not be covered or may be limited to a certain dollar amount. Usually, the restrictions on benefits coverage will cease after the patient has been covered under a contract for six months or longer. In 2014, preexisting conditions will no longer be allowed in insurance contracts.

Some contracts also have a treatment-free period. With this provision, if the patient can go without treatment for a specified period of time (often 12 months), then the insurance carrier will no longer consider the condition to be preexisting and will cover the illness or condition under the normal terms of the contract.

Remember that treatment includes any kind of contact in relationship with the illness, including the office visit or testing that was used to diagnose the illness. It also includes treatment of the condition, tests or office visits to monitor the condition, and filling of prescriptions related to the condition.

EXCLUSIONS. Every contract will have a list of **exclusions**, conditions or expenses for which no coverage is provided. It is important to check the list of exclusions before verifying benefits for services. If the procedures or treatments are not covered, the member will be responsible for the entire amount of the bill. Common exclusions are elective surgery, weight reduction plans, and alternative therapies.

ACTIVITY #2

Benefits

Directions: Answer the following questions after reviewing the material just covered. Write your answers in the space provided.

1. What are basic benefits? _____

_____

2. What is an accident? _____

_____

3. What is preadmission testing? _____

_____

4. What is outpatient surgery? _____

_____

5. What is a deductible? _____

_____

6. What is an individual deductible? _____

_____

7. What is coinsurance? _____

_____

8. What are mental health expenses? _____

_____

ACTIVITY #3

Contracts

Directions: Review the Winter Insurance Contract in Appendix A. Answer the following questions in the space provided.

1. What is the individual deductible amount? _____

_____

2. What is the dependent eligibility age limit? _____

_____

3. What is the family calendar year deductible? _____

_____

4. What is the individual coinsurance limit? _____

_____

5. What are the coinsurance percentages? _____

_____

6. How many hours must the employee work to be eligible?

_____

7. Does the contract include dental coverage? _____

_____

8. What is the family coinsurance limit? _____

_____

9. Is the family coinsurance aggregate or nonaggregate?

_____

10. Is there a carryover provision on the individual deductible? _____

_____

11. How many months must the employee work before coverage becomes effective? _____

_____

ACTIVITY #4

Deductibles

Directions: Read the relevant insurance contracts in Appendix A, and list the amounts for the following deductible provisions in the spaces provided.

	Winter	Ball	Summer
1. What is the individual deductible amount?	_____	_____	_____
2. What is the family calendar year deductible?	_____	_____	_____
3. What is the coinsurance percentage?	_____	_____	_____

Eligibility

When an individual has met the eligibility requirements, he or she is eligible for insurance. Therefore, as far as insurance is concerned, being **eligible** means meeting certain qualities or requirements to be covered by the plan. Do not confuse "eligible" with "effective." In insurance, these are two very different concepts. A person can be eligible for coverage without having the coverage ever become effective. (We will cover the concept of coverage becoming effective later in this chapter).

The definition of an eligible person varies from plan to plan. Most plans have separate definitions for eligible employees or subscribers and eligible dependents. The requirements for the insured can include a minimum number of hours that the employee has worked for the policyholder and a minimum number of months that the employee has been employed by the policyholder. The requirements for the dependents of the insured can include such things as being a lawful spouse, domestic partner, or dependent child of the insured; being under a certain age limit; or attending school full-time. The specific requirements vary by plan as well as by insurance company. Before verifying eligibility and benefits, be sure to review the plan definition of an eligible dependent and the company policy for covering domestic partners.

It is important for the medical biller and health claims examiner to understand the concept of eligibility and the eligibility requirements under each contract in order to process claims correctly.

Employee Eligibility

Most contracts define participants according to the minimum number of hours that the employee or subscriber must work per specified period of time, usually per week. Generally, part-time employees and full-time employees who work fewer than 30 hours per week are not considered eligible for coverage.

ACTIVITY #5

Exclusions

Directions: Read the following list of exclusions and place an E in the space provided if the service is excluded under the applicable contract (see Appendix A). Place an N/E in the space provided if the service is not excluded under the contract.

	Winter	Ball	Summer
1. Gender-altering treatments or surgeries or related studies.	_____	_____	_____
2. Work-related injuries or illnesses.	_____	_____	_____
3. Changes or services in excess of what is usual, customary, and reasonable (UCR).	_____	_____	_____
4. Charge made for failure to keep an appointment.	_____	_____	_____
5. Routine, preventative, or experimental services.	_____	_____	_____
6. Orthopedic shoes (medically necessary) following foot surgery.	_____	_____	_____
7. Radial keratotomy.	_____	_____	_____
8. Cosmetic surgery for breast following mastectomy.	_____	_____	_____
9. Services for which there is no charge in the absence of insurance.	_____	_____	_____
10. Surgical correction of cleft palate.	_____	_____	_____
11. Custodial care.	_____	_____	_____
12. Reversal of voluntary sterilization.	_____	_____	_____
13. Contraceptive materials or devices.	_____	_____	_____
14. Expenses resulting from self-inflicted injuries.	_____	_____	_____
15. Elective abortions.	_____	_____	_____
16. Charges for services not medically necessary.	_____	_____	_____
17. Experimental transplants.	_____	_____	_____

Membership Insurance

Other contracts define the subscriber in terms of membership in an organization, such as the Certified Public Accountants (CPA) Society or real estate societies. A minimum number of hours worked may also apply in these circumstances. Partners and proprietors are also considered participants as long as they engage in the conduct of business on a full-time basis or a minimum number of hours per week. Other organizations offer insurance plans based on the person's membership in said organization.

For example, refer to the XYZ Corporation contract (see Appendix A). As indicated therein, the employee must

- Routinely work a minimum of 30 hours per week.
- Be considered a full-time employee. (Even though the contract does not specifically indicate this, it is an industry standard.) Therefore, unless the booklet or contract says otherwise, full-time status is assumed.
- Work three consecutive months to be eligible. Coverage may become effective the first of the month following the completion of three months of work (assuming the employee has applied for coverage).

PRACTICE **PITFALLS**

Suppose an employee is hired on 3/2/CCYY (current year), works 40 hours per week, and is covered under the XYZ Corporation contract. This contract states that an employee is eligible for coverage the first of the month following three consecutive months of continuous employment. The three months would end on 6/2/CCYY. However, because 6/2/CCYY is past the first of the month, coverage will become effective the first of the month following the completion of the three-month waiting period. Therefore, coverage would become effective on 7/1/CCYY.

Under many union contracts, eligibility depends on the number of hours the member worked during the previous year or the previous month. A member of a union may work for multiple employers during a month or week. As long as both the employer and the employee are members of the union, the employee accumulates hours toward the satisfaction of the hourly requirement.

Consider this common type of wording for union contracts: If you are a bargaining unit employee, you will become eligible for benefits on the first day of the second month following any three consecutive months during which you worked for one or more contributing employers a minimum total of 300 hours. After eligibility has been established, you and your dependents will be covered for a minimum of three consecutive months.

For example, if you worked the following amounts:

January:	110 hr
February:	0 hr
March:	190 hr
Total:	300 hr

Your coverage will begin May 1 and will last at least through July.

In this example, the requirements are

- 300 hours in any consecutive three-month period,
- Eligibility begins on the first day of the second month following the three consecutive months, and
- Coverage will be for a minimum of three consecutive months.

It is not unusual for a plan to have different eligibility provisions for different classifications of employees. For example, separate provisions may be given for employees classified as Active Officers, Board Members, Management Employees, or Retired Employees. Special provisions may also be applicable to employees who are laid off or on leave. Therefore, it is very important to check the plan provisions to determine whether there are a variety of classifications and, if so, to know how to verify the specific classifications of the claimants whose claims you are handling.

Dependent Eligibility

The first step in determining whether a dependent is eligible is to verify whether the dependent fits the definition of an eligible dependent. Defining a dependent is much more difficult than defining an employee because of the complex family and social dynamics in our society. A plan must try as much as possible to define all the dependents that can exist and to place those definitions into either covered or noncovered categories.

In general, "dependent" means

1. The employee's legal spouse (either through marriage or through common-law status if recognized by the state in which they are residing). In order for the spouse to be covered as a dependent, the employee and spouse cannot be divorced or legally separated, even if there is a court decree stating that the employee is responsible for providing medical coverage.
2. Dependent, unmarried children up to age 26. The term "dependent" means that the child must rely on the employee for daily maintenance and care. The term "children" always includes one's biological children and may also include
    a. Adopted children for whom the final court order has been issued or for whom it is specified by the adoption agreement during any state-mandated waiting period that the adoptive parents provide all medical care.
    b. Stepchildren residing with the employee.
    c. Grandchildren residing with the employee who depend on the employee for more than 50% of their support.
    d. Foster children whose foster-child agreement specifies that the state is not responsible for their healthcare and that the foster parents are responsible. (The state usually maintains responsibility for the foster children's healthcare).
    e. Any other children related to the employee by blood or marriage, provided that they are living in a regular parent–child relationship and depend on the employee for support and maintenance. In the case of grandchildren, a regular parent–child relationship does not exist if either of the child's parents also reside with the employee.

Many states have enacted legislation concerning coverage for dependent children from birth. Although specific wording and intent are determined by individual state legislation, the laws generally provide that newborn children can be afforded the same eligibility for accident and health coverage as any other dependent and are covered from birth for treatment of a disease or injury. Preexisting limitations by definition cannot be applied to newborn children. This automatic coverage generally lasts for an initial 31-day period from the date of birth. In order to continue such coverage past the 31-day period, the employee must

- Complete any required enrollment form, and
- Make any required contributions, effective from the date of birth.

The law does not usually oblige insurance plans to pay for well-baby or custodial care. However, a few states require insured plans to have well-child care provisions (refer to the mandates listed later in this chapter).

Many plans also specify that a person who is eligible as an employee cannot be enrolled as a dependent on the same plan. Furthermore, if both husband and wife are covered under the same plan as employees, one or the other but not both may elect to cover their dependents. This rule prevents a particular child from being covered as a dependent under both parents. Some self-funded plans do permit dual coverage under the same plan for husbands, wives, and dependent children. Unless participants of a plan are specifically excluded from being covered as both employees and dependents or as dependents under both parents, dual coverage is permitted. Be sure to review the contract for the definition of dependent coverage.

Employee Enrollment

In order for an eligible employee's coverage or a dependent's coverage to become effective, the person is usually required to complete the necessary enrollment papers prior to the date of eligibility. The rules defining the effective date of coverage vary, depending on whether the plan is considered to be a contributory or noncontributory plan.

In a **contributory plan**, the employees contribute to the cost of the coverage, usually through payroll deductions. In a **noncontributory plan**, the employer bears the complete cost of the coverage and the employee does not contribute.

In a contributory plan,

- The employee must complete the enrollment application listing himself or herself and the dependents that he or she wants to be covered; usually, all eligible dependents must be listed.
- Such application must be received by the employer or by the plan administrator on or before the eligibility date of the coverage in order for coverage to become effective on that date.
- The employee must also authorize the applicable payroll deductions or make the necessary premium payments.

EXAMPLE:

Sammy Subscriber begins working on 1/15/CCYY for White Corporation, which offers the Winter Insurance. This insurance states that he will become eligible on the first of the month after 60 days of continuous employment.

Therefore, he will become eligible for coverage on 4/1/CCYY. If he has not completed the enrollment application, turned it in to the employer, and made arrangements for payment before 4/1/CCYY, his insurance will not become effective. Thus, he will not be insured.

If the enrollment application is not received on or before the eligibility date of coverage, but it is received within one month (or 30 or 31 days) after the date of eligibility, the employee is considered to be a late applicant. This employee's coverage will begin either on the date of application or on the first or fifteenth of the month following the date of application. The plan provisions must specify which of the time limitations applies.

ACTIVITY #6

Enrollment

Sammy thought he had finished all the paperwork and would be enrolled on 4/1/CCYY. However, on 4/2/CCYY, his employer informed him that they never received his enrollment application. Sammy discovered it in his desk at work and turned it in on 4/2/CCYY. What will happen to his coverage?

If the enrollment application is not submitted within one month (or 30 or 31 days) after the date of eligibility, the employee may be required to submit proof of good health. Also known as **evidence of insurability**, this proof is often a health questionnaire that must be filled out for the policyholder and all eligible dependents seeking coverage. The questionnaire will be submitted to the medical consultants of the insurer or plan administrator for review. If the participant appears to be a good "risk," that is, he or she does not appear to have any active illness or conditions, coverage may be approved. If the participant appears to be a poor risk because he or she has active illnesses, coverage may not be approved and the employee and dependents may not be able to obtain coverage under the plan at that time. (Some plans provide for open enrollment periods, which will be discussed later.) The employee's dependents cannot be covered unless the employee is covered. In other words, if the employee is not healthy, the employee's eligibility is denied. Thus, even though the dependents may be healthy, they will not be covered under the plan.

In a noncontributory plan in which the employer pays the full cost, a request for coverage is not necessary except for recordkeeping purposes and beneficiary designations. The person who would receive payment on a claim if he or she has not signed an assignment of benefits to the provider is a **beneficiary**. The beneficiary can also be the person who receives the benefit in the case of a deceased member. Coverage for employees and, in some instances, their dependents begins automatically on the employee's eligibility date, regardless of when the enrollment application is completed and submitted. If the insurer or administrator is not informed of an employee's eligibility on the appropriate date and a claim or an enrollment application is subsequently submitted, the insurer/administrator will automatically add the member and bill the employer for all back premiums due. After the back premiums are paid, the claim(s) will be paid. Evidence of insurability is not required in these cases and there are not considered to be any late applicants on the plan.

ACTIVITY #7

Health Assessment

Use the information covered thus far to answer the question at the end of this scenario. Patty Participant began working for White Corporation on 1/15/CCYY. This corporation offers the Winter Insurance Contract (see Appendix A). She chose not to enroll in the insurance program at that time. If she changes her mind on 6/1/CCYY and wants to enroll in the insurance program, what requirement will she have to meet, and when will her insurance become effective?

Be aware that a plan can be noncontributory for the employee and contributory for the dependents. Therefore, a combination of the above rules may apply. For example, a company provides free health insurance for its employees (noncontributory), but any employees who also want coverage for their spouse and children must pay for it (contributory).

Whether the group is contributory or noncontributory, the usual effective date of coverage is deferred if on the effective date the employee is absent from work because of illness or injury. Most plans stipulate that in order for coverage to become effective, the employee must have completed either a full day of active work on that date or a full day of active work on the last regularly scheduled work day and must be able to work on the date of eligibility. If the employee does not meet these requirements, the coverage will become effective on the date that he or she returns to active work.

Active work and actively-at-work usually means performing the regular duties of a full work day for the employer.

Dependent Effective Date of Coverage

The rules regarding the effective date of coverage for dependents are similar to the rules for employees. The rules depend on whether the plan is contributory or noncontributory.

In the case of an employee, the plan usually makes a stipulation that the employee must be actively at work. A similar provision is also made for dependents. However, because a dependent often does not work, policies usually state that if a dependent is in the hospital, the coverage for that dependent becomes effective on the day after the date of discharge, or the date on which the dependent is able to perform all the duties he or she usually performs. In other words, if the dependent is of school age, coverage might begin when the child returns to school. An exception would be made in the case of a newborn child, who is usually born in a hospital. In such a case, coverage begins immediately (see Figure 3-4 ●).

In a contributory plan, dependents are handled the same as employees regarding late enrollment. However, many contributory plans require that for dependents to be covered, all eligible dependents must be enrolled in the plan. This requirement prevents an employee from selectively putting sick dependents on one plan and healthy dependents on another plan.

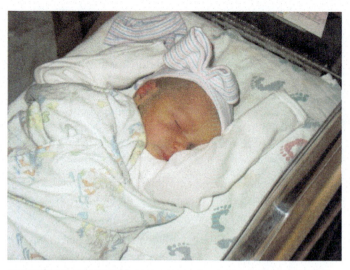

FIGURE 3-4   Effective date of coverage for newborns is immediately upon birth
Source: Bronwen Glowacki/Pearson Education/PH College

ACTIVITY #8

Eligible Dependents

Directions: Indicate whether the person listed would be considered an eligible dependent (ED) or a noneligible dependent (NED) under the general provisions. Assume that the first person in each case is covered under the general provisions, and the second person is applying as his or her dependent.

1. Natalie's legally married spouse. _____
   _____

2. Nathaniel's dependent child, age four. _____
   _____

3. Bryant's cousin Terrell. _____
   _____

4. Tabari's divorced ex-spouse. _____
   _____

5. Tiron's son, age 45, fully functional. _____
   _____

6. Kyra's dependent child, age 19, who is a full-time student. _____
   _____

7. Kayla's brother Kenneth. _____
   _____

8. Ann's dog Pepper. _____
   _____

9. Aaron's adopted daughter. _____
   _____

10. Brittany's mother-in-law. _____
    _____

Open Enrollment

Open enrollment is a process that allows late applicants to enroll in a plan without having to complete evidence of insurability. This enrollment process usually occurs on the anniversary date of the plan and when an employer has multiple plan options. For example, larger employers are required by law to offer their employees an HMO option. These employers often offer an HMO plan, a low-indemnity plan (which has higher deductibles and lower coinsurance payable by the plan), and perhaps a high-indemnity plan (which has a lower deductible and higher coinsurance payable by the plan). By having an open enrollment period, employees may switch from one plan to another without penalties or a gap in coverage and without having to complete a health statement.

Termination of Coverage

The provisions for terminating an individual's coverage vary according to the type of group and how the employer wants the plan administered. In a union or association group, for example, coverage ends when the employer terminates the group's membership in the union or association. The most common termination provisions are based on conditions pertaining to employment. Coverage is usually terminated under one of these conditions:

- The group policy terminates (e.g., a company terminates the policy).
- The policy is amended to terminate the eligibility of the class of employees to which the individual belongs (e.g., the employer decides they will no longer cover commissioned sales people).
- The employee transfers out of a class covered by the policy (e.g., an employee goes from full-time to part-time work hours).
- Active employment ceases (e.g., the employee quits).
- The employee ceases to pay the required contributions for the coverage.

When coverage ceases, regardless of the reason, some form of continuation of coverage may be available.

> ▶ **CRITICAL THINKING QUESTION:** What would you advise an employee who has been terminated recently to do to make sure that her health insurance continues?

Continuation of Coverage

Many plans allow benefits to extend beyond the normal date or terms of eligibility. These extensions can be of several types, depending on the reason for the continuation (e.g., disability, COBRA). We will discuss the main situations in which benefits are extended beyond normal eligibility and the requirements for continuing such coverage.

An employee or dependent losing coverage may qualify for continuation of benefits under more than one provision. The order in which these provisions apply is important. Continuation is first considered under COBRA (see the heading on COBRA) because it is premium-based and covers all conditions when the

insured makes the payments. The extension of benefits for disability is considered second because the only person eligible for coverage under this provision is the employee, and only the disabling condition is covered. The coverage usually lasts for 12 months and the premium contributions are waived. The conversion privilege is the last coverage option to be exercised.

ACTIVITY #9

Termination of Benefits

Directions: Answer the following questions after reviewing the material just covered. Write your answers in the space provided.

List the five conditions under which coverage is usually terminated.

1. _____
2. _____
3. _____
4. _____
5. _____

Extension of Benefits

Most plans contain an extension-of-benefits provision for totally disabled members. Basically, this provision continues benefits for a maximum of 12 months free of charge to a terminated employee, but only for the person on the policy who is totally disabled. This type of provision requires that

- The person was eligible and covered under the plan when his or her coverage terminated.
- As of the termination date, the person was totally disabled due to an injury or illness.
- Only covered expenses (as defined by the plan provisions) incurred for the illness or injury causing the disability are eligible for benefit consideration.
- Coverage will last only for the length of time specified in the policy.

The requirements indicate that first there must be documented proof that the person was totally disabled with an injury or illness when he or she terminated. Second, only eligible expenses incurred for the injury or illness that is causing the disability are covered after the termination date.

Refer to the three contracts in Appendix A. As indicated, the Winter and Ball contracts both have a standard extension-of-benefits provision. Coverage will continue for 12 months from the date of termination under the plan or until the person is no longer totally disabled, whichever interval is shorter. Summer Enterprises does not have an extension-of-benefits provision.

Therefore, to determine whether an extension-of-benefits provision is applicable, follow these steps:

1. Was the member eligible and effective under the plan when coverage terminated? If not, the investigation would end, because the member could not continue coverage if he or she was not eligible and effective on the plan when the coverage terminated.

2. If the member was eligible and effective when coverage terminated, was the member totally disabled at the time the coverage terminated? If not, extension of benefits would not apply.

3. If the member was eligible and totally disabled at that time, a letter from the attending physician must be obtained stating the condition or conditions causing the disability, the date that the member became totally disabled, and the anticipated end of the total disability.

4. If the employee is claiming disability, try to find out whether he or she is employed anywhere. Sometimes, members apply for this type of extension because it does not require premiums and the member wants coverage between jobs.

Conversion Policies

Most states have legislatively mandated that insurance policies contain a continuation of coverage provision known as **conversion**. Conversion permits employees and dependents to continue their insurance protection on an individual basis when their coverage under a group plan ceases for any of the following reasons:

- The employee's employment in the class of employees insured under the group policy terminates.
- The policy is amended to terminate coverage for the class to which the employee belongs.
- The employee terminates employment with the employer.
- A dependent child reaches the limiting age for the plan.
- The employee and spouse are divorced or legally separated so that the spouse is no longer considered eligible under the provisions of the plan.

Evidence of insurability is not required, but the person must apply in writing and pay the required premiums within a specified time period of the date of termination of coverage under the group plan (usually 31 days). Members who voluntarily discontinue their insurance coverage while they are still employed are not eligible to convert, nor is the conversion privilege available when the employer's complete policy is terminated.

As a rule, conversion policies are extremely expensive. The reason for the high cost is that usually only employees who are disabled and extremely ill convert their policies. Because of the high expenses on the conversion policy, the resulting premiums are also very high.

Unfortunately, if an individual is so ill that he or she must cease working, it is extremely difficult for that individual to afford the high premiums. Nevertheless, conversion is an available option.

ACTIVITY #10

Reason for Termination

Directions: Place a "yes" or "no" next to each of the following examples to show whether coverage would be terminated under the circumstances given. Assume that each person listed is the member on the plan. Do not be concerned about whether the person is entitled to continuation of coverage.

1. Nancy goes from full-time to 20 hours per week. _____
2. Alonzo is terminated by the company. _____
3. Kerri's company terminates the policy. _____
4. Sydney becomes self-employed but works on a contract basis for the same company. _____
5. Sean stops paying the premium for his insurance. _____
6. Thomas goes on vacation for two weeks. _____
7. Floree forgets to enroll during her company's open enrollment period. _____
8. Mia is transferred out of a class covered by the policy. _____
9. Mayra goes on maternity leave. _____
10. Carol gets married. _____

COBRA

In 1986, President Reagan signed into law HR3128, the **Consolidated Omnibus Budget Reconciliation Act of 1985 (COBRA)**, also referred to hereafter as continuation of coverage. Within this act, there is a very significant provision, Title X, which has had profound effects on employee welfare benefit plans.

Before COBRA took effect, employers were generally not required to provide continuation of group insurance coverage for individuals who ceased to be eligible for such coverage. The objective of Congress through Title X was to require employers to permit employees whose coverage was ending (and their dependents) to purchase transitional healthcare coverage at favorable group rates until the employees could obtain replacement coverage. The intended result was to reduce the number of people without healthcare coverage.

Title X is composed of the following amendments:

Section 10001	Amendments to the Internal Revenue Code (IRC).
Section 10002	Amendments to the Employee Retirement Income Security Act (ERISA).
Section 10003	Amendments to the Public Health Service Act (PHSA).

The effect of these amendments is to require virtually every type of group health plan, insured or self-funded, to provide the option of self-payment for continuation of coverage. Because the penalties for noncompliance are administered by the Internal Revenue Service, noncompliance is costly.

COBRA APPLICABILITY. COBRA applies to all private employers who regularly employ 20 or more employees (including both full-time and part-time workers) on a typical working day. It applies to single-employer health plans, multiple employer trust plans, collectively bargained plans, insured plans, and self-funded plans.

Under the amendment to the PHSA (Section 10003), certain state and local governmental employers of 20 or more employees are required to offer continuation of coverage even though these employers are exempt from both taxes and ERISA. The applicability of COBRA to state and local governmental employers is based on the receipt of funds under PHSA. If the state or local governmental employer received funds under PHSA, compliance is required.

In sum, all employee group health benefit plans are required to offer continuation of coverage, with the exception of the following:

- Any group health plan for any calendar year if the employer normally maintained fewer than 20 employees on a typical business day during the preceding calendar year.
- Certain church plans.
- Group health plans maintained by state or local governmental employers who do not receive funds under PHSA.
- Group health plans maintained for employees by the government of the District of Columbia or any territory or possession of the United States.

Governmental and nongovernmental group health plans that are not collectively bargained were subject to the COBRA requirements as of the first of the plan year, beginning subsequent to June 30, 1986.

QUALIFIED BENEFICIARIES. The option of self-payment continuation of coverage must be offered by the affected employers to certain individuals referred to as qualified beneficiaries. A **qualified beneficiary** is defined as anyone who, on the day before the relevant qualifying event, is covered under the health coverage plan as an employee, a dependent spouse, or a dependent child.

QUALIFYING EVENT. The term **qualifying event** refers to one of the following events which results in the loss of eligibility under the employer-sponsored health plan:

- Voluntary or involuntary termination of employment, with the exception of termination for gross misconduct.
- Reduction in work hours.
- Eligibility of the employee only for Medicare.
- Death of the employee.
- Divorce or legal separation.
- Disqualification of a dependent child as an eligible dependent.

Employers are required to offer the self-pay continuation of coverage option to the following individuals:

- Terminated or laid-off employees (except those who were terminated for gross misconduct), employees for whom a reduction in work hours would result in the loss of coverage, and retired employees who are not eligible for Medicare.
- The surviving spouse and dependent children of a deceased employee.

- Divorced spouses and their dependent children.
- Spouses and dependent children of employees who are eligible for Medicare.
- Dependent children who cease to meet the plan definition of a dependent child.

There are no length-of-service requirements associated with COBRA. As long as the employee was covered under the employer-sponsored health plan prior to the qualifying event, he or she has the right to elect continuation. This right also applies to the employee's spouse and dependent children, provided they were covered under the plan the day before the event.

The covered employee or spouse (when the spouse is the elector) may act as the agent for the entire family. It is not necessary for each family member to make an individual election.

DURATION OF COVERAGE. COBRA requires that affected employers permit employees and covered dependents, at the time their coverage would cease because of a qualifying event, to elect continuation of their insurance coverage for up to 18, 29, or 36 months, depending on the circumstances.

For employees and their dependents, a maximum of 18 months of continuation is allowed after one of the following events:

- Voluntary or involuntary termination of employment other than for gross misconduct.
- Reduction of work hours below the plan eligibility requirements.

For employees or dependents who are permanently disabled at the time of the event, coverage may be continued for up to 29 months rather than 18 months. The plan may use the Social Security standard of permanent disability as a qualifying condition of the extended coverage.

For covered dependents only, a maximum of 36 months of continued coverage is allowed after one of the following events:

- Death of the employee.
- Divorce or legal separation from the employee.
- The employee becomes eligible for Medicare.
- A child ceases to be an eligible dependent as defined by the plan provisions.

If a second qualifying event occurs during the time of the continuation of coverage for dependents, the maximum time allowed can be increased from 18 to 36 months if a qualifying event occurs as described. For example, an employee terminates and chooses to continue coverage through COBRA for 18 months. During these 18 months, the employee's child ceases to be an eligible dependent. That dependent may continue coverage, but other family members may not. Also, it may be possible to extend coverage from 18 to 29 months if an employee becomes totally disabled while he or she is covered. However, coverage cannot be extended beyond 29 months.

NOTIFICATION OF ELIGIBILITY. One of the most important aspects of the COBRA Act is the requirement that eligible members be informed of their eligibility for COBRA. Many employers have interpreted this to mean that when an employee terminates coverage, usually by terminating employment termination, the employer must inform the employee of the COBRA rights. However, this procedure addresses only a portion of those who are actually eligible for continuation of coverage; there may be a significant number of dependents who also are eligible.

Figure 3-5 ● is an example of a document that may be used to enroll the applicant for continuation of coverage. In

---

ABC Company
333 Whata Way
Hollywood, CA 91731

Continuation of Coverage Request

If you were eligible under your employer's group health insurance plan, you may be eligible to continue your coverage. In order to apply, this form must be completed and returned to the Administrator's office indicated above within 60 days of the date your eligibility under the group plan terminates. Within 14 days of our receipt of this request, you will be sent a copy of your Election Rights under the Consolidation Omnibus Reconciliation Act of 1985 (COBRA), Public Act 99-272, Title X.

EMPLOYEE NAME – LAST	FIRST	FACILITY	ID NO.

COMPLETE HOME ADDRESS	CITY	STATE	ZIP

Qualifying Event: Check off the event and give the event date.
□ Reduction in Work Hours. Effective: _____
□ Employment Termination (Except due to "gross misconduct"). Last Work Day: _____
□ Dependent Child Attained Maximum Age Defined by Plan. _____
□ Legal Separation and/or Divorce. Date: _____
□ Death of Covered Employee. Date: _____

CONTINUATION OF COVERAGE REQUESTED FOR: (Coverage(s) cannot be added. May be dropped only.)

□ Employee Only	□ Employee & Dependent(s)	□ Dependent(s) Only
□ Medical Only	□ Medical Only	□ Medical Only
□ Dental + Vision Only	□ Dental + Vision Only	□ Dental + Vision Only
□ Medical + Dental + Vision	□ Medical + Dental + Vision	□ Medical + Dental + Vision

ALL DEPENDENTS MUST BE LISTED BELOW. LIST THE SOCIAL SECURITY NUMBER OF THE EMPLOYEE'S SPOUSE AND OVER AGE DEPENDENT CHILDREN.

NAME	ID NO.	BIRTHDATE	RELATIONSHIP

Signature of Applicant/Date Signed

FIGURE 3-5 Sample COBRA enrollment form

addition, the employer must notify all employees and their dependents about the availability of COBRA. If the employer distributes reference materials about COBRA early, the employer can avoid liability for failure to notify affected employees or dependents, and the responsibility for timely application would be shifted entirely to the affected employee if (1) dependents become overage, (2) a divorce or separation occurs, or (3) the employee abandons or terminates employment without advance notification. The applicant has 60 days from the date that such coverage is terminated due to a qualifying event in which to submit the application for continuation to the administrator or insurance company, or 60 days from the date on which the notice of the right to elect COBRA continuation is sent to the employee. Therefore, if the employer or plan fails to send out notification of the election right for two years after the actual event date, the employee would have to be given 60 days from the two-year date in which to elect coverage. Mistakes like this can prove to be very costly to a plan.

PREMIUM PAYMENTS. After an individual has elected to continue coverage through COBRA, he or she has 45 days in which to pay the initial premium, including all retroactive premiums that were due since he or she terminated coverage as a regular employee. If the initial premium and all back premiums are not paid within this time, coverage will remain terminated and COBRA coverage will not become effective.

Normally, a monthly COBRA statement is provided to the employee, which reflects the premium due date for each month and the amount of the monthly premium according to the coverage elected by the applicant. However, the law permits a 30-day grace period from the premium due date. This grace period allows the applicant 30 additional days in which to pay the required premium amount. If the premium is not mailed within the 30-day grace period, coverage will automatically lapse back to the last premium paid date. The amount of the premium can be up to 102% of the premium costs for employees. The 2% is to cover administrative costs. For employees who are eligible for the 29-month extension, the premium can be up to 150% of the employee's premium cost for months 19 through 29.

Normally, claims are not paid until the member has paid the premium for the month in which the services were incurred or until the grace period has lapsed. Consequently, if the member consistently pays at the end of the grace period, claim payments may be consistently delayed. In other words, when the claim is processed, the incurred date of services will be compared with the paid-through date. If the premium for the month in which services were incurred has not been paid, processing will be delayed until the end of the grace period.

Bounced checks or any type of nonpaid check may result in lapse of coverage if the check is returned from the bank after the premium due date and a replacement check is not received prior to the end of the grace period. The mailing date of premiums should be strictly monitored with no exceptions. The date of receipt is not important. Judgment of whether or not a payment was received on time is based on the postmark on the envelope. By law, if the payment was mailed within the specified time, it must be accepted as being paid on time.

It is very important that all applicants and members be treated equitably regarding the premium payment policy, as deviations may set precedents and extend plan liabilities above acceptable limits.

TERMINATION OF COVERAGE. An individual may terminate the continuation of coverage before the completion of the 18-, 29-, or 36-month period. However, if coverage is terminated before the maximum period has elapsed, the employer is not required to offer a second election of extension. In other words, after continuation has been discontinued, coverage will not be reinstated or restarted.

If any of the following events occurs before the end of the 18-, 29-, or 36-month continuation period, coverage will cease at the end of the month following the date of the occurrence:

- Termination of all of the employer's sponsored group health plans.
- Failure to pay required premium contributions within 30 days of premium due date.
- Becoming covered under another group-sponsored health plan, unless the replacement plan exempts coverage for a preexisting condition affecting the member. Under this circumstance, the member may continue COBRA with the COBRA plan covering only those expenses incurred as a result of the preexisting condition. The replacement plan would cover all other expenses.
- Becoming entitled to Medicare coverage.

ACTIVITY #11

COBRA

Directions: Answer the following questions after reviewing the material just covered. Write your answers in the space provided.

1. To whom does the COBRA Act apply? _____
   _____

2. What is a qualified beneficiary? _____
   _____

3. What is a qualifying event? _____
   _____

4. What is the maximum time in which a dependent can continue COBRA? _____
   _____

5. What is the maximum time in which an employee can continue COBRA? _____
   _____

6. How long does a member have to apply for COBRA after termination of coverage? _____
   _____

ACTIVITY #12

Insurance Contracts

Directions: Read through the Ball Insurance Carrier contract and possible preexisting conditions (see Appendix A) and list the amounts for the following provisions in the space provided.

1. What is the individual deductible amount? _____
_____

2. What is the dependent eligibility age limit? _____
_____

3. What is the family calendar year deductible? _____
_____

4. What is the individual coinsurance limit? _____
_____

5. What is the coinsurance percentage? _____
_____

6. How many hours must the employee work in order to be eligible? _____
_____

7. Does the contract include dental coverage? _____
_____

8. What is the family coinsurance limit? _____
_____

9. Is the family coinsurance aggregate or nonaggregate?
_____

10. Is there a carryover provision on the individual deductible? _____
_____

11. How many months must the employee work before coverage becomes effective? _____
_____

General Plan Provisions

The following provisions affect most, if not all, insurance plans:

1. *Acts of third parties and subrogation.* These provisions allow a plan to be reimbursed for medical expenses that it has covered which should have been covered by another party.

2. *Preexisting conditions (as allowed by current law).* This policy is how insurance carriers attempt to limit amounts paid on behalf of people who were ill or injured before they obtained insurance. Disallowing preexisting conditions prevents someone from only getting insurance coverage when they need it to cover a serious illness or injury.

3. *State mandates.* Some states mandate that certain items, situations, or patients be covered or eligible for coverage within their state.

4. *Affordable Care Act of 2010.* This legislation is part of the Health Care Reform started by President Obama in 2009. This reform act includes mandated rights afforded to individuals who are obtaining insurance, options for insurance, insurance cost limitations, and the requirement that insurance companies cover certain preventative care services with no additional cost to the insured.

These common provisions can affect payment on certain claims. It is important for medical billers and health claims examiners to be aware of these provisions and apply them properly. If these provisions are not applied properly, an insurance carrier could end up making thousands of dollars of benefit payments on claims for which they are not responsible.

PRACTICE PITFALLS

A claimant is injured while on the premises of a grocery store. He submits the claims for his injuries to his benefit plan for payment. Subsequently, he also seeks recovery from the store. When recovery is successful, the claimant is required to reimburse the benefit plan for its losses.

Acts of Third Parties

Acts of Third Parties (ATP) and **subrogation** are provisions that are included in many benefit plans to allow a plan to recover money that the plan has paid on claims incurred as a result of a third party's act or acts for which that party is financially responsible.

ATP, also known as Third-Party Liability, and subrogation have some similarities, but they are actually different. Many older plans had subrogation (covered in more detail later), whereas many new plans have TPL. State laws affect general plan provisions. Although a plan may contain one of these provisions, it may not always be allowed to function if it is prohibited by a specific state statute or statutes.

THIRD-PARTY LIABILITY. Under **Third-Party Liability (TPL)**, the plan advances money to the injured person with the understanding that, if the claimant is successful in obtaining reimbursement from a third party, the plan will be reimbursed for its losses. The plan's interests lie with the claimant, not with the third party. An example of a third-party provision is as follows:

A special provision applies when you or your dependent covered under the plan is injured through the act or omission of another person. When this happens, the plan will advance the benefits under the policy only under the condition that you or your dependents agree in writing to the following items:

1. To repay the plan in full for any sums advanced to cover such claims paid by the plan, from the judgment or settlement you or a dependent receives.
2. To provide the plan with a lien to repay the plan to the extent of benefits advanced by the plan. The lien may be filed with the person whose act caused the injuries, his or her agent, the court, or the attorney of the person covered under the plan.

Thus, when an insurance carrier receives such a claim, the plan must send a repayment agreement to the claimant. This agreement requires the member to provide the information necessary to investigate the claim and subsequently, if appropriate, to file a lien with the member's attorney for reimburse-

ment against any settlement procured by the member. Usually, payment of losses is not made until the claimant has signed the repayment agreement and returned it to the administrator.

The plan may not demand reimbursement until the insured has been compensated for the loss by the third party. Filing a lien against such compensation protects the plan by making it mandatory that the plan be reimbursed before the claimant receives such compensation. Although the loss claimed by the claimant may include medical expenses, property damage, loss of earnings, pain and suffering, and even future medical expenses, the plan is permitted to recover only the amount actually paid out as a result of the injury. A sample of a payment demand is shown in Figure 3-6 ●. When any payments are received, they should be noted on a Right of Reimbursement Claims Log. A sample copy of such a log sheet is shown in Figure 3-7 ●.

ANY INSURANCE CARRIER, INC.
123 Any Drive, Anywhere, USA 12345 ● (800) 555-1234

Date:

Policyholder: _____

Control: _____

Employee: _____

Dependent: _____

Dear

This is to advise you that benefits totaling _____ have been paid to date to

_____ as a result of the accident on

_____.

Under the terms of _____ group health coverage, the insurance carrier is entitled to claim reimbursement from any third party liability coverage applicable to the same accident. Therefore, subrogation rights are claimed. Please advise as soon as possible when we might expect payment.

Sincerely,

Any Insurance Carrier

FIGURE 3-6   Sample Demand Payment Letter

ANY INSURANCE CARRIER, INC.
123 Any Drive, Anywhere, USA 12345 • (800) 555-1234

For Right of Reimbursement Claims

Claimant: _____   Policyholder: _____

Attorney: _____

Date of Accident: _____   Control No.: _____

Description of Condition/Diagnosis: _____

Type of Transaction	Payee/Receiver	Date	By	Amount of Payment	Total Paid to Date

FIGURE 3-7 Sample Reimbursement Claims Log

When a claim is received for expenses incurred as a result of an injury, determine how, when, and where the injury occurred. If this information is not indicated on the forms submitted, write to the member and request details. Samples of a letter and questionnaire are shown in Figures 3-8 ● and 3-9 ●.

If the injury occurred as the result of another party's acts and the plan has a TPL or subrogation provision, the plan should send the claimant a letter informing him or her about the appropriate provision and including an agreement. A sample copy of such letter is shown in Figure 3-10 ●. The claimant must sign the agreement indicating that if he or she receives monies from another source to cover these expenses, he or she is legally obligated to reimburse the plan. A sample copy of the agreement is shown in Figure 3-11 ●. This signed agreement is then kept on file with occasional follow-ups to track recovery; some payers file a lien against monies to which the claimant might be entitled. If the plan does not have either of these types of provisions, the plan cannot seek reimbursement from a third source.

As a rule, these provisions cannot be used to recover against the member's own auto liability carrier or home-owner's insurance carrier.

Administration of this provision tends to be long-term and time-intensive. Therefore, many plans retain special agencies to help track and recover TPL monies. In exchange, the agency is paid from the proceeds that they recover.

ANY INSURANCE CARRIER, INC.
123 Any Drive, Anywhere, USA 12345 ● (800) 555-1234

Re: Insured's I.D. No.

Dear

The claim that you recently submitted for accidental bodily injuries expenses is under review. Circumstances of the accident indicate that a third party may be liable for the payment of your medical or dental bills.

Accordingly, the policy in force between _____
and _____ contains a Third Party Liability exclusion, which provides that no medical or dental benefits are payable for injuries or illness caused by a third party if payment for such expenses has been or will be received from the third party or insurer. A copy of the entire provision is attached.

To assist us in evaluating the claim, please complete the enclosed questionnaire detailing particulars regarding the accident and parties involved. Any additional information would be greatly appreciated.

Additionally, if a third party is liable for your expenses, we have enclosed a Third Party Liability Reimbursement Agreement, to be signed, witnessed, and returned to us before benefits can be released.

If you have any questions regarding this matter, please do not hesitate to contact me.

Sincerely,

FIGURE 3-8 Sample letter requesting further information

ANY INSURANCE CARRIER, INC.
123 Any Drive, Anywhere, USA 12345 ● (800) 555-1234

TPL INVESTIGATION QUESTIONNAIRE

1. Name and address of responsible third party.

_____

_____

   City   State   Zip Code

2. Name and address of responsible third party's insurance company and policy number.

_____

_____

   City   State   Zip Code

3. If an accident, what were the circumstances?

_____

_____

_____

_____

_____

4. If Any Insurance Carrier, Inc. is to pay medical benefits under the terms of the contract, when is settlement expected or how often may we expect status reports?

_____

_____

_____

5. Is legal counsel involved? If yes, please give name and address.

_____

_____

   City   State   Zip Code

FIGURE 3-9 Sample TPL Questionnaire

Completion of the Right of Reimbursement Claims Log

To accurately track the reimbursement provided to/from third parties, most insurance plans keep a log. Most computer software programs will have a section for this purpose, but an example log is provided in Figure 3-7. The information in this log must be written or typed in a legible manner. This log is used to track all payments made on a particular case and all correspondence sent or received regarding the case.

COMPLETING THE LOG. This log is often printed (or created) on letterhead so that a copy of this form may be attached to any liens filed with the claimant's attorney. This log then becomes a statement of the amount due on the case, as of the date it is

sent (assuming the computer software program for electronic billing does not keep track of this information for you).

The fields on the Right of Reimbursement Claims Log Sheet are to be filled in as follows:

Claimant: Enter the name of the claimant (patient).

Policyholder: Enter the name of the policyholder or insured.

Attorney: Enter the name, address, and phone number of the attorney who is representing the claimant.

Date of Accident: Enter the date of the accident. If this claim pertains to an illness (i.e., an illness which may be covered under worker's compensation), enter the date the patient was diagnosed with this condition.

ANY INSURANCE CARRIER, INC.
123 Any Drive, Anywhere, USA 12345 • (800) 555-1234

Third Party Liability Exclusion Rider Effective _____
Attached to and made part of Group Insurance Policy No. _____
Issued by _____

to _____

No benefits will be paid under this policy to or on behalf of an insured individual
who has:

1. medical or dental charges, or
2. loss of earnings

If the insured individual has received payment, in whole or in part, from a third
party, or its insurer, for past or future medical or dental charges or loss of
earnings as the result of negligence or intentional acts of a third party.

If an insured party makes a claim to Any Insurance Carrier for medical, dental, or
loss of earnings benefits under this policy prior to receiving payment from a third
party, or its insurer, the insured individual (or legal representative of a minor or
incompetent) must agree in writing to repay Any Insurance Carrier from any
amount of money received by the insured individual from the third party, or its
insurer. The repayment will be to the extent of the benefits paid by Any
Insurance Carrier. However, the reasonable pro rata expenses, such as lawyer's
fees and court costs, incurred in affecting the third party payment may be
deducted from the repayment to Any Insurance Carrier.

The repayment agreement will be binding upon the insured individual (or legal
representative of a minor or incompetent) whether:

1. The payment received from the third party, or its insurer, is the result of:
   a. a legal judgment, or
   b. an arbitration award, or
   c. a compromise settlement, or
   d. any other arrangement, or
2. The third party, or its insurer, has admitted liability for the payment, or
3. The medical or dental charges or loss of earnings are itemized in the
   third party payment.

FIGURE 3-10   Third Party Liability Exclusion Rider

Control Number: Enter the control number assigned to this case. Each case will be assigned a control number to aid in tracking the case and all claims payments associated with it.

Description of Condition/Diagnosis: Enter the conditions or diagnoses associated with this situation. All conditions and diagnoses related to the accident or illness should be entered together on one sheet.

Type of Transaction: Enter the type of the transactions which occurred. This could be a claim which was processed, an agreement letter sent, a lien notice sent, correspondence sent, or any other transaction that occurred for this case.

Payee/Receiver: Enter the name of the person or facility that received payment on the claim. If the transaction was

a letter or other item sent through the mail, enter the name of the person to which the item was sent.

Date: Enter the date on which the item (such as a check) was sent out.

By: Enter the name of the person who sent the item or who processed the claim.

Amount of Payment: Enter the amount of the payment that was made on this claim. If the item is not a claim and no value is assessed (i.e., a lien notice or agreement was sent), enter N/A for Not Applicable.

Total Paid to Date: Add the amount paid with this transaction to the remaining balance (prior line of this column). This amount will show the total amount that the carrier should be reimbursed for claims paid out on this TPL case.

ANY INSURANCE CARRIER, INC.
123 Any Drive, Anywhere, USA 12345 ● (800) 555-1234

Third Party Liability Reimbursement Agreement

I, _____, an insured individual (or his or her legal representative) under group insurance policy number _____ issued by Any Insurance Carrier, Inc. to _____, the policyholder, pursuant to the terms of the group insurance policy, do hereby agree to reimburse Any Insurance Carrier for any medical or dental expenses or loss of earnings benefits which are paid by Any Insurance Carrier or will be paid by it, which expenses or benefits arise out of the accident or sickness commencing _____, 20_____, if payment is received from a third party, or its insurer.

I understand that this agreement to reimburse shall be binding on me regardless of whether:

1. the payment received from the third party, or its insurer, is the result of a legal judgment, arbitration award, compromise settlement or otherwise; or,
2. such third party, or its insurer, has admitted liability in connection with such payment; or,
3. such medical or dental expenses actually incurred or loss of earnings realized are itemized in such third party payment.

I further understand that the reasonable pro rata costs, including attorney fees, actually incurred by me in effecting the third party payment for such medical or dental expenses or loss of earnings may be deducted from any such reimbursement.

_____   _____
(Insured Individual or his or her Legal Representative)   Date

_____   _____
(Witness)   Date

FIGURE 3-11   Third Party Liability Reimbursement Agreement

Payments Received

If a payment is received by the insurance carrier for repayment of part or all of the case, also record this in the log. In this case, the following information would be entered:

Type of Transaction: Enter "Payment Received."

Payee/Receiver: Enter the name of the insurance carrier, and the name of the party sending the payment (e.g., Any Ins. Car. from Client's Attorney).

Date: Enter the date on which the payment was received.

By: Enter the name of the contact person or the person who sent the payment.

Amount of payment: Enter the amount of the payment.

Total Paid to Date: Subtract any payment amounts from the total amount shown on the previous line. This practice will allow you always to see the total amount due for this case on the last line.

Subrogation

An insurance company claims subrogation (a legal term that means substitution of) payment to them (versus the claimant) if the claim is paid by a third party after the insurance company has already paid on the claim. Under subrogation, the insurance carrier has an obligation to pay a benefit under the contract, but the carrier has a subrogated right for a portion of the recovery that the claimant may obtain from a third party. The insurance carrier has a direct interest with the third party.

For example, you are a subscriber and you or one of your dependents suffers an injury that requires hospitalization or other medical treatment. When benefits are paid under the terms of the plan, the plan shall be subrogate, unless otherwise prohibited by law, to your right of recovery or the rights of recovery of your dependent against any person who might acknowledge to be liable or might be found legally liable by a court of competent jurisdiction for the injury that necessitated the hospitalization or the medical or surgical treatment for which the benefits were paid.

Such subrogation rights shall extend only to the recovery by the insurance carrier of the benefits it has paid for such treatment, and the insurance carrier shall pay fees and costs associated with such recovery.

When a claim is received for expenses incurred as a result of any injury involving another party, a subrogation letter along with a subrogation statement should be sent to the claimant.

The subrogation statement requires the member to provide information necessary to investigate the claim. The form also requires the member to agree to allow the plan to file a lien against any settlement made by another party.

Although technically ATP and subrogation are not the same, from the health claims examiner's standpoint, the differences are moot. Do not be concerned about the differences. Instead, focus on the concepts behind them, the objective in each case, and how to obtain that objective.

ACTIVITY #13

Subrogation

Directions: Answer the following questions after reviewing the material just covered. Write your answers in the space provided.

1. Why are ATP and subrogation provisions included in many benefit plans? _____
_____
2. Under _____, the plan advances money to the injured person with the understanding that if the claimant is successful in obtaining reimbursement monies from a third party, the plan will be reimbursed.
3. Under _____, the plan has an obligation to pay a benefit under the contract, but has a subrogated right for a portion of the recovery that the claimant may obtain from a third party.

Preexisting Conditions

A preexisting condition is a condition for which the claimant was treated within a specified time period before the claimant became covered under the plan. This provision must be reviewed carefully because there are many variations and it will be eliminated in 2014. For example, it may apply to dependents only; time limits may be different for members

versus dependents; or the provision may be waived for all individuals who are covered on the effective date of the plan..

Whether the expense or expenses incurred are excluded completely or limited to a specific dollar benefit, most clauses provide that benefits will become payable after the member has been covered under the plan for a specific period of time and has not received any treatment for the preexisting condition during that time.

Handling Procedures

Improperly handled claims for preexisting conditions are a frequent source of complaints and lawsuits. A medical biller has an obligation to review insurance policies for preexisting conditions that are not covered and bill the individual when appropriate versus the insurance company. An examiner has an obligation to perform the following tasks:

1. Investigate each claim thoroughly, at the earliest appropriate time, preferably on the very first claim receipt. If the expenses result from an injury that was incurred after the effective date of the plan or from an illness that is not chronic, such as a cold or flu, the examiner should not make an inquiry. Always consider the specific plan provisions.
2. Notify the member and the provider, if appropriate, of the delay in writing.
3. Conclude the investigation as rapidly as possible by making a decision to pay or generating a fully documented denial.

Treatment-Free Provisions

To qualify for payment on the basis of having satisfied the treatment-free provision and the total limitation (no payment on preexisting conditions for 12 months), it must be determined that the patient did not receive any treatment for the preexisting condition from a doctor, hospital, clinic, or other medical practitioner. Receiving advice but no treatment from a practitioner may be considered treatment in the case of a preexisting condition. To determine whether a given condition is preexisting, follow these procedures:

1. Identify all potential preexisting conditions by noting the diagnosis and the length of time between the effective date of the plan and the first treatment documented on the claim form or in the claim file. Pay special attention to claims for chronic conditions or for major surgery with little or no preliminary diagnostic work or medical treatment.
2. Initiate the investigation as soon as appropriate by writing to the attending physician and all other consulting or referring physicians whose names can be determined. Figure 3-12 ● shows an example of a letter used to obtain additional information regarding a possible preexisting condition. Write to the following sources of information as well:

   • All hospitals involved to request a copy of hospital records, including the admitting history and physical, discharge summary, consultation, and operative reports.
   • Pharmacies to obtain drug names, dates filled, and names and phone numbers of prescribing physicians.

Any Insurance Carrier, INC.
123 Any Drive
Anywhere, USA 12345
(800) 555-1234

Re:

Control: _____

Insured: _____

Dear

We are presently processing a claim for the above patient. In order to give it full consideration, we need additional information. Please answer the questions outlined below. A pre-addressed envelope is provided for your convenience. Your cooperation will be appreciated and will help expedite the matter for your patient. (Authorization to release information is attached.)

Sincerely yours,

Claims Representative

Condition(s) described on claim form as: _____

_____

_____

1. Did you prescribe medication for, or treat the above condition or related symptoms from _____ through _____ ? ☐ Yes ☐ No If so, specify below:

Condition	Date Treated
_____	_____
_____	_____
_____	_____

2. | Drug | Date Prescribed | Drug | Date Prescribed |
|---|---|---|---|
| _____ | | _____ | |
| _____ | | _____ | |
| _____ | | _____ | |

3. Was the patient referred to you by another physician? ☐ Yes ☐ No If so, please provide name and address of referring doctor. _____

Dated _____   Signed _____

FIGURE 3-12 Preexisting Condition Form

- Attending physicians to request copies of treatment histories that detail the onset of the condition, referring physicians, and other pertinent information.
- Claimants to request the names, addresses, and phone numbers of all doctors seen and all medications taken during the appropriate time period stipulated in the plan.

Many insurance carriers have a standard form letter for requesting information regarding a preexisting condition.

3. Act immediately on leads or additional information supplied in response to the initial requests for information.

4. Bear in mind that the burden of proof lies with the plan to prove that a condition is preexisting. No matter how certain you may be that a condition is preexisting, a plan cannot deny a claim as such unless there is adequate documentation in the claim file.

5. If you do not receive answers to the inquiries, follow the administrator's guidelines for denying the claim. Do not deny the claim as preexisting. Instead, deny it pending receipt of previously requested information.

6. Determining whether a condition is a chronic illness or a new illness is essential in deciding whether the preexisting exclusion applies. For example, infectious conditions such as an upper respiratory infection, otitis media, bronchitis, or a urinary tract infection may occur repeatedly with resolution between episodes. If a period elapses between treatments, a new episode (and therefore, a new illness) may exist, in which the preexisting exclusion would not apply.

7. Related conditions and complications of existing conditions may make it difficult for you to determine whether an illness is preexisting. Certain diseases are progressive, and a different diagnosis may be assigned to the successive stages of the disease. The *Merck Manual* may be helpful in researching such conditions, but you should refer any questionable case to the supervisor, medical review department, or a consultant for review.

PRACTICE **PITFALLS**

A claimant is covered under the Winter Insurance Company contract, effective 07/01/CCYY. A claim is received for a diagnosis of diabetes for the date of service 08/01/CCYY. Diabetes is a chronic condition; therefore, it may be preexisting. An investigation must be pursued in a manner previously indicated so that the claim file can be properly documented to substantiate the claims decision. First, examine the claim form. Does it list the date of the first treatment of the condition? Was the treatment before the effective date? If so, the condition may be preexisting because some persons with diabetes require insulin injections or pills on a daily basis.

If the first treatment occurred after the effective date, is there a name of a referring physician? If so, write to that physician and request treatment information. If the first treatment date is not indicated, write to the physician who

submitted the claim and to the claimant, requesting the following information:

- The names of all physicians seen between 04/01/CCYY and 08/01/CCYY (this covers the 90-day period prior to the effective date of coverage, up to and including the current treatment date).
- The names and dates of all prescriptions written during this same period of time.
- The names of all other medical providers referred to or from and the dates of treatments during this period of time.

The objective of this questioning is two-fold:

1. To determine whether treatment commenced during the 90-day period of time before the effective date.
2. To determine whether a three-month period of time has occurred in which the claimant did not receive treatment (i.e., to determine whether the three-month treatment-free period provision applies).

Health Insurance Portability and Accountability Act

In 1996, a new law regarding health insurance, HIPAA, was signed by President Clinton. The most important changes to existing health insurance law involved preexisting limitations, prior coverage certification, and privacy issues. Here we will discuss preexisting limitations and prior coverage certification that will pertain only to claims filed before 2014.

This law has a direct impact on insurers, unlike other healthcare legislation, which primarily affects employers.

HIPAA restricts the circumstances and the period for which a group health plan may exclude coverage for a preexisting condition. The restriction has five parts:

1. A group health plan may not impose a preexisting condition limit unless the plan provides prior notice to the member of the existence and terms of the preexisting condition exclusion.
2. A group health plan may not impose a preexisting condition exclusion unless the member received treatment or advice from a state-licensed medical practitioner for the condition within the six-month period preceding the date of enrollment under the group health plan.
3. The group health plan must credit an individual's prior health coverage toward satisfaction of the preexisting condition limit unless that coverage was solely for excepted benefits, commonly called riders or waivers.
4. The maximum period allowed for a preexisting condition exclusion is generally 12 months (18 months in the case of an individual who does not enroll when he or she first becomes eligible).
5. The group health plan may not impose any preexisting condition exclusions for pregnancy or for a newborn or newly adopted child enrolled within 30 days.

Prior Notification

Unless the insurer gives the insured prior information regarding preexisting limitations, the insurer may not impose them. Most insurance carriers include preexisting clauses in their contracts. Placing the information within the contract satisfies the requirement of prior notification.

Preexisting Requirements

HIPAA limits the preexisting period (also called the look-back time) in determining whether a condition is preexisting to six months. A preexisting provision generally applies to medical advice, diagnosis, care, or treatment that is either recommended or received for a condition. The look-back period is the six-month period prior to the enrollment date in any new health plan. Some states use the prudent person standard in determining whether a condition is preexisting. This means that a condition is preexisting if a prudent person would have sought care or treatment. HIPAA rejects this standard and states that a condition is only preexisting if advice or care is actually sought.

Credit for Prior Coverage

HIPAA also states that an employee may receive credit for the period of time he was covered by his former employer, provided the coverage is considered "credible." Therefore, if an employee only had medical coverage with his former employer, the employee would be given credit for prior medical coverage, but preexisting exclusions could apply to dental, vision, and other services.

Credible Coverage

Credible coverage does not take into consideration the benefits of the old and new plan, only that both plans are medical coverage. A new insurance carrier may choose to enact the preexisting limitations on certain items that were not included in previous medical coverage. This allowance is limited to coverage for mental health, substance abuse treatment, prescriptions, dental care, and vision care. For example, if a participant's old plan did not include coverage for mental health benefits, then the new plan may elect to enact a preexisting limit on the mental health benefits that it normally offers in the plan.

Under the new law, preexisting exclusions are limited to a six-month look-back period, and credit must be given for prior coverage. Therefore, if a person is covered by insurance, and he or she transfers insurance coverage to a new company within 63 days of ceasing coverage at the old company, the new insurance carrier may not apply preexisting limitations to treatment. If there was a break of 63 days or more between termination of the old coverage and the available date of new coverage, preexisting exclusions are limited to six months.

If a person declines coverage under a new plan because he or she is covered under a previously existing plan, and then the person loses benefits under the old plan, he or she can enroll under a new plan without preexisting limitations. No preexisting limitation may be applied to those who transfer from one plan to another during a company's open-enrollment period.

Employees are no longer allowed to continue COBRA coverage on a policy if they are covered under a new policy. In the past, many employees would continue coverage on an old policy until the preexisting limitation had been satisfied on the new insurance. Because the new insurance is no longer allowed to apply preexisting limitations, the need for this coverage has been eliminated. Many people may still elect to continue coverage on the old policy until they have satisfied any length of employment (e.g., must be employed for 90 days) requirements. However, the waiting period is not considered a break in coverage for purposes of the 63-day break in coverage. Therefore, if an employee terminates at one company (and ceases coverage), and is hired at a second company within 63 days, the employee is considered to be continuously covered even if he or she must satisfy a 90-day waiting period before coverage begins with the new employer.

Employers are not allowed to discriminate against individuals who have higher medical costs in their hiring practices. This is true even though the higher costs will eventually show an increase in the company's insurance premiums. An **insurance premium** is the amount of money required for coverage under a specific insurance policy for a given period of time. Depending on the policy agreement, the premium may be paid monthly, quarterly, semiannually, or annually.

An employee leaving his or her employer should obtain a certificate of credible coverage which states that the employee was covered, describes what type of plan it was (e.g., dental only, medical), and states the length of coverage. This certificate of credible coverage is then applied to the new carrier's preexisting conditions clause.

Companies are also now required to provide written certification of all prior coverage for their employees. They must provide this information upon termination of coverage, and for up to 24 months after termination if the employee requests it. Certificates must include

- The date the certificate is issued.
- The name of the group health plan that provided the coverage described in the certificate.
- The name of the participant or dependent covered and identifying information for that person (e.g., social security number, identification number).
- A telephone number to call for further information regarding the certificate.
- Either
  a. A statement that the individual has had at least 18 months of creditable coverage, or
  b. The beginning date for any creditable coverage (and any waiting period).
- The ending date of coverage, or (in cases of COBRA) a statement that the participant or dependent is continuing coverage as of the date the certificate was issued.

If the information for a participant and the person's dependents is identical, the company may issue a single certificate, provided that all persons are properly named and identified on the certificate. If information is different for each individual (e.g., beginning and ending dates of coverage), then a plan administrator may either issue a separate certificate for each person, or detail the information for each person on one certificate.

Maximum Periods

For individuals who do not satisfy the continuous coverage requirements, preexisting exclusions are limited to conditions for which treatment was received within six months prior to coverage. Exclusions are only allowed to remain in effect for 12 months. Therefore, after 12 months the carrier must cover the condition, whether it was preexisting or not. If a person did not enroll when he or she first became eligible, then preexisting exclusions are allowed to continue for 18 months. This rule is because some people will not apply for coverage until they have a condition that they know is going to require extensive treatment. They will then attempt to get coverage for that condition.

HIPAA also states that if a preexisting condition exists, the 12-month period for imposing the preexisting exclusion is measured from the employee's enrollment date. The enrollment date is defined as the date of coverage in the plan or the first day of the waiting period before the coverage begins (usually the employment date), whichever is earlier. The waiting period rule does not apply when the enrollee is a late enrollee.

Some employers require a physical examination as a condition of employment as shown in Figure 3-13 ●. If that examination is done *after* the date of starting employment, any condition first identified during that examination cannot be applied to the preexisting condition exclusion clause. However, if the physical examination takes place *prior* to the employment date and the condition is first identified at that time, the preexisting condition exclusion clause can apply.

Pregnancies, Newborns, and Adopted Children under 18 Excluded

Preexisting limits are not allowed for pregnancy, newborns, or adopted children under 18 years of age. Therefore, if a woman transfers coverage while she is pregnant, the new insurance carrier must cover the costs associated with the pregnancy. Also, a preexisting condition exclusion cannot be applied to a newborn or adopted child under age 18 as long as the child became covered under the health plan within 30 days of birth or adoption.

HIPAA does much to reduce the burden placed on employees due to a preexisting condition. It does not eliminate the right of a carrier to investigate and impose the preexisting clause when applicable. This legislation is complex and all questions should be directed to your supervisor.

It is essential for you to have a good understanding of the preexisting condition clause in a plan in order to apply the rules under HIPAA.

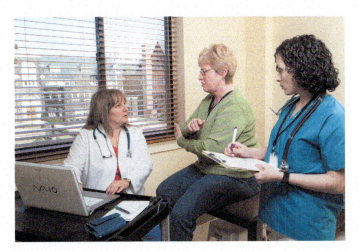

FIGURE 3-13   Patient in for a physical examination as part of the employment agreement

Source: Michal Heron/Pearson Education/PH College

ACTIVITY #14

HIPAA

Directions: Read each of the following scenarios and determine whether the certificate of prior insurance should be checked and why or why not.

1. Jennifer received treatment for a chronic ulcer on 7/1/CCYY and again on 8/1/CCYY. On 10/01/CCYY she quit her job and began working for a new employer two weeks later, on 10/15/CCYY. She immediately signed up for insurance and her coverage became effective after a 30-day waiting period, on 11/15/CCYY. On 1/15/CCNY, she was seen by the doctor for additional treatment for chronic ulcer. Do you need a copy of her coverage certificate with the 1/15/CCNY claim, and if so, why?

_____

_____

2. Mary received treatment for diabetes on 7/1/CCYY and again on 8/1/CCYY. On 10/1/CCYY, she quit her job and began working for a new employer two weeks later, on 10/15/CCYY. She immediately signed up for insurance and her coverage became effective after a 90-day waiting period, on 1/15/CCNY. On 10/15/CCNY, she was seen by the doctor for additional diabetes treatment. Do you need a copy of her coverage certificate with the 10/15/CCNY claim? Explain your answer.

_____

_____

3. Tom received treatment for kidney disease on 2/1/CCYY and again on 3/1/CCYY. On 10/1/CCYY, he quit his job and began working for a new employer two weeks later, on 10/15/CCYY. He immediately signed up for insurance and his coverage became effective after a 30-day waiting period, on 11/15/CCYY. On 12/15/CCYY, he was seen by the doctor for additional treatment for kidney disease. Do you need a copy of his coverage certificate with the 12/15/CCYY claim? Explain.

_____

_____

4. Betty had a routine visit for pregnancy on 7/1/CCYY and again on 8/1/CCYY. She did not have coverage at this time. On 10/1/CCYY, she began working for a new employer. She immediately signed up for insurance and her coverage became effective after a 30-day waiting period, on 11/1/CCYY. On 1/15/CCNY, she was seen by the doctor for an additional routine pregnancy visit. Do you need a copy of her coverage certificate for the 1/15/CCNY claim? If so, why?

_____

_____

5. Jessie received treatment for anorexia on 7/1/CCYY and again on 8/1/CCYY. On 10/16/CCYY, she quit her job and chose not to continue coverage under COBRA rules. On 12/15/CCYY she began working for a new employer. She immediately signed up for insurance and her coverage became effective after a 30-day waiting period, on 1/15/CCNY. On 1/25/CCNY, she was seen by the doctor for treatment of diabetes. Do you need a copy of her coverage certificate with the 1/25/CCNY claim? If so, why?

_____

_____

STATE Mandates

Mandates are laws enacted by states that require insurance carriers to cover certain services, dependents, or services provided by certain providers.

Mandates generally take one of two forms:

1. The insurance carrier is required to provide the coverage as part of all plans offered by the carrier, or
2. The insurance carrier within the state must offer the benefit. However, to the carrier is not required to include the benefit as part of a standard policy.

The second requirement is satisfied if the insurance carrier offers a second policy (often with a higher premium) that includes the benefit. Employers are not required to purchase them for employees. As most insurance coverage is offered as a benefit of employment, most employers will opt for the lower priced coverage that does not include the benefit. For that reason, many people whose health insurance coverage is provided through their employer are not covered by the benefit. Individuals who buy an individual insurance plan may choose to include these options or not.

There are over 1,000 mandates on the books as of this writing. However, special interest groups are constantly submitting bills to state legislatures requesting additional coverage. Each insurance carrier is required to obtain a copy of the mandates in any states where they sell coverage. Regardless of where the insurance carrier is located, if the policy is sold and coverage is offered in a state, then that state's mandates apply to the coverage offered in that state.

Some limitations may apply to these benefits (e.g., they apply to group insurance only). For more complete and current information for a state, contact that state's department of insurance.

Affordable Care Act of 2010

Healthcare reform started by President Obama in 2009 set forth several mandates, including removal of preexisting conditions clauses by 2014, coverage for preexisting conditions by the federal government until 2014, and 100% coverage of preventative services and women's services.

COVERAGE FOR PREEXISTING CONDITIONS. As of 2010, the Department of Health and Human Services offers coverage

TABLE 3-1 Mandated Women's Preventative Care Services

Well-woman visits.	Well-woman preventive care visit annually for adult women to obtain the recommended preventive services that are age and developmentally appropriate, including preconception and prenatal care. This well-woman visit should, where appropriate, include other preventive services listed in this set of guidelines, as well as others referenced in section 2713.	Annual, although HHS recognizes that several visits may be needed to obtain all necessary recommended preventive services, depending on a woman's health status, health needs, and other risk factors.
Screening for gestational diabetes.	Screening for gestational diabetes.	In pregnant women between 24 and 28 weeks of gestation and at the first prenatal visit for pregnant women identified to be at high risk for diabetes.
Human papillomavirus testing.	High-risk human papillomavirus DNA testing in women with normal cytology results.	Screening should begin at 30 years of age and should occur no more frequently than every 3 years.
Counseling for sexually transmitted infections.	Counseling on sexually transmitted infections for all sexually active women.	Annual.
Counseling and screening for human immune-deficiency virus.	Counseling and screening for human immune-deficiency virus infection for all sexually active women.	Annual.
Contraceptive methods and counseling.	All Food and Drug Administration approved contraceptive methods, sterilization procedures, and patient education and counseling for all women with reproductive capacity.	As prescribed.
Breastfeeding support, supplies, and counseling.	Comprehensive lactation support and counseling, by a trained provider during pregnancy and/or in the postpartum period, and costs for renting breastfeeding equipment.	In conjunction with each birth.
Screening and counseling for interpersonal and domestic violence.	Screening and counseling for interpersonal and domestic violence.	Annual.

for preexisting conditions as a bridge until 2014, when insurance companies will be prohibited from using preexisting conditions as part of the insurance policy. Some states have implemented such bridge plans already. Residents of states that have not implemented the bridge coverage are eligible for the federal program that covers preexisting condition coverage.

PREVENTATIVE CARE SERVICES. Healthcare reform includes a provision that insurance companies must cover certain preventative care services at 100%, generally including the following services:

1. Blood pressure, diabetes, and cholesterol tests
2. Many cancer screenings, including mammograms and colonoscopies
3. Counseling on such topics as quitting smoking, losing weight, eating healthfully, treating depression, and reducing alcohol use
4. Routine vaccinations against diseases such as measles, polio, or meningitis
5. Flu and pneumonia shots
6. Counseling, screening, and vaccines to ensure healthy pregnancies
7. Regular well-baby and well-child visits, from birth to age 21

Some of these preventative services have caveats associated with being a certain age, meeting an established criteria for needing the screening, and the timing of the insurance plan renewal.

WOMEN'S SERVICES. The healthcare reform program also includes a guideline for women's preventative services that are to be covered at no cost to the insured when the criteria and recommendations are met. (See Table 3-1 ● for women's services that became effective August 1, 2012.)

Prompt-Pay Laws

Prompt-pay laws require health plans to pay health insurance claims within a specified time period or face fines, added interest payments, and other penalties. Note that prompt-pay laws apply only to "clean claims" (claims without defect and with full information provided). If a state requires clean claims to be paid within a certain time, the state is listed under the appropriate time limit.

External or Independent Grievance Systems

External grievance systems allow claimants to take a dispute with their health plan to a doctor or review board unaffiliated with their health plan. Thus, both the claimant and their health plan receive an impartial ruling on its decision to deny coverage of services or treatment. In addition, claimants can file a complaint against their health insurer with their state's department of insurance.

The information in Table 3-2 ● identifies the grounds of the original denial where a claimant may appeal a health plan's unfavorable decisions and whether the panel's decision is binding or advisory. Information given applies to all health plans unless otherwise stated.

ACTIVITY #15

Mandates

Directions: Research your state's mandated insurance coverage online. (Hint: Go to the state department of insurance or .gov webpage for your state.) Write a 1–2-page summary of your findings.

TABLE 3-2 Common Reasons for Claim Denial

Reason	Explanation
Medical Necessity	The diagnostic codes and the service codes do not match; or they do not justify that the service was necessary; or it is an exclusion in the policy.
Experimental or Investigational Treatment	Most policies do not cover experimental services.
Termination of Coverage	The patient's policy was not intact at the time of the filing.
Untimely Filing	The claim is outside of the acceptable timelines for filing.
Elective Procedure	Something that had no medical necessity and the patient chose to have the procedure.
Incomplete Information	Patient may not be found in their system, blanks were left on the claim for, or there is a need for further information.

CHAPTER REVIEW

Summary

- The term "contract," in general, is an agreement among two or more persons that is enforceable by law. In order for a contract to be valid, the parties must agree on its terms. There must also be some form of offer and acceptance.
- When an offer has been properly communicated and accepted, a binding contract is formed.
- A group contract allows an insurance company to meet the financial security needs of a group of persons.
- It is vital that medical billers and health claims examiners understand how to interpret contracts. It will take practice to accurately understand the coverages provided under contracts and to pay benefits properly.
- Basic and major medical plans are generally classified as indemnity contracts.
- These plans indemnify or reimburse the insured for medical expenses incurred and typically require the insured to complete and file claims.
- These plans often also contain deductible and coinsurance provisions and may restrict coverage for certain types of medical care expenditures.
- The three contracts found in Appendix A will be used throughout the course to calculate benefits on sample claims and to clarify examples to demonstrate the application of plan provisions.
- These sample contracts are based on actual plans and should be used as examples of what is possible within the industry. There is no such thing as a definitive plan.

As you will discover, there are a multitude of possible contract provisions. Therefore, use these samples as learning tools only.

- Eligibility and effective dates of coverage are probably the most important factors to consider when you process a claim.
- Thus, the first things you should check when you receive a claim for payment are eligibility and effective date. If the patient is not eligible, no further action need be taken on the claim.
- Acts of Third Parties and subrogation can drastically alter the way a claim is paid and who is responsible for the claim payment.
- Preexisting conditions and lifetime limit benefits will be prohibited in 2014.
- Some preventative care services are now mandated to be covered at 100% by insurance.
- The health claims examiner and medical biller must understand these concepts and must know when they come into play.

Review Questions

Directions: Answer the following questions after reviewing the material just covered. Write your answers in the space provided.

1. True or False? Every health benefit plan, whether it is insured or not, is required by law to have a written document describing the plan benefits. _____

2. Define offer. _____

    _____

3. Define eligibility. _____

    _____

4. What is an exclusion? _____

5. _____ refers to the requirements that must be fulfilled for a person to be covered by the plan.

6. Most contracts define employees in terms of _____

    _____

7. What is a qualified beneficiary? _____

    _____

8. What is a qualifying event? _____

    _____

9. True or False? Improperly handled claims for preexisting conditions are a common source of complaints and lawsuits. _____

    _____

10. True or False? An examiner should not notify the member and the provider of the delay in processing a claim. _____

    _____

If you were unable to answer any of these questions, refer back to that section and then fill in the answers.

ACTIVITY #16

Eligibility Review

Directions: Place a "yes" or "no" next to each of the following people to show which would be eligible for coverage under the Ninja contract.

1. Kanika works 35 hours per week for Ninja. _____

2. Kenneth, Kanika's second husband, is self-employed. _____

3. Ryan, the 20-year-old son of Kanika and her first husband, is currently unemployed and is not a full-time student. _____

4. Ravyn, Ryan's twin, attends the local university full-time. _____

5. Jordan, Kanika's and Kenneth's 16-year-old daughter, is a high-school dropout. _____

6. Sheila is a 13-year-old foster child who lives with the family. _____

7. Sharon is a 10-year-old legally adopted child. _____

8. Paris is the three-year-old daughter of Ravyn. _____

9. Kytrena, Kanika's mother, has Alzheimer's disease and is listed as a dependent on Kanika's income tax form. _____

10. Caitlind is Kanika's mentally retarded sister. Kanika is not her legal guardian _____

Medical Benefit

Keywords and concepts you will learn in this chapter:

Accidental Injury

Accumulation Period

Allowed Amount

Automatic Annual Reinstatement (AAR)

Common Accident Provision

Concurrent Review

Conversion Factor

Covered Expense

Cumulative Benefit

Exclusive Provider Organization (EPO)

Extended Benefits

Fee Schedule

Gatekeeper PPO

In-Network Provider

Loss Date

Managed Care

Management Service Organization (MSO)

Mandatory Program

Maximum

Medical Case Management (MCM)

Nondisabling or Per-Visit Benefit

Out-of-Network Provider

Out-of-Pocket (OOP)

Out-of-Pocket Maximum

After completing this chapter, you will be able to:

▌ Define common terms relevant to dealing with benefits.

● Explain how coinsurance is calculated.

▌ Accurately calculate deductible amounts, given a contract and scenario.

● Discuss a common accident provision.

● Describe how to calculate basic benefits.

▌ Identify the various types of common basic benefits.

▌ Explain restrictions that apply to major medical benefits.

▌ Describe comprehensive major medical benefits

● Accurately calculate stop-loss.

● State the impact of UCR.

● Define relative value units.

● Define GPCI.

Per Period of Disability
Physician Hospital Organization (PHO)
Preauthorization
Precertification
Predetermination
Region
Relative Value Units (RVUs)
Retrospective Review
Three-Month Carryover (C/O) Provision
UCR Calculation
Unit Value
Unnecessary Surgery
Utilization Review (UR)
Voluntary Program

Explain the formula for determining physician fees.

Accurately calculate usual, customary, and reasonable fees.

Identify cost-containment programs and describe their implementation.

Describe the intent of managed care.

Discuss the purpose of medical case management.

Every healthcare plan is required by law to have a written description of the benefits available to the members of that plan. This plan document must indicate, in detail, and in layman's terms, the provisions of the coverage.

Three major types of indemnity coverage are currently available:

- Basic only
- Basic–Major Medical
- Comprehensive Major Medical

Within these types, there may be numerous variations. In addition, under managed care provisions there can be PPO and HMO contracts.

As the benefit payments calculated under each type of coverage can be identical, focus on the concept of the benefit being offered. Medical billers and health claims examiners should understand the type of benefit payments before submitting or processing claims. Accurate benefit payment calculation is essential to being a good biller or claims examiner. Inaccurate payments can cost providers or insurance carriers money.

▶ CRITICAL THINKING QUESTION: What is the purpose of making sure that all healthcare plans have a written description of the benefits available to the members of that plan?

Benefit Definitions

Here are some common terms relevant to dealing with benefits. The definitions in this section are not associated with calculations. Benefit definitions that require you to calculate items will be discussed in the Benefit Calculations section.

Accumulation Period

The period each year between the time when an insurance policy starts and when it renews is called the **accumulation period** (normally January 1 through December 31). During this time, all monies spent by the insured are accumulated to satisfy the deductible or count the number of visits for visit-specific benefits (e.g., an insured may see a chiropractor up to 12 times in the accumulation period).

Covered Expenses

An expense that is allowable under the insurance plan is referred to as a **covered expense**, covered service, or the allowed amount. Services that are specifically excluded by the plan or in excess of UCR fees are not considered to be covered expenses.

PRACTICE **PITFALLS**

EXAMPLE:
Surgery is billed at $500. The plan's UCR amount is $350; therefore, the covered expense would be $350. Any applicable deductible would be taken from the $350 allowed and the remaining amount would be paid at the Major Medical coinsurance percentage. The $150 difference between the submitted amount of $500 and the covered/allowable amount of $350 would be the member's responsibility, for a non-PPO provider.

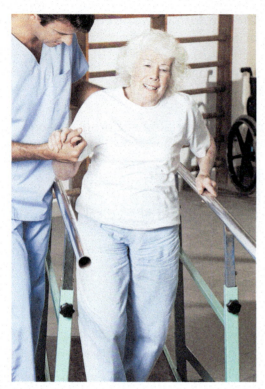

FIGURE 4-1 Expenses incurred for a disability can include obtaining physical therapy
Source: Tyler Olson/Shutterstock

Extended Benefits

Extended benefits are the continued entitlement of a member, under certain circumstances, to receive benefits after the coverage has terminated. Total disability is one reason that benefits may be extended. A doctor's certification of total disability is required before benefits can be extended. Usually, such coverage will continue only for expenses incurred from the condition that caused the disability (see Figure 4-1 ●) and for a maximum of 12 months following the date of disability or the date on which the member is no longer totally disabled, whichever is sooner.

Loss Date

The **loss date** is always the date of the accident or injury. Regardless of the date of service, the loss date remains the same.

Limit(s)

The **maximum** amount payable by the plan applies only to agreed-upon fees between the insurance company and the provider (i.e., managed care programs). As of 2014, annual and/or lifetime maximums are no longer written into insurance policies.

Out-of-Pocket Maximum

A yearly limit on the **out-of-pocket (OOP)** expenses that the insured is responsible for paying. When this limit or **out-of-pocket maximum** is reached, the plan pays subsequent covered expenses at 100% (or another specified percentage) instead of the usual percentage for the remainder of the policy year.

Per Period of Disability

Basic Benefit waiting periods and deductibles are referred to as **per-period disability**; these may be per illness or on a waiting period basis. In the case of per illness, for each new illness or injury a new benefit amount may be applicable or a new waiting period may apply. If there is a time period basis for renewal of the benefit, the patient must wait for a specified time period without receiving treatment for the specific illness or any illnesses. This situation most often applies to medical treatment while the patient is hospitalized or to office visit benefits. This is not a preexisting condition clause, which is no longer allowable under healthcare law.

Unit Value

A numerical value assigned by a relative value study (RVS) to a procedure code is the **unit value**. The unit value is multiplied by the **conversion factor** to determine the UCR allowance or a basic allowance. This may sound confusing, but luckily, the CMS figure these amounts for billers and examiners. The important piece of information here is to know why government-funded medical service fees in different locations vary.

> ▶ **CRITICAL THINKING QUESTION:** Why are the conversion factors based on geographic location? Hint: See www.cms.gov.

Benefit Calculations

Medical billers and claims examiners may need to calculate the items that follow in order to determine the proper benefit. Because not all items are needed on every claim, we will look at each item separately. Use this section as a resource for future work if you are unsure of a calculation. Note: Electronic billing software programs may complete the calculations for you.

When you reach the Medical Claims Administration chapter and the chapters which discuss the various types of claims, you will use these calculations to complete the Payment Worksheet.

Automatic Annual Reinstatement

Sometimes, an insurance policy gives credit for a contractually specified amount of money that may be added to the balance of available lifetime benefits, the **Automatic Annual Reinstatement (AAR)**. In the past, this applied to Major Medical Benefits when lifetime benefits were exhausted. Under the new healthcare laws, it is unclear how insurance companies will apply this principle.

Coinsurance

Coinsurance is calculated by multiplying the amount subject to Major Medical (after all Basic amounts, deductibles, and other benefits have been deducted) by the coinsurance amount that the plan provides. For example, if the amount subject to Major Medical is $120 and the plan pays 80%, the plan's Major Medical payment would be $96.

Out-of-Pocket

To calculate the **out-of-pocket (OOP)** expense, use the remainder not provided by coinsurance. Thus, if the insurance carrier pays 80% of the amount subject to Major Medical, the out-of-pocket amount would be 20% of the amount subject to Major Medical.

Copayment

The copayment is a fixed dollar amount (e.g., $20, $25) that is due to be paid by the insured each time a particular medical service is provided. For example, if the copayment is $25 for each office visit, the patient must provide this amount at each office visit.

Calculating the Deductible

A deductible must be paid by the member before benefits become payable by the plan under the Major Medical portion of the contract. Usually, this is a policy year deductible (which starts over on the policy renewal date year), but sometimes the deductible is calculated on a calendar year. The deductible is always taken out of the first eligible expense(s) submitted each year. The three common types of deductibles are individual, aggregate, and nonaggregate.

Individual Deductible

The individual deductible is only applicable to one insured's medical expenses (see Figure 4-2 ●).

PRACTICE **PITFALLS**

Billy Barton is covered under the Winter Insurance Company contract. The individual deductible amount is $100, and so far Billy has paid $0. Billy submits a claim for $25, of which $25 is considered covered expenses. Because Billy has not satisfied any portion of his individual deductible, the $25 that Billy pays will be applied toward his deductible.

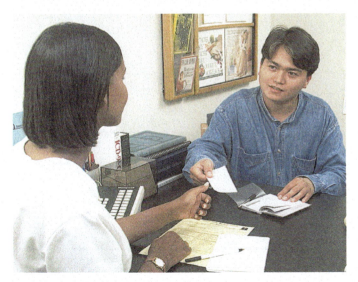

FIGURE 4-2 Patient paying his deductible at time of service
Source: Michal Heron/ Pearson Education/PH College

Aggregate Deductible

Aggregate deductibles are met by the group of people covered under the insurance policy accumulating medical expenses (usually a family). In these cases, large families can save money and not have to meet each individual deductible before they meet the overall deductible.

PRACTICE **PITFALLS**

The Barton Family is covered under the Winter Insurance Company contract and their family deductible is $200, aggregate.

Family Member	Amount of Deductible Satisfied
Billy	$25
Barry	$45
Bobby	$85
Betty	$ 0

Betty now submits a claim for $500 in covered expenses. She only needs to satisfy $45 toward her deductible, because with $45 is all that remains before the family reaches the $200 family deductible. Even though the family members have not met any of their individual limits, the family limit has been satisfied. Therefore, no more deductible will be taken from any family members for this deductible period.

Nonaggregate Deductible

Nonaggregate deductibles require both the individual deductible and the group or family amount to be met before the insurance plan will begin paying on claims.

PRACTICE **PITFALLS**

If the Barton family were covered under the Ball Insurance Carriers contract, the family deductible limit would be two family members satisfying their $125 individual deductibles.

Family Member	Deductible Satisfied
Billy	$25
Barry	$45
Bobby	$85
Betty	$ 0

Betty submits a claim for $500 in services. She must pay the full $125 toward her deductible. Even after she has paid it, the family deductible still has not been satisfied for this deductible period.

If the next claim is submitted by Billy for $75, the full $75 amount would be considered part of the deductible, thus bringing the amount Billy has paid toward his deductible to $100. However, the family deductible for this period still has not been met because only one family member (Betty) has reached the individual limit, and two family members must do so to satisfy the family deductible.

(Continued)

> Only when Billy, Barry, or Bobby has paid $125 toward his individual deductible during this deductible period will the family deductible be met. After the family deductible limit has been met, no more deductible will be taken from any member of the family for this deductible period.

Three-Month Carryover Provision

A **three-month carryover (C/O) provision** states that eligible charges incurred in the last quarter of the policy year (usually October, November, and December) that are applied toward the member's deductible will also carry over toward satisfying the following year's deductible. However, if the plan year is different from the calendar year, the last three months of the plan year will constitute the carryover deductible period. These monies may or may not be applied toward the family limit. (See the terms of the contract.)

PRACTICE **PITFALLS**

The deductible for John is $100 per year. The first claim submitted is $35 for services in June, CCYY, and the full amount is applied toward his CCYY deductible. The second claim submitted for John is for services dated November, CCYY. A $65 deductible was taken on this claim, thus satisfying the CCYY deductible. In addition, since $65 of the deductible was satisfied during the last three months of the CCYY, $65 of CCNY's deductible will also be considered satisfied.

Carryover deductibles reward a person who has been treatment-free for most of the year. If the individual is still paying his or her deductible during the last three months of the year, that individual has remained treatment-free for most of the year. Because deductibles are paid before the insurance carrier pays out any benefits, this means that the insurance carrier has not had to pay out any benefits during the year. The carrier is betting that the insured will not need benefits in the first three months of the next year, which is an additional benefit that can attract customers to the plan.

Common Accident Provision

A **common accident provision** states that only one deductible, under Major Medical, will be taken for all members of a family involved in the same accident (see Figure 4-3 ●). After the one deductible has been taken, remaining deductibles will be waived on all other members for expenses incurred for that accident only.

As a medical biller or health claims examiner, it is important for you to be aware of where each member of a family stands in relation to his or her deductible payments. The individual with the most charges during the year has probably gone the farthest toward meeting his or her deductible. Also, if the insurance carrier has previously made several payments, the deductible has usually (though not always) been satisfied.

If more than one member of a family is being treated, many insurance carriers will take the single deductible from the

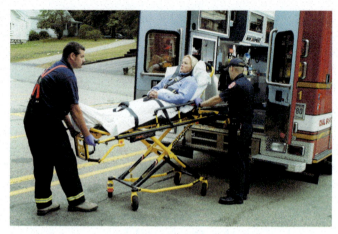

FIGURE 4-3 Based on the common accident provision, only one family involved in the accident must pay his/her deducible
Source: Michal Heron/Pearson Education/PH College

claim that comes in first. If several claims for the family come in at the same time, the insurance company takes the deductible from the patient who owes the most on his or her deductible.

PRACTICE **PITFALLS**

The entire Barton family was involved in an accident and they all visited the doctor on the same day. All claims were received by the insurance carrier at the same time. The family's policy has a common accident provision, a $125 deductible, and the following family deductible accumulations:

Family Member	Deductible Satisfied
Billy	$25
Barry	$45
Bobby	$85
Betty	$ 0

Most insurance carriers would take the full deductible amount from Betty and would then waive the deductible for the other family members.

ACTIVITY #1

Deductible

Directions: Calculate the amount of deductible which will be taken and answer the following questions. Write your answers in the space provided.

The Bear family is covered under the Ball Insurance Carriers. Their coinsurance payments and previous deductible are as follows:

	Brad	Bonnie	Barbara	Brian
Coinsurance paid	0.00	0.00	0.00	0.00
Deductible paid	10.00	0.00	5.00	55.00

1. What is the individual deductible limit on this contract?
   _____

2. What is the family deductible limit on this contract?
   _____

3. Is the family limit aggregate or nonaggregate? _____
   _____

4. How many people are needed to meet the family deductible for this year? _____

5. Bonnie incurs allowed charges of $55. How much will be applied to the deductible? _____

6. How much has Bonnie now met on her deductible?
   _____

7. How many people are now needed to meet the family deductible? _____

8. Brian incurs allowed charges of $85. How much will be applied to the deductible? _____

9. How much has Brian now met on his deductible?
   _____

10. How many people are now needed to meet the family deductible? _____

11. Barbara incurs allowed charges of $105. How much will be applied to the deductible? _____

12. How much has Barbara now met on her deductible?
    _____

13. How many people are now needed to meet the family deductible? _____

14. Brad incurs allowed charges of $60. How much will be applied to the deductible? _____

15. How much has Brad now met on his deductible?
    _____

16. How many people are now needed to meet the family deductible? _____

17. Bonnie incurs allowed charges of $35. How much will be applied to the deductible? _____

18. How much has Bonnie now met on her deductible?
    _____

19. How many people are now needed to meet the family deductible? _____

20. Brian incurs allowed charges of $35. How much will be applied to the deductible? _____

21. How much has Brian now met on his deductible?
    _____

22. How many people are now needed to meet the family deductible? _____

23. Barbara incurs allowed charges of $55. How much will be applied to the deductible? _____

24. How much has Barbara now met on her deductible?
    _____

25. How many people are now needed to meet the family deductible? _____

26. Brad incurs allowed charges of $60. How much will be applied to the deductible? _____

27. How much has Brad now met on his deductible?
    _____

28. How many people are now needed to meet the family deductible? _____

ACTIVITY #2

Calculations

Directions: Calculate the amount of deductible which will be taken and write your answers in the space provided.

The Carpenter family is covered under the Ball Insurance Carriers contract. Their coinsurance and previous deductible payments are as follows:

	Carrie	Connie	Cathy	Chris
C/O paid	0.00	5.00	10.00	55.00
Deductible paid	10.00	0.00	5.00	5.00

1. What is the individual deductible limit on this contract?
   _____

2. What is the family deductible limit on this contract?
   _____

3. Is the family limit aggregate or nonaggregate?
   _____

4. How many people are needed to meet the family deductible? _____

5. Connie incurs allowed charges of $35. How much will be applied to the deductible? _____
   _____

6. How much has Connie now met on her deductible?
   _____

7. How many people are now needed to meet the family deductible? _____

8. Carrie incurs allowed charges of $55. How much will be applied to the deductible? _____
   _____

9. How much has Carrie now met on her deductible?
   _____

10. How many people are now needed to meet the family deductible? _____

11. Chris incurs allowed charges of $60. How much will be applied to the deductible? _____
    _____

12. How much has Chris now met on his deductible?
    _____

13. How many people are now needed to meet the family deductible? _____

14. Chris incurs allowed charges of $35. How much will be applied to the deductible? _____

15. How much has Chris now met on his deductible?
    _____

16. How many people are now needed to meet the family deductible? _____

17. Connie incurs allowed charges of $95. How much will be applied to the deductible? _____

18. How much has Connie now met on her deductible?
    _____

(Continued)

19. How many people are now needed to meet the family deductible? _____

20. Carrie incurs allowed charges of $45. How much will be applied to the deductible? _____

21. How much has Carrie now met on her deductible? _____

22. How many people are now needed to meet the family deductible? _____

23. Cathy incurs allowed charges of $105. How much will be applied to the deductible? _____

24. How much has Cathy now met on her deductible? _____

25. How many people are now needed to meet the family deductible? _____

26. Carrie incurs allowed charges of $85. How much will be applied to the deductible? _____

27. How much has Carrie now met on her deductible? _____

28. How many people are now needed to meet the family deductible? _____

29. Chris incurs allowed charges of $85. How much will be applied to the deductible? _____

30. How much has Chris now met on his deductible? _____

31. How many people are now needed to meet the family deductible? _____

32. Cathy incurs allowed charges of $90. How much will be applied to the deductible? _____

33. How much has Cathy now met on her deductible? _____

34. How many people are now needed to meet the family deductible? _____

2. What is the family deductible limit on this contract? _____

3. Is the family limit aggregate or nonaggregate? _____

4. How much has been paid toward the family deductible? _____

5. Annie incurs allowed charges of $35. How much will be applied to the deductible? _____

6. How much has Annie now met on her deductible? _____

7. How much has now been paid toward the family deductible? _____

8. August incurs allowed charges of $55. How much will be applied to the deductible? _____

9. How much has August now met on his deductible? _____

10. How much has now been paid toward the family deductible? _____

11. April incurs allowed charges of $55. How much will be applied to the deductible? _____

12. How much has April now met on her deductible? _____

13. How much has now been paid toward the family deductible? _____

14. Adam incurs allowed charges of $60. How much will be applied to the deductible? _____

15. How much has Adam now met on his deductible? _____

16. How much has now been paid toward the family deductible? _____

17. Annie incurs allowed charges of $35. How much will be applied to the deductible? _____

18. How much has Annie now met on her deductible? _____

19. How much has now been paid toward the family deductible? _____

ACTIVITY #3

Copayment vs. Deductible

Directions: Calculate the amount of deductible that will be taken and write your answers in the space provided.

The Apple family is covered under the Winter Insurance Company contract. Their coinsurance and previous deductible payments are as follows:

	Annie	Adam	April	August	Ashley
C/O paid	0.00	5.00	10.00	55.00	0.00
Deductible paid	10.00	0.00	5.00	5.00	0.00

1. What is the individual deductible limit on this contract? _____

Basic Benefits

A Basic Benefit provides a specified allowance for a certain type of service. Usually, the allowance is 100% of either UCR charges (as defined by the plan) or some other amount based on the RVS and conversion factors.

A Basic Benefit usually has a stated dollar maximum, number of visits or treatments, or a combination of both for the policy year.

For example, refer to "Surgical" benefits in the Ball Insurance contract in Appendix A. As indicated, this Basic Benefit pays 100% of the UCR allowable expenses. A maximum of $1,600 is payable under the Basic Benefits only per surgery or operative session. Any money charged in excess of either the $1,600 or the allowable amount up to the UCR amount would be covered under Major Medical, subject to any limitations specified by that provision. Basic Benefits are always paid first. It is possible for a single expense to be covered under multiple Basic Benefits. In such a case, the first Basic Benefit would be computed, then any excess would be allowed under any other applicable Basic Benefit, and finally any remaining amount would be considered under Major Medical.

Here are some guidelines for calculating Basic Benefits:

1. Basic Benefits are always paid first, before applicable Major Medical Benefits are calculated.
2. Basic Benefits are usually paid at 100% of the stated amount. Any other applicable percentage must be specifically stated in the policy.
3. Basic Benefits usually have a dollar or number limit.

Under a Basic-only plan, any amount not paid by the Basic Benefit would not be covered at all. These charges would be the patient's responsibility.

Common Basic Benefits

There are several different types of Basic Benefits. The most common are listed here.

Preventative Service Benefits

Since the implementation of the Affordable Care Act in 2010, certain preventative services and/or screenings are mandated to be covered at 100% with no cost to the insured. Some of these services include women's annual screenings for cancer, annual examinations, and lab tests for cholesterol. The list of preventative services mandated changes as medical technology and research recommendations change (see Figure 4-4 ●). For example, if research finds that women who have normal Pap smears for a specific number of years have a lower risk of female organ cancers, the recommended preventative care for such a woman may be a Pap smear every two years, whereas a woman who is high risk for female organ cancers may qualify for a preventative Pap smear every year.

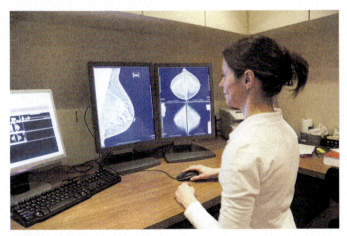

FIGURE 4-4 Preventative service benefits may include obtaining a mammogram on a yearly basis
Source: Juice Images/Fotolia

Accident Benefits

An **accidental injury** is a sudden and unforeseen event that occurred at a definite time and in a specific place. It includes trauma that happened involuntarily or as a result of a voluntary act entailing unforeseen consequences. The following terminology is related to accidental injuries:

AGGRAVATED PHYSIOLOGIC WEAKNESS. This term describes an injury caused when an individual has a physical weakness that is aggravated by some voluntary activity. Overexertion or unusual physical exertion is also considered an accident if there is a specific time and circumstance involved. Do not consider routine bodily movements to be an injury if there is a history of related illness, such as arthritis and chronic strain of the affected area. Strains or sprains resulting from an unknown cause are not considered an accident.

AGGRESSOR ACTS WHILE INTOXICATED. An aggressor may not be considered responsible for his or her actions. Therefore, resulting injuries may be covered under this provision. However, this rule is changing due to tougher intoxication laws and a push toward encouraging responsible drinking.

AGGRESSOR CLAIMS. If someone is the victim of an aggressor, his or her injuries are usually considered accidental. When an investigation does not clearly show who is the aggressor, the determination is usually made in the claimant's favor. As a rule, a person who is the aggressor or who is injured while committing a crime is not usually covered under an accident benefit.

FAMILY ALTERCATIONS. If an insured unintentionally injures a member of his or her family without provocation, the injuries are considered accidental. Cases of this sort need to be investigated to ascertain the facts.

INTERNAL REACTION WITH EXTERNAL TRAUMA. Injury that was incurred as the result of an internal condition (e.g., by falling after fainting; fainting is the internal condition) is considered accidental. There must be an external impact involved in the injury (e.g., falling on the floor; floor is the external impact).

REACTIONS TO EXTERNAL STIMULUS. Unforeseen consequences of voluntary acts, such as reactions to insect bites, allergic reactions to poison ivy or other foliage, food poisoning, and animal bites can be considered accidents.

Benefits under this provision usually pay the first charges submitted up to a specified limit at 100% for all expenses incurred within a specified time period of the date of the accident. Amounts that are over the dollar limit or that relate to injuries incurred after the time limit are likely covered under other plan provisions.

Note: Any complication involved in the treatment of what was originally deemed an "accident" would continue to be part of that accident. This includes reactions to drugs given as a result of the accident (e.g., a patient who was involved in a fall from the roof is given morphine and has an allergic reaction to the morphine).

Nonaccidental Injuries

Injuries received as a result of any of the following situations are usually not considered accidental and are therefore not covered under the accident provision:

- Injuries resulting from willful or reckless actions that are known to result in serious bodily injury, including extremes such as playing Russian roulette, parachute jumping, high-speed auto racing on city streets, and injuries sustained in the commission of a crime.
- Intentionally self-inflicted injuries, such as those sustained during an attempted suicide.

PRACTICE PITFALLS

Holly Hiker (who is covered under the Ball Insurance contract) was hiking along a mountain trail when a snake bit her. She ended up incurring allowable charges of $150 for the ambulance, $125 for the emergency room doctor, $225 for the second doctor, $1,100 in hospital fees, and $250 in lab fees. The total allowable amount is $1,850. Under the XYZ contract, the first $300 of an accident claim is covered at 100%. Therefore, if the bills were submitted in the order shown here, the ambulance charge ($150), the emergency room doctor's charge ($125), and $25 of the second doctor's charge would be paid at 100%. The remaining $200 for the second doctor, $1,100 for the hospital fees, and $250 for the lab fees would be paid under the Major Medical Benefit.

It is important to note that accident benefits usually have a date provision attached. Benefits may be limited to charges incurred within the first 90 days of the accident. Therefore, any treatments that occurred after the 90-day limit would not be allowed under Basic Accident benefits. They would only be paid under Major Medical Benefits.

- Injury sustained as a result of a family quarrel, unless the injured party takes legal action and receives a favorable court decision and it is the injured party who is the insured.
- Sunburn for any person over the age of 16. However, severe sunburn resulting from being stranded (e.g., in a desert) is covered as an accident for a person of any age.
- Any trauma resulting from the normal risks that a person takes when undergoing surgical or medical treatment for an illness. Examples that are included in this category would be experiencing the unintentional severing of a ureter during a hysterectomy, having a clamp or surgical instrument left in the operative field, and having allergic reactions to prescribed medications.
- Injuries sustained in a fight or brawl, if it is determined that the member was the aggressor.
- A "bad trip" as the result of voluntary injection, ingestion, or inhalation of illegal drugs in anyone over 16 years of age. In a person under 16 years of age, the first such experience may be considered accidental.
- Any injury when the patient cannot recall how it happened, with the exception of an obvious injury such as a fracture, burn, or laceration, or an injury to a small child who cannot be expected to remember.

Attempted Suicide

After HIPAA was enacted in 1996, insurance plans were no longer able to withhold payment for injuries incurred as a result of an attempted suicide. They can, however, cover it under only Basic or only Major Medical versus a special Accident insurance.

Diagnostic X-Ray and Laboratory

Benefits for diagnostic X-rays and laboratory (DXL) services can be handled in a variety of ways. In the past, it was not uncommon to have what was called a "scheduled benefit." This type of benefit specified that a set dollar amount was allowed for each test. Today, most Basic Benefit plans provide an alternative type of benefit called an "unscheduled" Basic Benefit, which limits payment under the Basic Benefit to a specified dollar amount per policy year based on UCR or based on a conversion factor and RVS units. After the policy year maximum has been paid, subsequent expenses are paid under the Major Medical Benefit.

If a Basic DXL benefit is provided by the plan, inpatient charges are usually excluded. That is, inpatient expenses are covered only under Major Medical Benefits. However, outpatient hospital claims would allow a Basic Benefit for DXL charges. Therefore, it is important to read the insurance plan before determining benefits. With the advent of electronic billing, it is likely that the computer software provided by the insurance company will determine the amount covered in various circumstances.

PRACTICE PITFALLS

Gen Gym is covered under Basic Benefit and Major Medical contracts. He had lab tests done and the billed and allowed amount is $25. The unit value for the lab tests is .96. The contract pays a Basic Benefit for laboratory charges, at a $7 conversion factor. Thus, the .96 unit value would be multiplied by $7, totaling $6.72. This $6.72 would be paid at the Basic Benefit rate of 100%, and the remaining $18.28 would be paid under Major Medical Benefits.

Hospital Benefits

This Basic Benefit may provide a per admission deductible that does not usually carry over to the Major Medical plan. This benefit usually applies not only to hospital expenses but also to outpatient surgery expenses (see Figure 4-5 ●) and charges incurred as a result of an accident within a specified time period (generally 24 hours).

This type of benefit usually has a dollar limit that is allowed per day for room and board and a separate allowance limit for ancillary expenses. As with other Basic Benefits, the provisions of this type of benefit vary widely from plan to plan.

Medical While Hospitalized

Inpatient hospital care is also called medical while hospitalized (MWH). The patient is admitted into a facility, and the physician visits him or her in the hospital.

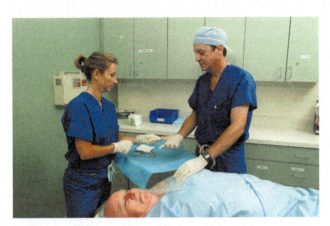

FIGURE 4-5   Hospital benefits can apply to outpatient surgery
Source: Michal Heron/Pearson Education/PH College

CUMULATIVE BENEFIT. Many types of MWH benefits are available. One of the more common types is called a **cumulative benefit**. To calculate benefits under this provision, multiply the number of days hospitalized by the benefit amount.

This amount is the maximum amount of Basic Benefit that can be paid out for this admission, regardless of how many doctors see the patient on a single day or the actual number of visits during the period. Some provisions allow multiple doctors to receive the benefit, but most plans limit the benefit to one, which may be split up and paid to multiple providers as long as it does not exceed the maximum as calculated. For an example of this benefit type, see the Ball Insurance Company contract in Appendix A.

PRACTICE **PITFALLS**

The Ball Insurance contract allows for an inpatient hospital Basic Benefit of room and board up to the semiprivate room charge (a stay in the intensive care unit or ICU is limited to $600 per day). Miscellaneous fees (all other hospital fees) are unlimited, but the Basic Benefit only allows 10 days per period of disability. This amount is also subject to a $50 deductible.

For example, if Emily Emerson was admitted to the hospital for 14 days, the Basic Benefit would pay the cost of her room and board up to the semiprivate room rate for the first 10 days. The additional four days would be paid under Major Medical. Likewise, the miscellaneous fees would be covered for the first 10 days under Basic Benefits and the remaining four days under Major Medical Benefits. Basic Benefits are paid at 100%, and Major Medical Benefits are covered at 80%.

The $50 hospital deductible would apply to the hospital charges. However, the patient would also have to pay the full $125 Major Medical deductible on any Major Medical charges, as the hospital deductible is separate from the Major Medical deductible. In addition, if Emily Emerson was hospitalized again at a later date, she would owe another $50 Basic hospital deductible for the hospital charges because the benefits (and deductible) in this case are per occurrence.

PRACTICE **PITFALLS**

Bobby Brainerd was hospitalized from 3/1/CCYY through 3/14/CCYY. His contract allows a $21 Basic Benefit for the first day of hospitalization and $7 per day thereafter.

The day of admission and the day of discharge are counted in the maximum allowance. To determine the cumulative Basic Benefit; multiply $7 by 13 days, which totals $91. Add this amount to the first day benefit of $21 for a total Basic Benefit payment of $112.

PER-VISIT BENEFIT. A second type of benefit has multiple names, which may include the terms **nondisabling or per-visit benefit**. For this type of benefit, there is a waiting period, a daily maximum, and a calendar year maximum. For example, the provision may indicate, "$10 per day payable after seven days and $200 per calendar year."

Applying this benefit to the same hospitalization scenario provides substantially different results. Count the day of admission and the day of discharge to determine the maximum allowance. Then subtract the seven-day waiting period from the 14 days, and multiply the remaining number of days (seven) by the daily benefit amount of $10 for a total of $70. Usually, this provision allows for the circumstance in which a patient is discharged and then readmitted within a specified period of time, without requiring another seven-day waiting period. It is important to check the plan provisions for this and any other exceptions.

Surgery While Hospitalized

If surgery is performed during the hospitalization, there are many ways to apply an inpatient visit provision, depending on the wording of the benefit and how the services are provided. Here is a summary of some of the more common circumstances. These rules apply to visits performed by the operating surgeon.

1. If surgery is performed, there should not be a charge for a visit on the same day as surgery, excluding diagnostic procedures such as proctosigmoidoscopy and other procedures with no follow-up days.
2. If the surgery has follow-up days listed but the surgery is not performed on the day of admission, the following rules apply:
   - Visits billed before the date of surgery are allowed. Calculate as indicated in the preceding examples, counting the date of admission and every day up to but not including the day of surgery.
   - Visits billed on the day of surgery are combined with the surgery charge. There should not be a separate charge for a visit on the same day of surgery. Allow up to the plan maximum for the surgery.
   - Visits billed on the days after surgery within the follow-up days listed are combined with the surgery charge. Visits billed after the follow-up days can be paid separately.

• If surgery is performed on the first day of admission, all visits occurring within the follow-up days should be combined with the surgery charge. An emergency consultation on the same day as surgery may be an exception to combining the visits with the surgery charge. The regular surgery benefit will be calculated in accordance with the plan provisions.

EXAMPLE:

Araceli Alejandro enters the hospital for treatment of a bone cyst (code 20615) on 3/1/CCYY. Surgery is performed on 3/2 and she is discharged on 3/12. The RVS lists 10 follow-up days for this procedure. Therefore, a physician visit benefit would be allowed on the first day, as surgery was not performed on that day. The visits for the next 10 days would be covered under the surgical charge. The visit for the last day would be paid because it occurred after the 10 follow-up days.

Office Visits

Like the MWH benefit, office visit benefits are usually based on a specified dollar limit per visit after a specified number of visits have been applied to the waiting period (see Figure 4-6 ●). The waiting period is often on a per-illness basis. That is, a specified number of visits are not covered under Basic Benefits for each illness. After the specified number of visits has been accumulated, Basic Benefits begin. The waiting period may be based on the illness, or it may be cumulative for all conditions based on a period of disability.

Surgery, Assistant Surgery, and Anesthesia

For surgery, assistant surgery, and anesthesia, determination of the Basic Benefit uses the RVS and plan-designated conversion factors. The assistant surgeon's allowance is almost always 20% of the surgeon's Basic allowance. Consequently, the conversion factors are the same for the surgeon and the assistant surgeon. The anesthesia benefit may have the same or

a different conversion factor. To get the Basic Benefit for all of these provisions, multiply the conversion factor by the RVS unit value. Usually, there is a maximum amount allowed per operative session and often also for a calendar year. After the member has reached these maximums, these services would be covered only under Major Medical unless excluded under that contract's provisions.

PRACTICE **PITFALLS**

Frank Fryeburger broke his arm while skateboarding. His Ball Insurance contract covers $17 for each visit after three visits. He sees the doctor five times during the treatment of his broken arm. Therefore, his first three visits to the doctor for treatment of the broken arm are not covered under Basic Benefits. However, the last two visits would be covered at $17 per visit under Basic Benefits. All remaining amounts on these visits would be processed under Major Medical.

PRACTICE **PITFALLS**

Terry Tucker had a cholecystectomy (code 47610) on 3/5/CCYY. The surgery involved an anesthesiologist, a surgeon, and an assistant surgeon. Terry's insurance has a unit value for the surgeon of 25.42 and 15.0 for the anesthesiologist.

The basic conversion factor in Terry's insurance policy for surgery is $8.50. Therefore, $216.07 (25.42 × $8.5) is payable under the Basic Benefit for the surgeon. Assistant surgeons are paid at 20% of the surgeon's amount. Therefore, $43.21 ($216.07 × 20%) is payable to the assistant surgeon.

The anesthesia conversion factor is $7.50. Therefore, $112.50 (15 × $7.5) is payable as a Basic Benefit for the anesthesiologist. Terry is responsible for amounts billed that are not covered.

Order of Basic Benefit Payments

To best use the funds available for Basic Benefits, apply benefits in the following order:

1. Hospital benefits
2. Surgery, assistant surgery, and anesthesia benefits
3. Physician's visits (in- or outpatient), including preventative services
4. DXL benefits
5. Supplemental accident benefits

Major Medical Benefits

With a Basic Benefits only plan, expenses not paid by the Basic Benefits would not be payable at all. With a Basic–Major Medical Plan, expenses not paid by the Basic Benefit portion of the contract may be payable under the Major Medical portion. Different limitations or restrictions may apply to Basic

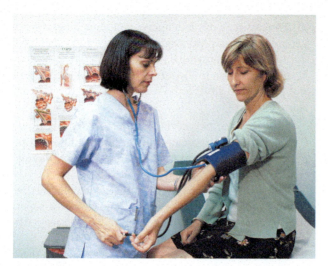

FIGURE 4-6   Office visit benefits are usually based on a specified dollar limit per visit
Source: DJW/Pearson Education/PH College

Benefits than to Major Medical benefits. Generally, the following guidelines apply:

1. Pay all applicable Basic Benefits.
2. Refer to the policy or plan document to see whether the excess amounts not paid under the Basic Benefit plan would be eligible under Major Medical.
3. Apply all Major Medical limitations, deductibles, UCR maximums, and other limitations.
4. Add the Basic Benefit allowance to the Major Medical allowance to determine the total claim payment.

PRACTICE PITFALLS

Assume that Terry Tucker in the previous example was visiting the hospital for the first time this year and has not satisfied any of his deductible. If the surgeon billed $1,500 for the surgery, and the allowed amount was $1,100, this is how the claim would be processed:

Billed amount	$1,500.00
Allowed amount	$1,100.00
Excluded amount	$ 400.00
Basic Benefit amount	$ 216.07
Major Medical amount	$ 883.93
Deductible amount	$ 125.00
Remaining amount	$ 758.93
Major Medical (payment at 80%)	$ 607.14
Payment (Major Medical + Basic)	$ 823.21

Usually, the Major Medical portion has a specified dollar deductible amount that must be satisfied yearly before any payments are made. In addition, expenses under Major Medical are not usually paid at 100%, at least not initially. Normally, payments are calculated at 80%, 70%, and so on (payments can be any percentage).

With a Basic–Major Medical plan, all Basic Benefits will have two limitations (assuming the services are covered under both the Basic Benefit provisions and the Major Medical provisions):

1. The Basic Benefit limitation
2. The Major Medical UCR or plan limitation

This process will become easier to understand as you gain practice billing and/or processing claims.

> ● **ONLINE INFORMATION:** To learn more about Basic Benefits offered by an insurance company, look up Blue Cross/Blue Shield in your area and determine the types of benefits offered by this plan.

Comprehensive Major Medical Benefits

The comprehensive Major Medical plan does not have Basic Benefits per se. However, there may be supplemental or built-in benefits that act the same as a Basic Benefit. In other words, some charges may be covered at 100%, the same as in a Basic Benefit plan. All of the definitions previously covered also apply to this type of plan.

All services would be subject to the Major Medical deductible (unless it is waived for certain types of services). After the deductible was satisfied, services would then be paid at the designated coinsurance rate.

Computing Stop-loss

Many Major Medical contracts have a provision that provides for a greater reimbursement percentage (usually 100%) after payment of a certain dollar amount for a policy year period. This provision limits the amount of money for which the member or patient will be responsible on allowable charges. Such a provision applies only toward "allowable" charges. Expenses that are not allowed under the plan would not be applied toward the stop-loss; these might include UCR excess amounts, noncovered expenses, and sometimes expenses that are not paid at the regular plan benefit level, such as 50% benefits. The patient would remain responsible for payment of these charges. An example of such contract wording would be "80% of the first $5,000, 100% thereafter."

To compute stop-loss:

EXAMPLE 1:

The plan coinsurance rate is 90%.

Stop-loss is $6,000.

Major Medical paid to date for the year is $5,200.

Claim: $2,225 eligible under Major Medical.

Step 1. Subtract the Major Medical amount paid to date for the year from the plan's stop-loss limit.

$$\begin{array}{r} \$6,000 \\ -5,200 \\ \hline \$ 800 \end{array}$$

$800 is 90% of the amount that must be considered by the payer to max the stop-loss for the year.

Step 2. Calculate the amount of which $800 is 90% to determine the amount of eligible charges subject to the coinsurance stop-loss limit. You may do this calculation by dividing the remaining amount by the coinsurance percentage.

$800 divided by .90 = $888.89

$888.89 will be covered at 90% to meet the stop-loss limitation.

Step 3. Subtract the amount covered at 90% ($888.89) from the allowable charges on the claim to determine the amount that will be paid at 100% because the stop-loss limit has been met.

Description	Allowed Amount	Paid at 90%	Paid at 100%
Visit	$ 100	$100.00	0
Lab Tests	$ 125	$125.00	0
Surgery	$2,000	$ 663.89	$1,336.11
Total	$2,225	$ 888.89	$1,336.11

Step 4. Calculate all remaining items normally. However, because the plan's stop-loss has now been met, all subsequent allowable charges will be payable at 100%. (There are some exceptions on some plans.) Some types of expenses, such as nervous and mental, remain at a specific coinsurance rate regardless of whether the coinsurance limit has been met.

EXAMPLE 2:

The plan's coinsurance rate is 80%. Stop-loss is $6,000.

Major Medical paid to date for the year is $5,700.

Claim: $2,000 eligible under Major Medical.

Step 1. Subtract the amount applied to the Major Medical stoploss limit to date.

$$\begin{array}{r} \$6,000 \\ -5,700 \\ \hline \$\ \ 300 \end{array}$$

Step 2. Calculate the amount of which $300 is 80% to determine the amount of eligible charges subject to the coinsurance stop-loss limit. You may do this calculation by dividing the remaining amount by the coinsurance percentage.

$$\$300 \text{ divided by } .80 = \$375$$

$375 will be covered at 80% to
meet the stop-loss limitation.

Step 3. Subtract the amount covered at 80% ($375) from the allowable charges on the claim to determine the amount that will be paid at 100% because the stop-loss limit has been met.

Description	Allowed Amount	Paid at 80%	Paid at 100%
Visit	$ 100	$100	0
Lab Tests	$ 75	$ 75	0
Surgery	$1,825	$200	$1,625
Total	$2,000	$375	$1,625

Step 4. Calculate all remaining items normally. However, since the plan's stoploss has now been met, all subsequent allowable charges will be payable at 100%. (There are some exceptions on some plans.) Some types of expenses, such as nervous and mental, remain at a specific coinsurance rate regardless of whether the coinsurance limit has been met.

EXAMPLE 3:

The plan's coinsurance rate is 70%.

Stop-loss is $5,000.

Major Medical paid to date for the year is $4,000.

Claim: $4,500 eligible under Major Medical. (Total submitted charges: $5,000.)

This is a Basic–Major Medical contract.

Step 1. Subtract the amount applied to the Major Medical stop-loss limit to date.

$$\begin{array}{r} \$5,000 \\ -4,000 \\ \hline \$1,000 \end{array}$$

Step 2. Calculate the amount of which $1,000 is 70% to determine the amount of eligible charges subject to the coinsurance stop-loss limit. You may do this calculation by dividing the remaining amount by the coinsurance percentage.

$$1,000 \text{ divided by } .70 - \$1,428.57$$

$1,428.57 will be covered at 70% to
meet the stop-loss limitation.

Step 3. Subtract the amount covered at 70% ($1,428.57) from the allowable Major Medical charges on the claim to determine the amount that will be paid at 100%, as the stop-loss limit has been met. Remember that Basic Benefits are paid first. Therefore, the amount of the Basic Benefits will be subtracted from the allowed amount to determine the Major Medical amount.

Desc	Allowed Amount	Basic Benefit	Paid at 70%	Paid at 100%
Visit	$ 100	$ 15.65	$ 84.35	0
Lab	$ 500	$110.78	$ 389.02	0
Surgery	$3,900	$232.16	$ 955.20	$2,712.64
Total	$4,500	$358.59	$1,428.57	$2,712.64

Even though the Basic Benefit and the stop-loss benefit are paid at the same amount (100%), they are broken into separate columns on the claim form. This practice allows anyone reviewing the payment worksheet to see the amounts paid under each benefit.

Step 4. Calculate all remaining items normally. However, because the plan's stoploss has now been met, all subsequent allowable charges will be payable at 100%. (There are some exceptions on some plans.) Some types of expenses, such as nervous and mental, remain at a specific coinsurance rate regardless of whether the coinsurance limit has been met.

The amount(s) paid at the coinsurance percentage will be placed in the Maj Med (Major Medical) column (the next-to-last column), and the amount(s) paid at 100% will be placed in the last column.

Usual, Customary, and Reasonable

Benefit plans define covered expenses as charges for the following services and supplies:

- Medically necessary expenses for the treatment or diagnosis of an injury or illness.
- Those expenses that are ordered or prescribed by a licensed provider.
- Those expenses that do not exceed the UCR fee generally charged by like providers in the same geographic area for the same procedure.

At one time, insurance companies covered a straight percentage of whatever the doctor charged. Over time, however, they found that some doctors were charging a much higher amount than other doctors for the same procedure. This was because doctors were setting their fees on the basis of their own perceived needs. For example, a doctor might set his fees according to the personal expenses he had to cover, rather than the actual costs of the procedures. Because of this, fees were increasing at an alarming rate. Eventually, insurance carriers decided to establish a system called Usual, Customary, and Reasonable (UCR) to limit their payments. Insurance carriers limit payment to a specified amount based on the UCR system. The **allowed amount** is what the insurance company considers to be a reasonable charge for the procedure performed, and it is often less than the amount that the doctor bills.

Another factor affecting costs is that costs in one area of the country or **region** are often much less than those in another area of the country. Thus, insurance carriers began compiling data on the usual amounts charged by doctors in different areas. They developed information on the average fees charged for a given service in a given area, and fee schedules (or lists of amounts for each procedure) were developed. The schedules based on geographic location are called the Geographic Practice Cost Index (GPCI).

Several sources compile and publish UCR data. Using this data or compiling their own data, third-party administrators and insurance carriers determine the **UCR calculation** or allowances for their plans or clients. Amounts in excess of UCR are not considered to be an allowable expense under the plan and are therefore excluded from all benefit calculations.

UCR is usually applicable only to professional services or to hospital billings that give CPT®/RVS codes. Not all procedures have a UCR fee. For instance, new procedures, experimental procedures, and very unusual and complex procedures may not have an established UCR amount. UCR can be established only when enough procedures of a particular type have been performed in a geographic area to allow an "average" or "usual" amount to be determined. Usually, a minimum of 50 operations is required to provide even a rough estimate of the amount that should be considered as usual.

Resource-Based Relative Value Studies

At one time, providers were paid not only on the basis of the procedure performed, but also according to the degree or title of the provider. For example, an M.D. and a D.C. would receive different amounts for performing the same procedure.

OBRA 90-Public Law 101-608 of 1987 brought major changes for physician payment. One change was the implementation of a fee schedule for physician payment. This fee schedule is based on relative value units that reflect the resources required to provide a service. The fee schedule is based on national uniform relative values for all physicians without respect to area of specialization. (See Table 4-1 ● for

TABLE 4-1 2012 CMS RVUs for Physician Fee Schedules

DATA RECORD			
HCPCS Code	1-5	X(5)	CPT or Level 2 HCPCS number for the service. NOTE: See copyright statement on cover sheet.
Modifier	6-7	X(2)	For diagnostic tests, a blank in this field denotes the global service and the following modifiers identify the components:
			—26 = Professional component
			—TC = Technical component
			—For services other than those with a professional and/or technical component, a blank will appear in this field with one exception: the presence of CPT modifier -53 indicates that separate RVUs and a fee schedule amount have been established for procedures which the physician terminated before completion. This modifier is used only with colonoscopy CPT code 45378, or with G0105 and G0121. Any other codes billed with modifier -53 are subject to carrier medical review and priced by individual consideration.
			—53 = Discontinued Procedure - Under certain circumstances, the physician may elect to terminate a surgical or diagnostic procedure. Due to extenuating circumstances, or those that threaten the well being of the patient, it may be necessary to indicate that a surgical or diagnostic procedure was started but discontinued.
Description	8-57	X(50)	
Status Code	58-58	X(1)	Indicates whether the code is in the fee schedule and whether it is separately payable if the service is covered. See Attachment A for description of values. Only RVUs associated with status codes of "A", "R", or "T", are used for Medicare payment.
Work RVU	60-65	999.99	Relative Value Unit (RVU) for the physician work in the service as published in the Federal Register Fee Schedule for Physicians Services for CY 2012.
Transitioned Non-Facility Practice Expense RVU	67-72	999.99	Relative Value Unit (RVU) for the transitioned resource-based practice expense for the non-facility setting, as published in the Federal Register Fee Schedule for Physicians Services for CY 2012.

(Continued)

TABLE 4-1 *(Continued)*

Transitioned Non-Facility NA Indicator	73-74	X(2)	An "NA" in this field indicates that this procedure is rarely or never performed in the non-facility setting.
Fully Implemented Non-Facility Practice Expense RVU	76-81	999.99	Relative Value Unit (RVU) for the fully-implemented resource-based practice expense for the non-facility setting, as published in the Federal Register Fee Schedule for Physicians Services for CY 2012.
Fully Implemented Non Facility NA Indicator	82-83	X(2)	An "NA" in this field indicates that this procedure is rarely or never performed in the non-facility setting.
Transitioned Facility Practice Expense RVU	85-90	999.99	Relative Value Unit (RVU) for the transitioned resource-based practice expense for the facility setting, as published in the Federal Register Fee Schedule for Physicians Services for CY 2012.
Transitioned Facility NA Indicator	91-92	X(2)	An "NA" in this field indicates that this procedure is rarely or never performed in the facility setting or is not paid under the Physician Fee Schedule in the facility setting.
Fully Implemented Facility Practice Expense RVU	94-99	999.99	Relative Value Unit (RVU) for the fully implemented resource-based practice expense for the facility setting, as published in the Federal Register Fee Schedule for Physicians Services for CY 2012.
Fully Implemented Facility NA Indicator	101-102	X(2)	An "NA" in this field indicates that this procedure is rarely or never performed in the facility setting.
Malpractice RVU	104-108	99.99	RVU for the malpractice expense for the service as published in the Federal Register Fee Schedule for Physicians' Services for CY 2012.
Total Transitioned Non-Facility RVUs	110-115	999.99	Sum of work, transitioned non-facility practice expense, and malpractice expense RVUs.
Filler	116-116	X(1)	
Total Fully Implemented Non-Facility RVUs	117-122	999.99	Sum of work, fully implemented non-facility practice expense, and malpractice expense RVUs.
Total Transitioned Facility RVUs	124-129	999.99	Sum of work, transitioned facility practice expense, and malpractice RVUs.
Total Fully Implemented Facility RVUs	131-136	999.99	Sum of work, fully implemented facility practice expense, and malpractice RVUs.
PC/TC Indicator	139-139	x(1)	See Attachment A for description of values.
Global Surgery	140-142	XXX	Provides time frames that apply to each surgical procedure. 000=Endoscopic or minor procedure with related preoperative and postoperative relative values on the day of the procedure only included in the fee schedule payment amount; evaluation and management services on the day of the procedure generally not payable. 010=Minor procedure with preoperative relative values on the day of the procedure and postoperative relative values during a 10 day postoperative period included in the fee schedule amount; evaluation and management services on the day of the procedure and during the 10-day postoperative period generally not payable. 090=Major surgery with a 1-day preoperative period and 90-day postoperative period included in the fee schedule amount. MMM=Maternity codes; usual global period does not apply. XXX=The global concept does not apply to the code. YYY=The carrier is to determine whether the global concept applies and establishes postoperative period, if appropriate, at time of pricing. ZZZ=The code is related to another service and is always included in the global period of the other service.
Preoperative Percentage	143-145	.99	Percentage for preoperative portion of global package.
Intraoperative Percentage	146-148	.99	Percentage for intraoperative portion of global package, including postoperative work in the hospital.
Postoperative Percentage	149-151	.99	Percentage for postoperative portion of global package that is provided in the office after discharge from the hospital.
Multiple Procedure (Modifier 51)	152-152	x(1)	Indicates applicable payment adjustment rule for multiple procedures: 0=No payment adjustment rules for multiple procedures apply. If procedure is reported on the same day as another procedure, base the payment on the lower of (a) the actual charge, or (b) the fee schedule amount for the procedure.

TABLE 4-1 (*Continued*)

			1=Standard payment adjustment rules in effect before January 1, 1995 for multiple procedures apply. In the 1995 file, this indicator only applies to codes with a status code of "D". If procedure is reported on the same day as another procedure that has an indicator of 1, 2, or 3, rank the procedures by fee schedule amount and apply the appropriate reduction to this code (100%, 50%, 25%, 25%, 25%, and by report). Base the payment on the lower of (a) the actual charge, or (b) the fee schedule amount reduced by the appropriate percentage.
			2=Standard payment adjustment rules for multiple procedures apply. If procedure is reported on the same day as another procedure with an indicator of 1, 2, or 3, rank the procedures by fee schedule amount and apply the appropriate reduction to this code (100%, 50%, 50%, 50%, 50% and by report). Base the payment on the lower of (a) the actual charge, or (b) the fee schedule amount reduced by the appropriate percentage.
			3=Special rules for multiple endoscopic procedures apply if procedure is billed with another endoscopy in the same family (i.e., another endoscopy that has the same base procedure). The base procedure for each code with this indicator is identified in the Endobase field of this file. Apply the multiple endoscopy rules to a family before ranking the family with the other procedures performed on the same day (for example, if multiple endoscopies in the same family are reported on the same day as endoscopies in another family or on the same day as a non-endoscopic procedure). If an endoscopic procedure is reported with only its base procedure, do not pay separately for the base procedure. Payment for the base procedure is included in the payment for the other endoscopy.
			4=Special rules for the technical component (TC) of diagnostic imaging procedures apply if procedure is billed with another diagnostic imaging procedure in the same family (per the diagnostic imaging family indicator, below). If procedure is reported in the same session on the same day as another procedure with the same family indicator, rank the procedures by fee schedule amount for the TC. Pay 100% for the highest priced procedure, and 50% for each subsequent procedure. Base the payment for subsequent procedures on the lower of (a) the actual charge, or (b) the fee schedule amount reduced by the appropriate percentage. The professional component (PC) is paid at 100% for all procedures.
			5=Subject to 20% of the practice expense component for certain therapy services (25% reduction for services rendered in an institutional setting - effective for services January 1, 2012 and after).
			9=Concept does not apply.
Bilateral Surgery (Modifier 50)	153-153	x(1)	Indicates services subject to payment adjustment.
			0=150% payment adjustment for bilateral procedures does not apply. If procedure is reported with modifier -50 or with modifiers RT and LT, base the payment for the two sides on the lower of: (a) the totat actual charge for both sides or (b) 100% of the fee schedule amount for a single code. Example: The fee schedule amount for code XXXXX is $125. The physician reports code XXXXX-LT with an actual charge of $100 and XXXXX-RT with an actual charge of $100. Payment should be based on the fee schedule amount ($125) since it is lower than the total actual charges for the left and right sides ($200). The bilateral adjustment is inappropriate for codes in this category (a) because of physiology or anatomy, or (b) because the code description specifically states that it is a unilateral procedure and there is an existing code for the bilateral procedure.
			1=150% payment adjustment for bilateral procedures applies. If the code is billed with the bilateral modifier or is reported twice on the same day by any other means (e.g., with RT and LT modifiers, or with a 2 in the units field), base the payment for these codes when reported as bilateral procedures on the lower of: (a) the total actual charge for both sides or (b) 150% of the fee schedule amount for a single code. If the code is reported as a bilateral procedure and is reported with other procedure codes on the same day, apply the bilateral adjustment before applying any multiple procedure rules.

(*Continued*)

TABLE 4-1 (*Continued*)

			2=150% payment adjustment does not apply. RVUs are already based on the procedure being performed as a bilateral procedure. If the procedure is reported with modifier -50 or is reported twice on the same day by any other means (e.g., with RT and LT modifiers or with a 2 in the units field), base the payment for both sides on the lower of (a) the total actual charge by the physician for both sides, or (b) 100% of the fee schedule for a single code. Example: The fee schedule amount for code YYYYY is $125. The physician reports code YYYYY-LT with an actual charge of $100 and YYYYY-RT with an actual charge of $100. Payment should be based on the fee schedule amount ($125) since it is lower than the total actual charges for the left and right sides ($200). The RVUs are based on a bilateral procedure because (a) the code descriptor specifically states that the procedure is bilateral, (b) the code descriptor states that the procedure may be performed either unilaterally or bilaterally, or (c) the procedure is usually performed as a bilateral procedure.
			3=The usual payment adjustment for bilateral procedures does not apply. If the procedure is reported with modifier -50 or is reported for both sides on the same day by any other means (e.g., with RT and LT modifiers or with a 2 in the units field), base the payment for each side or organ or site of a paired organ on the lower of (a) the actual charge for each side or (b) 100% of the fee schedule amount for each side. If the procedure is reported as a bilateral procedure and with other procedure codes on the same day, determine the fee schedule amount for a bilateral procedure before applying any multiple procedure rules. Services in this category are generally radiology procedures or other diagnostic tests which are not subject to the special payment rules for other bilateral surgeries.
			9=Concept does not apply.
Assistant at Surgery	154-154	x(1)	Indicates services where an assistant at surgery is never paid for per Medicare Claims Manual.
			0=Payment restriction for assistants at surgery applies to this procedure unless supporting documentation is submitted to establish medical necessity.
			1 =Statutory payment restriction for assistants at surgery applies to this procedure. Assistant at surgery may not be paid.
			2=Payment restriction for assistants at surgery does not apply to this procedure. Assistant at surgery may be paid.
			9=Concept does not apply.
Co-surgeons (Modifier 62)	155-155	x(1)	Indicates services for which two surgeons, each in a different specialty, may be paid.
			0=Co-surgeons not permitted for this procedure.
			1 =Co-surgeons could be paid, though supporting documentation is required to establish the medical necessity of two surgeons for the procedure.
			2=Co-surgeons permitted and no documentation required if the two-specialty requirement is met.
			9=Concept does not apply.
Team Surgery (Modifier 66)	156-156	x(1)	Indicates services for which team surgeons may be paid. 0=Team surgeons not permitted for this procedure. 1=Team surgeons could be paid, though supporting documentation required to establish medical necessity of a team; pay by report. 2=Team surgeons permitted; pay by report. 9=Concept does not apply.
Filler	157-157	x(1)	
Filler	158-158	x(1)	This field used to contain the Billable Medical Supplies indicator. Under resource based practice expense, all billable medical supplies have been incorporated into the practice expense relative values of individual services.
Filler	59-163	x(5)	
Endoscopic Base Code	164-168	X(5)	Code which identifies an endoscopic base code for each code with a multiple surgery indicator of 3.
Conversion Factor	169-176	999.9999	This is the multiplier that transforms relative values into payment amounts. This conversion factor reflects the MEI update adjustment. For 2002 and beyond, there is a single conversion factor for all services.

TABLE 4-1 (*Continued*)

Physician Supervision Diagnostic Proceduresof	178-179	X(2)	This field is for use in post payment review. 1 = Procedure must be performed under the general supervision of a physician. 2 = Procedure must be performed under the direct supervision of a physician. 3 = Procedure must be performed under the personal supervision of physician. 4 = Physician supervision policy does not apply when procedure is furnished by a qualified, independent psychologist or a clinical psychologist; otherwise must be performed under the general supervision of a physician. 5 = Physician supervision policy does not apply when procedure is furnished by a qualified audiologist; otherwise must be performed under the general supervision of a physician. 06 = Procedure must be performed by a physician or a physical therapist (PT) who is certified by the American Board of Physical Therapy Specialties (ABPTS) as a qualified electrophysiological clinical specialist and is permitted to provide the procedure under State law. 21 = Procedure may be performed by a technician with certification under general supervision of a physician; otherwise must be performed under direct supervision of a physician. 22 = May be performed by a technician with on-line real-time contact with physician. 66 = May be performed by a physician or by a physical therapist with ABPTS certification and certification in this specific procedure. 6A= Supervision standards for level 66 apply; in addition, the PT with ABPTS certification may supervise another PT, but only the PT with ABPTS certification may bill. 77 = Procedure must be performed by a PT with ABPTS certification or by a PT without certification under direct supervision of a physician, or by a technician with certification under general supervision of a physician. 7A = Supervision standards for level 77 apply; in addition, the PT with ABPTS certification may supervise another PT, but only the PT with ABPTS certification may bill. 09 = Concept does not apply.
Calculation Flag	180-180	X(1)	A Value of "1" indicates that an adjustment of 1.03 should be applied to the 2012 fee schedule amount ** NOTE WITH THE MARCH 1, 2012 RELEASE: THE EXTENDERS** ** PROVISION FOR THE MENTAL HEALTH ADD-ON WAS** ** DISCONTINUED IN THE MIDDLE CLASS TAX RELIEF AND** ** JOB CREATION ACT OF 2012. A VALUE OF "2" IS NO LONGER** ** BEING UTILIZED IN THE CALCULATION FLAG FIELD.** A Value of "3" indicates that an adjustment of 0.98 should be applied to the 2011 fee schedule amount for the following codes 98940, 98941, and 98942.
Diagnostic Imaging Family Indicator	182-183	X(2)	This field identifies the applicable diagnostic serrvice family for that HCPCS codes with a multiple procedure indicator of '4'.*For services effective January 1, 2011 and after, family indicators 01-11 will not be populated.* The values are: 01 =Ultrasound (Chest/Abdomen/Pelvis-Non-Obstetrical) 02=CT and CTA (Chest/Thorax/Abd/Pelvis) 03=CT and CTA (Head/Brain/Orbit/Maxillofacial/Neck) 04=MRI and MRA (Chest/Abd/Pelvis) 05=MRI and MRA (Head/Brain/Neck) 06=MRI and MRA (Spine) 07=CT (Spine) 08=MRI and MRA (Lower Extremities) 09=CT and CTA (Lower Extremities) 10=MR and MRI (Upper Extremities and Joints) 11=CT and CTA (Upper Extremities) 88 = Subject to the reduction of the TC diagnostic imaging (effective for services January 1, 2011 and after). 99=Concept does not apply

(*Continued*)

TABLE 4-1 *(Continued)*

Non-Facility Practice Expense Used for OPPS Payment Amount	188-193	999.99	The OPPS Payment Amount calculated using these values is compared to the Medicare Physician Fee Schedule to determine appicability of the OPPS Imaging Cap mandated by Section 5102(b) of the Deficit Reduction Act of 2005.
Facility Practice Expense Used for OPPS Payment Amount	195-200	999.99	The OPPS Payment Amount calculated using these values is compared to the Medicare Physician Fee Schedule to determine appicability of the OPPS Imaging Cap mandated by Section 5102(b) of the Deficit Reduction Act of 2005.
Malpractice Used for OPPS Payment Amount	202-207	999.99	The OPPS Payment Amount calculated using these values is compared to the Medicare Physician Fee Schedule to determine appicability of the OPPS Imaging Cap mandated by Section 5102(b) of the Deficit Reduction Act of 2005.

the 2012 Relative Value Units that were used to create the physician fee schedule published by the CMS.)

The **Relative Value Units (RVUs)** represent the total RVS for components of the schedule, which is revised every five years. Components for practice expenses are resource-based and include the following costs:

- **Direct Costs:** Determined by the Physicians Practice Information Survey (PPIS), direct costs include Physician Work RVUs (recommended by an American Medical Association committee), Practice Expenses (PE RVUs), and Malpractice costs (MP RVUs).
- **Indirect Costs:** These costs are calculated by supplementary survey data for hourly data.

Practice expense RVUs are further broken down by facility and nonfacility setting.

- **Facility Practice Setting:** inpatient or outpatient hospital, emergency room, skilled nursing facility, or ambulatory care center.
- **Nonfacility Practice Setting**—any other practice setting.

Geographical Practice Cost Index

GPCI is the determined fee usually charged by similar providers for the same procedure in the same geographic area during a specified period of time (these are often referred to as conversion factors). Table 4-2 ● shows the 2012 Surgery Fees by locality.

TABLE 4-2 2012 CMS Geographic Process Cost Index

Contractor	Locality	Locality name	2012	2012	2012
10102	00	Alabama	1.000	0.878	0.474
02101	01	Alaska**	1.500	1.067	0.661
03102	00	Arizona	1.000	0.978	1.015
00520	13	Arkansas	1.000	0.865	0.450
01192	26	Anaheim/SA	1.044	1.218	0.676
01192	18	Los Angeles, CA	1.036	1.154	0.642
01102	03	Marin/Napa/Sola	1.051	1.248	0.456
01102	07	Oakland/Berk	1.058	1.254	0.516
01102	99	Rest of California*	1.024	1.085	0.547
01192	99	Rest of California*	1.024	1.085	0.547
01102	05	San Francisco, CA	1.072	1.360	0.516
01102	06	San Mateo, CA	1.072	1.354	0.516
01102	09	Santa Clara, CA	1.077	1.337	0.516
01192	17	Ventura, CA	1.034	1.193	0.605
04102	01	Colorado	1.000	1.004	0.872
13102	00	Connecticut	1.024	1.110	1.235
12202	01	DC + MD/VA Subs	1.049	1.198	1.130
12102	01	Delaware	1.012	1.044	0.672
09102	03	Fort Lauderdale	1.000	1.051	1.982
09102	04	Miami, FL	1.000	1.054	2.815
09102	99	Rest of Florida	1.000	0.968	1.553
10202	01	Atlanta, GA	1.002	1.015	0.949
10202	99	Rest of Georgia	1.000	0.898	0.928
01202	01	Hawaii/Guam	1.000	1.154	0.700

TABLE 4-2 (*Continued*)

Contractor	Locality	Locality name	2012	2012	2012
02202	00	Idaho	1.000	0.894	0.603
00952	16	Chicago, IL	1.030	1.051	2.077
00952	12	East St. Louis, IL	1.000	0.936	1.934
00952	99	Rest of Illinois	1.000	0.909	1.336
00952	15	Suburban Chicago, IL	1.025	1.072	1.706
00630	00	Indiana	1.000	0.923	0.613
05102	00	Iowa	1.000	0.887	0.456
05202	00	Kansas	1.000	0.894	0.957
15102	00	Kentucky	1.000	0.871	0.752
00528	01	New Orleans, LA	1.000	0.976	0.921
00528	99	Rest of Louisiana	1.000	0.877	0.744
14102	99	Rest of Maine	1.000	0.904	0.676
14102	03	Southern Maine	1.000	1.024	0.676
12302	01	Baltimore/Surr.	1.027	1.097	1.206
12302	99	Rest of Maryland	1.011	1.035	0.987
14202	01	Metropolitan Boston	1.014	1.149	0.790
14202	99	Rest of Massachusetts	1.013	1.062	0.790
00953	01	Detroit, MI	1.022	1.023	1.814
00953	99	Rest of Michigan	1.000	0.923	1.069
00954	00	Minnesota	1.000	1.012	0.282
00512	00	Mississippi	1.000	0.866	0.761
05302	02	Metropolitan KC	1.000	0.953	1.233
05302	01	Metropolitan St Louis	1.000	0.964	1.064
05302	99	Rest of Missouri	1.000	0.851	1.023
03202	01	Montana ***	1.000	1.000	1.103
05402	00	Nebraska	1.000	0.904	0.322
01302	00	Nevada ***	1.000	1.058	1.232
14302	40	New Hampshire	1.000	1.044	0.860
12402	01	Northern NJ	1.044	1.186	1.045
12402	99	Rest of New Jersey	1.021	1.126	1.045
04202	05	New Mexico	1.000	0.916	0.997
13202	01	Manhattan, NY	1.062	1.162	1.271
13202	02	NYC Suburbs/Long I.	1.049	1.212	1.441
13202	03	Poughkpsie/N NYC	1.011	1.065	1.081
13292	04	Queens, NY	1.062	1.195	1.491
13282	99	Rest of New York	1.000	0.939	0.562
11502	00	North Carolina	1.000	0.927	0.695
03302	01	North Dakota ***	1.000	1.000	0.517
15202	00	Ohio	1.000	0.927	1.240
04302	00	Oklahoma	1.000	0.856	0.734
02302	01	Portland, OR	1.005	1.044	0.625
02302	99	Rest of Oregon	1.000	0.962	0.625
12502	01	Metropolitan PA	1.014	1.059	1.624
12502	99	Rest of Pennsylvania	1.000	0.913	1.123
09202	20	Puerto Rico	1.000	0.678	0.249
14402	01	Rhode Island	1.017	1.052	1.187
11202	01	South Carolina	1.000	0.909	0.520
03402	02	South Dakota***	1.000	1.000	0.432
10302	35	Tennessee	1.000	0.898	0.523

(*Continued*)

TABLE 4-2 *(Continued)*

Contractor	Locality	Locality name	2012	2012	2012
04402	31	Austin, TX	1.000	1.009	0.751
04402	20	Beaumont, TX	1.000	0.896	0.923
04402	09	Brazoria, TX	1.009	0.987	0.923
04402	11	Dallas, TX	1.009	1.017	0.834
04402	28	Fort Worth, TX	1.000	0.979	0.826
04402	15	Galveston, TX	1.009	0.996	0.985
04402	18	Houston, TX	1.009	1.002	0.923
04402	99	Rest of Texas	1.000	0.912	0.809
03502	09	Utah	1.000	0.916	1.102
14502	50	Vermont	1.000	1.008	0.554
09202	50	Virgin Islands	1.000	1.002	1.010
11302	00	Virginia	1.000	0.977	0.731
02402	99	Rest of WA	1.000	1.012	0.861
02402	02	Seattle, WA	1.025	1.144	0.881
11402	16	West Virginia	1.000	0.828	1.229
00951	00	Wisconsin	1.000	0.960	0.547
03602	21	Wyoming ***	1.000	1.000	1.233

ACTIVITY #4

Physician Fees for Surgery

Directions: Using the Surgery Physicians Fee Scale (see Table 4-2), list the payable amount for these codes in the indicated carrier locality.

Carrier Locality	Code 10022	Code 11056	Code 11471
1. 00740			
2. 00528			
3. 31143			
4. 00523			
5. 00805			
6. 00522			
7. 00910			
8. 00831			
9. 31146			
10. 00824			

Formulas for Determining Physician Fees

The Federal Register publishes the RVUs that allow the claims administrator to determine the allowable fees for the services provided.

> ● **ONLINE INFORMATION:** There are many conversion factors that affect the calculation of physician fees. Look up the current Federal Register and review the various conversion factors for your locality.

The 2012 *Nonfacility* Pricing Amount is calculated by multiplying the Work RVU by the Work GPCI, added to the Transitioned Nonfacility PE RVU, multiplied by the PE GPCI, added to the MP RVU, multiplied by the MP GPCI. This amount is then multiplied by the conversion factor to get the end result.

The 2012 *Facility* Pricing Amount is calculated by multiplying the Work RVU by the Work GPCI, added to the Transitioned Facility PE RVU, multiplied by the PE GPCI, added to the MP RVU, multiplied by the MP GPCI. This amount is then multiplied by the conversion factor to get the end result.

ACTIVITY #5

Physician Fee Schedule

Directions: Answer the following questions after reviewing the material covered previously. Write your answers in the space provided.

1. What does PE RVU mean? _____
   _____
   _____

2. On what is PE RVU based? _____
   _____
   _____

3. Explain why a geographical conversion factor is used for calculating the physician fee. _____
   _____
   _____

4. What other conversion factors are currently being used?
   _____
   _____

Amounts higher than the Major Medical physician fee allowance are not considered covered by the plan. The physician fee amount or the lesser amount (if the amount is lower than the UCR amount) is applied toward all of the plan limitations, including the deductible and coinsurance. The amounts not covered by the plan are the patient's sole responsibility.

Normally, if the provider's charge exceeds the physician fee allowance by more than 20% or 25%, a Peer Review (by a consultant) may be required.

ACTIVITY #6

UCR Conversions

Directions: Using the conversion factor for ZIP code 90820, calculate the UCR amounts for the following procedures.

Code	Description	Factor	Units	Amount
1. 15952	Excision Trochanteric Pressure Ulcer			
2. 93000	Electrocardiogram			
3. 27372	Removal of Foreign Body, Deep, Thigh			
4. 78811	Tumor Imaging			
5. 70250	Radiologic Exam, Skull			
6. 19125	Excision of Breast Lesion			
7. 36430	Transfusion, Blood			
8. 87040	Culture, Bacterial; Blood			
9. 40808	Biopsy, Vestibule of Mouth			
10. 20205	Biopsy, Muscle, Deep			

ACTIVITY #7

More UCR Conversions

Directions: Using ZIP code 36810, determine the physician fee for the following procedure codes.

Code	Description	Factor	Units	Amount
1. 15952	Excision Trochanteric Pressure Ulcer			
2. 93000	Electrocardiogram			

Code	Description	Factor	Units	Amount
3. 27372	Removal of Foreign Body, Deep, Thigh			
4. 78810	Tumor Imaging			
5. 70250	Radiologic Exam, Skull			
6. 19125	Excision of Breast Lesion			
7. 36430	Transfusion, Blood			
8. 87040	Culture, Bacterial; Blood			
9. 40808	Biopsy, Vestibule of Mouth			
10. 20205	Biopsy, Muscle, Deep			

Modifiers

Special rules govern the use of a modifier in coding. For example, if a patient receives two radiology tests in the same setting on the same day, a -59 modifier would be used to indicate that the second procedure was a distinct, separate, medically necessary procedure. The multiple imaging procedures would need clarification in order to administer payment on the claim. Continuing updates to the Federal Register show these clarifications (found at www.cms.gov). For this reason, it is important to stay up to date on the CMS guidance regarding physician fee allowances.

Fee Schedules

Some plans have established their own calculations of the amount payable for particular services. These amounts are listed on what is commonly called a **fee schedule** (see Table 4-3 ●). Fees are assigned according to the particular CPT code, and this is considered the allowable amount for that particular procedure.

If a fee schedule is used, the medical biller or health claims examiner looks up the appropriate code to obtain the allowed amount. This practice eliminates the need for numerous calculations and can speed up the process of claims examining. However, the compensation using these schedules are not the same in a large city as in outlying areas.

Cost Containment Programs

Until the tremendous growth in healthcare costs triggered the need for new approaches, plan sponsors had been primarily concerned with improving employees' access to quality medical care. As a result of the increased healthcare costs of the last 40 years, many employers have been struggling to provide adequate care for their employees at an affordable cost.

TABLE 4-3 Example Insurance Plan Fee Schedule

Common Illness	Our Charge	*Average Estimate Payment from Insurance
Allerigies (seasonal)	$108.00	$70.00
Bladder Infection	$108.00	$70.00
Bronchitis	$108.00	$70.00
Ear Infections	$108.00	$70.00
Flu Diagnosis (ages 10 through 65)	$108.00	$70.00
Rashes	$108.00	$70.00
Minor Skin Infections	$108.00	$70.00
Pink Eye and Styes	$108.00	$70.00
Sinus Infection	$108.00	$70.00
Strep Throat	$108.00	$70.00
Vaccines		
Chicken Pox	$97.00	$63.00
Dtap (Diptheria,Tetnus, Pertussis)	$64.00	$42.00
Hepatitis A	$138.00	$90.00
Hepatitis B	$147.00	$96.00
Hep B & Hib	$88.00	$57.00
Hib	$35.00	$23.00
Influenza	$33.00	$21.00
Polio	$62.00	$40.00
Meningitis	$130.00	$85.00
MMR (Mumps, Measles Rubella)	$76.00	$49.00
Pneumonia	$52.00	$34.00
Mantoux	$33.00	$21.00
Tetnus (adult)	$45.00	$29.00

Because of this problem, a variety of programs have been developed to slow down the rate of increase in both the premiums and the cost of healthcare.

Some of the more popular methods used in trying to slow down spiraling healthcare costs include the following:

- Preadmission Testing (PAT)
- Precertification of Inpatient Admissions
- Utilization Review (UR)
- Second Surgical Opinion Consultation (SSO)
- PPOs
- HMOs

Here are two other cost containment programs:

Preauthorization—A number of insurance carriers require that certain benefits be preauthorized before the services are received. Preauthorization means to gain approval of the services that are to be performed, as well as to find out whether the insurance carrier will cover these services.

Predetermination—This term is an estimate of maximum benefits that may be paid under the plan for the services. It is not, however, a guarantee that benefits will be paid.

Preadmission Testing

Preadmission testing (PAT) was designed to reduce the duration of elective hospital confinements. This benefit is appropriate for scheduled, nonemergency hospital admissions that require the standard prerequisite testing before surgery. As a rule, this type of testing is restricted to a period of three to seven days before admission. In addition, some plans limit the place of testing to either the hospital where the surgery is performed or the patient's regular provider of services (see Figure 4-7 ●).

No payments under PAT are made for preadmission tests that are performed during the hospitalization or those results that are rejected by the physician as unreliable. As preadmission testing generally serves to reduce costs, most plans offer an incentive to the member to use PAT by paying these charges at a higher coinsurance level than regular testing or hospital-related services.

EXAMPLE:

Outpatient diagnostic tests performed prior to inpatient admission were paid at 100%, regardless of whether they were conducted by a network provider.

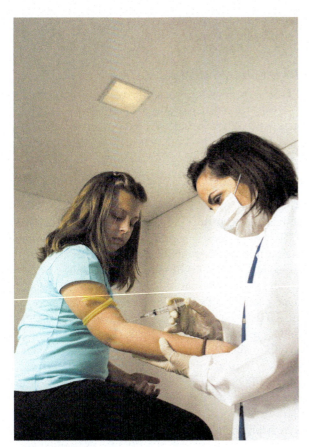

FIGURE 4-7   Preadmission testing (PAT) was designed to reduce the duration of elective hospital confinements
Source: Orange Line Media/Shutterstock

Precertification of Inpatient Admissions

Precertification means preapproval for admission on an elective, nonemergency hospitalization. The member should contact either the plan administrator or some other entity sanctioned to determine the necessity of the admission. Most often, these entities are composed of a specialized group of nurses working under the direction of a physician. The nurses deal directly with the physician's office and the facility to determine whether the admission is necessary and whether the number of days of care is medically necessary. If the patient stays longer than the approved number of days, the additional days of care may not be covered, or the usual payment may be reduced by a percentage specified in the plan document. The objective of this program is to prevent unnecessary hospital admissions and to get the patient out of the hospital as soon as it is medically appropriate.

Some programs provide for precertification only prior to or on the day of hospitalization. Other programs provide for a complete approach to managing the care, which entails a utilization review program.

As part of HIPAA, the federal government has mandated that no precertification can be required on maternity confinements. The law stipulates that a confinement for a normal delivery cannot be limited to less than 48 hours (two days) or in the case of a cesarean section 96 hours (four days). The law, however, does not state that a concurrent review cannot be required. Therefore, if the patient stays hospital-confined beyond the two days for a normal delivery or four days for a cesarean section, and the plan has concurrent review and extended stay provisions, applicable penalties can be imposed on those extra days.

Utilization Review

As previously indicated, precertification or a prospective review determines the need for and appropriateness of the recommended care. **Utilization review (UR)** is a process whereby insurance carriers review the total treatment of a patient and determine whether the costs will be covered. A complete UR program contains the following three components:

1. Precertification (prior to) or prospective review.
2. Concurrent review (during the confinement).
3. Retrospective review (after termination of confinement).

CONCURRENT REVIEW. A **concurrent review** determines whether the estimated length of time and scope of the inpatient stay are justified by the diagnosis and symptoms. This review is conducted periodically during the projected length of stay. If the length of stay exceeds the criteria or if there is a change in treatment, the matter is referred to the medical consultant for review. This consultant at no time dictates the method of treatment or the length of stay. Such decisions are left entirely to the patient and the attending physician. However, the consultant is entitled to inform the patient, physician, and facility that the continued stay exceeds the approved number of days and may not be covered by the plan as medically necessary. It is then the patient's responsibility to decide what action to take.

RETROSPECTIVE REVIEW. A **retrospective review** is used to determine after discharge whether the hospitalization and treatment were medically necessary and covered by the terms of the benefit program. This type of review may be used as a substitute for admission and concurrent reviews when the failure to notify the UR program of an admission prevents the regular review procedures. The main drawback to the retrospective review is that the patient and providers are not notified about the services that will not be covered until after they have been provided. It is more effective to notify the patient beforehand that he or she will be primarily responsible for payment of services. This approach deters the member from incurring unanticipated expenses.

Second Surgical Opinion Consultations

Surgical claims represent the second highest categorical cost to benefit plans, after hospitalization. The United States has the world's highest rate of surgical treatment because neither the physician nor the patient has any financial incentive to consider less expensive alternatives.

About 80% of all surgeries can be considered "elective." That is, they are not required because of a life-threatening situation. The objective of a Second Surgical Opinion Consultation (SSO) is to eliminate elective surgical procedures that are classified as unnecessary.

UNNECESSARY SURGERY. Unnecessary surgery is recommended as an elective procedure when an alternative method of treatment may be preferable for a number of reasons, including the following:

- The surgery itself may be premature, taking into consideration all pathologic indications.
- The risk to the patient may not justify the benefits of surgery.
- An alternative medical treatment may be superior for both medical and cost-effective reasons.
- A less severe or no surgical procedure may be preferable under the circumstances.

In an SSO, the plan participant consults an independent specialist to determine whether the recommended elective surgical procedure is advisable. This process is not intended to interfere with the patient–physician relationship or to prevent the participant from receiving necessary elective operations. This program may be administered in one of two ways:

1. A **mandatory program** requires the patient to obtain an SSO for specific procedures or face an automatic reduction or denial of benefits. For an example of this type of program, see the Ninja Enterprises contract in Appendix A.
2. A **voluntary program** encourages participants to have an SSO, but there is no automatic reduction of benefits if the patient does not comply.

In both approaches, the SSO and related tests are usually paid at 100% so that the patient will not have any out-of-pocket expenses for conforming to the program.

The SSO program has met with much criticism because it has not effectively reduced the number of elective surgeries. One of the main reasons for this ineffectiveness is that physicians may be reluctant to tell a patient that a surgery is not necessary. This attitude stems from the growing number of malpractice lawsuits. For example, if a physician indicates that a patient does not need surgery and a sudden emergency situation arises that is related to the original need for surgery, the physician may be held liable under a malpractice suit. Consequently, many plans are abandoning the SSO plan provision.

Managed Care

Managed care is a strategy for reducing or controlling healthcare costs by closely monitoring and restricting the use and cost of services. Using this system, the insurer manages the delivery of healthcare and controls costs by emphasizing primary and preventive care services. Managed care plans use quality assurance and utilization review to ensure the appropriate delivery of care. PPOs, HMOs, and POS plans are examples of managed care plans. An **in-network provider** is a physician or other service provider who is contracted with a managed care plan. An **out-of-network provider** is a healthcare provider with whom the specified managed care organization does not have a contract to provide healthcare services.

Preferred Provider Organizations

A PPO is a group of healthcare providers who agree to provide services to a specific pool of patients for an agreed fee (contractual). PPOs include doctors, dentists, hospitals, and any provider group that contracts with another entity to provide services at competitive fees.

PPO packages may involve contractual agreements for a limited number of healthcare services or for a full range of inpatient and outpatient medical services. Because the PPO group has agreed to specific benefits, they usually have their own UR committees or guidelines to reduce the amount of testing performed, hospitalizations, and other services.

In some cases, a health plan may continue to offer standard indemnity coverage but may also offer special PPO arrangements in which the PPO provider is paid more quickly and at a higher rate than non-PPO providers. In such a case, the plan participant saves money because out-of-pocket expenses are also reduced. The Summer Insurance contract in Appendix A is an example of a PPO contract.

Many PPO providers are available. The benefits of a PPO provider over a non-PPO provider vary greatly from plan to plan. However, generally both the patient and the plan reduce costs by being members of a good PPO.

Some of the advantages of a PPO for the patient are

- Reduced healthcare costs with no restriction (or with only minimal restrictions) of freedom of choice of providers. Reduced healthcare costs mean reduced out-of-pocket expenses.
- Less paperwork in filing claims because the PPO submits the claim directly to the payer and payment is made directly to the PPO.
- Treatment only for services that are medically necessary because there is usually a formal UR program.

Some of the advantages of a PPO to the provider are

- Increased patient volume.
- Prompt claim payment.
- Reduced financial risk due to automatic assignment of benefits.
- Active participation in local cost-containment efforts.

Some of the advantages of a PPO to the benefit plan are

- Reduced healthcare cost.
- Better utilization control.

Health Maintenance Organizations

An HMO is a type of prepayment policy in which the organization bears the responsibility and financial risk of providing agreed-on healthcare services to the members enrolled in its plan, in exchange for a fixed monthly membership fee. This fee can be paid by the member, or it can be paid on members' behalf by their employer or government-sponsored plan.

If services are available through the HMO but the insured does not go through the HMO provider, either the benefit will be reduced or the member will be entirely responsible for the payment of care received. Any services provided outside the HMO network must be preapproved for coverage by the HMO. If services are not approved, the HMO usually will not pay the charges.

The main difference between a PPO and an HMO is that an HMO provider receives a monthly fee based on capitation (number of covered plan members), whereas a PPO provider is paid only when a member is treated. A disadvantage of the HMO arrangement is the limitation of the patient's freedom of choice of physicians. In addition, the location of the HMO facilities may be limited or inconvenient for many plan members.

Exclusive Provider Organizations

In the **Exclusive Provider Organization (EPO)**, the patient must select a primary care provider and can only use physicians who are part of the network or who are referred by the primary care physician. EPO physicians are paid as services are rendered, after which they receive a capitation or utilization bonus from the carrier.

Gatekeeper PPO

In the **Gatekeeper PPO** scenario, the member chooses a family provider or physician and must see him or her before being referred to a specialist. The specialist may or may not be within the network. In essence, the family physician is the "gatekeeper" to specialized services and can choose to refer the patient or not.

Physician Hospital Organizations

A **Physician Hospital Organization (PHO)** is an organization of physicians and hospitals that bands together for the purpose of obtaining contracts from payer organizations. The PHO bargains as an entity for preferred provider status with various payers. The organization also refers clients to one another.

Management Service Organizations

A **Management Service Organization (MSO)** is a separate corporation set up to provide management services to a medical group for a fee. Individual physicians and providers contract with the MSO for services. An MSO may be owned by a single hospital, several hospitals, or investors.

Medical Case Management

Medical Case Management (MCM) is the process of evaluating the effectiveness and frequency of medical treatments by reviewing services to determine whether the care that is being rendered or that is going to be rendered is appropriate. When a situation arises in which the potential for high claims payment exists, due to the diagnosis or the type of services needed by the claimant, the case is generally referred to the MCM Department. In some instances, an outside company performs this function. The MCM reviews these cases and tries to minimize the company's loss by finding alternative solutions for patient care. Solutions may involve providing the patient with equipment or care that is normally not covered under the plan if it is more cost-effective for the plan and also beneficial to the patient to make these provisions. MCM usually focuses on high-dollar claims involving inpatient hospital confinements. It explores less costly alternatives, such as hospice, nursing home, and home healthcare with discounted nursing or equipment.

An important goal of MCM is to save costs for the insured, the patient, the plan, the healthcare providers, and the administrator. This process also can result in higher quality care.

Under most plans, MCM is a voluntary process. To be successful, it is important to have the cooperation of the patient and family.

Situations that may indicate possible claims for MCM are included in Appendix C. The health claims examiner should watch carefully for the following factors that may indicate that a claim file is a good candidate for MCM:

1. Pattern of repeated hospital admissions (or two admissions within six months)
2. Outpatient therapies of more than six weeks (including nursing services)
3. Home care by an RN of more than four hours per day
4. Skilled nursing care in an extended care facility of more than six weeks
5. Any hospital interim bill (reflecting an excessive length of stay)
6. Any terminal or progressive disease requiring long-term skilled care (see Figure 4-8 ●).

Use experience and common sense to identify claims that are unusual and that may become "catastrophic" by virtue of chronicity or immediately high cost.

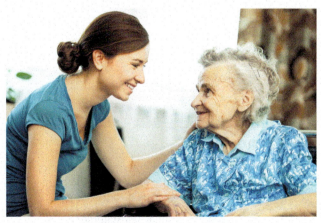

FIGURE 4-8   A good candidate for MCM is an individual receiving care in an extended care facility
Source: Alexander Raths/Fotolia

CHAPTER REVIEW

Summary

- The three major types of indemnity coverage currently available are
  1. Basic Benefit
  2. Basic–Major Medical
  3. Comprehensive Major Medical.
- It is important to understand the terminology associated with contracts and to know how benefit payments are calculated under each type of coverage.
- Quick and accurate benefit payments make a health claims examiner a valuable employee.
- The concept of UCR charges allows a payer to determine allowable charges on the basis of what is considered to be a usual and reasonable charge for a given service performed in a given area.
- This practice prevents the paying of excessive benefits to doctors who may charge high fees on their bills.
- Physician fee schedules allow insurance carriers to pay higher rates in areas where there is a higher cost of doing business (e.g., building costs, personnel) and lower rates in areas in which there is a lower cost of doing business.
- The cost of healthcare coverage in general has increased over the past decade.
- Cost containment provisions are likely to continue for the survival of the health insurance industry.

Review Questions

Directions: Answer the following questions after reviewing the material just covered. Write your answers in the space provided.

1. Name the three major types of coverage which are currently available.

   a. _____

   b. _____

   c. _____

2. _____ are the expenses that are covered under the plan.

3. True or False: Expenses not paid by the Basic Benefit portion of the contract may be payable under the Major Medical portion. _____

4. Define accumulation period. _____

   _____

5. Define Automatic Annual Reinstatement. _____

   _____

6. Explain the three-month carryover provision. _____

   _____

7. _____ means to get preapproval for an admission on an elective, nonemergency hospitalization.

8. List the two ways that second surgical opinion programs may be administered.

   a. _____

   b. _____

If you were unable to answer any of these questions, refer back to that section and then fill in the answers.

ACTIVITY #8

Matching

Directions: Match the following terms with the proper definition by writing the letter of the correct definition in the space next to the term.

1. _____ Automatic Annual Reinstatement
2. _____ Common Accident Provision
3. _____ Exclusive Provider Organization
4. _____ Health Maintenance Organization
5. _____ Management Service Organization
6. _____ Medical Case Management
7. _____ Nondisabling or Per-Visit Benefit
8. _____ Out-of-Network
9. _____ Physician Hospital Organization
10. _____ Preferred Provider Organization
11. _____ Relative Value Units
12. _____ Three-Month Carryover Provision
13. _____ Usual, Customary, and Reasonable

a. Eligible charges incurred in the last quarter of the calendar year and applied toward the member's deductible will also count toward the following year's deductible.

b. A healthcare provider with whom a managed care organization does not have a contract to provide healthcare services.

c. Insurance carriers limit payment to a specified amount using this system.

d. This type of benefit features a waiting period, a daily maximum, and a calendar year maximum.

e. Represent the total RVS for components of the schedule.

f. A group of healthcare providers who agree to provide services to a specific pool of patients for an agreed fee.

g. An organization of physicians and hospitals that bands together for the purpose of obtaining contracts from payer organizations.

h. A corporation set up to provide management services to a medical group for a fee.

i. A type of prepayment policy in which the organization bears the responsibility and financial risk of providing agreed-on healthcare services to the members enrolled in its plan, in exchange for a fixed monthly membership fee.

j. The process of evaluating the effectiveness and frequency of medical treatments by reviewing services to determine whether the care that is being rendered or that is going to be rendered is appropriate.

k. A contractually specified amount of money that may be added to the balance of available lifetime benefits.

l. The patient selects a primary care physician and can use only physicians who are part of the network and who are referred by the primary care physician.

m. A provision whereby only one deductible is taken for all members of a family involved in the same accident.

CHAPTER 5
Medical Claims Administration

CHAPTER 6
Physician's, Clinical, and Hospital Services Claims

CHAPTER 7
Surgery and Anesthesia Claims

CHAPTER 8
Medicare and Medicaid

CHAPTER 9
Workers' Compensation

CHAPTER 10
Managed Care Claims

Medical Claims Administration

Keywords and concepts you will learn in this chapter:

Adjustment

Allowable Expense

Assignment of Benefits

Batch Files

Claim Determination Period

Claim Files

Claim Investigation

Claim Processing

Coordination of Benefits (COB)

Credit Reserve (CR)

Documentation

Electronic Claims

Electronic Claims Submission

Explanation of Benefits (EOB)

Family Financial Files

Full-Credit Adjustment

Global COB

Group Plan

Insurance Coordination of Benefits

Member Files

Normal Liability (NL)

Order of Benefit Determination (OBD) Rules

Overinsurance

Partial-Credit Adjustment

After completing this chapter, you will be able to:

- Describe the way claim files are organized.

- List the rules for proper documentation in claim files.

- Explain the process of claims investigation.

- Identify claims that require referral from the PCP or to technical examiner specialists.

- Define pending claims.

- Describe the steps taken in performing a claims analysis.

- Discuss the practice of unbundling.

- Identify the use of separate procedure codes.

- Identify the major guidelines for claims processing.

- Properly process a claim using a payment worksheet.

- Explain the parts of a payment worksheet.

- Discuss the quick reference formulas used to help process a payment worksheet.

Patient Protection and Affordable
Care Act of 2010
Pended Claims
Primary Plan
Rebundling
Referral
Secondary Plan
Statistical Adjustment
Supplemental Adjustment
Unbundling

▌ Recognize tracking forms used by the medical biller or claims examiner.

▌ Explain the criteria used to determine whether a prescribed medication is covered by insurance.

▌ Properly process a drug or prescription claim using a payment worksheet.

▌ Explain the purpose of coordination of benefits (COB).

● Define terms related to COB.

▌ Properly determine primary, secondary, and tertiary payers, using the order of benefit determination rules (OBD).

▌ Recognize when a request or release of information is required.

▌ Explain the guidelines as related to the right of recovery.

▌ Determine COB benefits as they apply to HMO plans.

▌ Determine COB benefits as they apply to PPO plans.

● Discuss TRICARE coverage.

▌ Review how to determine the presence of dual coverage.

● Explain the various types of adjustments.

The job duties of medical billers and claims examiners include a wide variety of administrative duties to ensure proper handling of claims. In this chapter, we will cover the importance of verifying coverage and eligibility, how to accurately document in the claim file, and how to handle investigation, referrals, and approval of claims. Company guidelines vary from payer to payer, so review company guidelines when you are making claim submission and/or status determinations.

Maintenance of Claim Files

The electronic medical billing software will likely keep track of claims sent to insurance companies for payment. However, it may be necessary for you to group claims into files on the computer by date or insurance provider. The database capabilities are endless in the electronic world, so it is important to become familiar with the capabilities of the software being used.

On the insurance company side of claim files, the computer keeps track of claims received, approved, denied and/or sent back for more information. The software assigns a claim number and indicates the date and time that the claim was received.

The date and time are important because this information is used to keep claims received in chronological order. The claims that were received first are processed first. After the claim has been received, it is routed to the claims examiner for handling.

Claim files or batches in the provider office contain the information indicating which claims have been submitted, which ones have been returned to insurance companies with supplemental information, and which have been denied. The insurance company organizes the claims into similar files or batches that contain groups of submitted claims, processed claims, claims requiring further information, and denied claims. Some providers and payers print summaries of electronic data interchange each day or keep some type of hard copy as a checks-and-balances system for information sent and received.

Tracking Family Claims

Because deductibles may be aggregate in a family situation, in these situations there may be special handling or oversight to ensure that the claims are properly billed for appropriate amounts. Generally, the insurance company does the figuring and sends back to the provider an explanation of benefits (EOB). It is important for you, as a medical biller, to understand this process so that you can answer questions from patients about billing.

Insurance claims examiners have the responsibility to ensure that families are billed appropriately according to their deductible status.

Member Files

Each patient will have an electronic file at the provider office or facility. Likewise, the insurance company will have **member files** for those who are insured. Depending on the software capabilities, there will be an individual financial file or a **family financial file**. If hard copy correspondence is received, the information is entered or scanned into the appropriate computer file or hard copy file, according to company policy.

Batch Files

Batch files are groups of claims that are categorized for the convenience of the biller or examiner, whichever is the case (see Figure 5-1 ●).

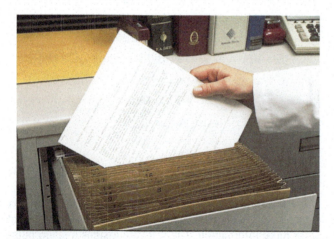

FIGURE 5-1 Keep claims in order by claim number
Source: Michal Heron/Pearson Education/PH College

When electronic billing methods are used, batches are searchable, so it is easy to refer back to earlier activity on the claim.

ACTIVITY #1

Claim File Maintenance

Name the three ways that a claim file is maintained.

1. _____
2. _____
3. _____

▶ **CRITICAL THINKING QUESTION:** What has been your experience at a provider office or in gaining information from a claims representative? Has it been simple or difficult to obtain information? Write a reflection about your most recent experience with billing or claims personnel.

Documentation to Substantiate a Claim

Documentation is the substance of a claim. Claims should be orderly and should contain important facts that furnish decisive evidence to support claims billing or processing. Most computer software systems will have a place for documenting in the claim file pertinent conversations with patients, providers, or insurance representatives. If more information is needed before the claim can be processed, the claims examiner should indicate the disposition of the claim in the notes. It is the responsibility of the medical biller or claims examiner to document the information requested and the date of the request. In addition, the date that a follow-up letter is required (in the event that the information is not received within a certain amount of time) should also be included in the documentation.

This documentation enables work to be done on a claim at a future date. You may not be the person who follows up on the claim or receives the information requested, so be sure that the documentation is understandable and that it provides concise, informative, and pertinent information. Proper documentation should have the following attributes:

1. *Professional.* Keep personal remarks out of documentation. Keep your information objective. Do not bold, highlight or otherwise mark any sections, passages, or words of a narrative report or claim form. As innocent as it may seem, a judge, jury, or plaintiff's attorney may see such markings as singling out a patient, acting in bad faith, or being discriminatory and arbitrary.
2. *Evidence based.* The representations made in documentation must not only be fair and reasonable but must also create a file that shows fairness, reasonableness, and factual accuracy when it is read by a jury. Correctly record the basis for all coding or claims decisions. Double check to ensure that your documentation is objective and your decisions are correct.
3. *Language.* Words or phrases may be taken out of context and used to give a bad connotation to your documentation.

Be particularly aware of words that may have a double meaning, especially if they are taken out of context. Some programs have built-in checklists that help the biller or examiner use specific approved language.

4. *Communication with an Attorney.* If you are communicating with an attorney who is representing the claimant, give only initial, factual information. If the attorney requests further information concerning the extent and nature of the factual information provided, discuss your response with a member of your company's legal department or a supervisor before responding. All information or printouts of documents provided should be clearly documented in the file.

Some companies retain specialists to handle attorney-posed claim questions. In such instances, the case should be referred directly to the specialist. Nothing should be said or sent to the attorney regarding the case unless you are directed

to do so by the authorized specialist. Because the handling of these claims differs significantly from company to company, always request clarification on the handling of such claims before taking any action. The following guidelines deal with communications about a claim:

1. *Be thorough.* All information regarding a claim should be documented in the database or electronic practice management program. This includes phone conversations, which should be summarized in the file. You can use a Telephone Information Sheet to record these communications and enter them after each phone call. (See Figure 5-2 ● for a sample of a Telephone Information Sheet.)

2. *Be conscientious.* Information furnished by a doctor or provider with regard to a claim may be privileged. When a patient requests medical information from the biller or examiner, advise him or her to speak to the provider directly.

ANY INSURANCE CARRIER, INC.
123 Any Drive
Anywhere, USA 12345
(800) 555-1234

TELEPHONE INFORMATION SHEET

Date: _____

Claim Identification: _____

Person making inquiry: _____
Person supplying information: _____
Telephone Number: _____
Briefly state information received or desired: _____

Indicate additional handling, if any: _____

This form, when completed should be placed in the claim file.

FIGURE 5-2 Telephone Information Sheet

Claims Investigations

Claims investigations can be accomplished on the provider side or the insurance side. A provider may investigate a claim to inquire about the status of a claim, track down a lost or denied claim, or proceed with obtaining payment on the claim.

When an insurance claims examiner investigates a claim, it is likely due to a question regarding validity of a claim for payment. Reasons for investigation may also include suspected fraud, injuries that are not clearly defined as nonwork related or nonautomobile related, and Coordination of Benefits (COB).

When you make a request for information, be specific about the type of information required. Ask questions that require a statement, rather than a yes or no answer. Avoid sending multiple requests for different information to the same provider or member. Request all information at once so that you will have all the necessary information to review the claim. Attach an Authorization to Release Information to your request.

Referrals

The term **referral** is different for the medical biller and the claims examiner. The medical biller ensures that required referrals from PCPs were obtained before the service was provided. Meanwhile, a claims examiner will verify such a referral was made (if required), but the term referral is also used when the claim is referred to a technical specialist for review.

Medical Billing Referrals

As discussed in the contracts chapter, a patient may need preauthorization or a referral before he or she can be treated. The medical biller must be aware of the insurance contracts that require preauthorizations or referrals. If the medical biller cannot find the required referral or preauthorization, he or she must seek a duplicate copy from the PCP. Billing without the referral or preauthorization could result in denial of the claim.

Claims Examiner Referrals

Upon receipt of a claim, the examiner first verifies that the referral or preauthorization was obtained as required by the insurance contract. When reviewing claims in general, the claims examiner may find that the claim decision is beyond his or her expertise or authorization. When this occurs, the examiner should refer the claim to a technical specialist: a lead examiner, supervisor, medical review person, or consultant (see Figure 5-3 ●). This referral process ensures that there is a consistent approach to unusual situations and maintains an avenue of communication to higher levels for cases with sensitive issues. The following types of claims normally are referred to more technical personnel:

1. *Lawsuits, legal actions, or legislative issues.* Examples include an attorney letter demanding payment or making reference to insurance law, a summons, a Notice of Complaint, or other lawsuit notification correspondence.

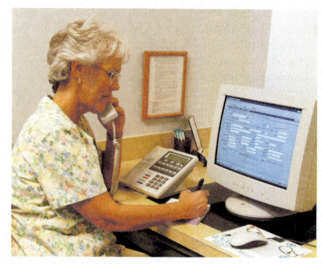

FIGURE 5-3 Medical professional obtaining information on a claim
Source: Michal Heron/Pearson Education/PH College

2. *Flagged providers.* Flagged providers have been identified as questionable; therefore, special handling is required. Providers may be flagged for having questionable billing practices, overusing certain benefits (e.g., chiropractic services, biofeedback), being new providers who are pending state approval to perform qualified services (e.g., surgi-center), or other issues.
3. *Fraud.* If a claim has indications of fraud and is pending for verification, it should be referred to a specialist. (For more information on fraud see Chapter 1.

When claims fit these situations, the medical biller or examiner should complete a referral form and rout it (via email or other company system) to the appropriate department. It is important that copies of all documents, letters, and forms be routed with the referred claim. Figure 5-4 ● is an example of a claim referral form.

Pending Claims

Pended claims are on hold awaiting further information. These claims may require follow-up investigation so that correct and prompt liability decisions can be made to comply with legislative or regulatory requirements for fair claims handling.

When you are requesting information for a claim, request all the information you need to complete the processing of the claim to ensure that additional delays do not occur. Send a letter notifying the claimant and the provider that additional information is needed before the claim can be processed. Many companies use a standard form letter requesting further information. Figures 5-5 ● and 5-6 ● are examples of standard request forms.

The first follow-up date is scheduled three to four weeks after the original request. If the requested information has not been received within the scheduled follow-up period, send a second notice letter with follow-up scheduled for three to four weeks. If the requested information is not received within 60 days of the second notice, it may be necessary to close the

---

Claim Office Referral Sheet

To   From   Date

Policy #   Soc. Sec. #   Employee's Name   Dependent's Name

Eff. Date   Term. Date   Patient's Age   Provider of Service

Reason for Referral:

_____
_____
_____
_____
_____
_____

Attachments:

( ) □ Denial/□ Attorney Letters ( ) Preop Photos   ( ) □ Policy/□ Booklet Page
( ) Special Correspondence   ( ) Op/Anesthesia/Path Report ( ) Billings
( ) □ Hospital/ □ Dr. Records   ( ) X-rays   ( ) Other:
                                                            _____

Please make sure that all materials referenced in any appeal letter (insured/provider/attorney) are enclosed with this file.

Reply:

_____
_____
_____
_____
_____

_____   _____
      Signature   Date

ANY INSURANCE CARRIER, INC.

FIGURE 5-4   Claim Referral Form

claim. Send a final letter advising the claimant and the provider that because the information requested has not been received, the claim is being closed. Indicate that if the requested information is received within a reasonable length of time, you will reconsider the claim. If the company has a statute of limitations on filing a claim, indicate this information as well in the letter.

Claim Processing

All healthcare claims are submitted electronically to insurance carriers. These claims are called **electronic claims**. **Electronic claims submission** is a process whereby insurance claims are submitted via an Electronic Data Interchange (EDI) directly from the provider to the insurance company.

The Administrative Simplification and Compliance Act of 2001 (ASCA) required Medicare claims to be submitted electronically, beginning in January 2012. The Health Information Technology for Economic and Clinical Health Act of 2009 (HITECH) also requires healthcare claims to be submitted electronically for standardization of the insurance billing process (see Figure 5-7 ●).

Claims submitted electronically usually contain fewer errors because they eliminate the need for data entry personnel to reenter the information, and payment is generated more quickly. In addition, by using electronic claims, insurance carriers reduce their management and overhead costs.

From the provider end, electronic claims submissions are performed on a routine basis. The medical biller reviews the claims that are ready to submit and sends them to the insurance

ANY INSURANCE CARRIER, INC.
123 Any Drive
Anywhere, USA 12345
(800) 555-1234

Control No.: _____

Name: _____

Please refer to the paragraph checked below.

☐ Careful attention is being given to this claim. We will write you further about it in a short time.

☐ As you requested, we are returning the _____

_____

☐ Please let us know whether this claimant has returned to work and if so, when _____ If not, does total disability still exist? _____ Will proofs of claim be submitted? _____ Information as to the claimant's present condition will be appreciated.

☐ Please have the _____ statement completed and return the attached form to us.

☐ Consideration of further benefits can be given only after we receive the _____

_____

_____

_____

_____

☐ The attached furnished our first knowledge of this claim. Will you please arrange for submission of the required proofs of claim if this is properly covered under our insurance.

FIGURE 5-5   Request For Additional Information Letter

company via the insurance company portal (via an EDI). Because electronic claims submission does not allow the opportunity for the physician to sign the claims, a physician's signature on the agreement with the insurance company is accepted in lieu of a signature on the claim form. It is imperative to also have the patient's signature on an Authorization to Release Information form and an Assignment of Benefits form in the patient file. In both of these cases, indicate on the claim form signature lines "authorized signature on file."

From the insurance company end, **claim processing** is a process of determining benefit amounts and paying, pending, or denying a claim. In passage that follows, we will discuss coverage and guidelines for processing claims. These guidelines are generalized, and company guidelines will always supersede the guidelines discussed here. Use these guidelines when processing the claims activities described in this text.

> ● **ONLINE INFORMATION:** Conduct an online search for the HITECH Act. Review the four categories of privacy and security violations. Hint: see www.cms.gov.

Claim Analysis

A good medical biller or claims examiner has a thorough systematic process for reviewing claims for appropriateness. He or she uses the same process for each claim, regardless of the claim's complexity. This is how consistency and accuracy are maintained. To develop this type of system, first identify the issues involved in the claim. Follow these steps to identify the issues:

1. Confirm eligibility:
   a. Has the policy lapsed for nonpayment of premiums?
   b. At the time of service, was the patient enrolled under the plan?

ANY INSURANCE CARRIER, INC.
123 Any Drive
Anywhere, USA 12345
(800) 555-1234

Request Form
□ Medical □ Dental

Please return requested information to: _____

□ **First Request**   □ **Second Request**   □ **Third and Final Request**

Insured: _____   Date: _____

Patient: _____

**BEFORE WE CAN PROCESS YOUR CLAIM, WE NEED THE ADDITIONAL
INFORMATION CHECKED BELOW:**

□ Please complete in full the member portion of the claim form. Dental (employee section).

□ Itemized Statements from: _____
_____

□ Copies of other Insurance Payments from: _____
_____

□ Full-time Student Eligibility Form Request: Please have the Registrar of the College or
University that _____ attends complete the attached Student Eligibility
Form for the _____ Semester/Quarter.

□ Other: _____

□ THE FOLLOWING EXPENSES WILL BE HELD UNTIL THE ABOVE REQUESTED
ITEMS ARE RECEIVED IN THIS OFFICE _____

□ We have attempted on _____ to obtain the above necessary information to
properly process your claim. As of this date, it has not been received. The file will **now** be
considered **closed** until the information is received and proper evaluation can be given
to your claim.

Thank you,

FIGURE 5-6   Request For Additional Information Letter

c. If the patient is a dependent, is the patient within the allowable age limit?

d. Have all eligibility requirements set forth in the policy been met?

e. Was any material misrepresentation made in the original application for coverage (for insurance company analysis only)?

2. Check for possible other coverage:

a. Is an injury involved? If so, do you have the date, place, and circumstances of the injury on file?

b. Is there evidence of other insurance? Could TPL be involved?

c. Is the injury work-related? If so, has a Workers' Compensation claim been filed?

d. Does the patient have other insurance that might cover these services?

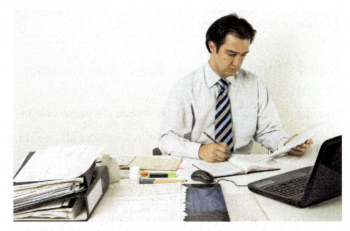

FIGURE 5-7   Reviewing patient for proper submission is the responsibility of health care providers
Source: mim/Fotolia

3. Examine the policy or plan language:

   a. What is the definition in the policy or plan of total disability?

   b. What is the contract definition of accident and sickness?

   c. What plan provisions could apply to this claim? What plan limitations and maximums could apply to the claim? (Be aware of the current annual and lifetime limits as set forth by the **Patient Protection and Affordable Care Act of 2010**. The Act prohibits *lifetime* limits on most benefits in any health plan or insurance policy issued or renewed on or after September 23, 2010. By 2014, *annual* maximums will be phased out. Annual maximums are $1.25 million for a plan year or policy year starting on or after September 23, 2011, but starting before September 23, 2012; $2 million for a plan year or policy year starting on or after September 23, 2012, but starting before January 1, 2014. No annual dollar limits are allowed on most covered benefits beginning January 1, 2014.

   d. Is there a preexisting limitation on the plan and, if so, how is it applied? Effective 2014, people with preexisting health conditions cannot be denied health insurance. Since 2010, children under the age of 19 cannot be denied health insurance due to a preexisting condition.

4. Determine whether there is any information missing from the claim which is necessary for determination of payment (e.g., diagnosis, patient, provider licensing).

5. Obtain all relevant facts. Request all missing information or documentation at one time. Thoroughly investigate all available data. Do not pend a claim again to request information that you should have requested initially.

6. Make an honest evaluation of the facts and the plan benefits. Seek assistance from supervisors when necessary.

7. Keep the patient or claimant informed. Each time a claim is pended or denied, the insurance claims examiner should send an EOB. Each time an EOB is received, the provider should send an updated statement.

8. No decision is final. If the benefits are denied, there is always an opportunity to reevaluate or appeal the claim if new or different information is received.

Good Claim Practices for the Insurance Claims Examiner

Consider the following five guidelines when you process claims:

1. *Fully analyze the claim initially.* Consider all possible reasons for acceptance or denial. Look for a way to pay a claim, not deny it. Often an initial review of a claim will reveal clear and obvious grounds for denial. Sometimes the obvious grounds disappear later when the denial is questioned. Always clearly document the grounds for denial. Resist the natural temptation to deny a claim without a complete investigation and without considering all other possible grounds for acceptance. Keep in mind that for health plan years beginning on or after September 23, 2010, the Affordable Care Act of 2010 makes it illegal for insurance companies to rescind coverage on the basis of an error or technicality.

2. *Thoroughly investigate and document the facts within the claim file.* This may be one of the most important steps that each examiner needs to take before paying or denying a claim. The lack of a proper investigation or documentation has probably resulted in more bad faith lawsuits than any other individual factor.

   a. Investigate and thoroughly document all aspects under investigation before taking a position on the status of a claim.

   b. After investigation, evaluate the facts in an impartial and objective manner. If the facts are technical, seek assistance from a lead examiner or supervisor.

   c. Verify the authenticity of the information. Is the person providing the information a qualified provider or other qualified person?

   d. Never rely on incomplete or ambiguous claim forms or inspection reports.

   e. Consider all policy provisions.

3. *Handle claims promptly and keep claimants informed.*

   a. Give priority to delayed or pended claims.

   b. Resolve conflicting evidence or information promptly.

   c. Do not withhold or delay payments in hope of a compromise.

   d. Be sure to indicate the date and other documentation when claims are received or processed, when correspondence is received or sent, and when telephone calls are received or made.

4. *Make proper use of medical evidence.*

   a. Always contact the doctor to clear up any medical questions concerning the claimant.

   b. When a second medical opinion is required, the proper selection of an independent medical examiner is very important. Choose a specialist for the specific disease or injury. The specialist must always be provided with all the claimant's relevant medical information and records, whether they are favorable or unfavorable. Remember that you cannot reach the correct conclusion unless you ask the correct questions. Sometimes asking the correct questions is the most difficult part of preparing a case for review.

5. *Be observant in looking for excessive charges.* Some providers indicate a long list of diagnoses to match up the wide variety of tests given, so that the claim will be covered by the insurance carrier. Watch for the following situations:

   a. High charges, a long list of diagnoses, and no subsequent visits.

   b. Multiple diagnoses involving multiple bodily functions.

   c. Services described in very technical and nonstandard medical terminology, especially in connection with exotic extensive medical testing.

   d. Vague or ambiguous diagnoses.

e. Diagnoses involving extensive testing, beginning with hyper- or hypo- (e.g., hypoglycemia, hypercholesterolemia, hypomineralism).

f. Claims or bills that appear to be preprinted or that are wordy descriptions of services.

These are only a few of the instances that should alert the attention of a good claims examiner. If necessary, request medical records to investigate the patient's history and chief complaints, the tests performed, and their results.

In questionable cases, use common sense and seek advice early. Often a second opinion or different point of view can clarify the situation. Do not hesitate to seek the opinion of your supervisor or lead examiner. Two areas in which help is often needed are questioning preexisting conditions and determining usual and customary charges. Keep in mind that payment or coverage cannot be denied for preexisting conditions in children under 26 years of age, and, effective 2014, no one can be denied payment or coverage due to preexisting conditions. Your responsibility is to make decisions, but prudent decisions come with time and experience. Until you have experience, consider asking questions to be a part of your learning and training.

Unbundling of Services

Medical billers should avoid **unbundling** (also called fragmentation or code splitting), the practice of billing multiple procedure codes for a group of procedures that are covered by a single comprehensive code. It can occur in charges for surgery, pathology and lab, radiology, and medical services. Coding manipulations such as unbundling are often used to inappropriately increase claim reimbursements. The claims examiner should only allow charge determination based on the single comprehensive code which includes the entire procedure.

If unbundling has occurred, the claims examiner should deny the component parts of the procedure because they are already included within the allowable charge for the single procedure. This process is referred to as **rebundling**.

Here are some examples of unbundling:

- Fragmenting one service into component parts and coding each component part as if it were a separate service. For example, the correct CPT® comprehensive code to use for upper gastrointestinal endoscopy with biopsy of stomach is 43239. Separating the service into two component parts, using CPT code 43235 for upper gastrointestinal endoscopy and CPT code 43600 for biopsy of the stomach, is inappropriate and is considered fraudulent.

- Reporting separate codes for related services when one comprehensive code includes all related services. An example is coding a total abdominal hysterectomy with or without removal of tubes, with or without removal of ovaries (CPT code 58150), plus salpingectomy (CPT code 58700), plus oophorectomy (CPT code 58940), rather than using the comprehensive CPT code 58150 for all three related services.

- Breaking out bilateral procedures when one code is appropriate. For example, bilateral mammography is coded correctly using CPT code 76091. It is incorrect to submit

CPT code 76090-RT for the right mammography and CPT code 76090-LT for left mammography.

- Downcoding a service in order to use an additional code when one higher level, more comprehensive code is appropriate. A laboratory should bill CPT code 80048 (basic metabolic panel), when coding for a calcium, carbon dioxide, chloride, creatinine, glucose, potassium, sodium, and urea nitrogen performed as automated multichannel tests. It would be inappropriate and fraudulent to report CPT codes 82310, 82374, 82435, 82565, 82947, 84132, 84295 and/or 84520 in addition to the CPT code 80048 unless one of these laboratory tests was performed at a different time of day to obtain follow-up results, in which case a modifier -91 would be utilized.

- Separating a diagnostic approach from a major surgical service. For example, a provider should not bill CPT code 49000 for exploratory laparotomy and CPT code 44150 for total abdominal colectomy for the same operation because the exploration of the surgical field is included in the CPT code 44150.

> ● **ONLINE INFORMATION:** Find a reputable website and read why CMS considers unbundling to be fraudulent activity.

Mutually Exclusive Code Pairs

Medical billers should avoid mutually exclusive code pairings. These codes represent services or procedures that, according to either the CPT definition or standard medical practice, would not or could not reasonably be performed at the same session by the same provider on the same patient. Codes representing these services or procedures cannot be submitted together.

Examples of mutually exclusive code pairs include the following:

- Two different methods for repairing an organ. The surgeon must choose one method to repair the organ, and that is the code that must be used.

- The billing of an "initial" service and a "subsequent" service. A service cannot be initial and subsequent at the same time. If a physician reports "mutually exclusive" coding combinations, the carrier will pay for the procedure with the lowest work relative value unit and deny the other code(s).

- A vaginal hysterectomy (procedure code 58260) and a total abdominal hysterectomy (procedure code 58150)—either one or the other, but not both procedures, is performed.

- CPT codes 13100 and 13101 for the complex repair of the trunk. If multiple wounds of the trunk are repaired in the same operative session, coding is based on the total length of all the repairs.

- Complex Treatment Device CPT Code 77334 billed on the same date of service (DOS) as the Simple Treatment Device Code 77332. Only one treatment device code should be paid because they are mutually exclusive on the same date of service. If these codes are billed on the same DOS, many payers will deny the major code as a duplicate and pay only the lesser code.

Separate Procedures

Although certain CPT codes are identified as *separate procedures*, it has been determined that these codes occasionally may be provided as part of a more comprehensive procedure. Under such circumstances, the more comprehensive procedure code should be used for billing.

Note: Separate procedure codes can only be billed when the separate procedure is the only procedure performed or when it was performed on a different site. For example, if two procedures are conducted on the right arm through the same incision, they are included together. If the same procedure is performed on both arms, they should be billed as two separate procedures.

Payment Worksheet

Although electronic billing and claims software programs may compute these figures for you, the instructions provided here will help you understand the formation of a claim charge. You can use a payment worksheet like the examples found in Figures 5-8 ● and 5-9 ● to explain to a patient how the benefits on the claim were calculated. Although worksheets vary from company to company, the general format and requirements remain the same.

Header Information

The header area includes the patient and plan identification information. It is composed of the following fields:

Eligible Employee. The full name of the insured or employee.

Company. The name of the employer or company.

Insured's Identification Number. The social security number or other identification number for the insured or employee.

Patient. The name of the patient or claimant.

Relationship. The relationship of the patient to the insured.

The following information should be filled in after the claim payment worksheet has been completed:

Accident Benefit. Amount of accident benefit, year to date.

Deductible. Amount of deductible, year to date.

Carryover Deductible. Amount of deductible carried over from the previous year.

Coinsurance. Amount of coinsurance paid, year to date.

Claim Data Information

The body of the worksheet is where the billed services are itemized, indicating the amount allowed for each service, the amount excluded, and the percentage at which the amount allowed is payable. This section includes the following fields:

Procedure/Type of Service. The applicable CPT code or English-language description of service.

Dates of Service. The date of service for this particular single line of coding.

Billed Amount. The total amount of charges for the services indicated on this single line of coding.

Excluded Amounts. The amount of charges for this single line of coding that is not allowable under the plan. An explanation should be placed under Denial Reasons.

Allowed. The amount remaining after the excluded expenses are subtracted from the billed amount.

Basic 100%. The amount of the allowed expense that is payable at 100%. If there are multiple applicable plan percentages for a single charge, the allowed expense should be broken up according to the amount payable at each specific percentage.

Major Med %. The Major Medical amount allowed after any higher benefits such as Basic have been subtracted from the allowed expense.

%. Any additional applicable percentage rate that may apply to an allowed amount. This can be due to OOP maximums, SSO Consultations that were not performed, and so on.

Totals. The total of all amounts within each column.

Deductible. The amount of the charges applied to the plan deductible.

Amount Subject to Coinsurance. Amount payable at the plan coinsurance rate after any deductible is taken.

Coinsurance. The coinsurance rate that is the patient's liability.

Amount Subject to Adjustment. The amount that needs to be adjusted because of COB, overpayment, or any other type of adjustment.

Adjustment. The actual adjustment being made.

Payment Amount. The payment amount that is expected for this claim.

Remarks. The type and reason for any adjustments being made. This space is also used to detail any other patient information related to the handling of this claim.

Claims examiners can also complete the following fields:

Denial Reasons. The reason for the denial must be explained to the member whenever a charge or portion of a charge is not covered under a plan. The reason should be entered in this area and referenced by line item.

Payees. The amount of the claim payment and who is to be paid.

The Examiner Processing of a Claim

After you have determined that the claim is properly completed, the patient is covered, the provider is appropriate, there is no other insurance, and that the services are covered, it is time to begin processing the claim.

The claim information is taken from the sample CMS-1500 seen in Figure 5-10 ●. This information is shown on the claim form and on the description in parentheses. The information shown in brackets is either the calculation used to

Payment Worksheet

Eligible Employee:	Nancy Normal	Accident Benefit:	$ 0.00	(CCYY)
Company:	XYZ Corporation			
Insured's ID Number:	777 77 XYZ	Deductible:	$ 125.00	(CCYY)
Patient:	Normal Nancy	Carryover Ded:	$ 0.00	(CCNY)
Relationship:	Self	Coinsurance:	$ 11.74	(CCYY)
Provider's Zip Code:	89578	Date of Injury:		

Procedure Type of Service	Dates of Service	Billed Amount	Excluded Amounts*	Allowed	Basic/ Accident 100%	Maj. Med. ___%	___%	UCR Calculations
1. 99201	2/5/CCYY	$ 220.00	$ 24.48	$ 195.52	$ 48.75	$ 146.77		6.5 x 30.08
2. 85025	2/5/CCYY	$ 40.00	$ 19.38	$ 20.62	$ 5.60	$ 15.02		0.8 x 25.78
3. 87040	2/5/CCYY	$ 30.00	$ 0.00	$ 30.00	$ 8.40	$ 21.60		1.2 x 25.78
4.								
5.								
6.								

⇩Remarks:	Totals:	$ 290.00	$ 43.86	$ 246.14	$ 62.75	$ 183.39	
Deductible has been satisfied.	Deductible:				$ 0.00	$ 125.00	
	Amount Subject to Coinsurance:				$ 62.75	$ 58.39	
	Coinsurance:				$ 0.00	$ 11.68	
	Amount Subject to Adjustment:				$ 62.75	$ 46.71	
	Adjustment (See Remarks):				$ 0.00	$ 0.00	
	Payment Amount:		$ 109.46		$ 62.75	$ 46.71	

*Denial Reasons
1. $ 24.48 not covered — Exceeds amount allowed by your plan.
2. $ 19.38 not covered — Exceeds amount allowed by your plan.
3.
4.
5.
6.

Payees
1. $ 90.00 — Dee N. Aee, M.D.
2. $ 19.46 — Nancy Normal
3.
4.
5.
6.

If you disagree with our decision on your claim, you have the right by law to request that your claim be reviewed by your plan administrator. This request must be made in writing within 60 days of receipt of this notice. If you wish, you may submit your written comments and views. Please consult your plan's claim review procedures. See your employer regarding any other ERISA questions.

FIGURE 5-8 Payment Worksheet

Payment Worksheet

Eligible Employee:	Betty Bossy	Accident Benefit:	$	0.00	(CCYY)
Company:	Ninja Enterprises				
Insured's ID Number:	999-99 NIN	Deductible:	$	0.00	(CCYY)
Patient:	Self	Carryover Ded:	$	0.00	(CCNY)
Relationship:	Self	Coinsurance:	$	1,250.00	(CCYY)
Provider's Zip Code:	12890	Date of Injury:			

Procedure Type of Service	Dates of Service	Billed Amount	Excluded Amounts*	Allowed	Basic/ Accident 100%	Major Medical 80 %	___ %	UCR Calcula-tions
1. R&B	02/06/YY-02/14/YY	$3160.00		$ 3160.00		3160.00		
2. MISC	02/06/YY-02/14/YY	$7086.00		$ 7086.00		7086.00		
3.								
4.								
5.								
6.								

⇩Remarks:	Totals:	$10246.00	$	$10246.00	$	$10246.00	
Network Provider paid at 80%	Deductible:				$	$ 150.00	
	Amount Subject to Coinsurance:				$	$10096.00	
Precertification performed.	Coinsurance:				$	$ 1250.00	
	Amount Subject to Adjustment:				$	$ 8846.00	
	Adjustment (See Remarks):				$	$	
	Payment Amount:		$ 8846.00		$	$ 8846.00	

*Denial Reasons
1.
2.
3.
4.
5.
6.

Payees
1. $8846.00—Abe Domin, M.D.
2.
3.
4.
5.
6.

If you disagree with our decision on your claim, you have the right by law to request that your claim be reviewed by your plan administrator. This request must be made in writing within 60 days of receipt of this notice. If you wish, you may submit your written comments and views. Please consult your plan's claim review procedures. See your employer regarding any other ERISA questions.

FIGURE 5-9   Payment Worksheet

1500

HEALTH INSURANCE CLAIM FORM

APPROVED BY NATIONAL UNIFORM CLAIM COMMITTEE 08/05

BALL INSURANCE CARRIERS
3895 BUBBLE BLVD STE 283
BUXWOOD CO 85926

☐☐☐ PICA   PICA ☐☐☐

1. MEDICARE MEDICAID TRICARE CHAMPVA GROUP FECA OTHER CHAMPUS HEALTH PLAN BLK LUNG	1a. INSURED'S I.D. NUMBER (For Program in Item 1)
☐(Medicare #) ☐(Medicaid #) ☐(Sponsor's SSN) ☐(Member ID#) ☒(SSN or ID) ☐(SSN) ☐(ID)	777 77 XYZ

2. PATIENT'S NAME (Last Name, First Name, Middle Initial)	3. PATIENT'S BIRTH DATE SEX	4. INSURED'S NAME (Last Name, First Name, Middle Initial)
NORMAL NANCY N	MM DD YY 07 02 CCYY-28 M☐ F☒	SAME

5. PATIENT'S ADDRESS (No, Street)	6. PATIENT RELATIONSHIP TO INSURED	7. INSURED'S ADDRESS (No, Street)
707 NATIONAL STREET	Self ☒ Spouse ☐ Child ☐ Other ☐	

CITY	STATE	8. PATIENT STATUS	CITY	STATE
NANDO	NV	Single ☒ Married ☐ Other ☐		

ZIP CODE	TELEPHONE (Include Area Code)		ZIP CODE	TELEPHONE (Include Area Code)
89577	(775) 555 3377	Employed ☒ Full-Time Student ☐ Part-Time Student ☐		

9. OTHER INSURED'S NAME (Last Name, First Name, Middle Initial)	10. IS PATIENT'S CONDITION RELATED TO:	11. INSURED'S POLICY GROUP OR FECA NUMBER 62958XYZ
a. OTHER INSURED'S POLICY OR GROUP NUMBER	a. EMPLOYMENT? (Current or Previous) ☐YES ☒NO	a. INSURED'S DATE OF BIRTH SEX MM DD YY M☐ F☐
b. OTHER INSURED'S DATE OF BIRTH SEX MM DD YY M☐ F☐	b. AUTO ACCIDENT? PLACE (State) ☐YES ☒NO	b. EMPLOYER'S NAME OR SCHOOL NAME XYZ CORPORATION
c. EMPLOYER'S NAME OR SCHOOL NAME	c. OTHER ACCIDENT? ☐YES ☒NO	c. INSURANCE PLAN NAME OR PROGRAM NAME BALL INSURANCE CARRIERS
d. INSURANCE PLAN NAME OR PROGRAM NAME	10d. RESERVED FOR LOCAL USE	d. IS THERE ANOTHER HEALTH BENEFIT PLAN? ☐YES ☒NO If yes, return to and complete item 9 a-d

READ BACK OF FORM BEFORE COMPLETING & SIGNING THIS FORM.

12. PATIENT'S OR AUTHORIZED PERSON'S SIGNATURE I authorize the release of any medical or other information necessary to process this claim. I also request payment of government benefits either to myself or to the party who accepts assignment below.

SIGNED *SIGNATURE ON FILE*   DATE_____

13. INSURED'S OR AUTHORIZED PERSON'S SIGNATURE I authorize payment of medical benefits to the undersigned physician or supplier for services described below.

SIGNED *SIGNATURE ON FILE*

14. DATE OF CURRENT ILLNESS (First symptom) OR INJURY (Accident) OR PREGNANCY (LMP) MM DD YY 02 03 YY	15. IF PATIENT HAS HAD SAME OR SIMILAR ILLNESS, GIVE FIRST DATE MM DD YY	16. DATES PATIENT UNABLE TO WORK IN CURRENT OCCUPATION MM DD YY MM DD YY FROM TO
17. NAME OF REFERRING PHYSICIAN OR OTHER SOURCE	17a. 17b. NPI	18. HOSPITALIZATION DATES RELATED TO CURRENT SERVICES MM DD YY MM DD YY FROM TO
19. RESERVED FOR LOCAL USE		20. OUTSIDE LAB? $ CHARGES ☐YES ☐NO

21. DIAGNOSIS OR NATURE OF ILLNESS OR INJURY (Relate Items 1,2,3 or 4 to Item 24E by Line)

1. |_079 . 3_____| 3. |_____|
2. |_____| 4. |_____|

22. MEDICAID RESUBMISSION CODE   ORIGINAL REF. NO.
23. PRIOR AUTHORIZATION NUMBER

24. A. DATE(S) OF SERVICE   B.   C.   D. PROCEDURES, SERVICES, OR SUPPLIES   E.   F.   G.   H.   I.   J.

From			To			B. PLACE OF SERVICE	C. EMG	D. CPT/HCPCS MODIFIER	E. DIAGNOSIS POINTER	F. $ CHARGES	G. DAYS OR UNITS	H. EPSDT Family Plan	I. ID. QUAL.	J. RENDERING PROVIDER ID. #
MM	DD	YY	MM	DD	YY									
02	05	YY	02	05	YY	11	1	99201	1	220 00	1		NPI	
02	05	YY	02	05	YY	11	1	85025	1	40 00	1		NPI	
02	05	YY	02	05	YY	11	1	87040	1	30 00	1		NPI	
													NPI	
													NPI	
													NPI	

25. FEDERAL TAX ID NUMBER SSN EIN	26. PATIENT'S ACCOUNT NO.	27. ACCEPT ASSIGNMENT? (For govt. claims, see back)	28. TOTAL CHARGE	29. AMOUNT PAID	30. BALANCE DUE
70 7759777 ☐☒	NANNR001 737	☒YES ☐NO	$ 290 00	$ 200 00	$ 90 00

31. SIGNATURE OF PHYSICIAN OR SUPPLIER INCLUDING DEGREES OR CREDENTIALS (I certify that the statements on the reverse apply to this bill and are made a part thereof) SIGNED *Dee N Aee MD* DATE 02/18/YY	32. SERVICE FACILITY LOCATION INFORMATION a. b.	33. BILLING PROVIDER INFO & PH. # DEE N AEE MD 2577 NONE STREET STE 575N NOLTY NV 89578 (775) 555 0077 D44444 a. b.

NUCC Instruction Manual available at: www.nucc.org   PLEASE PRINT OR TYPE   APPROVED OMB 0938-0999 FORM CMS-1500 (08/05)

FIGURE 5-10 Front of CMS-1500 with patient information provided

arrive at an amount or the block on the CMS-1500 that contains the information. We will be using the Ball Insurance Company from Appendix A and the RVS Schedule and UCR Conversion Factor Report from Appendix C.

Completing the Payment Worksheet

The claim payment worksheet is equivalent to an EOB. A copy of this worksheet will be sent to the insured member to explain the benefit payment for the claim. Therefore, each section should be filled out accurately and completely.

The claim payment worksheet used in this chapter is intended to be an example only. It contains the information in much the same format as most insurance carriers' EOBs. This worksheet and the guidelines for completing it are to be used for training and reference purposes only, as the particular company or plan worksheets and guidelines may differ.

The following information will explain how to complete the sections of the payment worksheet.

Step 1.   Complete the information regarding the patient and insured first. This information is contained in the box in the upper left-hand corner of the payment worksheet.

Payment Worksheet Field	CMS-1500	CMS-1500 Block Number	UB-04	UB-04 Form Locator
Eligible Employee	Nancy Normal	Block 4	Betty B. Bossy	FL 58
Company	XYZ Corporation	Block 11b	Ninja Enterprises	FL 65
Insured's Identification Number	777-77-WXYZ	Block 1a	999-99 NIN	FL 60
Patient	Nancy Normal	Block 2	Betty B. Bossy	FL 12
Relationship	Self	Block 6	18 (self)	FL 59
Provider's ZIP Code	89578	Block 33	12890	FL 1

Step 2.   Next, each CPT code should be listed in the "Procedure Type of Service" column. Only codes that are the same should be combined together. Otherwise, list one code per line, even if this means using more than one payment worksheet.

Procedure Type of Service	1. 99201 2. 85025 3. 87040	Field 24D	111 (inpatient hospital claim)	FL 4

Step 3.   List the date(s) of service in the "Dates of Service" column.

Dates of Service	1. 02/05/ CCYY 2. 02/05/ CCYY 3. 02/05/ CCYY	Field 24A	02/06/ CCYY through 02/14/ CCYY	FL 6

Step 4.   Enter the amount the provider billed in "Billed Amount" column.

Billed Amount	1. $220.00 2. $40.00 3. $30.00	Field 24F	$10,246.00	FL 55

Step 5.   Determine the allowed amount for the service or procedure. Using the Relative Value Scale shown in Appendix C, locate the unit value for the CPT code that is assigned to each service provided. The unit value for the procedure is located in the right-hand column titled "Total RVUs." Next, determine the conversion factor for the procedure from the UCR Conversion Factor Report (see Appendix C).

Using the first three numbers of the provider's ZIP code, locate the type of service. Four categories are listed next to the ZIP code location:

1. Surgery
2. Medicine
3. X-ray/Lab
4. Anesthesia

Multiply the appropriate conversion factor by the unit value for the procedure. The appropriate category is determined by the CPT code, not the description of service. This total is the allowed amount. If the billed amount is less than the allowed amount, the billed amount is considered to be the allowed amount.

Thus, in this example the amounts are 195.52, 20.62, and 30.94.

6.5 [RVS] × 30.08 [Medicine Conversion factor for
ZIP codes starting 895] = 195.52

0.8 [RVS] × 25.78 [X-ray/lab conversion factor]
= 20.62

1.2 [RVS] × 25.78 (X-ray/lab conversion factor)
= 30.94

Because the billed amount for line three is less than the UCR amount, the allowed amount will be the billed amount.

Skip to the Allowed column and enter the allowed amounts as just figured.

Payment Worksheet Field	Calculation		UB-04 Input	UB-04 Form Locator Field
Allowed	1. $195.52 2. $20.62 3. $30.00		1. $3160.00 2. $7086.00	

Step 6.   Next, subtract the allowed amount from the billed amount. The resulting figure is the excluded amount that should be placed in the Excluded Amounts column. Remember, if the allowed amount is greater than the billed amount, the billed amount will be the allowed amount. Therefore, the excluded amounts will be $24.48, $19.38, and 0.00.

$220.00 [billed amount] − $195.52 [allowed amount]
= $24.48

$40.00 − $20.62 = $19.38

$30.00 − $30.00 = $0.00

Excluded Amounts	1. $24.48			
	2. $19.38			
	3. $0.00			

Step 7. Each EOB must list any amounts that are denied and the reason for the denial. Skip to the Denial Reasons section and enter a denial reason on the corresponding line. Usually, a brief explanation such as "$24.48 not covered—charge exceeds amount covered by your plan" is sufficient. If the service is not covered, list the corresponding code (or description) and an explanation in the same manner (e.g., "$300.00 not covered—cosmetic services are not covered by your plan"). (See Appendix C for a list of denial reasons to use.)

Denial Reasons	1. $24.48 not covered — Exceeds amount allowed by your plan			
	2. $19.38 not covered — Exceeds amount allowed by your plan.			

Step 8. If the plan has a Basic allowance, multiply the unit value by the Basic allowance listed in the contract. For example, if the contract stipulates that the Basic allowance for an office visit is $7.00 and the CPT has a unit value of 1.0, then the Basic allowance would be $7.00. The Basic allowance amount would be placed in the Basic/Accident 100% column. The amounts are $48.75, $5.60, and $8.40.

$7.50 [Outpatient physician visits Basic conversion factor from contract] $\times$ 6.5 [RVS units] = $48.75

$7.00 [X-ray and laboratory Basic conversion factor from contract] $\times$ 0.8 [RVS units] = $5.60

$7.00 [X-ray and laboratory Basic conversion factor from contract] $\times$ 1.2 [RVS units] = $8.40

Basic/Accident 100%	1. $48.75			
	2. $5.60			
	3. $8.40			

Step 9. The Basic allowance is subtracted from the allowed amount and the remainder is placed in the Major Medical column. The remainder amounts are $146.77, $15.02, and $21.60.

$195.52 [Major Medical allowed amount] − $48.75 [Basic amount] = $146.77

$20.62 [Major Medical amount] − $5.60 [Basic amount] = $15.02

$30.00 [Major Medical amount] − $8.40 [Basic amount] = $21.60

Major Medical	1. $146.77		1. $3160.00	
	2. $15.02		2. $7086.00	
	3. $21.60			

Step 10. After all the charges have been figured individually, add the total for each column and place it at the bottom of the column in the "Totals" row. The totals are $43.86, $246.14, $62.75, and $183.39.

Check your totals for accuracy by adding the Major Medical amount to the Basic amount. These two amounts should total the Allowed Amount. Then add the Allowed Amount to the Excluded Amount. The total of these two figures should match the Billed Amount column and the total amount of the claim.

If the contract allows different percentages based on the type of service (e.g., Basic Benefits at 100%, Major Medical at 80%, Accidents at 100%), then each different type of benefit (i.e., Basic, Major Medical, Accident) should be placed in a different column. If there are not enough columns on the payment worksheet, you may place all services paid at the same percent together in a single column. There is also an additional untitled column to allow for varying percentages.

Totals	1. $43.86		1. $3160.00	
	2. $246.14		2. $7086.00	
	3. $62.75			
	4. $183.39			

Step 11. Now it is time to calculate the actual benefit payment. At the top of each payment column (Basic/Accident, Major Medical and Untitled), place the coinsurance percentage amount that applies to the figures in that column if it is not indicated (e.g., 100%, 80%).

Step 12. Check the contract for the deductible amount and the Beginning Financials, if applicable, for any previously paid deductible amounts. Also, answer the following questions:

- Is there a deductible amount for Basic benefits?
- Has the deductible for this individual been satisfied?
- Does the deductible combine the medical plan with a dental plan (i.e., are the plans integrated)?
- If so, has the deductible been satisfied under the medical or dental portion of the contract?
- Has the family deductible been satisfied?
- Is there any carryover deductible from the previous year that should be applied?

Using this information, calculate both the Basic and the Major Medical deductible amounts. Usually, the deductible amount on the Basic portion of a plan is only for hospital services.

Deductible	1. $0.00		$150.00	
	2. $125.00			

Step 13. To calculate the Basic Benefits, first enter the amount of the deductible in the "Deductible" row in the Basic Benefits column. In this case, there is no Basic deductible on the services for Nancy Normal. The only Basic deductible stated in the contract is a $50 inpatient hospital deductible. However, this claim is not for inpatient hospital services.

Deductible	$0.00			

Step 14. Next, subtract the deductible amount from the total of the column and place the resulting amount in the "Amount Subject to Coinsurance" row. As the deductible amount is $0.00, the amount to be placed here is $62.75.

$$\$62.75 - \$0.00 = \$62.75$$

Amount Subject to Coinsurance	$62.75			

Step 15. Next, multiply the amount subject to coinsurance by the insured's portion of the coinsurance amount (the remaining amount needed to reach 100%). For example, if the plan's coinsurance amount is 80%, then the insured's responsibility is 20%. For this column, the payment amount is 100%, so there is no coinsurance amount for the patient.

$$\$62.75 \times 0\% = \$0.00$$

Coinsurance	$0.00			

Step 16. Subtract the coinsurance amount from the amount subject to coinsurance. The remaining balance is the amount subject to adjustment and goes in the next column.

$$\$62.75 - \$0.00 = \$62.75$$

We will cover the rows "Adjustment (See Remarks)," and "Payment Amount" in Steps 23 and 24

Amount Subject to Adjustment	$62.75			

Step 17. To calculate the Major Medical benefits, first, calculate the Major Medical deductible that should be applied on this claim. Since this treatment is for a new patient visit at the beginning of the year, we will conclude that Nancy Normal has not yet paid any of her deductible. Therefore, we will place $125.00 in the "Deductible" row of the Major Medical column.

Note: If any individual or family deductible or coinsurance amounts are met on this claim, place an asterisk beside the deductible or coinsurance amount and make a notation in the remarks box (e.g., CCYY individual deductible has now been met).

Deductible	$125.00			

Step 18. Next, subtract the deductible amount from the total of the column and place the resulting amount in the "Amount Subject to Coinsurance" row.

$$\$183.39 - \$125.00 = \$58.39$$

If the amount in the "Deductible" field equals the amount in the "Totals" field, then the "Amount Subject to Coinsurance" would be $0, and no Major Medical payment will be made on the claim.

Amount Subject to Coinsurance	$58.39		$10096.00	

Step 19. Next, multiply the amount subject to coinsurance by the insured's portion of the coinsurance amount (the remaining amount needed to reach 100%). For example, if the plan's coinsurance amount is 80%, then the insured's responsibility is 20%.

$$\$58.39 \times .2 = \$11.68$$

Coinsurance	($11.68)		($1250.00)	

Step 20. Next, ask the following questions:
- What is the maximum coinsurance amount listed in the contract?
- Has this coinsurance limit been met?
- If the individual coinsurance limit has not been met, has the family coinsurance limit been met?

If any coinsurance limits have been met, the coinsurance amount should be adjusted accordingly. For example, if the individual coinsurance limit is $1,500 and $1,495 has been paid by the individual, the coinsurance amount would be $5.

Step 21. Subtract the coinsurance amount from the amount that is subject to coinsurance. The remaining balance is the amount that is subject to adjustment and it goes in that row.

$$\$58.39 - \$11.68 = \$46.71$$

Amount Subject to Adjustment	$46.71		$8846.00	

Step 22. Ask the following questions:
- If there is other insurance, what is the amount paid by the other insurance company?
- Are there any other reasons why there would be an adjustment to this claim?
- If so, what is the proper adjustment amount?

If there is an adjustment, place the amount of the adjustment in the row "Adjustment (See Remarks)," and place an explanation in the "Remarks" box to the left. (See Appendix C for a list of remarks to use.) Many claims will not have an adjustment amount. If there is an adjustment amount, the amount of the adjustment cannot be more than the amount shown in the "Amount Subject to Adjustment." For example, if there was an adjustment of $100 on Nancy's claim, you would place $62.75 in the first column and $37.25 in the second column. As there is no adjustment on this claim, we will place $0.00 in these boxes for both the Basic and Major Medical columns.

Adjustment (See Remarks) Remarks	1. $0.00 2. $0.00		$ 0.00	

Step 23. The adjustment amount if any, should then be subtracted from the amount subject to adjustment, and the resulting amount would be placed in the "Payment Amount" row. For the Basic Benefits column, this amount is $62.75, and for the Major Medical column, this amount is $46.71.

Payment Amount	1. $62.75 2. $46.71		$8846.00	

Step 24. Add up the payment amount from all columns. The resulting payment amount should be placed in the box immediately to the right of the words "Payment Amount." This is the amount of the benefits being paid by the insurance carrier for this claim.

$$\$62.75 + 46.71 = \$109.46$$

Payment Amount	$109.46		$8846.00	

Step 25. In this case, Nancy has paid $200 on the claim, leaving a balance of $90 owed to the provider. As the provider should not be paid more than he or she has charged, the payment must be split. $90 will be paid to the provider and the remaining $19.46 will be reimbursed to Nancy. This information is placed in the "Payees" section.

Payees	1. $90.00—Dee N. Aee, M.D. 2. $19.46—Nancy Normal		1. $8846.00 — Abe Domin, M.D.	

Step 26. In this case, this is the first claim for Nancy. Thus, the following amounts are listed in her updated history:

Accident Benefit: $0.00 (CCYY) [This was not an accident claim, so no accident benefits were paid.]
Deductible: $125.00 (CCYY) Nancy paid $125 in deductible on this claim. She has now met the CCYY deductible.]
Carryover Ded: $0.00 (CCNY) [This claim was not paid in the last three months of the year, so there is no carryover deductible.]
Coinsurance: $ 11.74 (CCYY) [This is the amount of Nancy's copayment on this claim.]
Date of Injury: [This would not apply because this claim is not an accident.]

Accident Benefit	$0.00		$0.00	
Deductible	$125.00		$150.00	
Carryover Ded	$0.00		$0.00	
Coinsurance	$11.74		$1,250.00	
Date of Injury	N/A		N/A	

Employment Retirement Income Security Act

Federal Employment Retirement Income Security Act of 1974 (ERISA) requirements affect all claim denials. The ERISA Right of Review statement must be included with every claim denial and on every EOB where all or part of a claim is denied. The following wording may be used on the EOB or statement:

If you disagree with our decision on your claim, you have the right by law to request that your claim be reviewed by your plan administrator. This request must be made in writing within 60 days of receipt of this notice. If you wish, you may submit your written comments and views. Please consult your plan's claim review procedures. See your employer regarding any other ERISA questions.

Payees

Now the only remaining tasks are to determine whom to pay and to update the financial history. Look at the claim form. Benefits may be assigned to the provider of services by the member. The assignment must bear the member's written signature on an **Assignment of Benefits** form that authorizes benefits payable directly to the provider of service. Alternatively, the provider must accept assignment for that insurance company, in which situation the insurance company will automatically direct the payment to the provider.

When you are reviewing a claim, note whether an assignment has been made. If payment is made because of failure to honor an assignment and benefits are released to the member, the provider of service can also request payment, and payment must be made to the provider as well. The incorrect payment made to the member will have to be recouped. (This will be covered later in the section on Adjustments.) Ensuring that all valid assignments are honored is a basic part of good claim handling.

When you are processing a claim, ask whether the insured authorized payment directly to the provider of services or whether there is a mandatory assignment of benefits.

- If neither case is true, the payee would be the insured.
- If payment was authorized or there was a mandatory assignment of benefits, check the billed amount from the claim and the amount (if any) that the patient/insured has already paid. If the difference between the billed amount and the amount that the patient or insured paid (balance due) is less than the benefit payment amount, the payee is the provider of services up to the balance due. Any remaining funds should then be paid to the insured.

Updating History

Updating the payment history is vitally important because it ensures that proper benefit payments are calculated. The answers to each of the questions related to previous payments of deductibles, coinsurance amounts, satisfaction of individual or family limits, accident benefits, and other accumulated amounts will change with each claim. On our payment worksheet, the updated history appears in the upper left-hand corner of the sheet. If claims are processed by computer, the computer should handle the updating of the history for you.

If accident benefits were paid on this claim, add the payment amount of the accident benefits to any previous accident benefit amounts paid on this individual for this accident. This amount goes on the first line. The amount paid on all accidents in this calendar year should be placed to the right of this amount, along with the current year (in parentheses).

The amount of the benefits paid under Major Medical should be added to all previous Major Medical benefits paid. If the plan has a calendar year maximum, the amount of the benefits paid should be added to all previous benefits paid during that calendar year. (Remember that annual maximums will be prohibited starting in 2014.) Check the contract to see whether there is an annual maximum for Basic and Major Medical payment amounts.

The amount of any deductibles calculated on this claim should be added to any previously paid deductible amounts, and the result should be placed in the deductible space with the current year.

If any of the dates of service on this claim fall within the last three months of the calendar year and the contract includes a carryover provision, the amount of deductible paid on these services should be placed on the line labeled "carryover deductible," along with the year. If there is more than one date of service and some fall in the last three months while others do not, the deductible amount should be taken from the amount or amounts of the services in the order in which they are received.

EXAMPLE:

An exam on 9/18/CCYY found two moles, which were removed on 10/10/CCYY. The allowed amount was $40 for the exam and $120 for the mole removal. The patient had previously satisfied $25 of the $100 deductible. The total paid deductible amount is $75 on this claim. So $40 dollars of the deductible is for the first service and $35 is for the mole removal. Therefore, the carryover deductible amount is $35.

Finally, add the amount listed on the coinsurance line to any previous coinsurance amounts for the calendar year. The total, along with the year, should be placed on the coinsurance line of the financial history box. You have now completed payment on this claim.

Quick Reference Formulas

The following quick reference formulas will help you remember the calculation included on a payment worksheet.

PLAN UCR. Unit value × plan conversion factor = plan UCR

Anesthesia: Time units + procedure unit value × plan conversion factor

$$(TU + UV) \times CF = ANES. \ ALLOW.$$

Multiple Surgery: 100% of the Basic or UCR allowance for the primary procedure.

NONCOVERED CHARGES. Total charges minus allowable amounts (UCR)

$$TC - UCR = NC$$

BASIC ALLOWANCE. Procedure unit value × Basic conversion factor

$$UV \times BCF = BASIC$$

MAJOR MEDICAL ALLOWANCE. Plan UCR allowance minus Basic allowance

$$UCR - BASIC = MM \ ALLOWABLE$$

MAJOR MEDICAL PAYMENT. Plan UCR minus Basic allowance minus applicable deductibles multiplied by plan coinsurance rate

$$(UCR - BASIC) - DEDS \times \% = MM \ PAYMT$$

TOTAL PAYMENT. Major Medical payment plus Basic payment

$$MM + Basic = TP$$

Billing or Claims Management Office Administration

Several forms can help the medical biller or claims examiner in tracking important information. Using the Inventory/Production Sheet (Figure 5-11 ●), the medical biller records all claims submitted. Using this same form, the claims examiner records all the claims processed or pended, the finished correspondence, phone calls, all the received claims that are not yet processed, and all unfinished correspondence for that work week. (This information may be available as a report from the computer software.)

The Family Benefits Tracking Sheet (Figure 5-12 ●) is a form designed to keep track of the benefits that have been paid to date on each member of a family so that a medical biller or claims examiner may quickly calculate any remaining aggregate deductible, nonaggregate deductible, and coinsurance limits on a given family contract.

Prescription Drug Claims

Many health plans cover expenses for prescription drugs. However, in order to be covered, these drugs must often meet the following three criteria:

1. They must be prescribed by the patient's physician. This physician must be duly licensed and able to prescribe medications in the state in which the prescription was issued.
2. They must be prescription medications (i.e., they must, by law, require a prescription from a licensed physician for their dispensation).
3. They must be prescribed to treat a disease, bodily injury, or a mental or nervous disorder.

Some insurance plans may cover prescriptions that do not meet the preceding criteria. These can include antacids, eye and ear medications, compounded dermatalogic preparations, or other medications. If these drugs are covered, they will be specifically indicated in the policy.

Nonprescription drugs generally are not covered under the provisions of a contract. In addition, some prescription drugs may not be covered. These can include the following:

- Dietary supplements, health foods, or vitamins (including prenatal vitamins)
- Appetite suppressants

Consult the *Physicians' Desk Reference* to determine whether a drug is a prescription or a nonprescription drug.

"Red Book" and "Blue Book"

Some plans have separate drug subcoverage. These plans often pay for drugs according to a set price schedule, regardless of the amount charged by the pharmacy or dispensing physician. The schedules are often based on the *Blue Book* or the *Red Book*, two books that list wholesale prices of drugs. Often the plan provisions will specify payment at 150% or 175% of the *Blue Book* or *Red Book* price.

Inventory/ Production Sheet

Name: _____

Department: _____

Week of: _____

	Medical Claims Processed	Hospital Claims Processed	Dental Claims Processed	Pended Claims	Correspondence Handled or Written	Phone Calls Made	Downtime
Day 1							
Day 2							
Day 3							
Day 4							
Day 5							
TOTALS							

	Unprocessed Medical Claims	Unprocessed Hospital Claims	Unprocessed Dental Claims	Pended Claims	Unfinished Correspondence
Day 1					
Day 2					
Day 3					
Day 4					
Day 5					
TOTALS					

FIGURE 5-11   Inventory / Production Sheet

143

FAMILY BENEFITS TRACKING SHEET

FAMILY DEDUCTIBLE

Patient Name	Document #	Amount	Total

Contract: _____

Ind. Ded.: _____

Family Ded.: _____

    Aggregate   Nonaggregate

Coins. Limit: _____

Family Coins. Limit: _____

    Aggregate   Nonaggregate

Document #	Individual Deductible		Coinsurance	
	Amount	Total	Amount	Total

Patient Name:

Prior C/O	-------		-------	

Patient Name:

Prior C/O	-------		-------	

Patient Name:

Prior C/O	-------		-------	

Patient Name:

Prior C/O	-------		-------	

FIGURE 5-12   Family Benefits Tracking Sheet

To find the correct payment amount, first determine the manufacturer of the drug. If the drug manufacturer is not listed, look up the information using the *Physicians' Desk Reference*. Use the least expensive generic drug to calculate benefits.

Determine the charge for the smallest quantity listed, and then determine the price per unit. The unit may be indicated in quantification by tables, by ounces, or by some other measurement. If the drugs are listed in metric units and the prescription is issued in Imperial (nonmetric) units, the metric units must be converted to Imperial units (or vice versa). Metric conversion tables can be found in most medical dictionaries.

Multiply the price per unit by the number of units dispensed. This is the wholesale price for the drug. This wholesale price should be multiplied by the percentage (150% or 175%) indicated by the plan. Then add any amount indicated as $A ($1.35, $1.50, or $1.65). If this amount is more than the amount charged, use the amount charged. If not, this amount is considered the allowable amount. This allowed amount is then paid at the percentage at which benefits are payable (50%, 75%, or 100%).

Claims Examiner Handling of Prescription Drug Claims

Prescription drugs can be issued on an outpatient or inpatient basis. For the guidelines regarding payment for inpatient drugs (including those issued for take-home drugs), see Chapter 6, Physician's, Clinical, and Hospital Services Claims.

For outpatient drug claims, follow certain guidelines, including the following:

1. A valid claim form must be on file showing the eligible diagnosis for which the drugs are being prescribed. This form shows that the patient was under the care of a physician for the covered diagnosis when the prescription was issued. After a valid claim form has been accepted, it is not necessary for a new claim form to accompany each drug claim, as long as the patient is still under the doctor's care and the diagnosis is still valid. For example, if the diagnosis is of a chronic nature, drugs will often be refills of earlier prescriptions.
2. The pharmacy bill, receipt, or pharmacy statement for each prescription must accompany the request for payment.
3. All drug receipts or pharmacy bills must show the prescription number, the name of the physician, the name of the patient, the date of issuance, and the amount charged. If any of these items is omitted, check the validity of the prescription before paying the claim. Some receipts may also list the type of drug. This is helpful for determining whether the drug is a prescription drug or an over-the-counter drug.
4. The drugs must be appropriate for the condition being treated, the amount of time since the first diagnosis of the condition, and the amount of drug prescribed. For example, persons who are suffering from a serious heart disease or diabetes may require large amounts of drugs over an extended period of time, whereas a patient suffering from an ear infection requires a small amount of drugs over a much shorter period of time.

5. If prescriptions are questionable, obtain further information from the prescribing physician, not from the patient. The following scenarios are cause for review:
   a. The cost of the prescription expense or amount of medication prescribed is not appropriate to the condition being treated.
   b. The drugs are generally used to treat conditions that are not covered under the policy (e.g., exogenous obesity, male-pattern hair loss).
   c. The drugs are contraceptive medications. Since August 1, 2012, most new and renewed health plans have been required to cover these services without cost sharing for women across the country.
   d. Many prescription claims are submitted at one time. This may indicate that claims are being submitted for prescriptions that were issued to more than one person.
   e. The prescription or information on any claim appears to have been altered.
6. If a receipt or statement is received for more than one drug, take care to determine which drugs are covered and which are not. Often, several types appear on the same claim.
7. Check the plan provisions to determine which drugs are covered and which are not. Drugs issued for a noncovered diagnosis should be denied as not covered.

   EXAMPLE:
   Morphine is covered for heart surgery but not for cosmetic surgery.

8. Check the licensure of the prescribing doctor. In many states, physicians, dentists, podiatrists, and psychiatrists are allowed to prescribe medications. However, chiropractors, naturopaths, optometrists, and psychologists are not. These doctors may suggest or dispense nonprescription medications, food supplements, or vitamins, but as these items are not generally covered under the plan, no benefits would be payable. If the drug appears to be a prescription drug, but the person listed as the physician is not a physician, dentist, podiatrist, or psychiatrist, further investigation is warranted.
9. Finally, check the appropriate coverages for drug claims. Most prescription drugs are covered under Major Medical benefits and would be processed according to the general guidelines provided in the Major Medical plan. However, there may be specific plan provisions on medications. Take care to check the exclusions listed in the policy because this is usually where the exclusions to types of drugs and diagnoses are listed.

Coordination of Benefits

Both medical billers and claims examiners must be aware of the **coordination of benefits (COB)** process. The need for COB occurs when two or more plans provide coverage on the same person. Coordination between the two plans is necessary to allow for payment of 100% of the allowable expense but no more. This process was developed in response to a growing problem of overinsurance.

Overinsurance occurs when a person is covered under two or more policies and is eligible to collect an accumulation of benefits that actually exceeds the amount charged by the provider. The purpose of COB is to allow coverage and usually payment of 100% of allowable expenses without allowing the covered member or members to "make money" over and above the total costs for care. For example, imagine a patient has two insurance policies. The first will pay for everything except the copayment, deductible, or coinsurance. The second insurance will cover the copayment, deductible, and coinsurance, but cannot duplicate the payment already made by the first insurance company.

In response to the diversity of handling procedures used by various carriers and administrators in coordinating coverages, the National Association of Insurance Commissioners (NAIC) developed a standardized model for COB administration. Most benefit plans follow this model, but it is not mandatory. Therefore, you must check the plan provisions before you send or process COB claims, as the handling procedures may vary according to whether the NAIC guides are used.

Definitions

To process COB claims correctly, you must understand the following definitions:

Group plan: A form of coverage that allows coordination of benefits. A plan may be any of the following:

1. Group, blanket, or franchise insurance policy or plan if not individually underwritten.
2. HMO, hospital, or medical service prepayment policy available through an employer, union, or association.
3. Trustee policy or plan, union welfare policy or plan, multiple employer policy or plan, or employee benefit policy or plan.
4. Government programs (Medicare) or policies or plans required by a statute, except Medicaid or Medi-Cal.
5. "No-fault" auto policy or plan. (Applies to some plans only. The plan must specify whether or not this is applicable.)

Primary plan: The benefit plan that determines and pays its benefits first without regard to the existence of any other coverage.

Secondary plan: The plan that pays after the primary plan has paid its benefits. The secondary plan takes into consideration the benefits of the primary plan and may reduce its payment so that only 100% of allowable expenses are paid. A copy of the first insurance payment must be sent at the time of billing the second insurance.

Allowable expense: Any necessary, reasonable, and customary item of a medical or dental expense that is at least partly covered under at least one of the plans covering the claimant. Items that are excluded by the secondary plan, such as dental services and vision care services, are not considered allowable. However, the entire charge of amounts that are limited under the secondary plan are allowable. Consider the following examples:

1. Each plan provides a limit of $35 per visit for outpatient psychiatric care. The psychiatrist charges $50 per

visit. As both plans limit payment to $35 per visit, only $35 is considered an allowable expense under COB.
2. According to the primary plan's UCR guidelines, the amount allowable for surgery is $1,200. The secondary plan's UCR for the same surgery is $1,000. When coordinating benefits, the secondary plan would allow the greatest amount allowed by at least one of the plans. Therefore, the allowable amount when coordinating benefits would be $1,200. Bear in mind that this amount has nothing to do with how the secondary plan calculates its usual payment. The secondary insurance may not pay anything because the maximum is not met. You will see how the two amounts interact later.

Claim determination period: Usually a calendar year. It does not include any part of a year before the effective date of duplicate coverage under the secondary plan. It does not include any remaining amount during a calendar year after the termination date of the primary plan. As long as the secondary plan is not terminated, COB continues to be performed even though there are no longer multiple coverages.

Normal liability (NL): The amount payable under the secondary plan's provisions without regard to any other coverage (what would regularly have been paid if there were no other insurance). This is not necessarily the amount that will actually be paid.

EXAMPLE:
The secondary plan pays 80% of UCR after a $100 deductible. The first claim is paid as follows:

Charge	$200
Deductible	$100
Other insurance payment	$160
Secondary plan's NL	$80
Secondary plan's actual payment	$40

Credit reserve (CR): Also called benefit credit or credit savings, this is a cumulative amount within a claim determination period that is derived from the amount of funds that a plan has saved by being the secondary carrier. The credit reserve does not carry over from one calendar year to another. Each year, the balance begins at $0. A running total is kept for each separate determination period (calendar year).

EXAMPLE:
Same benefits as the preceding example.

Charge	$200
Deductible	$100
Other insurance payment	$100
Secondary plan's NL	$80
Secondary plan's actual payment	$40

CR = NL − AP, or $80 − $40 = $40 in savings.

Insular COB: COB applied separately to medical and dental charges. All savings are kept separately.

Global COB: COB applied to both medical and dental charges combined. All savings are kept intermingled.

EOB: An EOB letter from a payer indicates how a member's benefits have been applied in response to the submission of a claim for services. The EOB indicates deductibles, coinsurance amounts, nonallowable amounts, UCR limitations, and other pertinent information. An EOB is required by law to be generated on each claim submission showing the disposition of the claim (i.e., how it was paid, reason for denial, pending for additional information; see Figure 5-13 ●).

EXPLANATION OF BENEFITS

Today's Date

Payer's Name and Address

Aetna Insurance Company
P.O. Box 15999
New York, NY 12345

Provider's Name and Address

J.D. Mallard, M.D.
1933 East Frankford Road
Carrollton, TX 12345

This statement covers payments for the following patient(s):
Claim Detail Section (If there are numbers in the "REMARKS" column, see the Remarks Section for explanation)

Patient Name: Hughes, Patsy   **Patient Account Number:** Hugan0
Patient ID Number: **Insured's Name:** Andrew Hughes
Group Number: 55216
Provider Name: J.D. Mallard, M.D.   **Inventory Number:** 44562   **Claim Control Number:** 28971

Service Date(s)	Procedure	Charges	Adjustment	Allowed	Copay	Deduct/Not Covered	Coins	Paid Amt.	Provider Paid/Remarks
02/16/CCYY	97039	$50.00	$	$49.00	$0.00	$	$	80%	
02/16/CCYY	97042	65.00	65.00		0.00	00.00			
02/19/CCYY	97039	50.00		50.00	0.00			80%	
02/21/CCYY	97039	50.00		50.00		50.00		80%	03
TOTALS									

BALANCE DUE FROM PATIENT: PT'S DED/NOT COV $_____

PT'S COINS. $_____

03 Met Maximum Limit

PAYMENT SUMMARY SECTION (TOTALS)

Charges	Adjustment	Allowed	Copay	Deduct/Not Covered	Coins	Total Paid

Remarks: 03-Met Maximum Limit

FIGURE 5-13   Explanation of Benefits Form

TABLE 5-1 Order of Benefit Determination

Rule #	Description
1	The plan without a COB provision will be primary to a plan with a COB provision.
2	When a plan does not have OBD rules, and as a result the plans do not agree on the OBD, the plan without these OBD rules will determine the order of payment.
3	The plan that covers an individual as an employee will be primary to a plan that covers that individual as a dependent.
4	If an individual is an employee under two plans, the primary is the one under which the employee has been covered the longest.
5	If an employee is an active employee under one plan and a retiree (or laid off) under another, the active plan will pay as primary.
	**The parent birthday rule, explained in #6 and #7, affects the OBD for dependent children of parents who are living together and married (not divorced or legally separated).**
6	The plan of the parent whose birthday (based on month and day only) occurs first during the calendar year, is the primary plan.
7	When both parents' birthdays are the same (based on month and day), the plan that covered one parent the longest is the primary plan.
	**For dependents of legally separated or divorced parents and those whose parents have remarried, the order of benefits determination is based on the following rule:**
8	The plan of the parent specified as having legal responsibility for the healthcare expense of the child is the primary plan.
	**For dependents of separated parents with no court decree:**
9	The plan of the parent with custody is prime.
10	The plan of the step-parent (if any) with whom the child resides is secondary.
11	The plan of the natural parent without custody is tertiary.
12	The step-parent (if any) who does not reside with the child has no legal right to declare dependency. Therefore, no coordination should be performed because the child is probably not an eligible dependent under the plan.
13	For joint custody, with no additional responsibility designation, the plan of the parent whose coverage has been in effect the longest would be the primary payer. However, this rule may vary by administrator. Some parents pay costs on a 50/50 basis, thereby sharing equally in the healthcare risk.
14	A few rare plans do not use the birthday rule as previously described. These plans generally use the **gender rule**; which states that the plan covering the male employee is primary, and the plan covering the female employee is secondary.

Order of Benefit Determination Rules

The **Order of Benefit Determination (OBD) Rules** were established to provide standardized rules for coordination among health plans. Because each plan would prefer to pay as the secondary payer, it became necessary to develop rules to determine when a plan should pay as primary, secondary, or tertiary.

The 14 rules determining the order of payment are the OBD rules (see Table 5-1 ●).

ACTIVITY #2

Coordination of Benefits

1. Define COB. _____
   _____

2. What is the purpose of COB? _____
   _____

3. The _____ is the benefit plan that determines and pays its benefits first without regard to the existence of any other coverage.

4. The _____ is the plan that pays after the primary plan has paid its benefits.

Right to Receive and Release Information

Certain information is needed about a member's policy in order to determine and apply the appropriate COB rules. Plan representatives have the right to decide which facts are required and to obtain the needed facts from, or give the facts to, any other organization. The plan should get the insured's consent to do this. In addition, each person claiming benefits under a plan must give the facts required to properly process a claim. It is also important to realize that most providers of care do not release any information to a payer without a signed release from the member. Information should be requested or released to others only when absolutely necessary to determine benefits under the plan. The unnecessary request or release of information is a violation of the patient's right to privacy, which is punishable by law. Therefore, request only what is necessary, and routinely request a written authorization from the member to release information.

Right of Recovery

If the amount of the payments made by the plan is more than the plan should have paid under the COB provision, the plan may recover the excess from one or more of the following:

1. The person or persons it has paid or on behalf of whom it has paid.
2. Other insurers/plans.
3. Other organizations.

The "amount of the payments made" includes the reasonable cash value of any benefits provided in the form of services.

PRACTICE **PITFALLS**

The following guidelines on allowable expenses and COB may be helpful to you:

- The difference between the cost of a private and a semiprivate hospital room is not considered an allowable expense unless the patient's stay in a private room was medically necessary, either as generally accepted medical practice or as specifically defined in the plan.
- Items of expense under coverages such as dental care, vision care, prescription drug, or hearing aid programs may be excluded from the definition of allowable expense. A plan that provides only benefits for such items may limit its definition of allowable expense to like items.
- A medical plan may have COB with medical expenses only, and a dental-only plan may limit COB to other dental plans only.
- An item of expense covered under the primary plan may be considered an allowable expense under the secondary plan, even though that plan does not provide such a benefit. For example, if the primary plan covers routine examinations and the secondary plan excludes routine examinations, routine exams may be considered an allowable expense by the secondary carrier in this instance.
- The COB rule varies widely from payer to payer. As previously indicated, some payers do not consider excluded expenses to be allowable; others do. Therefore, you must verify the COB provisions and administrative handling rules. (Remember that we are talking about the amount considered as an allowable expense under COB, not the amount used to determine the secondary plan's normal liability.)

Health Maintenance Organizations

An HMO is a type of prepayment plan in which providers agree to charge members for their services according to a fixed schedule of rates. The HMO member (insured) usually pays a specified copayment at the time the service is rendered. The patient and the doctor usually are not involved in completing the claim forms for submission to a payer. Instead, the HMO is billed directly, or the HMO pays a monthly retainer fee (capitation) to the physician for membership plus other specified fees.

If the required medical services are available through the HMO but the insured does not go to an HMO provider for the treatment, he or she may be held entirely responsible for all the expenses.

Prepayment plans are included in the definition of the type of policies to which COB provisions apply. Many HMOs do not have COB provisions, although more are starting to incorporate the COB concept because of the spiraling costs of medical care.

An example of an HMO is Kaiser Permanente. Kaiser provides a prepayment policy for hospital and professional medical services at no cost or for a small fee, as long as the member goes to a Kaiser facility. Subsequently, the HMO provides the member with a "reasonable cost statement," which represents the amount that would have been charged to a nonmember. If the HMO does not have the COB provision, the HMO is considered the primary payer. To coordinate benefits, a request must be made for receipts or statements showing the actual "out-of-pocket" expense. The secondary plan will pay no more than the amount that is considered the allowable expense. If the HMO does have a COB provision, the regular OBD rules should be applied.

Preferred Provider Organizations

As previously described, PPOs have special arrangements in which members are responsible for expenses according to specific contractual UCR arrangements. Some services may be covered at a higher rate than others, and some may not be covered at all. Usually, COB will apply to PPO claims. The main difference between going to a regular provider and going to an out-of-network provider is reflected in the patient's liability. That is, if the member goes to a PPO (in-network) provider, the member is not responsible for any amounts in excess of the PPO contractual UCR amount.

In addition, depending on the payer, the plan, and the PPO, the secondary payer may not be held responsible for any amounts that exceed the contractual PPO amount, even though the secondary payer is not a party to the contract. This handling is based on the premise that if the member is not responsible for anything over the PPO rate, then neither is the secondary plan. Once again, this handling varies among plans.

A PPO's EOB usually specifically states the member's responsibility. By referring to the appropriate field on the EOB, the secondary carrier can tell what amount to use to determine the allowable expense. Anything in excess of the patient's liability amount is not considered allowable.

If the member does go to a non-PPO (out-of-network) provider, the member is responsible for all the charges, including the amounts in excess of the primary plan's UCR. In addition, most plans penalize their members for not going to PPO providers by reducing the plan's payment (e.g., the coinsurance percentage paid by the plan is reduced from 80% to 70%, or even lower). An exception to this rule is when the member is traveling outside the United States for business or pleasure. In this case, eligible expenses for medically necessary emergency and urgent care services are covered at the in-network level. Other medically necessary care is covered at the out-of-network level.

TRICARE

TRICARE (formerly CHAMPUS) provides a comprehensive program of healthcare benefits for active duty and retired services personnel, their dependents, and the dependents of deceased military personnel. TRICARE is secondary to all other insurance or health policies except Medicaid and TRI-CARE supplemental insurance. However, because many services are provided free of charge or for only a minimal fee, many examiners never see a TRICARE EOB.

ACTIVITY #3

Health Maintenance Organizations

1. What is a PPO? _____
   _____
2. What does HMO stand for, and what is an HMO? ___
   _____
3. What is TRICARE? _____
   _____

▶ **CRITICAL THINKING QUESTION:** Given the option, why would a person choose an HMO over a PPO, or vice versa?

Recognizing the Presence of Dual Coverage

The following two examples deal with the possibility that a claimant has dual coverage:

1. The greatest likelihood of dual coverage occurs when the spouse is employed. Claim forms usually request the name of the employee's spouse and the name and address of the spouse's employer. The claim form defines what is meant by other group insurance and asks the claimant to designate which type of other insurance exists.
2. Even when the claimant states that there is no other coverage, additional inquiries should be made in some cases:

   - The claim involves a married employee or his or her dependents. Often the spouse also has group coverage on the family.
   - The claim form indicates that the spouse is not employed. The spouse may have extended benefits or COBRA under the policy held by the spouse's previous employer.
   - The claim is for a dependent child, but the area on the form requesting other insurance information has been left blank.
   - Notations on the hospital bills or claim papers show that some other insurer or plan has paid benefits or that there is other employment within the family.
   - The claimant does not assign hospital benefits. This may indicate that the claimant has used other benefits to pay the provider and thus does not want a duplicate payment to be made (to the provider).
   - It is known from a group's local sources that a patient is covered under another plan.
   - Photocopies of bills are submitted. Usually, the original is submitted as part of the claim and the member

keeps a copy. If copies are submitted, the originals may have been submitted to another payer.
   - The provider charges for the completion of a claim form, but the submitted form was not received from the provider. The charge may have been for completing a form for another payer.
   - Requests for information are received from other policyholders, plans, or insurers.
   - The occupation of the claimant, spouse, or dependent suggests that he or she may have coverage through a union or other professional affiliation.
   - A hospital or surgeon's bill refers to other coverage.
   - A bill shows a substantial credit or adjustment to the account.
   - The claim submitted is the first maternity bill for the subscriber's spouse. In such a case, the wife may have been regularly employed until her pregnancy, and she may have benefits through the extension of benefits provision of her previous policy.
   - The claim is submitted on another carrier's claim form, or an EOB is attached.
   - A duplicate coverage inquiry is received. This is an industry-approved form designed to establish the existence of other coverage.
   - An HMO requests reimbursement for the value of service provided to one of their patients.
   - Claim history shows that COB payments or secondary carrier payments were made in the past, but claims are now being paid as primary with no explanation.

You may pursue the details pertaining to other coverage through a variety of sources. If the claim form indicates that the insured's spouse is employed and includes the name and address of the spouse's employer, contact that employer to determine whether there is other group coverage. If the claim form does not indicate the name and address of the spouse's employer, request the missing information from the subscriber.

Additional sources of information regarding the existence of dual coverage include

- Files from hospital admissions.
- City directories listing members of a family, their occupations, and places of employment.
- Information cards compiled by the Benefits Office for local employer plans.

ACTIVITY #4

Dual Coverage

1. True or False: A plan without a COB provision is secondary to a plan with a COB provision. _____
2. Define Global COB. _____
   _____
3. _____ applies separately to medical and dental charges. All savings are kept separate.

COB Worksheet

The COB worksheet is used to help calculate the proper benefits when there is COB between more than one health plan. Figure 5-14 ● is a sample COB worksheet. To begin, calculate the allowable amount that would be paid on this claim if there was no other insurance. Then, follow the instructions on the bottom of the COB Calculation Worksheet.

Coordination of Benefits Calculation Worksheet

Patient's Name: _____   Year: _____

Payment Calculation:

1. Total allowable amount for this claim is the higher of either the primary plan's allowable amount or the secondary plan's allowable amount.   _____

2. Total primary insurance carrier payment for this claim.   _____

3. Difference between Line 1 and Line 2.   _____

4. Secondary insurance carrier's normal liability for this claim.   _____

5. The lesser of Line 3 or Line 4.
   This is the amount of the secondary insurance carrier actual payment on this claim.   _____

Credit Reserve:

6. Normal liability for this claim (Line 4 above).   _____

7. Actual payment for this claim (Line 5 above).   _____

8. Subtract Line 7 from Line 6.   _____

9. Credit reserve on all previous claims for this patient.   _____

10. Total credit reserve (add Line 8 and Line 9).   _____

Instructions:
Place the patient's name and the year that services were rendered in the box on the top of the COB calculation sheet.
1. Enter the total allowable amount on this claim. The total allowable amount is the greater of either the primary plan's allowable amount or the secondary plan's allowable amount.
2. Enter the total amount that other insurance companies have paid on this claim.
3. Subtract Line 2 from Line 1.
4. Enter the normal liability amount for this insurance company for this claim.
5. Enter the lesser of either Line 3 or Line 4. This is the actual amount of the secondary insurance payer on this claim.

To Calculate Credit Reserve:
6. Enter the normal liability amount for the secondary insurance carrier for this claim.
7. Enter the actual payment for the secondary insurance carrier for this claim.
8. Subtract Line 7 from Line 6. This is the amount of money the secondary carrier has saved by paying secondary on this claim. This amount becomes part of the credit reserve.
9. Enter the credit reserve amount for all previous claims for this patient.
10. Add Line 8 and Line 9. This is the total credit reserve for this patient.

FIGURE 5-14   COB Worksheet

Adjustments

An **adjustment** in the medical billing world is really a write-off. For a claims examiner, it is the reprocessing of a claim to correct prior errors. Although the terminology may vary from company to company, the concepts behind each type are basically the same. There are four basic types of adjustments:

1. *Statistical Adjustment*—An adjustment that changes the claim data (e.g., procedure coding, type of benefit paid, diagnosis) but does not increase or decrease the original claim payment.
2. *Supplemental Adjustment*—An adjustment that increases the original claim payment. A statistical adjustment is often also involved (but not always), as the original claim coding may have caused the incorrect payment.
3. *Full-Credit Adjustment*—An adjustment that completely reverses a claim payment because the original submission should not have been paid at all.
4. *Partial-Credit Adjustment*—An adjustment that partially reverses a claim payment. The original claim was overpaid.

Statistical Adjustment

A **statistical adjustment** changes claim data but does not increase or decrease the claim payment. As the name implies, this type of adjustment is required to correct historical data only. The original payment is not affected by the corrected data.

The following are some of the more common reasons for requiring a statistical adjustment:

1. The claim was processed under an incorrect member identification (ID) number.
2. The claim was processed under the correct ID number but on an incorrect claimant.
3. The claim payment was issued to an incorrect provider of service. The provider's tax ID number or social security number was entered incorrectly, or a totally wrong provider was paid. If the provider paid was in the same medical group, a statistical adjustment may be sufficient. However, if a completely separate and unaffiliated provider was paid, a full-credit adjustment is probably required with a new payment issued to the correct provider.
4. The payment was the correct amount but the claim was processed under an incorrect group number.
5. The claim was erroneously denied; charges should have been applied to the deductible. (No payment will be made even when the claim is processed correctly.)
6. Charges were applied to the deductible but should have been denied.

Supplemental Adjustment

A **supplemental adjustment** is performed to increase an original claim payment. Often, a supplemental adjustment is required because the original claim was coded incorrectly. Therefore, a statistical adjustment is usually involved, but the changes usually result in a payment or an additional payment.

The following are some of the more common reasons why a supplemental adjustment may be required:

1. The original claim was erroneously denied when benefits should have been paid.
2. Charges were applied to the deductible in error; benefits should have been paid. This situation usually occurs when the deductible applies to specific types of expenses, but not to all types.
3. Some benefits were paid, but additional benefits should have been paid.
4. Late charges are received.
5. Corrected billing or other information is received.
6. The claims examiner or adjuster applied incorrect benefits.
7. The examiner coded the diagnosis or procedure incorrectly, thus causing an incorrect UCR allowance or other limitation.

Whenever an underpayment is found, an adjustment should be performed for the corrected amount. Either a letter or full explanation on the new EOB should be sent to the proper parties.

Full-Credit Adjustment

A **full-credit adjustment** completely reverses the original claim payment. Usually, this type of adjustment is not performed until the original monies paid out have been returned in full to the payer. When an incorrect provider is paid and the money is returned, many companies consider this to be a full-credit adjustment with a subsequent payment remitted to the correct provider. Regardless of whether a subsequent corrected payment is issued, the original payment is received back in the claims office and is reversed in the system. The following are some reasons why full-credit adjustments may be required:

1. A duplicate claim is received and paid in error.
2. The member is not eligible for benefits under the plan.
3. Claim benefits are paid incorrectly, or the benefits paid did not adhere to plan limitations.
4. An incorrect provider is paid who is unaffiliated with the correct provider of service.

Partial-Credit Adjustment

A **partial-credit adjustment** partially reverses a claim payment. In this case, part of the original payment is correct and part is incorrect. The following are common reasons that partial-credit adjustments are performed:

1. A greater payment was made on a claim than should have been made according to the plan provisions and limitations.
2. The claims examiner applied benefits incorrectly by performing incorrect coding, duplication of payment, inappropriate application of benefits, or some other error.

Collecting Overpayments

Even the best claims examiners make errors. When this happens, an overpayment of benefits may occur. Under most circumstances, every attempt should be made to recover overpayments when they are discovered. Most insurance companies have a standard adjustment form letter to send the member in order to inform them of an adjustment to their claim; see Figure 5-15 ● for an example. However, there are

Any Insurance Carrier, Inc.
123 Any Drive
Anywhere, USA 12345
(800) 555-1234

Dear Member:

An error was inadvertently made during the processing of your claim. The attached explanation of benefits shows the corrected payment amount.

The reason for the adjustment is:

☐ Incorrect deductible taken.
☐ Allowed amount figured improperly.
☐ Benefits are not allowed for this procedure.
☐ Incorrect coinsurance amount was applied.
☐ The patient was listed incorrectly.
☐ Other: _____

_____
_____

The following action will be taken to correct this error:

An underpayment was previously made on your claim.
☐ A check is enclosed for $_____ .
☐ Benefits were assigned on this claim. A check in the amount of $_____ has been forwarded to the provider of services.

An overpayment was previously made on your claim and a check was issued to you.
☐ Please remit payment of $_____to our office immediately.
☐ Payment will be subtracted from our next payment to you.

An overpayment was previously made on your claim. Benefits were assigned on this claim and therefore payment was made to the provider of services. Your provider may bill you for amounts refunded to us.
☐ A request for repayment had been sent to your provider.
☐ Payment will be subtracted from your next payment to this provider.
☐ Other: _____

_____

We are sorry for any inconvenience this may have caused.

Sincerely,

FIGURE 5-15 Adjustment Form Letter

times when the recovery of overpayments is not feasible or cost effective. The following are guidelines only for situations in which overpayment recovery should not be attempted:

- The overpayment is under $25.
- The overpayment occurred more than 12 months ago and is under $200.
- The claimant is deceased and the overpayment is under $200.

There are normally three ways to recover an overpayment.

1. Deduct the overpayment from the future benefits for the family member for whom the overpayment occurred. You cannot deduct an overpayment on one family member's claim from benefits that are due on another family member's claim unless specifically requested to do so by the insured and confirmed in writing. It is not necessary to obtain permission to deduct benefits for the member for whom the overpayment occurred, but advise the claimant of the circumstances of the overpayment and the method that will be used for recoupment.
2. Have the insured make a lump sum payment or establish a payment plan to recoup the overpayment.
3. Obtain reimbursement from a third party, usually another carrier when COB is involved.

   Remember that benefits cannot be taken from charges that have been assigned to the provider of services. When a refund is received or offered, accept or pursue all such refunds, regardless of the amount of overpayment or the time that has elapsed since the overpayment occurred.

ACTIVITY #5

COB Worksheet

1. List the four basic types of adjustments.

    a. _____

    b. _____

    c. _____

    d. _____

2. A _____ adjustment changes claim data but does not increase or decrease a claim payment.
3. A _____ adjustment is performed to increase an original claim payment.
4. A _____ adjustment reverses the original claim payment.
5. A _____ adjustment partially reverses a claim payment.

ACTIVITY #6

COB Calculation Worksheet

Directions: Using the following information, complete a COB calculation worksheet for each of the cases. Worksheets are provided in Appendix B.

1. Patient's Name: Betty Bossy. Year: CCYY. Total submitted expenses: $1,600.

    Primary plan, A, considers the allowable amount to be $1,450 and has made a payment of $1,160 on this claim. Secondary plan, B, considers the allowable amount to be $1,495. Both calculate benefits at 80%. Neither plan has made any previous payments or had any previous allowable amounts. Prior credit reserve amount is $487.

2. Patient's Name: Danny Dingbat. Year: CCYY. Total submitted expenses: $1,200. Primary plan, A, considers the allowable amount to be $1,000 and has made a payment of $800 on this claim. Secondary plan, B, considers the allowable amount to be $1,200. Both calculate benefits at 80%. Prior credit reserve amount is $595.

3. Patient's Name: Patty P. Patient. Year: CCYY. Total submitted expenses: $1,400. Primary plan, A, considers the allowable amount to be $1,400 and has made a payment of $1,120 on this claim. Secondary plan, B, considers the allowable amount to be $1,200. Plan A calculates benefits at 80%. Plan B limits payment to 50% of the allowable amount up to a calendar year maximum of $500; $450 has already been paid. Prior credit reserve amount is $740.

CHAPTER REVIEW

Summary

- The claims examiner has many important responsibilities.
- By applying basic guidelines, the examiner will establish a practice that will enable him or her routinely to make clear and concise claim decisions.
- Coordination of benefits is necessary to ensure that when charges are covered by more than one carrier, the total payment does not exceed 100% of the bill.

- These guidelines should be considered whenever there is the possibility of dual coverage or a third-party payer.
- Learn to identify the possible existence of another payer by applying guidelines and rules.
- Remember that most adjustments affect the monies that the subscribers, members, or providers receive. Adjustments are always a sensitive situation. Therefore, always be sure that an adjustment is necessary and that it is performed correctly so that a second or third adjustment is not required.

- Follow the procedures established by the payer for handling adjustments, and give the affected parties adequate notification.
- Failure to follow such procedures significantly increases the likelihood of subsequent ill will or legal action. If in doubt, request assistance before making an adjustment.

Review Questions

Directions: Answer the following questions after reviewing the information presented in this chapter. Write your answers in the space provided.

1. If the claim cannot be processed upon receipt, the claim file must be

_____

_____

2. Referrals should be made for which three types of claims?

a. _____

b. _____

c. _____

3. What is electronic claims submission? _____

_____

4. Briefly explain the pended claim follow-up procedure. __

_____

_____

_____

5. Why is it important to update payment history? _____

_____

If you were unable to answer any of these questions, refer back to that section and then fill in the answers.

ACTIVITY #7

Find the Terms

Directions: Find and circle the words listed in this activity. Words can appear horizontally, vertically, diagonally, forward, or backward.

```
C  R  F  A  E  V  X  M  O  K  L  K  D  L  W  C  R  C  R  T  R  M
H  R  Z  M  L  W  P  L  T  G  W  O  M  L  H  R  W  L  P  U  U  O
C  D  M  O  X  L  O  Z  D  I  C  D  U  F  T  E  X  T  X  K  B  A
C  S  O  M  B  L  O  C  Z  U  M  N  Z  J  O  D  V  O  I  T  K  W
T  X  U  G  F  Y  R  W  M  R  S  J  W  X  S  I  I  I  E  M  R  N
W  L  Q  H  W  C  J  E  A  M  N  X  X  E  N  T  R  M  F  P  Z  U
Q  R  C  V  R  C  N  R  Y  B  W  E  L  T  N  R  H  I  V  F  O  N
J  V  P  G  Z  T  O  R  G  E  L  K  Y  F  P  E  V  D  K  S  N  G
Y  Y  Q  U  A  V  S  D  Y  Q  N  E  Z  O  H  S  D  Y  Q  M  K  W
U  O  C  T  M  E  W  W  H  P  F  A  E  G  I  E  G  A  O  D  X  E
E  G  I  X  F  N  K  Z  O  F  N  M  L  X  S  R  W  L  L  D  F  L
S  O  S  G  A  A  U  F  Z  C  E  E  Q  P  P  V  D  N  N  Y  M  U
N  E  C  N  A  R  U  S  N  I  R  E  V  O  Y  E  E  V  N  S  S  R
T  O  L  F  M  W  I  J  P  A  Y  X  J  L  D  R  N  R  A  X  R  R
M  Q  L  E  W  Z  A  V  C  D  U  V  D  M  D  V  A  S  D  R  G  E
S  T  A  T  I  S  T  I  C  A  L  A  D  J  U  S  T  M  E  N  T  D
U  P  E  H  K  S  R  H  U  O  U  X  W  A  L  Y  C  M  I  V  Q  N
K  M  J  S  G  T  X  L  W  D  P  M  N  G  J  I  Y  K  X  R  V  E
J  K  I  R  R  F  V  K  A  Z  N  T  X  S  O  I  K  Q  O  H  P  G
V  P  F  P  F  W  I  C  R  W  Q  K  I  P  O  L  B  A  P  S  F  R
I  P  Q  T  N  U  T  H  O  J  K  L  Y  R  I  M  K  Q  K  N  X  R
V  A  T  C  D  P  O  D  P  R  A  W  N  R  Z  G  Q  R  I  Q  P  B
```

1. Allowable Expense
2. Credit Reserve
3. Documentation
4. Gender Rule
5. Overinsurance
6. Primary Plan
7. Statistical Adjustment
8. TRICARE

ACTIVITY #8

Matching

Directions: Match the following terms with the proper definition by writing the letter of the correct definition in the space next to the term.

1. _____ Assignment of Benefits
2. _____ Claim Determination Period
3. _____ Claim Investigation
4. _____ Coordination of Benefits
5. _____ Explanation of Benefits
6. _____ Full-Credit Adjustment
7. _____ Order of Benefit Determination Rules
8. _____ Partial-Credit Adjustment
9. _____ Supplemental Adjustment

a. A letter from a payer, indicating how a member's benefits have been applied.

b. An adjustment that increases the original claim payment.

c. An adjustment that completely reverses a claim payment.

d. An adjustment that partially reverses a claim payment.

e. Fourteen rules determining the order of payment.

f. A process that occurs when two or more group plans provide coverage on the same person, intended to prevent the insured from making money from an illness or injury.

g. A period in which COB is determined, usually a calendar year.

h. Making a detailed inquiry to verify facts pertaining to a submitted claim.

i. A statement, usually included on the claim form, which permits the member to authorize the administrator to pay benefits directly to the person or institution that provided the service.

Physician's, Clinical, and Hospital Services Claims

After completing this chapter, you will be able to:

Demonstrate the ability to correctly code evaluation and management services.

Explain the service covered in the Medicine section of the CPT manual.

Describe modifiers used with evaluation and management and medicine CPT codes.

Discuss how to code X-ray and laboratory services.

Explain how the Radiology section of the CPT is arranged.

Identify modifiers appropriate for use with Radiology CPT codes.

Recognize CPT codes used to describe pathology and laboratory services.

Outline how component charges are calculated.

Discuss modifiers appropriate for use with pathology (lab) CPT codes.

Discuss common types of hospital services.

Keywords and concepts you will learn in this chapter:

Acupuncture
Air Ambulance
Alternative Birthing Centers (ABCs)
Ambulance Expenses
Ambulatory Surgical Centers (ASCs) (also called surgi-centers)
Ancillary Expenses
Biofeedback
Computed Tomography (CT) Scan
Consultation
Convalescent Facilities
Custodial Care
Day Care Centers
Diagnostic Charges
Diagnostic X-rays
Dialysis
Durable Medical Equipment (DME)
Emergency Medical Technicians (EMTs)
Facility Services
Hospice Care
Hospital Services
Inpatient Care
Laboratory Examinations
Medical Management

Explain the use of the UB-04 billing form. ●

Identify ambulance services charges. ●

Describe durable medical equipment (DME) billing codes. ●

Identify types of durable medical equipment. ●

Identify common criteria for equipment covered under the DME provisions. ●

Medically Oriented Equipment
Miscellaneous Services
Mobile Intensive Care Unit
Necessity
Night Care Centers
Nuclear Medicine
Nursing Homes
Office or Other Outpatient Visits
Ophthalmology Care
Orthoptics
Osteopathic Treatment
Outpatient
Panel Tests
Papanicolaou or "Pap" Smear
Paramedics
Personal Items
Physical Medicine
Professional Component
Professional Services
Prosthetic Devices
Radiation Oncology
Reasonableness
Rehabilitation Facilities
Speech Therapy
Stat Fees
Take-Home Prescriptions
Technical Component
Telemetry Charges
Ultrasonography
Urgent Care Center
Van Transportation Units
X-rays

The most common services billed by a physician are office and hospital visits. This chapter reviews and discusses some specific physician's services and basic guidelines and coverage for these services. There are three basic categories of medical services:

1. Professional services
   a. Surgical
   b. Nonsurgical

2. Facility services

3. Miscellaneous services

Professional services are performed by a licensed individual, such as a medical doctor, physician's assistant, advanced nurse practitioner, or chiropractor. **Facility services** are provided at a "place"—for example, a hospital or clinic. Equipment usage and room fees (e.g., X-ray equipment, operating room) are considered facility expenses.

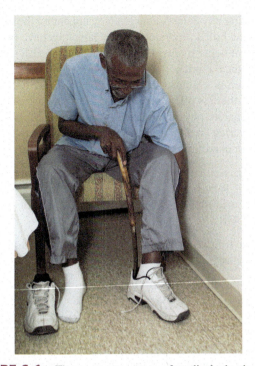

FIGURE 6-1   There are many types of medical adaptive devices including the stocking holder being used here
Source: Pat Watson/Pearson Education/PH College

TABLE 6-1 Evaluation and Management Codes

Office or Other Outpatient Services	99201–99215
Hospital Observation Services	99217-99226
Hospital Inpatient Services	99221-99239
Consultations	99241-99255
Emergency Department Services	99281-99288
Critical Care Services	99291-99292
Nursing Facility Services	99304-99318
Domiciliary, Rest Home, or Custodial Care Services	99324-99337
Home Services	99341-99350
Prolonged Services	99354-99360
Case Management Services	99363-99368
Care Plan Oversight Services	99374-99380
Preventive Medicine Services	99381-99429
Non-Face-to-Face Physician Services	99441-99444
Special E/M Services	99450-99456
Newborn Care Services	99460-99480
Other Evaluation and Management Services	99499

Miscellaneous services are all other types of services not included in the first two categories. For example, prescriptions, medical equipment (e.g., wheelchairs, crutches), and ambulance charges are all considered to be miscellaneous types of expenses. (See Figure 6-1 ●.)

Coding Evaluation and Management

In this chapter we will discuss each of the sections of the CPT® and any guidelines for that section. Refer to the CPT for additional information.

The first section of the CPT includes the 99201–99499 series of codes for evaluation and management (E/M) of a patient. (See Table 6-1 ●.) The Medicine section of the CPT is usually found toward the back of the book and includes codes 90281–99602.

Office or Other Outpatient Services (99201–99215)

This section is used to report **office visits** or other encounters between a physician and patient that occur outside a hospital setting.

There are different codes for new and established patients. In general, codes for new patients (99201–99205) carry a higher unit value because the physician is expected to spend additional time completing initial paperwork on the patient and performing a more in-depth history and physical than for a returning patient. Because of this difference, medical billers and claims examiners should determine whether a patient has previously seen the physician before they process a claim for a new patient. A new patient is one who has not received any

services from this provider, or from another provider of the same specialty and subspecialty who belongs to the same group practice, for the last three years. If the patient sees a provider who is on call or is covering for another provider, the patient is classified as he or she would be for the "regular" provider who is not available (i.e., the one being covered for).

Hospital Observation Services (99217–99226, 99234–99236)

These codes denote that the patient was kept in the hospital "for observation." This situation generally happens when there is a chance that the patient's condition may worsen and the doctor wants to be sure that immediate medical help is available if that should happen. The first set of codes is for initial episodes of observation encounters. Codes 99224–99226 are for subsequent episodes of observation encounters. Subsequent encounters include reviewing the medical record, results of diagnostic studies, and changes in the patient's condition since the last assessment.

Hospital Inpatient Services (99221–99239)

Hospital inpatient services are visits that a patient makes during the course of a hospital stay. These visits are billed separately from other hospital charges.

An initial hospital visit is the first encounter with the patient by the admitting physician. Everything after this first visit is classified as a subsequent visit, regardless of whether the additional visit is performed by the admitting physician or by a different physician.

If a physician performs admit services at a location other than the hospital (e.g., his office), this information should be reported with the claim.

Consultations (99241–99255)

Usually, a **consultation** is provided by a specialist who has been requested to provide an opinion only. The consultation can be done either for an outpatient (99241–99245) or inpatient (99251–99255). The specialist examines the patient at the request of another physician. He or she may request diagnostic services and may make therapeutic recommendations to the referring physician. However, the specialist does not usually take over the day-to-day treatment or management of the patient. In fact, in order for the visit to qualify as a consultation, the consulting physician cannot be responsible for the regular management of the patient.

If the physician subsequently assumes responsibility for the routine care of the patient, the services should be coded as visits, not consultations, even if they are billed as consultations. (The initial visit could be billed as a consultation.) If the consultant continues to see the patient in addition to the regular attending physician, 99231–99233 should be used for inpatient and outpatient codes.

Modifier -32 is used to indicate that the consultation is rendered at the request of a third party (e.g., the insurer).

Confirmatory Consultations

A **second opinion or confirmatory consultation** is designed as a benefit to the patient by confirming the need for surgeries that have a reputation for being done needlessly. Chapter 5 described SSO Consultations, which provide 100% payment on services provided by a second, independent specialist whom the patient consults before scheduling an elective, non-emergency surgery. Normally, for an SSO Consultation benefit to be payable, the following requirements must be satisfied:

1. The second or third opinion physician must be totally uninvolved with the original recommending physician. Therefore, he or she cannot be part of the same medical group and will often be picked by the administrator, medical management firm, or payer.
2. The consultation must be completed before the surgery is scheduled.
3. The second opinion physician cannot perform the recommended surgery.

Depending on the plan, failure to obtain an SSO Consultation may result in the following penalties:

1. Denial of all charges for the surgery and related services.
2. Application of a special, reduced coinsurance. For instance, instead of paying 80% of the allowed amount, the plan may pay only 50%.
3. No change of benefits. In this case, the SSO Consultation is considered to be a benefit for the member and there is no penalty for noncompliance.

> ▶ **CRITICAL THINKING QUESTION:** Why are insurance companies so willing to pay for an SSO Consultation when normally they are looking for ways to cut expenses?

Emergency Department Services (99281–99288)

When a patient goes to the outpatient or emergency department of a hospital, a physician is usually in attendance who has a contract to provide professional care at the facility. The

contracting physician's charges may appear on the hospital bill or may be billed separately. Many hospitals have two types of outpatient departments: the emergency room (ER), and outpatient medical clinics.

When a claim is received from a hospital for clinic charges, there is often a room charge for the use of the facility and a separate physician charge. The coding of these types of claims varies greatly from payer to payer; however, there are two main handling procedures:

1. CPT services are coded separately and are subject to UCR fees.
2. Generic or UB-04 codes are used and are not subject to UCR.

The following rules provide some common handling suggestions:

1. If a hospital is billing for professional component charges separately from the actual lab or X-ray charges, combine the two together because they represent one total service.
2. Physician treatment charges (professional fees) may be coded separately from other fees. How they are coded depends on whether the payer is cost conscious. If they are coded separately, the charge is usually subject to UCR, whereas if they are not coded separately, the charge will not be subject to UCR.
3. **Stat fees**, a charge for DXL services performed on an expedited priority basis, should also be combined with the actual laboratory or X-ray charges.

These guidelines vary from payer to payer, so be sure to verify the procedures.

If the patient in a hospital wants to have his or her regular physician in attendance and the physician is called in from outside the hospital to provide services, use code 99056. If the patient visits the outpatient clinic of a facility, use regular office visit coding, as a clinic is conceptually the same as an office. That is, in a clinic the same doctors see the same patients, visits are scheduled the same way as in the office, and the treatment provided is the same as what would be provided in an office. In essence, the physician is using the facility as his or her office.

For ER services, the facility must accept emergency patients 24 hours a day, seven days a week. No distinction is made between the first visit and subsequent visits. If the care provided is critical, then the critical care CPT codes should be used, rather than the ER codes.

Critical Care Services (99291–99292)

Critical care involves the care of critically ill patients during a medical emergency that requires the constant attention of the provider. The coding in this section is time-dependent. The first 30–74 minutes are coded as 99291. Each additional 30-minute segment is coded as 99292. Critical care services include the monitoring of the patient. Additional services, such as suturing lacerations, setting fractures, or most other procedures, are reported and allowed separately from the critical care services.

Nursing Facility Services (99304–99318)

These codes are used to report services in nursing facilities, intermediate care facilities, long-term care facilities, or psychiatric facilities.

A patient may be transferred from an inpatient hospital to a nursing facility for supervised care when the patient no longer requires the skill levels of the inpatient hospital. Patients may also come directly from their homes or any other environment.

If a patient is admitted to the nursing facility after receiving services in the physician's office or hospital emergency room, all E/M services are considered inclusive in that visit. No separate allowance is made for an additional E/M at the skilled nursing facility.

Except for hospital discharge services, any E/M provided on the same day as admission to the nursing facility (whether it is provided at the facility or at a different location) is considered to be the initial admission evaluation.

Domiciliary, Rest Home, or Custodial Care Services (99324–99337)

Custodial care is primarily performed to meet the personal daily needs of the patient and can be provided by personnel without medical care skills or training. Custodial care includes assistance with walking, bathing, dressing, eating, and other activities. Skilled nursing personnel are not required for this nonmedical type of care, which is commonly referred to as "meeting the daily living needs" of the patient. Most plans do not provide coverage for these types of services and for those that do, payment is very limited. If it is not clear whether care is custodial, request copies of the provider's nursing notes or the admission and discharge reports.

Home Services (99341–99350)

These codes are used to bill for services provided to a patient in his or her home. Home services are often provided in lieu of hospitalization. For example, a patient who has suffered a heart attack may need extensive bed rest, with medications provided once or twice a day. If a nurse visits the home to provide the medications, there may be no need to hospitalize the patient.

Codes 99341–99350 are used by physicians to report E/M procedures that are provided in the private residence of the patient. These services are considered Medicare Part B services. Plans will often cover this type of care, especially if it represents an overall cost savings.

Prolonged Services (99354–99360)

These codes are used to bill for prolonged or standby service that is beyond the usual service for inpatient or outpatient services. The service must last at least 30 minutes before it is considered a prolonged service. These codes are reported in addition to the original service. Services which involve face-to-face contact are coded according to the amount of time the provider spent with the patient, regardless of whether that time is continuous or not (e.g., a physician may check in on his or her patient several times during a day). Keep in mind that these codes must first meet the highest E/M code criteria to be used.

Code 99360 is used to report physician stand-by service (e.g., operative standby, standby for frozen section, high-risk delivery).

Case Management Services (99363–99368)

These codes are used to bill for coordinating or managing healthcare services and for team conferences or phone calls made by a provider in the treatment of a patient. These services can include consulting with other providers, coordinating the patient's care with other professionals who are assigned to the patient (e.g., nurses, therapists), and contacting other medical professionals in any way regarding the care of the patient.

Codes 99363 and 99364 are used to bill for anticoagulation management. For example, when a physician orders a PT/INR lab to check the level of a patient taking Coumadin (an anticoagulant medication). The results come from the lab and the physician reviews them and adjusts the dose as needed. This process is anticoagulation management and involves restrictions on the number of times the codes may be used.

Codes 99366–99368 are used to bill for a Medical Team Conference, either with direct or indirect contact. Medical Team Conferences can be billed when a physician, patient or family of the patient, or other healthcare professionals are present. They may occur at the skilled nursing facility, assisted living facility, hospital, or physician office.

Care Plan Oversight Services (99374–99380)

Care plan oversight is the reviewing of a patient's medical care and records, usually for a patient who is under the care of a home health agency, hospice, or nursing home. The time spent on such services is not considered to be face-to-face time with the patient.

Care plan oversight is reported according to the amount of time per month (or per 30-day period) that the physician spends reviewing the patient's treatment plan and records. Only one provider is allowed to bill for this service each month.

Preventive Medicine Services (99381–99429)

These codes are used to bill for the E/M of patients who do not have an illness or injury (e.g., who are visiting the doctor for an annual checkup). The patient's age is often a factor in the codes in this section (checkup for an infant, shown in Figure 6-2 ●, is

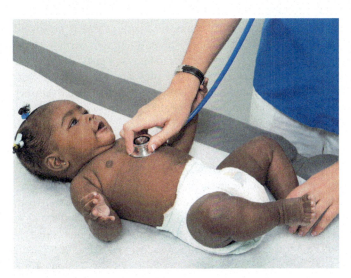

FIGURE 6-2 Checkup on an infant is conducted as a preventative measure

Source: Michal Heron/Pearson Education/PH College

different from a checkup for an older person). This section also includes codes for risk factor assessment (e.g., suicidal tendencies, weight problems, substance abuse).

> ▶ CRITICAL THINKING QUESTION: Why is a patient's age a factor in determining which code to use for preventive medicine?

Non-Face-to-Face Physician Services (99441–99444)

These codes are for E/M services that are provided either by telephone or online (i.e., via e-mail). For example, a physician receives an email from a patient related to potential side effects from a medication that the physician recently prescribed. The physician calls the patient and discusses the options for changing the medication. This interaction can be billed as a non-face-to-face service.

Special Evaluation and Management Services (99450–99456)

These codes are used to bill for basic life or disability evaluations (e.g., follow-up evaluation for a work-related disability patient). They are used to establish baseline information when the main purpose of the visit is to evaluate the patient, not to provide treatment.

Coverage for these services can vary widely by payer. Check with your supervisor before processing these claims. The report compiled for this evaluation is attached to the claim submission.

Newborn Care Services (99460–99480)

These codes are used to bill for services provided by a physician to a newborn infant, including the immediate postpartum exam, preparation of birth and other medical records, and stabilization of a newborn infant.

Codes 99477–99480 are specific to intensive care services of the infant.

Other Evaluation and Management Services (99499)

This code is used to bill for any E/M service that is not listed elsewhere. For example, a nurse practitioner may visit a patient in the hospital and leave notes for the physician to address, and the physician may visit the same day and also make notes. Both providers would code 99499 and the insurance examiner would determine which party would be paid.

CPT Coding Medicine

The Medicine section of the CPT contains evaluation, therapeutic and diagnostic procedures, and services that are generally not invasive. The Medicine section has multiple subsections. It is important to read the subsection information and instructions that pertain to the group codes that will follow. The codes in this section range from 90281 to 99607 and may be used in conjunction with all other CPT sections. (See Table 6-2 ●.) Codes in this section do not include supplies used in the testing, therapy, or diagnostic treatments, unless specifically stated in the code description.

TABLE 6-2 Medicine Codes

Immune Globulins	90281-90399
Immunization Administration for Vaccines/Toxoids	90460-90474
Vaccines, Toxoids	90476-90749
Psychiatry	90801-90899
Biofeedback	90901-90911
Dialysis	90935-90999
Gastroenterology	91010-91299
General Ophthalmology Services	92002-92499
Otorhinolaryngologic Services	92502-92700
Cardiovascular	92950-93998
Pulmonary Services	94002-94799
Allergy and Clinical Immunology	95004-95199
Endocrinology	95250-95251
Neurology and Neuromuscular Procedures	95800-96020
Central Nervous System Assessments/Tests	96101-96125
Health and Behavior Assessment/Intervention	96150-96155
Chemotherapy Administration	96401-96549
Photodynamic Therapy	96567-96571
Special Dermatological Procedures	96900-96999
Physical Medicine and Rehabilitation Services	97001-97799
Medical Nutrition Therapy	97802-97804
Acupuncture	97810-97814
Osteopathic Manipulative Treatment	98925-98929
Chiropractic Manipulative Treatment	98940-98943
Education and Training for Patient Self-Management	98960-98962
Non-Face-to-Face Non-Physician Services	98966-98969
Special Services, Procedures, and Reports	99000-99091
Qualifying Circumstances for Anesthesia	99100-99140
Moderate (Conscious) Sedation	99143-99150
Other Services and Procedures	99170-99199
Home Health Procedures/Services	99500-99600
Home Infusion Procedures/Services	99601-99602
Medication Therapy Management Services	99605-99607

Immune Globulins (90281–90399), Immunization Administration for Vaccines/Toxoids (90460–90474), and Vaccines and Toxoids (90476–90749)

An immunization is the administration of a vaccine or toxoid (a weakened form of a toxin) to stimulate the immune system to provide protection against a certain disease or condition. The actual immunization administration (codes 96365–96368, 96372, 96374, or 96375 as appropriate) is coded in addition to the immune globulins (90281–90399) and/or vaccine or toxin (90476–90749) which has been injected. Remember, this means that two codes are required.

Immunizations are considered preventive treatment. As of September 23, 2012, enrollees in a health plan are required to be covered for this preventive service as part of the Affordable Care Act.

When an immunization is the only service provided, the E/M code for a minimal service exam is also allowed. If the vaccine is provided by the government, the provider cannot bill for the product.

Even though these services take a prolonged period of time, these codes are not to be used with the codes for prolonged services. The prolonged amount of time has been included in the RVS amount for these codes.

Psychiatry (90801–90899)

The care and treatment of psychiatric or mental/nervous problems includes the treatment of the following issues:

- Psychotic and neurotic disorders
- Organic brain dysfunction
- Alcoholism
- Chemical dependency

The language description on the claim form generally indicates "psychotherapy," "individual therapy," or "group therapy." The providers of service are usually medical doctors (typically psychiatrists) or clinical psychologists.

If one of the following providers is indicated, most benefit plans require a referral by an M.D.:

1. Marriage, Family, and Child Counselor (MFCC)
2. Licensed Clinical Social Worker (LCSW)
3. Master of Social Work (MSW)

These CPT codes are used only when psychiatric counseling or therapy is provided. If such therapy is not provided, even if the service is performed by one of the preceding licensed providers, use a different code range. This category includes both individual and group therapy by these providers.

Most plans pay a reduced benefit for mental/nervous and psychiatric treatment. There may be a limit on the number of visits per year and a dollar limit per visit or per calendar year. Also, many plans only cover certain provider licensing. Therefore, read the plan document carefully before processing these types of claims and determine whether a referral or prior approval for services is required.

> ● **ONLINE INFORMATION:** Find a reputable online source that discusses HIPAA and mental health. Consider the privacy rules and additional safety measures that apply to psychotherapy notes but not to general medical records.

Biofeedback (90901–90911)

Biofeedback is training an individual to consciously control automatic, internal bodily functions. For example, through conscious control, some body rhythms that control the constriction of blood vessels or the beating of the heart can be increased or decreased. This type of treatment can be used for a variety of illnesses or symptoms. A common use is for the control of intractable pain.

Biofeedback is controversial in that its effectiveness is very hard to prove or disprove. In addition, it does not cure anything. Instead of treating a condition, it is used as a tool in dealing with the symptoms. Most plans do not cover biofeedback treatment, or if it is covered, it is very limited and only for certain diagnoses.

Dialysis (90935–90999)

Dialysis is a treatment given to patients who have suffered acute kidney failure and rely on artificial handling of their kidney functions. Notice that this is not really a treatment because it is only handling the functions that are normally performed by the body. (However, it is still referred to generically as "treatment.") In order for a patient with this condition to survive, the blood cleansing function must be performed artificially by one of these processes currently available:

- Hemodialysis
- Hemofiltration
- Continuous Ambulatory Peritoneal Dialysis (CAPD)
- Transplantation of a new kidney

Most hemodialysis is performed at private dialysis centers. A small percentage of the patients have a machine in their homes. Dialysis is usually billed on a monthly basis. The bill should indicate either the actual dates of service or a monthly from/through date. Normally, the only time you see these bills is during the first 30 months of treatment. After 30 months, Medicare becomes the primary payer (refer to the Medicare and Medicaid chapter for additional information). If the dialysis is performed in an acute facility, you may be billed separately for the facility fees and the physician fees. Remember, the CPT codes are used only for physician's services.

Hemofiltration is usually given to critically ill patients with renal disease and is generally performed in an intensive care unit. It is a slow process that occurs over 10–12 hours and requires a central venous catheter.

CAPD is performed by the patient at home. The peritoneum of the stomach is used to cleanse the blood. Surgery is required to implant catheters and construct the internal bag (made of the peritoneum) to hold the dialysate fluids. Monthly supplies must be purchased, and the attending physician assesses monthly examination charges.

A kidney transplant is the only cure for end-stage renal disease. Transplants are coded in accordance with the surgery section of the CPT.

All E/M services on the day of dialysis are considered to be part of the dialysis treatment. No separate allowance is made for an E/M visit, unless the E/M visit is for treatment that is unrelated to dialysis.

Gastroenterology (91010–91299)

Gastroenterology services deal primarily with the esophagus, stomach, and intestines. These codes are used to bill for diagnostic services of the digestive system. The RVS allowance for these codes is for the diagnostic procedure only. The claim should also list an E/M code for the visit. No modifiers are used in this instance.

General Ophthalmological Services (92002–92499)

Ophthalmology care is eye care provided either by an optometrist (O.D.) or an ophthalmologist (M.D.). Most health plans do not cover routine vision care services related to the refraction of the eye and subsequent prescription of glasses or contact lenses. If these services are covered, the benefits are

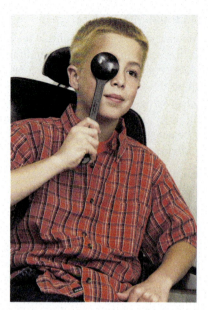

FIGURE 6-3 A vision test being performed on a child
Source: GWImages/Shutterstock

usually very limited in both the dollar allowance and frequency of services, and they are often provided under a separate vision care plan or benefit. Therefore, always be sure to verify plan benefits before processing a vision claim. Also be aware that not all vision care is routine. Some vision care is essential for the proper care and treatment of eye disease. Most payers have a list of payable diagnoses. However, prescription services for glasses or contact lenses may still be considered routine (except possibly if the lens of the eye has been removed, as in cataract surgery). (See Figure 6-3 ●.)

Orthoptics is the retraining of the muscles that control vision. Some plans allow for this therapy for certain conditions such as strabismus and binocular vision. If the plan does allow therapy, it is usually very limited and may only be covered if the patient has obtained a second opinion from an ophthalmologist.

Otorhinolaryngologic Services (92502–92700)

Otorhinolarygological services are associated with the head, or more specifically, the ear, nose, and throat (ENT). This section is for the billing of special services that are not part of a routine examination, such as checking the speaker system on cochlear implants.

Speech therapy (codes 92507–92508) is usually provided to correct speech that has been impaired because of sickness or injury that occurred while the individual was insured under the plan. The services must also be performed by a qualified practitioner. Conditions such as restoration of speech ability after a stroke or throat surgery are covered. However, speech therapy for conditions such as stuttering or congenital deafness usually is not covered.

If you are unsure whether there is an underlying need for the speech therapy services, refer the claim to a specialist for further review.

Cardiovascular (92950–93998)

Cardiovascular services treat the heart, arteries, and veins. Vascular studies (93875–93981) are diagnostic procedures to determine the condition of or blood flow through an artery or vein. All cardiovascular codes should be listed in addition to the E/M services code describing the visit.

This is a very large section, and it is heavily used by medical billers and examiners. The following codes are some of the more commonly billed services:

93000	Electrocardiogram (EKG or ECG)
93010	EKG Interpretation and Report Only
93015	Cardiovascular Stress Test
93224	24-hr EKG Monitoring

As a rule, the codes from 93000 through 93350 and 93600 through 93981 are considered to be DXL expenses. New codes 93452–93461 are for catheterization and cover contrast injection(s), imaging supervision, interpretation, and reports for typically performed imaging.

Pulmonary Services (94002–94799)

These codes are used to bill procedures of the lungs and airways. These are most often diagnostic procedures for determining air flow, blood gases, and the conditions of the respiratory system. These procedures include performing the procedure and interpreting the results. If the physician only provided the interpretation of the results, use modifier -26.

Pulmonary procedures should be coded separately from the appropriate E/M code for the visit.

Allergy and Clinical Immunology (95004–95199)

These codes are used to bill for services that were performed to determine whether a patient is allergic or sensitive to certain substances and the treatment of those allergies.

These codes should be reported in addition to the appropriate E/M code for the visit. Use codes 99241–99245 to report consultations with the patient or the patient's family regarding the management of their condition.

Endocrinology (95250–95251)

These codes are used for the glucose monitoring of a patient. These codes should not be used with the code for collection and interpretation of physiologic data (99091).

Neurology and Neuromuscular Procedures (95800–96020)

These codes are used to bill for procedures of the nervous system and are often reported in conjunction with consultations. Make a separate allowance for the test and the consultation.

Electroencephalogram (EEG) or EKG services include both the taking of the test and the interpretation of the results. Use modifier -26 may be used with EEG or EKG codes to report that the physician only provided the interpretation of the results.

Central Nervous System Assessments/Tests (96101–96125)

These codes are used to bill for services to test the response of the central nervous system, including psychological testing, aphasia (lack of speech) testing, and developmental testing.

Health and Behavior Assessment/Intervention (96150–96155)

These codes are used to bill for health and behavior assessment or intervention performed by a physician. Time is the major component for determining the correct code for these procedures. For example, a brief behavior assessment of 30 minutes would be coded differently than a behavior assessment and intervention such as a personality test, interview, and report that took three hours.

Chemotherapy Administration (96401–96549)

Codes 96360 and 96361 are used to report hydration IV infusion only (e.g., normal saline, D5 half-normal saline); they are not used to report infusion of drugs or other substances.

Codes 96365–96379 are used to report IV infusion of drugs or other substances, other than hydration fluids.

Chemotherapy is the treatment of cancer using chemicals introduced to the body. Codes 96401–96549 are for the administration of chemotherapy agents by a physician or by a qualified person under the direction of a physician.

These codes should be reported in addition to the appropriate E/M code for the visit. If the physician places an intra-arterial catheter to facilitate the administration of the chemotherapy drugs, add the appropriate code from the cardiovascular surgery section.

If chemotherapy is administered by more than one technique, report each technique separately.

Photodynamic Therapy (96567–96571)

Photodynamic therapy is a treatment method for some types of cancer. It uses light and a light-sensitive agent. For example, laser therapies delivered through endoscopic procedures can affect or stop viruses.

Special Dermatological Procedures (96900–96999)

These codes are used to bill for treatment to the skin, including acne and other dermatologic disorders. The underlying cause for treatment must be determined before you can identify whether these services are covered, as many dermatological procedures are considered cosmetic.

Physical Medicine and Rehabilitation Services (97001–97799)

Physical medicine is the manipulation and physical therapy associated with the nonsurgical care and treatment of the patient. The most common form of physical medicine is chiropractic manipulation of the spine. (Theoretically, any joint can be involved.) The chiropractor's scope of practice is limited in most states. For instance, in some states, chiropractors are not allowed to draw blood and can only prescribe over-the-counter medications. The limitations vary by state.

Chiropractic care and billing used to be limited to manipulation of the spine and X-rays. Now, chiropractors use many different physical therapy modalities. Consequently, an intense monitoring and restricting of payment for chiropractic services has developed. Such restrictions may limit the number of visits per year, per month, or per condition; specify daily reimbursement maximums; or limit the number of modalities that may be performed in a single visit. A wide variety of techniques have emerged to handle the overutilization of chiropractic care. As a result, it is important to check the coverage, as the payment policies vary from payer to payer.

Many chiropractors use accident diagnosis 84x.xx series for billing purposes. Unless an accident or injury has actually occurred and the date, place, and circumstances are indicated, the coding should be changed to reflect a noninjury skeletal condition, 72x.xx. (This varies by payer.) Situations that should warrant further review include

- Possible overutilization of the code
- More than three physical medicine visits in a week
- More than 12 visits in a month
- At least 34 physical medicine visits that span more than three months
- Second provider of physical medicine on the same day
- More than four physical medicine codes per day
- More than one initial office visit by the same physician
- Claims when the only physical medicine charges are for modalities or massage (97010–97039 procedure codes). Modalities are a method of therapy, usually physical (e.g., a massage).
- Claims for use of an orthion table or for orthion therapy

If a particular claim appears to be excessive, you should contact the attending physician and obtain the following information:

- An outline of the therapy program recommended
- A list of goals to be achieved through the program
- A narrative description of how each procedure being performed is required to achieve one or more of the goals listed

If the physician's reply justifies the use, frequency, and duration of therapy, process the claim accordingly. It takes time and skill to be able to interpret or determine the necessity of services rendered. Therefore, if you are not sure what action should be taken after you have compiled the information necessary to make a claim determination, refer the information to a claims specialist. Any limitations depend on the health plan and the payer's policy.

Medical Nutrition Therapy (97802–97804)

These codes are used to bill for services to assess, counsel, and treat patients regarding their nutritional needs. The services can include taking body measurements and histories, providing nutritional counseling, and administrating medical foods or tube feedings. The diagnoses for these codes can involve weight issues, nutritional deficiency issues (whether they are caused by diet or by a medical condition), and diseases or conditions that require a modification in the patient's normal nutritional routine (e.g., diabetes).

As many plans do not cover obesity or other weight issues, you should check the patient's diagnosis and the plan guidelines before processing the claim.

Acupuncture (97810–97814)

Acupuncture is the ancient Chinese practice of inserting fine needles into various points in the body to relieve pain, induce anesthesia, and regulate and improve body functions. The codes in this section are used to report acupuncture services. Acupuncture codes report 15-minute increments. Use the time the provider spends face-to-face with the patient, not the amount of time that the needles are in place. There are different codes for needles used with and without electrical stimulation.

Osteopathic Manipulative Treatment (98925–98929)

Osteopathic treatment is based on the idea that the body can cure itself if it is in a normal state and provided with the proper environmental conditions. The appropriate code is determined by the number of body regions involved in the treatment. This therapy is often considered controversial and is not covered by many plans.

Chiropractic Manipulative Treatment (98940–98943)

These codes are used to bill for treatment of the body's bones and muscles, especially in the back. The codes in this section are often used in the treatment of patients who were involved in auto accidents or work-related injuries. Any manipulation treatment includes a patient assessment.

Due to the high amount of abuse in this area, consider the diagnosis before you process chiropractic codes. Often the patient will need to submit documentation of a proposed treatment plan, and only a specific number of treatments will be preauthorized. If the patient does not obtain preauthorization prior to obtaining treatment, many plans limit or deny payment for the claim.

Education and Training for Patient Self-Management (98960–98962)

These codes are used to report educational and training services prescribed by a physician and provided by a qualified nonphysician healthcare provider (for example, training for management of diabetes or weight loss education).

Non-Face-to-Face Nonphysician Services (98966–98969)

These codes are used to report non-face-to-face encounters (via telephone or Internet communication) between a nonphysician and an established patient or the patient's guardian. If a decision is made to see the patient within 24 hours, the code is not reported and the encounter is considered part of the preservice workup. Likewise, if the communication is for a service that was performed in the previous seven days, the code is not reported, and the encounter is considered part of that previous service.

Special Services, Procedures, and Reports (99000–99091)

These codes are used to bill for special circumstances regarding services performed, such as the handling of a laboratory specimen. These codes are used in addition to the normal code that describes the procedure performed.

Proper use of this code can increase the reimbursement allowance. However, as the normal allowance for a laboratory test includes both performing the test and interpreting the results, it is important to verify the procedures performed by each provider prior to processing the claim, in order to make sure the extra allowance is appropriate.

Qualifying Circumstances for Anesthesia (99100–99140)

Anesthesia is sedation used for surgery and/or pain management. The coding of this service depends on what part of the procedure is completed by an anesthesiologist. (This topic is explored further in the Surgery and Anesthesia Claims chapter).

Moderate (Conscious) Sedation (99143–99150)

This section covers the billing of conscious sedation (with or without analgesia) when both the sedation and the actual procedure are provided by the same physician. If the physician who is performing the conscious sedation is not the physician who is performing the procedure, use the appropriate anesthesia code. Some of these codes include several procedures. Note the bull's eye symbol next to some codes; it means that the additional listed codes are included in that particular code.

Many plans will limit additional payments for sedation provided by the physician who performs the actual procedure. For further information, see the Surgery and Anesthesia Claims chapter.

Other Services and Procedures (99170–99199)

This section is used for reporting services that do not fit under any of the other categories. It includes codes for physician attendance at hyperbaric oxygen therapy, assessment of a child for possible sexual abuse, hypothermia treatment, and many other conditions.

As the circumstances for these procedures are widely varied, check the diagnosis to determine whether the therapy is covered by the plan.

Home Health Procedures/Services (99500–99600)

These codes are used to bill for services provided in the patient's home by nonphysician healthcare professionals, such as midwives, nurse practitioners, and physicians' assistants. For example, if a midwife delivers a baby in the home, use these codes.

Home Infusion Procedures/Services (99601–99602)

These codes are used to report per-diem home visits for the purpose of administering infusions, such as IV antibiotics or pain medication.

Medication Therapy Management Services (99605–99607)

These codes are used to report face-to-face assessment and intervention by a pharmacist. For example, use these codes to report when a physician calls on a pharmacist to meet with a patient to determine the best pharmacological interventions.

Category II and III Codes

Category II codes are classification codes which allow the collection of data for performance measurement. These codes are four digits followed by the letter F.

Category III codes are for "emerging technologies," new procedures whose value may not yet be fully realized. Many insurance carriers consider these to be experimental procedures and exclude them. These codes are four digits followed by the letter T. For example, 0291T describes an intravascular optical coherence tomography (coronary native vessel or graft) during diagnostic evaluation, and/or therapeutic intervention, including imaging supervision, interpretation, and report, for an initial vessel. This code is used in conjunction with cardiac catheterization codes 92975, 92980, 92982, 92995, 93454–93461, 93563, and 93564. Category II and III codes are electronically updated twice a year.

ACTIVITY #1

Evaluation and Management Codes

Directions: Write the codes for each section in the space provided.

Section	Codes
1. Consultations	_____
2. Emergency Department Services	_____
3. Domiciliary, Rest Home, or Custodial Care Services	_____
4. Prolonged Services	_____
5. Preventive Medicine Services	_____
6. Therapeutic, Prophylactic, or Diagnostic Injections	_____
7. Psychiatry	_____
8. Biofeedback	_____
9. Gastroenterology	_____
10. Ophthalmology	_____
11. Otorhinolaryngologic Services	_____
12. Allergy and Clinical Immunology	_____
13. Neurology and Neuromuscular Procedures	_____
14. Chemotherapy Administration	_____
15. Physical Medicine and Rehabilitation Services	_____
16. Medical Nutrition Therapy	_____
17. Home Health Procedures/Services	_____

Modifiers for Evaluation and Management and Medicine Codes

The following modifiers are used with E/M and Medicine CPT codes. This is not an exhaustive list of modifiers, only a list of the most commonly used ones.

Evaluation and Management

-24 Unrelated Evaluation and Management Service by the Same Physician during a Postoperative Period

-25 Significant, Separately Identifiable Evaluation Management Service by the Same Physician on the Same Day of the Procedure or Other Service. This modifier indicates that a completely separate visit was performed by the same provider.

EXAMPLE:
A patient visits a general practitioner for an earache. On the way home, he is involved in a car accident. He returns to the same doctor for treatment of a broken arm sustained in the car accident.

-32 Mandated Services

-52 Reduced Services. These services were less intensive than the services normally associated with this code. This modifier often warrants a reduction in the payment made to the provider.

-57 Decision for Surgery. This procedure was necessary to determine the need for a subsequent surgical procedure. Depending on the amount of time which lapses between the visit and the subsequent surgery, the visit may be considered part of the overall surgical procedure. Claims with this modifier often require the addition of a report detailing the circumstances. The report and claim should be forwarded to a claim specialist.

ACTIVITY #2

Evaluation and Management Review

Directions: After reviewing the previous material, answer the following questions in the space provided.

1. True or False: If the diagnosis is for psychiatric care, regardless of the service provided, use codes 90801 to 90899. _____
2. What are dialysis services? _____
3. True or False: Custodial care is usually a covered service. _____
4. List the three types of end-stage renal disease treatments.
   a. _____
   b. _____
   c. _____
5. What is biofeedback? _____
6. Consultations are usually provided by a _____
7. True or False: In order for psychiatric services to be payable, a clinical psychologist requires a referral from an M.D. _____
8. What type of care does a Skilled Nursing Care Facility provide? _____
9. True or False: A second-opinion physician can be in the same medical group as the surgeon. _____
10. What type of care is usually provided by an MFCC? _____

Medicine:

-22 Increased Procedural Services

-26 Professional Component

-51 Multiple Procedures

-52 Reduced Services

-76 Repeat Procedure by Same Physician

-77 Repeat Procedure by Another Physician

-90 Reference (Outside) Laboratory

PRACTICE PITFALLS

The following are examples of incorrect unbundling of medical services:

- Billing of a rhythm strip in addition to an electrocardiogram. The rhythm strip should not be billed separately.
- Billing of an upper extremity (brachial) doppler study in addition to a lower extremity doppler study in order to obtain an "ankle-brachial index." The upper extremity doppler should not be billed separately.
- Billing of an electrocardiogram as part of a cardiac stress test. The electrocardiogram should not be billed separately.

X-Ray and Laboratory Services

Radiology and laboratory charges may be billed by a physician, an independent laboratory, or a freestanding radiology facility. Here we will discuss some of the basic guidelines used to determine whether billed DXL services are covered. We will also cover the guidelines for processing laboratory and radiology charges.

Laboratory examinations analyze body substances to determine their chemical or tissue make-up. Body fluids or tissues are either run through analyzing machines or examined under a microscope. (See Figure 6-4 ● to identify any abnormal substances or tissues.)

There are basically two types of X-ray and laboratory charges: DXL and medical management X-ray/lab. **Diagnostic charges** are for initial testing to confirm a diagnosis or to rule out other diagnoses. **Medical management** X-ray/lab charges are incurred to control or manage a diagnosis (i.e., monitoring blood glucose levels on a patient with diabetes).

Laboratory tests that are medically necessary are usually covered expenses and may be payable under an X-ray and laboratory benefit. This benefit pays for the X-ray and laboratory test up to the policy maximum necessary to diagnose or manage a condition, as long as the expense is not payable under another Basic Benefit (e.g., inpatient hospital, preadmission testing, accident). The laboratory benefit usually does not cover any unnecessary examination or test that contributes to the diagnosis of an injury or illness.

The Ball Insurance Company plan has a Basic Benefit that covers a maximum of $200 per calendar year for X-ray/lab charges.

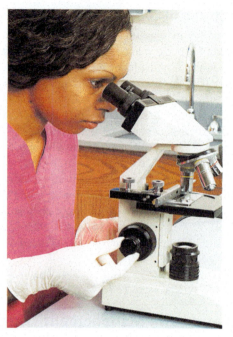

FIGURE 6-4 Examining a laboratory specimen
Source: Michal Heron/Pearson Education/PH College

Radiology (X-Ray)

The radiology section of the CPT is arranged according to anatomic position (i.e., by body part, starting at the head and moving downward toward the feet). Radiology service codes, listed in Table 6-3 ●, range from 70010 to 79999. The following subsections appear in the radiology section of the CPT:

Diagnostic Radiology (70010–76499)

Diagnostic X-rays are flat or two-dimensional pictures of a particular body part or organ. **X-rays** are created by sending low-level radiation through the body and capturing the resulting image on a sheet of film. X-rays are most useful for looking at bones and dense tissue, as softer tissue is not clearly defined in the images. A patient might undergo a diagnostic X-ray to evaluate kidney damage, gallstones, or bone loss.

Computed tomography (CT) scans are made by a process that uses multiple X-ray images to create three-dimensional images of body structures. These scans are used to help identify tumors and cancers located in an organ. CT scans are much more definitive than X-rays.

Diagnostic Ultrasound (76506–76999)

Ultrasonography provides a more definitive type of picture than X-rays. Instead of using radiation, ultrasonography

TABLE 6-3 Radiology Codes

Diagnostic Radiology	70010-76499
Diagnostic Ultrasound	76506-76999
Radiation Oncology	77261-77799
Nuclear Medicine	78000-79999

bounces sound waves off the desired structure to form a picture of the organ. This type of viewing is less potentially damaging than X-rays, which is why ultrasound scanning can be used during pregnancy, whereas X-rays cannot.

Radiation Oncology (77261–77799)

Radiation oncology is the use of radiation in conjunction with chemotherapy to treat malignant cancers. Normally, radiation therapy is composed of multiple treatments and does not generate a "picture" of the body part. It is done for treatment purposes only, not for diagnostic reasons. The radiation treatments are different for different stages of cancer.

Nuclear Medicine (78000–79999)

Nuclear medicine combines the use of radioactive elements and X-rays to image organs or body parts. Certain radioactive elements collect in different organs. The purpose of nuclear medicine is to determine whether an organ is working effectively or whether it is enlarged. A radioactive element is injected into the patient, and then pictures are taken of the organ at specified intervals to see how, where, and how much of the element collects in a specific organ.

Modifiers for Radiology (X-Ray) Codes

The following modifiers are appropriate for use with Radiology (X-ray) CPT codes. This is not an exhaustive list of modifiers, only a list of the most commonly used ones.

- **-22** Increased Procedural Services
- **-26** Professional Component
- **-32** Mandated Services
- **-51** Multiple Procedures
- **-52** Reduced Services
- **-76** Repeat Procedure by the Same Physician
- **-77** Repeat Procedure by Another Physician
- **-LT** Left Side of Body
- **-RT** Right Side of Body

Pathology and Laboratory (80047–89398)

It is important to establish whether laboratory tests are being done as part of a routine check-up or because the patient has symptoms of a condition that the physician is attempting to diagnose. Also, you should check that the testing is appropriate for the reported symptoms. Some tests are routine for some diagnoses but not for others. You will learn this type of discrimination through experience and time. (Pathology service codes are listed in Table 6-4 ●.)

The following sections cover the subsections of the laboratory portion of the CPT.

TABLE 6-4 Pathology Codes

Organ or Disease-Oriented Panels	80047-80076
Drug Testing	80100-80104
Therapeutic Drug Assays	80150-80299
Evocative/Suppression Testing	80400-80440
Consultations (Clinical Pathology)	80500-80502
Urinalysis	81000-81099
Chemistry	82000-94999
Hematology & Coagulation	85002-85999
Immunology	86000-86849
Transfusion Medicine	86850-86999
Microbiology	87001-87999
Anatomic Pathology	88000-88099
Cytopathology	88104-88199
Cytogenetic Studies	88230-88299
Surgical Pathology	88300-88399
In Vivo (eg. Transcutaneous) Laboratory Procedures	88720-88749
Other Procedures	89049-89240
Reproductive Medicine Procedures	89250-89398

PRACTICE **PITFALLS**

The following are examples of incorrect unbundling of radiology services:

- CPT code 72110 (Radiologic examination, spine, lumbosacral; minimum of four views) was billed with CPT code 72114 (Radiologic examination, spine, lumbosacral; complete, including bending views; minimum of six views). However, reimbursement of services for CPT 72110 is included in the reimbursement of 72114, so the codes should not have been submitted together.
- The 3D simulation CPT code 77295 "bundles" or includes the complex isodose plan CPT code 77315, which means that 77315 should not be billed in addition to the 77295 code.

Organ or Disease-Oriented Panels (80047–80076)

Panel tests are multiple tests that are combined and run from one or two specimens. These tests cost substantially less than several tests that are ordered separately from separate specimens. These services are very sophisticated, highly computerized, and usually very reliable. CPT codes 80047–80076 refer to various types of panel tests. The number of tests performed determines the code to use. For example, there is a different code for a Basic Metabolic Panel and a Comprehensive Metabolic Panel, even though the Basic Metabolic Panel is a part of the Comprehensive Metabolic Panel. Providers are allowed to bill for the collection of the specimen, for a venipuncture if the specimen is blood, and for the handling or packaging of the specimen. It is important to ensure all the tests within the panel were completed before you use a panel code.

Drug Testing (80100–80104)

These codes are used to bill for the testing of bodily fluids to identify a specific class of drugs (e.g., amphetamines). It is important to check the diagnosis when you process these types of claims, as overdoses may fall into the category of accidents (which may have additional benefits) or attempted suicide or self-inflicted injury (for which benefits may be reduced or denied). It is important to note that some qualitative drug tests indicate a positive or negative result (+ means that the drug is present, and − means that the drug is not present). In contrast, some quantitative drug tests show how much of the drug is in the person's system, and may indicate how often or how much of a drug is being used.

Therapeutic Drug Assays (80150–80299)

These codes are used to bill for monitoring the therapeutic levels of a specific drug (e.g., a drug prescribed by a physician). Some drugs work at a certain level in the person's blood and therefore an assay is used to determine if the level is therapeutic, after which the physician can alter the dose accordingly. Examples include Coumadin, Depakote, lithium, and other anticoagulant, antiseizure, and medications for mental/behavioral disorders.

Evocative/Suppression Testing (80400–80440)

These codes are used to report panel tests that help providers determine whether the patient has a condition creating insufficient or excessive hormones or chemicals in the body. These tests often confirm or rule out a diagnosis.

Consultations (Clinical Pathology) (80500–80502)

These codes are used to report consultations or evaluation of a patient's condition using clinical results (lab tests). Clinical pathology includes review of a biopsy, several blood tests, and other readings that would indicate disease of the organ or body system being tested.

Urinalysis (81000–81099)

Analysis of the urine can provide a wide range of information for the provider. This is one of the most common laboratory tests performed. For example, a urinalysis can detect infection, sugars, protein, and several other indicators of body systems' functioning.

Chemistry (82000–84999)

This section lists the codes that are used to bill for the testing of a specific substance within the patient's body (e.g., a chemical, a vitamin, a mineral, a hormone). The results of these tests can often help to confirm or deny a diagnosis or to provide information regarding a patient's condition or behavior.

Hematology & Coagulation (85002–85999)

These codes are used to report the testing of blood for its components (e.g., hemoglobin count). These tests can allow a provider to track a patient's condition and determine whether there are any possible contraindications for surgery (e.g., slow blood clotting time).

Immunology (86000–86849)

These codes are used to report tests done on body fluids to determine prior immune responses (i.e., check whether the body has antibodies to fight a specific disease). These tests can help a provider determine whether a disease is currently present in a patient's body or whether the patient has been exposed to a disease.

Transfusion Medicine (86850–86999)

These codes are used to bill for tests performed prior to a transfusion or other procedures, when a patient may be given fluids or cells from a donor (e.g., the patient may have blood typing done before receiving a transfusion to ensure that the patient receives a compatible blood type).

Microbiology (87001–87999)

Microbiology is the study of microorganisms. These codes report the culture of microorganisms to determine their presence in the human body. Microbiology testing is used for determining pathogens in a specimen. For example, a urinalysis may detect bacteria in the urine, but in order to know which antibiotic to use, the lab must culture the urine to see what kind of bacteria grow.

Anatomic Pathology (88000–88099)

These codes are used to bill for examinations on a deceased person to assist in determining the cause of death. For example, if a person died of an apparent heart attack, an anatomic pathology test of the heart muscle would show what type of heart disease or other significant damage led to the heart attack.

Cytopathology (88104–88199)

Cytopathology is the study of changes in a cell or the ability of an agent (e.g., virus, bacteria) to destroy a cell. These codes are used to bill for cells removed from a person through smears (e.g., Pap smear), scrapings, or other forms of cell collection.

Cytogenetic Studies (88230–88299)

Cytogenic refers to the production of cells. These codes report procedures associated with the collection or growing of cells within the lab (e.g., growing a skin graft for a burn patient).

Surgical Pathology (88300–88399)

The codes in this section report tests done in preparation for or during surgery. For example, during a surgical removal of skin cancer, a pathologist will look at the removed skin to make sure the entire cancer has been removed. It is helpful for surgeons to know whether they need to remove more skin. The important piece of information for medical billers is how many dissections were taken so that they can code the correct number of procedures.

In Vivo (e.g., Transcutaneous) Laboratory Procedures (88720–88749)

The codes in this section are used to report transcutaneous (secreted through the skin) bilirubin, hemoglobin, and other unlisted *in vivo* laboratory services.

Other Procedures (89049–89240)

This section lists lab procedures that did not fit under any of the other headings.

Reproductive Medicine Procedures (89250–89398)

The codes in this section report services associated with reproductive procedures (e.g., cryopreservation of embryos and sperm, *in vitro* fertilization).

PAPANICOLAOU (PAP) SMEAR. A **Papanicolaou or "Pap" smear** is a diagnostic laboratory test for detecting the absence or presence of infection, viruses, trauma, or cancer. Under the Affordable Care Act, Pap smears are covered for women over 40.

PRACTICE PITFALLS

Following are some general guidelines regarding the processing of DXL claims.

Automated Laboratory Charge

Automated laboratories offer their services primarily to doctors' offices. Usually, the doctor's office is furnished with all the necessary supplies for securing samples of blood and urine and lab sheets indicating which tests are to be performed on which specimens. The laboratory performs the tests and returns the lab reports to the doctor's office, usually within approximately three days. The doctor is usually billed monthly for this service.

Unbundling

Some providers will unbundle codes by billing separately for each test performed, even though all the tests came from the same specimen and were done simultaneously. If the claim was processed as billed, the provider would be paid significantly more money without doing any additional services. When a bill is received "unbundled," the examiner needs to rebundle it. An example of unbundling is shown in Table 6-5 ●. Medical billers should know which laboratory and pathology panels should be coded as one procedure rather than being unbundled and billed as several procedures.

In Table 6-5, all the billed charges should be combined and coded under one panel code. Benefits would then be determined on the basis of the one code.

TABLE 6-5 Unbundling

Bill from Doctor	CPT® Code	Charge	Coding by Examiner	Charge
Calcium	82310	$20.00	80048	$95.00
CO₂	82374	15.00		
Chloride	82435	25.00		
Creatinine	82565	15.00		
Glucose	82947	10.00		
Potassium	84132	15.00		
Sodium	84295	15.00		
BUN	84520	30.00		
		$145.00		$95.00

PRACTICE PITFALLS

One of the most common places to find unbundling of CPT codes is in the area of laboratory procedures. The following are examples of unbundling of laboratory services:

CPT code 80058 (TORCH antibody panel) includes the following tests:
CPT code 86644: Antibody – cytomegalovirus
CPT code 86694: Antibody – herpes simplex
CPT code 86762: Antibody – rubella
CPT code 86777: Antibody – toxoplasma

When all four tests are ordered and are medically necessary, the panel test must be billed in place of the individual tests.

Some other laboratory codes that may also be subject to unbundling include the following:

- General Health Panel (80050)
- Electrolyte Panel (80051)
- Lipid Panel (80061)
- Renal Function Panel (80069)

It is also important to review ER charges to be sure that services and supplies which are supposed to be included in the basic emergency room or trauma charge are not billed separately.

Component Charges

Whenever a lab test or an X-ray is performed, the provider actually performs two distinct services:

1. The first service is the taking of the specimen or X-ray. This charge should include the expense for the personnel who perform the test and the cost of the necessary equipment. This is called the **technical component (TC)**. In other words, the provider who owns the equipment bills for the service.
2. The second service is the interpretation or the reading of the results of the test. This is called the **professional component (PC)** and it is denoted by adding modifier -26 to the CPT code.

An independent pathologist or radiologist often bills separately for the interpretation of the report. This interpretation-only charge is a PC fee. To figure the cost of an X-ray or lab test, add the PC charge (if it is billed separately) to the base or TC charge (the charge for performing the test). Sometimes, both the TC charge and the PC charge are billed by the same provider but are broken out separately. This is common on hospital bills. When you code the claim, combine the two charges and code them as one charge. The exception to this rule is when the professional component and the technical component are performed by different providers. In that case, do not combine and code them as a single expense, but code and pay the charges separately.

A PC's value ranges from 25% to 40% of the UCR value of the actual test. The TC's value ranges from 60% to 75% of the UCR value of the test. (For training purposes, contracts that do not state a professional component percentage should be computed at 40% of UCR.)

Modifiers for Pathology (Lab) Codes

The following modifiers are appropriate for use with Pathology (Lab) CPT codes. This is not an exhaustive list of modifiers, only a list of the most commonly used ones.

-22 Unusual Services

-26 Professional Component

-32 Mandated Services

-52 Reduced Services

-GG Screening and Diagnostic Mammography Completed on the Same Day

-UN Portable X-Ray Two Patients

-UP Portable X-Ray Three Patients

-UQ Portable X-Ray Four Patients

-UR Portable X-Ray Five Patients

-US Portable X-Ray Six Patients

-90 Reference (Outside) Laboratory

ACTIVITY #3

Component Charges

Directions: Answer the following questions without looking back at the material just covered. Write your answers in the space provided.

1. What two distinct services are actually performed whenever a lab or an X-ray test is performed?

   a. _____

   b. _____

2. Define the two services that are performed.

   a. _____

   _____

   b. _____

   _____

Hospital Services

Hospital services are those services performed in a hospital setting, as shown in Figure 6-5 ●. The term is used generically to refer to charges billed by a hospital, urgent care center, surgi-center, alternative birthing center, or similar institution. This section deals with the various types of facilities available, their billing formats, and general handling guidelines.

To qualify as a hospital, a facility must meet most of the following criteria:

1. It must mainly provide medical treatment to inpatients.

2. It must provide treatment only by or under a staff of physicians.

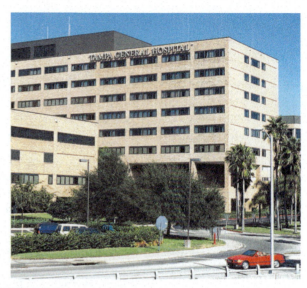

FIGURE 6-5 A general hospital
Source: Michal Heron/Pearson Education/PH College

3. It must provide care by registered nurses 24 hours per day.

4. It must maintain facilities for diagnosis.

5. It must maintain a daily medical record for each patient.

6. It must comply with all licensing and other legal and regulatory requirements.

7. It must maintain permanent facilities for surgery.

Most carriers have a file of established hospitals, surgicenters, skilled nursing facilities, or birthing facilities that are licensed to treat patients in the state where they practice business. Occasionally, a new facility opens and, when you receive claims for that facility, you must request and verify information to determine whether the facility is eligible for payment.

Hospital services are covered under the hospital benefits portion of the contract. Whether the contract is a Basic/Major Medical plan or a Comprehensive Major Medical plan, hospital charges are usually a covered benefit. The following are typical hospital expenses:

- Daily room and board
- Outpatient emergency treatment of illness and injuries
- Outpatient surgery
- Medical services and supplies during confinement, excluding private duty nursing
- Administration of anesthesia
- Ambulance care if billed through the hospital
- Lab tests and other services performed by an outside facility at the hospital's request

UB-04 Billing Form

Before you process a UB-04 form, you must review it to determine whether inpatient or outpatient benefits apply. An inpatient billing will usually have a room-and-board charge, and the from and to dates on the statement will correspond with the number of room-and-board days billed. Outpatient bills will usually have an indicator such as 131 in field locator four, the same date for from and to on the statement, the same date for admission and discharge, and no charge for room and board. Some hospitals do not put the discharge time on the outpatient bill; however, you may want to request this information if the billing appears excessive or if it appears that the patient might have stayed overnight in an extended stay or observation room.

Inpatient Hospital Claims

On inpatient hospital claims, the provider of service is a facility that provides inpatient care. This may be a hospital, an acute care facility, a skilled nursing facility, a custodial care facility, or a similar facility.

For **inpatient care**, the patient must be admitted into the hospital and stay for a period of time, usually a minimum of 24 hours. There must be a room-and-board charge. A hospital room-and-board charge is similar to that for staying in a hotel. The claim includes a room-and-board charge for the day the patient is admitted but not the day that he or she is discharged, as long as the discharge time is before the required checkout time. The UB-04 form should always indicate admission and discharge dates.

When you are coding inpatient hospital claims, do not use the CPT or RVS books unless the billing has itemized some charges according to valid CPT/RVS codes. Each payer has their own coding guidelines. Therefore, before a claim can be coded for processing, you must obtain the payer-specific codes. Most payers break up the bills according to

- Room-and-board charges
- Ancillary charges
- Take-home prescriptions
- Professional fees for exams, surgery, etc.

Providers of service use revenue codes in field locator 42 of the UB-04 form to indicate or identify the specific accommodation, ancillary service, or billing calculation.

ROOM AND BOARD. Hospitals have a variety of rooms available, including but not limited to

- *Private*—A single-occupancy room. The extra cost for a private room is not covered by most plans unless the room was medically necessary due to the patient's illness (e.g., highly contagious disorder).
- *Semiprivate*—A double-occupancy room. Most plans cover the cost of a semiprivate room. The cost may vary according to the type of floor on which the room is located. That is, a semiprivate room in a burn ward may cost more than a semiprivate room in a maternity ward because of the increased level of care required.
- *Ward*—A room with three or more beds. A ward is also covered by most plans. Except for county hospitals, most facilities no longer offer this type of room.
- *Nursery*—A large room for newborn babies. A nursery may have 20 or 30 babies.
- *Specialized Units*—Areas in which special monitoring equipment and a higher ratio of nurses to patients are required. These units are established for extremely ill or terminal patients with different illnesses or injuries that require more acute, intensive care. Specialized units tend to be considerably more expensive than other units. This type of room may cost $1,000 or more per day. Examples are the Intensive Care Unit, Coronary Care Unit, and Definitive Observation Unit.

Note: When you are calculating claim benefits, the normal UCR for Intensive Care Unit rooms is three times the semiprivate room rate.

Telemetry charges (specialized observation equipment) may be billed separately from the base room-and-board amount. In addition, nursing charges may also be billed separately. If they are billed separately, the telemetry and nursing charges should be combined with the base room-and-board amount to obtain the actual room-and-board charge.

To code the room-and-board amount, first determine the number of days in the hospital by counting the day of admission but not the day of discharge. If there is a charge for the day of discharge, you will need to contact the facility to determine why the last day is being charged. Usually, the charge will be for a late discharge. In this case, the late discharge is covered if it was caused or ordered by the attending physician. A late discharge for the patient's convenience, however, is not usually a covered expense.

Each type of room accommodation is coded on a separate line, and the quantity (number of days) applies to that type of room only. In addition, if either the type of room (semiprivate, private, or other) or the per-day charges are different, even if the room type is the same, separate lines of coding are required. For instance, consider the following claim:

5/1/CCYY–5/2/CCYY	Semiprivate $650 per day
5/3/CCYY–5/4/CCYY	Semiprivate $675 per day

In this case, the two different semiprivate room rates must be coded on two different lines, with two services shown on each line (unless 5/4 is the discharge date). If the charge per day was the same for all of the semiprivate rooms, only one line of coding would be required and the number of services would be four.

ANCILLARY EXPENSES. **Ancillary expenses** are miscellaneous services or supplies that are provided by the hospital on an inpatient or outpatient basis, which are necessary for the medical care or treatment of an individual. The most common charges include X-rays, lab fees, pharmacy, med-surgical supplies, operating room expenses, surgery room supplies, recovery room time, anesthesia supplies, occupational therapy, and inhalation therapy. All these expenses can be combined under a single line of coding for ancillary expenses. The only items that may be separated and coded on separate lines are charges for personal items, noncovered items, doctor's ER examination charges, other professional exam charges, or other expenses that may be limited by the plan. This list does not include PC charges (unless specified by the plan).

TAKE-HOME PRESCRIPTIONS. Often doctors in a hospital prescribe **take-home prescriptions**, medications to be taken after the patient is released from the hospital. These medications may be dispensed by the hospital pharmacy and the charges may be included on the hospital bill. The medications are often covered under Major Medical benefits rather than standard hospital benefits. For this reason, these items are usually billed and coded separately, as they are not considered to be hospital expenses and may be subject to other plan provisions. Sometimes the plan has a separate payer for prescriptions, in which case the take-home drugs should be denied.

PROFESSIONAL FEES. Bills for doctors, anesthesiologists, technicians, and other hospital professionals are often included on the hospital bill rather than being billed separately on a CMS-1500. These bills are broken out from the regular hospital bill and paid under the normal plan provisions as if they had been billed on a CMS-1500. Therefore, it is important to go through the itemized billing and determine whether the charges were for materials, equipment, and overhead (rendered by the hospital), or for professional services (rendered by a provider).

PERSONAL ITEMS. Personal items are those items that are primarily for the comfort of the patient and that are not medically necessary. Personal items are not usually covered by a benefit plan. These charges may need to be coded separately, or they may be combined with other ancillary charges and then denied with an appropriate explanation indicating that they are not covered under the plan. Handling procedures vary from payer to payer. Personal items can include

- Barber expenses
- Personal hygiene kit
- Videotaping of birth
- Birth certificate and photos
- Cot rental
- Room transfer as requested by patient
- Lotion
- Television
- Telephone
- Toothbrush and toothpaste
- Guest trays
- Mouthwash
- Gift shop expenses
- Slippers

Most hospitals automatically issue an admission kit to incoming patients. An admission kit usually includes an emesis basin, carafe, cup, lotion, tissue, and mouthwash. Some plans administratively allow for one kit and do not cover additional kits. This type of kit may also be called a maternity kit, Ob-Gyn kit, hygiene kit, or patient comfort kit. Therefore, if items such as mouthwash and toothpaste are billed separately in addition to a kit, they are not usually considered covered charges. (Even if a kit is not billed, these types of charges are not usually allowable.) It is important to consider whether there is a medical necessity for an item prior to denying it. For example, the hospital bill may list a razor. If the patient was scheduled for surgery and the nurse shaved the operative area, the razor would be considered medically necessary.

Outpatient Hospital Claims

The **outpatient** provider of service is a hospital facility (the title may be Hospital, Medical Center, Surgi-Center, or Birthing Center) in which there are no room-and-board charges. Commonly, "come-and-go" or outpatient surgery is performed in the outpatient department because an inpatient admission is not medically necessary. An outpatient hospital facility may have two departments:

1. The ER
2. Outpatient Clinics

There may be facility charges, such as ER usage fees, examination room usage charges, operating room expenses, and recovery room expenses. In an outpatient setting, ancillary expenses include everything except professional fees for examinations, surgery, and other professional services. Clinic charges should be treated as an office visit when you code for the physician. The actual facility usage fee is coded separately; it is not coded with or considered a professional fee.

Other commonly submitted outpatient charges may be for lab or X-ray services, pharmacy, or Durable Medical Equipment.

Miscellaneous Facilities

Many other types of treatment centers may be classified as facilities. Usually, they are designed to handle specialized treatment programs such as psychiatric care, addiction, and emergency care. The following is a sampling of other types of facilities in existence.

DAY CARE/NIGHT CARE CENTERS. As the name implies, **day care centers** provide treatment during the daylight hours and the patient is released at night. **Night care centers** allow the patient to pursue a normal routine during the day such as working, and be treated at the center and cared for overnight. Generally, these types of centers are for treatment of mental or nervous disorders.

There is a great disparity in the handling of these claims from payer to payer. Usually, medical biller or health claims examiner requires a complete review of the facility to determine whether the treatment or the facility are eligible for benefits. The review covers

- Staffing—the type of licensing required for the staff
- Type of billing—how the bills are broken down, and whether they are inclusive, itemized, and so on
- Type of state or federal licensing the facility has
- The facility's primary purpose (custodial care, active treatment, or other).
- Detailed description of the type of treatment, including length of each treatment, licensing of the person who is actually performing the treatment, ancillary services, and other pertinent data.

Often, experienced medical billers or senior examiners may handle daycare claims to ensure that the proper correspondence is prepared and mailed. They also review the documentation when a reply is received. Before any benefits are denied, all plan provisions and limitations must be verified.

URGENT CARE CENTERS. An **urgent care center** is a facility that follows professionally recognized standards to provide urgent or emergency treatment. Many plans have specialized benefits to handle this type of center. An urgent care center generally meets these eight criteria:

1. Mainly provides urgent or emergency medical treatment for acute conditions
2. Does not provide services or accommodations for overnight stays
3. Is open to receive patients every day of the calendar year
4. Has a physician trained in emergency medicine, nurses, and other supporting personnel who are specially trained in emergency care on duty at all times
5. Has X-ray and laboratory diagnostic facilities, emergency equipment, trays, and supplies available for use in life-threatening events
6. Has a written agreement with a local acute care inpatient facility for the immediate transfer of patients who require more intensive care than can be furnished at an outpatient facility, has written guidelines for stabilizing and transporting such patients, and has immediate and reliable direct communication channels with the acute care facility.
7. Complies with all state and federal licensing, regulatory requirements, and other legal requirements.
8. Is not the office or clinic of any physician.

Generally, a medical emergency exists when the following are true:

• Severe symptoms occur. The symptoms must be severe enough to cause a person to seek immediate medical aid regardless of the hour of the day or night.
• The severe symptoms must occur suddenly and unexpectedly. A chronic condition with subacute symptoms that have existed over a period of time usually does not qualify as a medical emergency. However, symptoms that become severe enough to require immediate medical aid may qualify.
• Immediate care was secured. Usually, a situation is not considered to be a medical emergency unless medical care was received immediately after the appearance of acute symptoms. A telephone call to a doctor does not fulfill this requirement if the actual examination and treatment are deferred until the next day.

The administration of the urgent care benefit varies greatly. Therefore, refer to the plan provisions prior to taking any action on such claims.

Some patients seek urgent care treatment for nonemergency reasons (e.g., the patient is suffering from flu symptoms and does not want to take time off to see a doctor). Some payers will deny or reduce payment on these claims, using the reasoning that the level of care obtained was not consistent with the situation.

SURGI-CENTERS. **Ambulatory surgical centers (surgi-centers)** are equipped to allow the performance of surgery on an outpatient basis. These centers may be freestanding or attached to a major acute care facility. Surgi-centers provide financial savings for insureds by eliminating the need for admission into an inpatient facility. An ambulatory surgical facility is a specialized facility that meets all eight of the professionally recognized standards indicated here:

1. Provides a setting for outpatient surgeries
2. Does not provide services or accommodations for overnight stays
3. Has at least two operating rooms and one recovery room; all the medical equipment needed to support the surgery being performed; X-ray and laboratory diagnostic facilities; and emergency equipment, trays, and supplies for use in life-threatening events
4. Has a medical staff that is supervised full-time by a physician, including a registered nurse when patients are in the facility
5. Maintains a medical record for each patient
6. Has a written agreement with a local acute care facility for the immediate transfer of patients who require greater care than can be provided on an outpatient basis
7. Complies with all state and federal licensing and other legal requirements
8. Is not an office or clinic for any physician

Usually, plans provide benefits on a global basis, covering the facility room usage charge and supplies (e.g., anesthesia gases, medications, trays) on the same basis as inpatient hospital services. However, as with other benefits, coverage provisions vary greatly.

ALTERNATIVE BIRTHING CENTERS. **Alternative birthing centers (ABCs)** are outpatient care centers that provide special rooms for routine deliveries. As a rule, these centers provide quiet, nontraditional types of home-like rooms which are designed to allow the parents to be together and participate in the birthing experience.

Often, a nurse practitioner or certified nurse midwife, rather than a physician, is in attendance. The mother normally goes home within five to 12 hours after the delivery. As with other types of outpatient facilities, the following six or similar requirements are necessary for a facility to qualify as a birthing center:

1. Does not provide services or accommodations for overnight stays.
2. Has a medical staff that is supervised full-time by a physician. A registered nurse is also in attendance when patients are in the facility.
3. Maintains a medical record for each patient.
4. Has a written agreement with a local acute care facility for the immediate transfer of patients who require greater care than can be provided on an outpatient basis.
5. Complies with all state and federal licensing, regulatory, and other legal requirements.
6. Is not an office or clinic for any physician.

Most confinements at an ABC should not exceed 24 hours without a transfer to an acute care facility. If the stay exceeds 24 hours, refer the charges for investigation to determine why the continued stay was medically necessary.

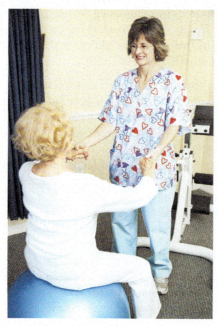

FIGURE 6-6   Post-injury care being provided at a rehabilitation facility
Source: Lisa F. Young/Shutterstock

REHABILITATION FACILITIES. Rehabilitation facilities specialize in long-term, postsickness, or postinjury care. Rehabilitative treatment, rather than active medical care, is the primary focus. This treatment is designed to return a patient to a normal or more normal state. Rehabilitative care is designed for those who are left paralyzed, deformed, handicapped, or otherwise not totally functional as a result of an accident, injury, or illness, such as a stroke or spinal cord injury. (See Figure 6-6 ●.)

Although care at a rehabilitation facility is more aggressive than care provided in a convalescent facility, it is generally very similar to convalescent care.

Many plans provide for some type of rehabilitative care. The limitations of coverage are usually based on a point at which progress ceases and the condition or status of the patient is stabilized. However, some plans do not provide any benefits for rehabilitative treatment.

CONVALESCENT HOSPITALS. Convalescent facilities are usually considered to be midrange facilities that provide non-acute care for persons who are recovering from an acute illness or injury. Usually, admission into a convalescent facility must commence within a specified number of days following a discharge from an acute care facility. The care provided must be active treatment, not custodial care.

The institution generally must meet all seven of the following requirements to be considered an eligible convalescent facility:

1. Is primarily engaged in providing skilled nursing care to sick or injured persons as inpatients under 24-hour supervision of a physician or registered nurse.
2. Has a registered nurse, licensed vocational nurse, or skilled practical nurse on duty at all times. A registered nurse must be on duty at least eight hours a day.

3. Is not, other than incidentally, a treatment facility for drug addicts, alcoholics, mentally ill persons, or senile or mentally deficient persons.
4. Maintains a medical record for each patient.
5. Has a written agreement with a local acute care facility for the immediate transfer of patients who require greater care than can be provided in a nonacute care facility.
6. Complies with all state and federal licensing, regulatory, and other legal requirements.
7. Is not an office or clinic for any physician.

Many plans provide very limited convalescent care benefits. Always verify that the care being provided is not custodial. The care may include some rehabilitative services that may be billed separately or included on a global basis (no breakdown).

NURSING HOMES. Nursing homes specialize in custodial care (that is, care that is primarily to meet the personal needs of the patient and that could be provided by personnel without professional skills or training). Custodial care may include assistance with walking, bathing, dressing, eating, and other activities of daily living. Most plans do not provide custodial care coverage or, if they do, payment is limited. If you are uncertain whether care is custodial, request copies of the provider's nursing notes and admission or discharge summary.

HOSPICE CARE. Hospice care is a healthcare program that provides coordinated services in a home setting. Sometimes care is provided in the patient's home by visiting specialists, and sometimes patients are admitted to a hospice facility. Usually, such care is provided only for persons who are suffering from a terminal condition and who generally have a life expectancy of six months or less. The hospice concept is based on the following principles:

- The beneficiaries of the program are the terminally ill person and his or her family.
- An interdisciplinary team is required to serve the patient, including nurses, social workers, psychologists, clergy, volunteers, and other professionals.
- The facility emphasizes the alleviation of pain and suffering rather than the treatment of the illness.
- Support is provided for all family members to help offset emotional pain.

Hospice care is billed in a variety of methods. If the patient is in a hospice facility, the facility will submit a single bill for all charges. If the patient is receiving treatment in his or her own home, the billing may be provided by a hospice agency which is then responsible for paying other providers. Another method may be to submit separate bills from the various providers. Usually, such services include the rental of beds, commodes, and other equipment, along with the purchase of various medications and supplies required to care for a terminally ill person. For hospice care to be covered, the contract usually specifies such benefits.

> ● **ONLINE INFORMATION:** To learn more about the hospice philosophy and the rise of the modern hospice healthcare system in the United States, conduct online research.

ACTIVITY #4

Hospital and Miscellaneous Facility Charges

Directions: Answer the following questions without looking back at the material just covered. Write your answers in the space provided.

1. Define hospital services. _____
   _____

2. What type of claim form is used to bill for hospital services? _____

3. Name the two types of outpatient hospital facility departments.
   a. _____
   b. _____

4. What is the difference between an inpatient and an outpatient provider service? _____
   _____

5. Name the eight examples given as miscellaneous facilities that use the UB-04 Billing Form to file claims.
   a. _____
   b. _____
   c. _____
   d. _____
   e. _____
   f. _____
   g. _____
   h. _____

6. Name the four categories of hospital charges that most payers use.
   a. _____
   b. _____
   c. _____
   d. _____

Ambulance Services

Ambulance expenses are charges billed for transporting an injured or ill person to a medical facility. Ambulance services are not considered professional or hospital services.

There are four types of ambulance services that are in common use:

1. Air Ambulance
2. Paramedics
3. Mobile Intensive Care Unit
4. Van Transportation Unit

When you receive a claim for ambulance services, you must initiate an investigation to determine whether the charges are eligible for coverage under the insured plan. Under most plans, charges must be from a professional ambulance service; private automobiles, taxicabs, or similar vehicles are usually not covered.

The plan provisions will indicate which limitations apply. Major Medical plans usually designate a maximum allowable or payable amount for each trip, following usual and customary guidelines. Expenses commonly billed by an ambulance service include

- Base call charge. This is the amount automatically charged for the ambulance to respond to a call, even if the patient is not subsequently transported.
- Oxygen and oxygen supplies
- Mileage
- Linens
- Emergency response charge. This is an extra expense in addition to the base charge, which may be added if the patient's condition is severe enough that resuscitation efforts or other types of stabilization measures are required.
- Paramedic response charge. If the responders are paramedics, rather than emergency medical technicians (EMTs), an extra expense may be added.

Air Ambulance

An **air ambulance** is a helicopter or other flight vehicle used to transport severely injured or ill persons to a hospital. Air medical transport may be covered if

1. The facility in the area where the patient is injured cannot manage the patient's condition and it is medically necessary to transfer the patient by air to another facility that is better equipped to treat the patient, or
2. Ground transport time would be prolonged, and would thus compromise the patient's medical status.

Coverage is limited to the regular air ambulance charge for transportation to the nearest facility in the area that can handle the case.

PRACTICE **PITFALLS**

Benefits are usually payable for transfer to another hospital when medically necessary. For example, if one hospital does not have the facilities to treat the patient's medical condition, the patient may be transferred to the closest hospital that has appropriate facilities.

An ambulance expense is covered under Major Medical, Basic ambulance, and Basic hospital benefits under the following conditions:

1. The ambulance must be medically necessary rather than being for the patient's convenience.
2. Transportation must be provided by a professional ambulance or paramedic service.
3. Transportation must be to the nearest facility capable of treating the patient.
4. Transportation must be provided from one facility to another when the first hospital can provide the necessary treatment.

(Continued)

5. Transportation from a facility back home is provided if the patient is unable to travel in an upright position. Exceptions to this policy vary by plan, so refer to the plan provisions before you process the claim.

6. Charges for ambulance services are covered when the claim also includes either emergency room or inpatient hospital charges. An exception would be an insured who is dead on arrival at the hospital.

7. Transportation must be to a facility if the claimant is dead on arrival, even though no treatment or charges are incurred at the facility.

Basic Benefits usually designate a maximum allowable or payable amount for

1. Each trip to and from a facility.
2. All trips made during a period of disability.
3. All expenses incurred during a calendar year.

Under a Basic plan, all trip or per disability limitations apply. A few Basic plans may have a special allowance designated to cover air medical transport. However, many plans do not cover this type of service, regardless of the reason required. The cost of air ambulance ranges upward from a base charge of about $1,200 and is usually based on an hourly rate.

When a person becomes ill while traveling, he or she may want to be transferred to a hospital near home or to be treated by a particular specialist in another city, even though the city that he or she is visiting has qualified specialists in the field. In these instances, ambulance expenses are not covered, regardless of whether the patient uses an air ambulance or a conventional ambulance. This policy is because the transportation is not considered "medically necessary."

Charges for commercial or private airplane transportation, regardless of the reason required, are usually not covered.

Paramedics

Paramedics are specially trained emergency medical personnel who render emergency treatment at the scene of the injury or illness. They are trained in advanced life support, whereas **Emergency Medical Technicians (EMTs)** are trained only in basic life support. There are significant differences in the educational and certification requirements of a paramedic and an EMT. Consequently, when a paramedic is required, an additional fee is usually charged.

Paramedic fees may be covered under a Basic Benefit or may be strictly allowable under Major Medical. The plan provisions should stipulate the handling of this expense.

Mobile Intensive Care Unit

A **mobile intensive care unit** is a life-support vehicle equipped to provide care to critically ill patients who require transportation to a hospital or from one hospital to another. It is designed to serve as an extension of an intensive care unit at a hospital.

The unit is typically staffed by a registered nurse and several other allied health professionals. The fees are in the same range as that for an air ambulance. Such charges may be covered if they are determined to be medically necessary in lieu of regular ambulance services.

Van Transportation Unit

Many companies provide nonemergency transportation of disabled patients to doctors' offices or hospital facilities. **Van transportation units** are specially equipped to handle wheelchairs and patients who are unable to get in and out of a regular vehicle. As a rule, it is required that the patient be able to sit in an upright position. The driver may have very basic medical training, such as knowledge of cardiopulmonary resuscitation, but he or she is generally not able or equipped to handle acutely ill patients. This type of transportation is not covered by most plans because it is not considered medically necessary.

> ● **ONLINE INFORMATION:** CMS provides a list of appropriate diagnoses that can be used for billing ambulance transportation costs. This list is found at http://www.cms.gov/Regulations-and-Guidance/Guidance/Manuals/downloads/clm104c15.pdf.

Durable Medical Equipment Billing Procedures

Durable Medical Equipment (DME) codes are found in the HCPCS manual. These codes are usually a letter followed by a series of numbers. For example, E0105 is the code for a cane of quad or three prong with adjustable or fixed abilities with tips, and E0186 is the code for an air pressure mattress. Both of these are DME equipment that may be prescribed by a physician to aid a patient in rehabilitation or healing. DME must meet a certain criteria to be considered for payment by an insurance company. DME must be an item that can be used for an extended period of time without significant deterioration (i.e., it can stand repeated use). Therefore, an item that can be rented and returned for reuse would meet the requirement for durability. Medical supplies of a disposable nature, such as incontinence pads and surgical stockings, do not qualify as durable. (However, these items may be covered under the plan as medical supplies.)

Medically oriented equipment is primarily and customarily used for medical purposes (i.e., it is designed to fulfill a medical need). Therefore, it is generally not useful in the absence of an illness or injury. For example, a heart patient may use an air conditioner to lower room temperature and reduce fluid loss. However, as the primary and customary use is nonmedical in nature, an air conditioner cannot be considered medical equipment. If a person could use the item in a regular manner in the absence of a medical diagnosis, it is probably nonmedical in nature. Crutches are a good example of DME equipment that is rarely used by a person without a diagnosis.

Most plans allow for patients to purchase or temporarily rent equipment and supplies when they are prescribed by a physician. However, the items must satisfy certain requirements before you can authorize payment.

Apply the following three tests to items billed as DME to determine whether the items are covered under a plan:

1. Does the item satisfy the definition of DME?
2. Is the item reasonable and necessary to treat an illness or injury or to improve the functioning of a malformed body part?
3. Is the item prescribed for use in the patient's home?

Only when all three conditions are met will the item be covered by the plan.

Evaluating Reasonable and Necessary

An item may meet the definition of DME and yet not be covered by the plan. Consider the following criteria:

1. **Reasonableness.** This concept evaluates the soundness and practicality of the DME approach to therapy.
   a. Is the need for the unit based on failures of other, less costly approaches? For example, if the patient tried using an inexpensive transfer board to get out of bed and was unsuccessful, then a trapeze, which is more expensive, would be a better option for the patient to transfer himself or herself out of the bed.
   b. Have more conservative means been attempted? A conservative type of DME might be a hot pack for muscle relaxation, whereas a less conservative method would be an electrical stimulation unit.
   c. What benefits will be derived from the unit? If DME will restore the patient's functioning to the previous level, it is usually considered beneficial. However, if the equipment is just a trial but is not likely to really help the patient progress in functioning, it is not considered a benefit.
   d. Do the benefits justify the expense?
2. **Necessity.** Equipment is necessary when it is expected to make a meaningful contribution to the treatment of the patient's illness or injury or to significantly improve the functioning of a malformed body part. Physicians tend to prescribe equipment for a variety of reasons:
   a. Familiarity. The physician is familiar with a particular piece of equipment. Other, less expensive, more effective means of treatment or equipment may be available.
   b. Current popularity. As with clothing fashions, treatment and equipment popularity runs in cycles. Patients may even request a certain piece of equipment because it is hyped by the news media or some other medium. The particular equipment may not be the best or least expensive treatment available.
   c. Monetarily beneficial. Some equipment suppliers provide monetary inducements to physicians who use their equipment. Therefore, some physicians may routinely prescribe certain equipment due to this factor.

Even if the claim includes a physician's prescription, it may be necessary to refer the claim to a consultant for review prior to issuing payment or approval for purchase.

DME for Patient's Home Use

In order for DME to be purchased or temporarily rented, the equipment must be prescribed for use in the home. Therefore, DME is excluded from coverage if the patient is staying at any facility that meets at least the minimum requirements of a hospital or skilled nursing facility. As many nursing homes are also skilled nursing facilities, DME is covered there if the patient is receiving skilled services (e.g., Physical Therapy, Occupational Therapy) to prepare him or her to return home. If the patient is transferring from the skilled service to the long-term care part of the nursing home, then the nursing home would have to purchase the DME.

A patient's home may be, but is not limited to being:

- His or her own home, apartment, or dwelling
- A relative's home
- A home for the elderly
- A nursing home.

PRACTICE **PITFALLS**

All claims for DME should be documented with the following information:

1. A description of the equipment prescribed by the physician. If the item is a commonly used item, a detailed description may not be necessary. However, if the equipment is new, it is important to try to obtain a marketing or manufacturer's brochure that indicates how the item is constructed and how it functions.
2. A statement of the medical necessity of the equipment. This statement should be in the form of a prescription showing the imprinted name, address, and telephone number of the prescribing physician and the relevant diagnosis.
3. An indication of whether the item is to be rented or purchased and the rental or purchase price.
4. The estimated length of time that the equipment will be needed. This information will aid in the analysis of whether a rental or a purchase is more economical.
5. An indication of where the equipment will be used and for how long.

Rental Versus Purchasing Determinations

The following four steps will assist you to determine the most cost-efficient means of reimbursement for DME.

1. Determine the period of time, in months. for which the item will be medically required, using the information provided by the attending physician.
2. Multiply the number of months by the monthly rental fee. (This fee must be obtained from the supplier. Do not include the costs of perishable supplies, batteries, electrodes, and other items). Estimated length of use in months × monthly rental fee = total estimated equipment rental fee.
3. Request the supplier's purchase price for the equipment. Compare the purchase price with the calculated total estimated rental fee obtained in step #2.

4. If the total estimated rental fee is less than or equal to the purchase price, allow the rental. If the rental fee is greater than the purchase price, rental is allowed up to but not exceeding the purchase price. The member is not required to purchase the item. However, both the member and the supplier need to be notified that a rental expense which is higher than the purchase price will not be allowed under the plan.

Repairs, Replacement, and Delivery

Repairs are covered when they are necessary to make the equipment functional. If the expense for repairs exceeds the estimated cost of purchasing or renting new equipment for the remaining period of medical need, payment is limited to the lower amount. Verify manufacturer's warranties before you pay repair fees.

Replacements are usually covered in cases of irreparable damage or wear or when the patient's physical condition has changed. Replacements due to wear or changes in the patient's physical condition must be supported by a current physician's order. Replacements due to loss may be covered, depending on the circumstances. Usually, replacement is not covered when disrepair or loss results from a patient's carelessness. Other reasons for repair or replacement may be covered according to the plan provisions.

Charges for delivery of the DME and oxygen are usually covered.

ACTIVITY #5

DME Billing

Directions: Answer the following questions without looking back at the material just covered. Write your answers in the space provided.

1. What are the three tests (questions) that you must apply to items billed as DME to determine whether the items may be covered under a plan?

    a. _____

    b. _____

    c. _____

2. Will a plan cover a billed DME if two out of the three conditions are met? _____

    _____

Types of Durable Medical Equipment

Oxygen

Many plans cover the use of oxygen under DME benefits. Even though the oxygen itself is not durable, the canister in which the oxygen is contained and transported is durable, and it therefore falls under the category of DME. The provider of the oxygen will bill the patient, or, if the patient is in a facility, the provider will bill the facility and the facility in turn will include oxygen on the bill to the insurance.

Remember that these are general guidelines only. The specific guidelines may vary from payer to payer.

Prosthetic Devices

Prosthetic devices are designed to replace a missing body part or to restore some function to a paralyzed body part. These devices are covered when the prosthetic is expected to improve life function. The physical therapist must make a case for the expected improvement and usually orders the prosthetic with the assistance of a supplier. Insurance plan coverage of prosthetics varies, so read the contract carefully before billing.

Prosthetic devices include the making and application of an artificial part that is medically necessary to replace a lost or impaired body part or function, such as an artificial arm or leg, or a urinary collection and retention system.

Covered expenses associated with prosthetics include

- Shipping and handling as part of the purchase price
- Temporary postoperative prostheses
- Replacement charges when replacement is due to a change in the patient's physical condition. (Children often need replacement prostheses every six to 12 months, depending on their growth rate and other factors.) Replacement is not covered for wear and tear.

Medical/Surgical Supplies

Perishable medical/surgical supplies may be covered under the plan if the items can be used only by the patient and are medically necessary in the treatment of the illness or injury. Medical and surgical supplies include

1. Disposable, nondurable supplies and accessories that are required to operate medical equipment or prosthetic devices.
2. Necessary drugs and biological items that are put directly into equipment (such as nonprescription nutrients).
3. Initial and replacement accessories that are essential for operating medical equipment. For example, the delivery and setup of an oxygen concentrator is an initial expense and the water bottle attached to it may need to be replaced periodically, so these accessories both fall into this category.
4. Supplies that are furnished and charged by a hospital, surgical center, or physician as part of active therapy, such as ace bandage, cast, or cervical collar.

Do not include items or supplies that could be used by the patient or a member of the patient's family for purposes other than medical care.

Refer any questionable items to your supervisor or other designated person and give the following information:

- Patient's diagnosis
- Prescription from attending physician
- Product description, literature, and prices.

See Appendix C for a list of DME coverage guidelines. This list is provided as a guide only. Actual administration may vary from company to company.

CHAPTER REVIEW

Summary

- Physician's services include a wide array of services, from treating a patient in the office to providing services in an ER setting or at a skilled nursing facility.
- Charges for physician's services may be billed by a variety of practitioners.
- It is important to learn to identify the covered providers, and use these guidelines to determine whether the charges billed are covered services.
- X-ray and laboratory services are essential in determining the patient's problems, ruling out conditions, and managing illnesses or injuries. It is now possible for patients to have certain tests performed in the privacy of their own homes (e.g., pregnancy and glucose level tests).
- There are rules and guidelines for processing charges received for laboratory and radiology services.
- These guidelines should enable you to identify covered services and determine the correct processing procedures for these services.
- Hospitals provide a sterile environment where patients may receive medically necessary services and treatments, surgical or otherwise. They also provide a controlled environment in which patients may recover.
- Most plans and payers have specific handling guidelines; check these guidelines before you process a claim.
- Ambulance expenses are incurred to transfer an injured or sick person to a medical facility. These expenses are not considered professional or hospital services.
- Charges for an ambulance, air ambulance, paramedics, or a mobile intensive care unit are often payable under Basic or Major Medical if the services are considered medically necessary.
- Durable Medical Equipment includes medical-surgical equipment that can stand repeated use, is not useful in the absence of illness or injury, and is prescribed by a physician. In addition, to qualify as DME the item must be necessary and reasonable for the treatment of the illness or injury or to replace an injured or lost bodily part or function, and it must be appropriate for home use.
- In addition to the cost of the item, the insurance typically covers charges for shipping, handling, and postage, which are considered part of the purchase price.
- Necessary repairs to purchased equipment (if the equipment is not covered under warranty) are also covered. However, the cost of repairs is usually not covered for rented equipment.

Review Questions

Directions: Answer the following questions without looking back at the material just covered. Write your answers in the space provided.

1. What is the numeric range of the CPT laboratory panel codes? _____

2. What are panel tests? _____

3. What is unbundling? _____
_____
_____

4. What are professional and technical components? _____
_____
_____
_____

5. What does modifier -26 denote? _____
_____

6. Name the five varieties of hospital rooms.
   a. _____
   b. _____
   c. _____
   d. _____
   e. _____

7. What are ancillary expenses? _____
_____

8. List at least three items that may be considered personal items. _____
_____

9. What are urgent care centers? _____
_____

10. What are surgi-centers? _____
_____

11. What does the abbreviation ABC stand for and what is it?
_____

12. Name the three different types of benefits that may cover ambulance expenses.
   a. _____
   b. _____
   c. _____

13. The base call charge is _____
_____

14. True or False: If a person is injured while he or she is on vacation, most plans will pay to have the patient transported to the nearest facility to his or her home, even if there is no other reason for the transfer. _____

15. True or False: In an emergency, taxicab fees are covered because the transportation was medically necessary. _____

16. Name the two circumstances in which air ambulance charges may be covered under a plan.

   a. _____

   b. _____

17. What documentation should be included with all DME claims?

   a. _____

   _____

   b. _____

   _____

c. _____

_____

d. _____

_____

e. _____

_____

18. Repairs are covered when they are necessary to make the equipment _____

19. Replacements are usually covered in cases of irreparable damages or because of _____

_____

20. _____ are designed to replace a missing body part or to restore function to a paralyzed part.

If you were unable to answer any of these questions, refer back to that section and then fill in the answers.

ACTIVITY #6

Find the Terms

Directions: Find and circle the words listed below. Words can appear horizontally, vertically, diagonally, forward, or backward.

```
M  S  S  Z  S  K  I  C  U  V  I  O  U  T  Q  S  K  E  A  Y  P  A  H  O  T
M  I  C  E  P  E  I  Z  H  N  J  G  S  S  E  Q  R  J  M  G  R  D  O  X  A
T  W  S  N  C  T  M  T  C  R  B  Z  E  C  X  U  G  A  J  O  O  W  G  C  Q
Y  E  T  C  U  I  K  O  K  D  R  U  I  V  T  C  I  R  O  L  F  Y  S  Z  E
V  H  L  Z  E  G  V  N  H  O  G  V  N  C  S  N  R  W  K  O  E  C  W  H  C
H  V  A  E  S  L  N  E  G  G  R  S  N  D  T  X  K  M  O  C  S  Z  P  Z  F
S  I  G  I  M  M  L  Z  D  E  N  U  Q  E  L  U  T  M  M  N  S  H  B  G  K
C  H  Y  O  K  E  G  A  S  C  P  I  N  J  J  I  V  X  D  O  I  H  R  S  A
Z  W  M  Z  O  X  T  Y  N  U  I  A  S  E  J  D  N  A  D  N  O  E  U  T  O
B  T  J  U  L  T  T  R  C  E  N  T  G  R  I  Y  I  G  W  O  N  I  O  C  N
L  O  O  Z  U  I  V  A  Y  C  O  H  E  A  U  R  F  Z  U  I  A  N  A  V  V
F  Y  G  E  L  Q  N  H  E  C  H  U  L  H  A  N  A  R  J  T  L  P  L  S  F
A  U  G  I  H  Q  J  T  I  N  H  Y  S  M  T  G  I  V  D  A  S  A  O  N  Z
O  I  C  M  T  B  H  M  B  D  S  A  B  S  C  S  H  H  T  I  E  T  C  E  L
U  A  H  M  J  E  Y  O  T  I  L  U  R  K  E  I  O  B  Y  D  R  I  I  C  Y
F  V  V  K  R  Q  V  N  S  E  L  V  V  G  Z  R  R  R  Y  A  V  E  N  E  Y
X  S  Y  A  R  X  O  Q  H  A  U  D  J  W  E  Y  V  H  P  R  I  N  A  S  C
E  W  P  M  D  M  S  W  N  N  F  G  Y  E  Q  S  Y  I  I  Z  C  T  P  S  Q
D  Y  N  I  G  H  T  C  A  R  E  C  E  N  T  E  R  S  C  R  E  C  A  I  L
W  T  B  A  I  B  E  N  O  I  T  A  T  L  U  S  N  O  C  E  S  A  P  T  I
P  S  X  B  B  O  T  L  O  U  T  P  A  T  I  E  N  T  K  H  S  R  N  Y  P
W  N  H  B  I  V  L  O  D  P  X  D  X  D  U  D  X  C  G  C  J  E  C  M  E
F  P  B  J  B  C  Q  R  K  N  O  S  Z  S  D  K  R  P  Y  A  B  G  J  S  M
S  E  S  N  E  P  X  E  E  C  N  A  L  U  B  M  A  Z  L  Q  H  V  D  A  Z
M  G  B  E  E  Q  N  Y  R  A  C  O  F  K  B  X  K  J  W  F  F  U  E  Y  L
```

1. Acupuncture
2. Air Ambulance
3. Ambulance Expenses
4. Consultation
5. Dialysis
6. Facility Services
7. Inpatient Care
8. Miscellaneous Services
9. Necessity
10. Night Care Centers
11. Nursing Homes
12. Outpatient
13. Papanicolaou
14. Professional Services
15. Prosthetic Devices
16. Radiation Oncology
17. Telemetry Charges
18. X-Rays

ACTIVITY #7

Matching

Directions: Match the following terms with the proper definition by writing the letter of the correct definition in the space next to the term.

1. _____ Alternative Birthing Centers
2. _____ Ambulatory Surgical Centers
3. _____ Ancillary Expenses
4. _____ Convalescent Facilities
5. _____ Day Care Centers
6. _____ Durable Medical Equipment
7. _____ Emergency Medical Technician
8. _____ Laboratory Examinations
9. _____ Medical Management
10. _____ Medically Oriented Equipment
11. _____ Mobile Intensive Care Unit
12. _____ Office or Other Outpatient Visits
13. _____ Professional Component
14. _____ Rehabilitation Facilities
15. _____ Speech Therapy
16. _____ Take-Home Prescriptions
17. _____ Technical Component
18. _____ Van Transportation Units

a. Vehicles specially equipped to handle wheelchairs and patients who are unable to get in and out of a regular vehicle.

b. Collection of a specimen or taking of an X-ray.

c. Medications to be taken after the patient is released from the hospital.

d. Office visits or other encounters between a physician and patient that occur outside a hospital setting.

e. Therapy to correct speech impairments.

f. The reading or interpreting of lab results or X-rays.

g. Specialize in long-term, postsickness, or postinjury care.

h. A life support vehicle equipped to provide care to critically ill patients during transportation to a hospital.

i. The analysis of body substances to determine their chemical or tissue make-up.

j. A person trained in basic life support.

k. X-ray and laboratory charges that are incurred to control or manage a diagnosis (e.g., monitoring blood glucose levels on a patient with diabetes).

l. Items primarily and customarily used for medical purposes.

m. A center equipped to allow for the performance of surgery on an outpatient basis. These centers may be free-standing or attached to a major acute care facility.

n. Provide treatment during the daylight hours; the patient is released at night.

o. Items that can be used for an extended period of time without significant deterioration.

p. Usually considered to be midrange facilities that provide nonacute care for persons recovering from an acute illness or injury.

q. Miscellaneous services or supplies that are provided by the hospital on an inpatient or outpatient basis, which are necessary for the medical care or treatment of an individual.

r. Outpatient care centers that provide special rooms for routine deliveries.

CHAPTER 7

Surgery and Anesthesia Claims

Keywords and concepts you will learn in this chapter:

Abortion

Anesthesia

Arthroplasty

Assistant Surgeon

Bilateral Procedures

Block Procedures

Bone Spur

Bunion

By Report (BR)

Capsulotomy

Chromosomal Analysis

Cosmetic Procedure

Cosmetic Surgery

Cosurgeons

Diagnostic Procedures

Dorsal Osteotomy

Dwyer Procedure

Endogenous Obesity

Epidural Anesthesia

Exogenous Obesity

False Nail

Flat Feet

Followup Days

After completing this chapter, you will be able to:

- List the four general classifications of surgery.

- Describe procedures covered in the surgical section of the CPT manual.

- Explain the general guidelines that relate to processing surgery claims.

- Apply surgical guidelines as they relate to maternity procedures.

- Apply surgical guidelines as they relate to cosmetic procedures.

- Explain the general guidelines that relate to processing obesity surgery.

- Explain the general guidelines that relate to processing assistant surgery.

- Discuss the use of modifiers to indicate co-surgeons.

- Define podiatry.

- Identify the guidelines for proper surgical coding of podiatric services.

Ganglions
General Anesthesia
Global Approach
Hammertoes
Heel Spur
High-Arched Feet
Hospital Staff Anesthesiologist
Hypnosis
In Vitro Fertilization
Incidental Procedure
Independent Anesthesiologist
Infusion Pump
Ingrown Toenail
Intractable Pain
Intravenous (IV) Sedation
In Utero Fetal Surgery
Joints
Ligaments
Local Anesthesia
Matrixectomy
Metatarsal Plantar Callus
Monitored Anesthesia Care (MAC)
Multiple Procedures
Nerve Block Anesthesia
Neuroma
Optional Modifiers
Orthosis
Orthotic Devices
Physical Status Modifiers
Podiatry
Positional Bunion
Reconstruction
Regional Anesthesia
Saddle Block
Serial Surgery
Spinal Anesthesia
Structural Bunion
Surgery
Tenotomy
Therapeutic Procedures
Topical Anesthesia
Unusual Services
Warts

- Identify common foot conditions and treatment procedures.

- Identify modifiers frequently used with surgical procedures.

- Describe the four methods of anesthesia administration.

- Identify codes which fall within the anesthesia range of the CPT.

- Discuss anesthesia handling procedures.

- Calculate anesthesia benefits using both basic and time units.

- Identify anesthesia modifiers.

- Explain monitored anesthesia care.

- Discuss how to code for care provided by an Anesthesia Assistant and CRNA.

- Recognize considerations to billing procedures related to pain control.

- Explain processing guidelines for epidural anesthesia.

Surgery is the branch of medicine that treats diseases, injuries, and deformities through operative or invasive methods. Although surgery usually involves cutting, cutting does not have to be involved for a procedure to be considered surgical. Surgery is anything that involves removing, altering, repairing, entering, or carrying out any other invasion of the body. Therefore, inserting a tube into a person's throat does not involve cutting but is considered surgical in nature because it invades the body. Many laser procedures are also considered surgical.

Most benefit plans cover only surgeries that are necessitated by disease or injury. In other words, the procedure must be considered medically necessary to repair or improve function or diagnose an illness. In addition, just because a procedure is listed in the surgery section of the CPT® does not mean that the procedure is allowable under a benefit plan, nor does it mean that it will necessarily be coded as a surgical procedure. The coding of procedures varies from company to company.

Surgical Procedures

In general, surgical procedures can be classified as one of the following types:

- Diagnostic
- Therapeutic
- Reconstructive
- Cosmetic

Diagnostic procedures are performed to determine the presence of disease or the cause of the patient's symptoms. Two of the most common forms of diagnostic surgery are endoscopy and diagnostic laparoscopy. An endoscopy involves inserting a very small instrument called a scope through a single incision or orifice and examining the interior of a hollow organ or cavity of the body. A diagnostic laparoscopy involves making one or more small incisions on the exterior part of the patient's abdomen in the area near the organ or space being examined. (Laparoscopy is used only for the abdominal area.) Then a scope is inserted through the incision into the body cavity. The surgeon can then look through the scope and see the interior of the examination area. If desired, the surgeon may take pictures or a video of the area. Examples of diagnostic procedures include bronchoscopy (31622), gastrointestinal endoscopy (43234), sigmoidoscopy (45330), and diagnostic laparoscopy (49320). (See Figure 7-1 ●.)

Therapeutic procedures are performed to remove or correct the functioning of a body part that is diseased or injured. Failure to perform a therapeutic procedure could cause the patient to enter a progressive functional decline or to lose his or her life.

A removal, repair, or manipulation may be performed to correct the abnormally functioning organ. Some cutting is usually required. However, as continual medical advances are made, more procedures are being performed without cutting or with minimal incisions. Examples of therapeutic procedures are liver transplant (47135), craniectomy (removal of tumor of the brain) (61510), and appendectomy (44950).

Reconstruction is performed to rebuild or aesthetically restore a part of the body that was damaged or defective as a result of an illness or injury. Reconstruction is necessary to return the body to its normal or near-normal appearance and may or may not affect the functioning of the organ or area. Even though reconstruction may be necessary for purely cosmetic reasons, it is covered under most plans as long as it is necessitated as a result of a disease or injury that occurred while the claimant was covered under the plan. If the injury or illness occurred before the claimant was covered under the plan, the repair may be considered cosmetic, not reconstructive. Examples of reconstructive procedures are rhinoplasty (surgical correction of the external appearance of the nose, 30400–30462) and breast augmentation or reconstruction (after mastectomy resulting from breast cancer, 19324–19396).

Cosmetic procedures are performed solely to improve the appearance of a body part and are not usually covered by benefit plans unless the procedure is functional in nature. For example, a scar revision is performed as a result of a contracture of a scar received in an accident. The release of the contracture is considered functional in nature, although the procedure might also significantly improve the appearance of the scar.

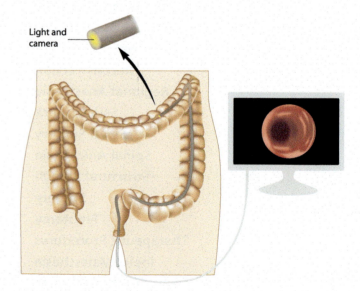

Light and camera

FIGURE 7-1   Flexible colonscope
Source: Alila Sao Mai/Shutterstock

In some situations, it is difficult to ascertain whether a procedure should be considered cosmetic or reconstructive. In these instances, seek a professional opinion.

> ▶ CRITICAL THINKING QUESTION: Why do you think cosmetic procedures are generally not a covered benefit under most insurance plans? Do you agree that they should not be covered? Why or why not?

Surgery and the CPT

For all procedures in the surgical section, codes are listed by body system (e.g., integumentary, digestive), then in order by body part, from the head downward. Surgery CPT codes, shown in Table 7-1 ●, range from 10040 to 69990. The following list provides an introduction to each section, along with a note of any special handling required for that section.

Integumentary System (10040–19499)

These codes are used to bill for procedures done on the integumentary system or skin.

LESIONS. Lesions are coded according to the overall size of the lesion that is removed (not necessarily the size that is sent for biopsy). If a lesion's measurements are covered by several size ranges (e.g., a lesion that is 3 cm × 2 cm × 1 cm deep), the highest measurement should be used (i.e., 3 cm). The other indicator for lesion coding is the malignant or benign nature of the lesion. Be sure to code each lesion separately.

REPAIRS. As with lesions, repairs are coded according to the length of the wound being repaired. However, there is an additional consideration for the depth and complexity of the wound. If multiple wounds are closed during the same operative session within a specific region (e.g., head), the total length of the repaired wounds should be added together, and one code should be used for all repairs to that part of the body.

SKIN GRAFTS. Skin grafts should be coded according to the size of the recipient area, not the donor area. The skin graft should be coded separately from the closure (repair) of the donor site. For example, a 64-year-old woman with a 4 cm × 4 cm full-thickness chronic ulceration of the plantar aspect of the left heel is debrided and a tissue-cultured allogeneic skin substitute equaling 25 square cm was grafted to the excised surface and secured with interrupted sutures. The code 15430 would be used because the tissue is nondermal (not taken from a person) and debridement is included in this code set.

Musculoskeletal System (20005–29999)

These codes are used to bill for procedures done on the muscles and bones of the body. In this section, *complicated* refers to an infection, delayed treatment, or an extraordinary amount of time for a surgery. In the case of complicated codes, the claim and an operating report often must be sent for medical review.

Repair of the wound site, casting, and/or initiation of traction are integral parts of musculoskeletal surgery and are not reported separately.

BONE, CARTILAGE, AND FASCIA GRAFTS. The codes for bone, cartilage, and fascia grafts include the acquisition of the donor graft. If a different physician acquires the grafts, that additional physician should bill using modifier -80 (assistant surgeon).

Respiratory System (30000–32999)

These codes are used to bill for procedures done on the organs of the respiratory system. For example, use codes 33255 for operative tissue ablation and reconstruction of atria, extensive (e.g., maze procedure); without cardiopulmonary bypass removal of a lung.

Cardiovascular System (33010–37799)

These codes are used to bill for invasive procedures on the heart, veins, and arteries. Codes for minor procedures involving the veins and arteries (e.g., injection), and cardiac catheterization are not included. These procedures are found in the Medicine section. (See the Physician's, Clinical, and Hospital Services Claims chapter for more information.)

Hemic and Lymphatic Systems (38100–38999)

These codes are used to bill for procedures of the spleen and lymph nodes, as well as bone marrow transplants.

BONE MARROW/STEM CELL TRANSPLANTS (38207–38215). Codes in this section may be reported once a day, regardless of the number of cells that are transplanted during any given session. It is acceptable to code for each procedure performed. For example, the procedures for codes 38206 ("Blood-derived hematopoietic progenitor cell harvesting for transplantation, per collection; autologous"), 38207 ("Transplant preparation

TABLE 7-1 Surgery CPT® Codes

Integumentary System	10040–19499
Musculoskeletal System	20005–29999
Respiratory System	30000–32999
Cardiovascular System	33010–37799
Hemic and Lymphatic Systems	38100–38999
Mediastinum and Diaphragm	39000–39599
Digestive System	40490–49999
Urinary System	50010–53899
Male Genital System	54000–55899
Intersex Surgery	55970–55980
Female Genital System	56405–58999
Maternity Care and Delivery	59000–59899
Endocrine System	60000–60699
Nervous System	61000–64999
Eye and Ocular Adnexa	65091–68899
Auditory System	69000–69979
Operating Microscope	69990

of hematopoietic progenitor cells; cryopreservation and storage"), and 38212 ("Transplant preparation of hematopoietic progenitor cells; red blood cell removal") might be done in one day and billed as separate procedures.

Mediastinum and Diaphragm (39000–39599)

These codes are used to bill for procedures of the mediastinum and diaphragm. For example, excision of a mediastinal cyst is coded 39200 and an endoscopy of the mediastinum with a biopsy is 39400.

Digestive System (40490–49999)

These codes are used to bill for procedures performed on all the organs of the digestive system, from the lips (mouth) down to the anus.

ENDOSCOPIES. The appropriate code for endoscopies is determined by the organs through which the endoscope is passed. An endoscope that is only passed into the esophagus would receive one code, and an endoscope passed through the esophagus to the duodenum would receive a different code. Remember that if an endoscopy turns into a surgery, the endoscopic procedure is not coded.

APPENDECTOMIES. The reason for an appendectomy must be documented (e.g., appendicitis). If an appropriate diagnosis code (one which requires an appendectomy) is not given, and the appendectomy is performed in conjunction with another surgery, the appendectomy should be considered incidental to the other surgery performed.

HERNIA REPAIR. The age of the patient is one of the prevailing factors in choosing the correct code for a hernia repair. Billers and claims examiners should be sure that the age of the patient matches the code given.

Urinary System (50010–53899)

These codes are used to bill for procedures performed on the kidneys, ureters, bladder, and urethra and include prostate resections. This section often combines several procedures together under one code. If an included procedure requires significant additional time or effort, use modifier -22 (increased procedural services) and submit an operative report so that the claim may be sent for review.

Male Genital System (54000–55899)

These codes are used to bill for procedures performed on the male genital system, including all male reproductive organs.

Intersex Surgery (55970–55980)

These codes are used to bill for procedures performed to transform a patient from one gender to another. These procedures are often excluded by most health plans.

Female Genital System (56405–58999)

These codes are used to bill for procedures performed on the female genital system. They include all female reproductive

organs but do not include maternity care, which is covered under the next subsection.

PELVIC EXAMINATIONS. Pelvic examinations should not be coded separately when another pelvic region procedure is performed. A dilation and curettage is considered to be an integral part of a pelvic exam; therefore, it is also not coded separately when another pelvic region procedure is performed.

LAPAROSCOPY/HYSTEROSCOPY. The codes in this section often combine several procedures under one code. If an included procedure requires significant additional time or effort, use modifier -22 (increased procedural services) and add the operating report to the claim so that it may be sent for review.

Maternity Care and Delivery (59000–59899)

See the section that follows regarding maternity care.

Endocrine System (60000–60699)

These codes are used to bill for procedures on the thymus, adrenal glands, thyroid, and parathyroid. Pituitary glands and pineal glands are included in the Nervous System codes.

Nervous System (61000–64999)

These codes are used to bill for procedures on the organs of the nervous system, including the nerves, brain, and spinal cord. Procedures on the pituitary glands and pineal glands are also included in this section, as they are both located in the brain.

Eye and Ocular Adnexa (65091–68899)

These codes are used to bill for surgical procedures on the eye and ocular adnexa. Diagnostic procedures for the eye and ocular adnexa are reported using the Medicine section of the CPT. Procedures performed only on the eyelid are coded using the surgical codes in the integumentary system.

CATARACT SURGERY. Any injections performed during cataract surgery are considered to be an integral part of the procedure and are not allowed separately. Lens and refraction services are also included as part of the surgery.

Auditory System (69000–69979)

These codes are used to bill for procedures performed on the organs of the auditory (hearing) system. This section includes surgical procedures only; use the Medicine section of the CPT to report diagnostic procedures. Repairs to the outer ear are included in the surgery codes for the integumentary system.

Operating Microscope (69990)

This code is used to bill for the use of an operating microscope during a surgical procedure. It is reported in addition to the actual surgical procedure that is performed.

> ● **ONLINE INFORMATION:** Go to www.entusa.com/surgery_videos.htm and view one of the endoscopic surgery videos. Identify the procedure performed and the CPT code. Be sure to include any applicable modifiers.

ACTIVITY #1

CPT Codes

Directions: Write the codes for each section and the procedures that are listed under each section in the space provided.

Section	Codes
1. Integumentary System	_____
2. Musculoskeletal System	_____
3. Cardiovascular System	_____
4. Hemic and Lymphatic Systems	_____
5. Digestive System	_____
6. Female Genital System	_____
7. Eye and Ocular Adnexa	_____

General Guidelines

The following guidelines will assist you in the processing of surgery claims.

Surgery in a Physician's Office

Claims for surgery performed in a physician's office, as in Figure 7-2 ●, are often itemized for each charge incurred, such as the surgery, local anesthesia, medication, surgical trays, and dressings.

Generally, the charge by the physician for surgery should include performing the surgical procedure, administering local anesthetic (if required), and providing all routine followup care. The charge for surgery always includes

- The immediate preoperative visit.
- The surgical procedure.
- Local anesthesia (e.g., topical, digital block).
- Routine followup care (visits) provided within the followup days listed in the *RVS*.

Nonroutine followup visits due to complications or other reasons may be billed and considered separately from the original surgical charge. Medical supplies, medications, X-rays, facility fees, and other services are usually considered separately.

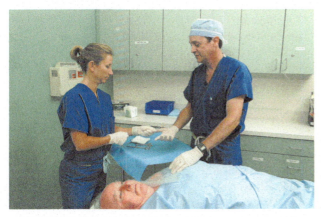

FIGURE 7-2   Surgery being performed in a physician's office
Source: Michal Heron/Pearson Education/PH College

Preoperative Care

An immediate preoperative visit in the hospital or elsewhere is generally necessary to examine the patient, complete the hospital records, and initiate the treatment program. Charges for these procedures are included in the surgical allowance. However, a separate allowance may be warranted for preoperative services in the following circumstances:

1. When the preoperative visit is the initial visit (i.e., in an emergency room), and prolonged detention or evaluation is required to prepare the patient or to establish the need for the surgery.
2. When the preoperative visit is a consultation. Be sure that the physician has not "upcoded" a preoperative visit to increase benefits. An example is a surgeon billing for a consultation prior to surgery, when in fact the visit was a simple preoperative visit.
3. When procedures that are not usually part of the basic surgical procedure (e.g., bronchoscopy prior to chest surgery) are provided during the immediate preoperative period.
4. When a procedure could normally be performed in the office, but under certain circumstances related to the patient's age and condition it requires hospitalization. See modifier code -22 in the CPT.

Followup Days

Followup days are the days immediately following a surgical procedure during which a doctor must monitor a patient's condition. The *RVS* lists unit values for surgical procedures that include the surgery, local anesthesia, and the normal, uncomplicated followup care associated with the procedure for the period indicated in the section titled Followup Days. Complications or other circumstances requiring additional or unusual services concurrent with the procedure or procedures, or during the listed period of normal followup care, may warrant additional charges on a fee-for-service basis. However, unless the physician specifically indicates unusual circumstances, assume that the followup care is routine. Regardless of how the physician bills the visits, all visits occurring within the listed followup days should be combined with the surgical charge. The following are categories of followup care:

1. Followup care for diagnostic procedures (e.g., endoscopy, injection procedures for radiology) includes only care that is related to recovery from the diagnostic procedure itself. Care of the underlying condition for which the diagnostic procedure was performed or other accompanying conditions is not included and may be charged separately in accordance with the services rendered.
2. Followup care for therapeutic procedures generally includes all normal postoperative care. Complications, exacerbations, recurrence, or the presence of other diseases or injuries requiring additional services concurrent with the surgical procedure(s) or during the indicated period of normal followup care may warrant the coding of additional charges that are allowable separately.

3. When additional surgical procedure(s) are carried out within the listed period of followup care for a previous surgery, the followup periods will run concurrently through their normal termination.

Combine the charges for routine followup care with the surgical charge and compare the total with the UCR fee for the procedure performed. Some plans follow this approach, and others deny the visit as being within the followup period, if they are billed separately.

EXAMPLE:

Procedure: 40808, biopsy, 10 followup days

Description	Date	CPT Code	Charge
Office Visit	4/1/CCYY	99213	$ 25
Surgery	4/3/CCYY	40808	$350
Followup Hospital Visit	4/4/CCYY	99221	$ 25
Followup Hospital Visit	4/5/CCYY	99231	$ 25
Followup Office Visit	4/10/CCYY	99213	$ 30
			$455

According to administrative practices, you may or may not include the preoperative visit with the surgical charge. In the example, and unless you are told otherwise, assume that the preoperative visit is part of the surgery charge. Therefore, compare $455 against the plan's UCR limitation for the surgery.

By Report Procedures

Some procedures are so unusual or variable that it is impossible to determine a standard UCR or unit value allowance for them. These procedures are called **By Report (BR)** procedures. The *RVS* may refer to these procedures as Relative Value Not Established (RNE). You should refer BR and RNE procedures to a professional review unit, a supervisor, or a consultant for review to determine the allowance. For proper review, include a copy of the operative report. You may also need to send the anesthesia record. If you do not have the operative report with the claim, pend the claim and request a copy of the report before you refer the claim.

Multiple or Bilateral Procedures

Multiple procedures are more than one surgical procedure performed during the same operative session. These surgeries are denoted by adding modifier -51 to the CPT code. **Bilateral procedures** are surgeries that involve a pair of similar body parts (e.g., breasts, eyes). Bilateral procedures are denoted by using the modifier -50. There are two main types of multiple or bilateral procedures: same time but different operative field, and same time and same operative field.

SAME TIME, DIFFERENT OPERATIVE FIELD. When more than one surgery is performed during the same operative session but through a different orifice (opening) or incision or in a different operative field, 100% of the UCR is allowable for the major procedure, and 50% of the UCR (or actual charge, whichever is less) is allowed for the second procedure. 25% of the UCR (or actual charge, whichever is less) is allowed for each additional procedure. Some insurance carriers, however, do not apply the 25% rule; instead, they allow 100% for the primary procedure and 50% thereafter.

Bilateral procedures follow the same rules as multiple procedures performed through different incisions. Multiply the UCR allowance for the single procedure by 150% or 1.5. If there is an established bilateral CPT code, that code would be allowable at 100% only because the units have already been assigned at 150% of the unit value for the single procedure.

There are two ways to identify a bilateral procedure. The provider will list the CPT and use modifier -50 to denote a bilateral procedure. Or the provider will identify LT (left) or RT (right) next to each procedure. When you are not sure whether a procedure was bilateral, obtain an operative report.

SAME TIME, SAME OPERATIVE FIELD. When multiple procedures are performed during the same operative session through the same incision, orifice, or operative field, the additional procedures are usually considered to be incidental.

An **incidental procedure** does not add significant time or complexity to the operative session. In such a case, the allowed amount will be that of the major procedure only.

However, if the additional procedures are not incidental, the rules for handling multiple procedures previously explained would apply. That is, the major procedure would be considered at 100% of UCR and the lesser at 50%.

In comparison with incidental procedures, integral procedures are performed as part of a more complex primary procedure.

EXAMPLE:

A provider submits the following bill:

	Billed Amount	UCR
Tonsillectomy (42821)	$600	$600
Eustachian tube inflation (69400)	$300	$200

Following the rules previously indicated, 100% of the major procedure plus 50% of the lesser procedure would be allowed. Therefore, the allowed amount in this example would be

100% of $600	$600
+50% of $200	$100
Total Allowance	$700
Total Billed Amount	$900
Less Allowed Amount	−$700
Member's Responsibility	$200

Gender Designated Surgery

Certain CPT codes are designated for male or female patients. Ensure that the submitted code designation accurately reflects the gender of the patient.

- CPT code 53210 is used for total urethrectomy, including cystostomy, in a female, whereas CPT code 53215 is used for the comparable procedure in a male.

Global UCR

It is important to look at the total billing and not to penalize the claimant for the way the physician bills. Thus, you should use the total amount allowed for UCR, even if the physician misallocates the billing for the procedures.

EXAMPLE:

Assume the same procedures as previously described were billed in the following way:

	Billed Amount	UCR
Tonsillectomy (42821)	$300	$600
Eustachian tube inflation (69400)	+$600	+$100
Total Billed Amount	$900	$700

Normal UCR would be

1st procedure—100% of $600 up to the actual charge amount	$300
2nd procedure—50% of $200 or the actual charge, whichever is less	+$100
Total Allowance	$400

By referring to the *RVS*, you can determine that the major procedure is the tonsillectomy, which allows 16.39

units, whereas eustachian tube inflation allows only 1.39 units. However, the physician billed the tonsillectomy as the minor procedure.

This billing would be financially detrimental to the claimant solely because the physician's office did not properly allocate the expenses. To avoid this problem, nearly all multiple surgery claims are calculated using a "**global approach**." In a global approach, the medical biller compares the total billed amount with the total UCR amount. In our example, the total UCR amount is $700 versus the total billed amount of $900. The objective is to deny amounts that exceed the global UCR.

EXAMPLE:

Assume the same procedures previously described were billed in the following way:

	Billed Amount	UCR
Tonsillectomy (42821)	$300	$600
Eustachian tube inflation (69400)	+$600	+$100
Total Billed Amount	$900	$700

Global UCR would be

Major procedure UCR—Tonsillectomy	$600
Minor procedure UCR—Eustachian tube inflation	+$100
Total Global Allowance	$700

This billing is more favorable to the claimant.

Some insurance companies use CMS guidelines. When multiple surgeries are performed and the additional procedures are not incidental, CMS guidelines are as follows:

Major procedure: 100% of UCR or the billed amount, whichever is less.

Second through fifth procedure: 50% of UCR or billed amount, whichever is less.

Multiple procedures (more than two) are often referred to consultants or professional review departments, which consist of medical doctors and nurses, for analysis before payment is made. The consultants or review department may give alternative instructions after seeing the actual operative report.

Block Procedures

Block procedures are multiple surgical procedures performed during the same operative session, in the same operative area. The objective of these codes is to handle multiple repetitions of the same service. A block procedure consists of a primary code and subsequent modifying codes.

EXAMPLE:

11100	is for biopsy of skin, subcutaneous tissue or mucous membrane, single lesion.
11101	is for each separate/additional lesion.

Therefore, if a bill was received for the removal of five lesions, the total allowance would be based on the following unit factors:

1.24	Units for the lesion
2.60	Units total for lesions 2, 3, 4, and 5 (4 × .65)
3.84	Total units allowed

For another example of a block procedure or add-ons, refer to Moh's surgery in the CPT. The CPT is now a great source for identifying add-ons and procedures that are exempt from the multiple surgery rule. Usually you will see either a "+" or "0" next to the CPT code, indicating that the procedure is not subject to multiple surgery reduction.

Unbundling

As briefly discussed in the Physician's, Clinical, and Hospital Services Claims chapter, some physicians practice what is known as "unbundling." The surgeon is considered to have "unbundled" when he bills separately for procedures that are a part of the major procedure. For example, a hysterectomy can be performed with or without the removal of the ovaries and/or the fallopian tubes. The code for hysterectomy surgery includes the removal of these other body parts. Therefore, a physician who bills for a hysterectomy and also bills for removal of the ovaries has unbundled the surgery. The maximum allowance is the UCR for the hysterectomy. An extreme example is a surgeon billing for the removal of a gallbladder and also billing for the repair of an open wound. Of course the repair is not covered separately, as it is inherently part of the gallbladder surgery. Take care in processing multiple surgeries to ensure that there is no unbundling and that the minor procedures are reduced accordingly.

Maternity Expenses

Most plans provide coverage for maternity-related expenses on the same basis as any other illness. The services normally provided in maternity cases include all routine, antepartum (prior to delivery) care, delivery, and all routine, postpartum (after delivery) care. The maternity CPT codes are based on this premise unless the specific code indicates otherwise. Therefore, if a physician itemizes charges for different segments, the charges should be combined and lumped together under the single appropriate code. This rule applies unless the patient sees different doctors for antepartum care and for delivery or for any other combination during gestation. In such a case, the benefits would be allowed in a way to compensate the physicians appropriately for their services.

Antepartum care (prenatal) includes

- Taking an initial and subsequent history.
- Performing physician's exams, usually one per month for the first eight months, then weekly during the ninth month.
- Checking weight and blood pressure and performing urinalysis (monthly or weekly).
- Listening to fetal heart tones (as shown in Figure 7-3 ●)
- Providing maternity counseling on food requirements, vitamins, and related items.

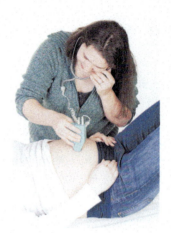

FIGURE 7-3 Listening to fetal heart tones
Source: Beth Van Trees/Shutterstock

Delivery includes

- Assisting vaginal delivery (with or without episiotomy, forceps, or breech delivery).
- Performing Cesarean delivery.

Postpartum care (after delivery) includes

- Conducting postdelivery hospital visits.
- Conducting postdelivery office visits (usually one or two routine check-ups) during the first six weeks following delivery.

Maternity Billing Procedures

Maternity cases are usually billed in a unique manner. Some physicians require full payment from the patient before the delivery date. But most benefit plans will not process the claim for any benefits until after the delivery. Therefore, the patient often has a substantial, initial out-of-pocket expense. The following are some of the more common maternity billing procedures:

1. *Lump sum billings:* When a lump sum charge (a single, all-encompassing charge) is made for total obstetric care, the charge should be coded and processed under the appropriate *CPT®/RVS* code for total obstetric care.
2. *Itemized billings after delivery:* When charges for antepartum care, delivery, and postpartum care are itemized by the physician, the charges should be combined into one charge and processed under the CPT code for total obstetric care. Charges for routine ultrasonography may or may not be covered by the plan. Usually, these charges are considered and coded separately from obstetric care. Charges for lab studies, especially urinalysis, are usually considered part of the complete care; in addition, the physician may indicate medical necessity for services beyond routine care. (Routine lab expenses may be coded and allowed separately. This varies by payer.)
3. *Predelivery billings:* Some physicians bill for the total obstetric care prior to delivery (splitting it into monthly installments, for example, the physician may bill 80% of the charge by the seventh month). In this situation, the plan may deny the claim and ask the doctor to rebill after delivery.

Other plans may consider payment on the services that have been provided as of the date of the billing. Request clarification for how to handle predelivery billings.

4. *Two or more physicians (unrelated, not in the same medical group):* Sometimes two or more physicians are involved in the total obstetric care of a patient; usually one performs the delivery and the other provides the antepartum or postpartum care. In this case, each physician's charge should be processed separately for the services rendered. CPT code 59409 is for a vaginal delivery only. For antepartum care only (up to three office visits), use the appropriate office visit code range of 99201–99205 for the initial visit and 99211–99215 for subsequent visits. Antepartum care beyond three visits should be billed using CPT code 59425 or 59426. Use 59430 for postpartum care only.

5. *Multiple Births:* After coding the global diagnosis for the first birth, you should multiple the delivery code by the number of other births.

> ▶ **CRITICAL THINKING QUESTION:** Why might a pregnant woman have two or more physicians (unrelated, not in the same medical group) during her pregnancy?

Other Maternity-Related Procedures

You may encounter the following other types of maternity claims.

1. **Artificial insemination** is the introduction of semen into the vagina or cervix by artificial means. Some plans consider this to be a covered expense, and some do not, as it is not performed to treat a disease or injury.

2. **Amniocentesis** or **chromosomal analysis** involves the transabdominal perforation of the uterus and withdrawal of amniotic fluid surrounding the fetus. The chromosomal analysis is the diagnostic study performed on the fluid to study the number and structure of the chromosomes to determine whether any abnormalities are present.

   An amniocentesis/chromosomal analysis is performed

   • To identify genetic defects of the fetus.
   • To determine whether the fetus has attained an adequate state of gestation.
   • To determine the sex of the fetus.

   Charges for amniocentesis and chromosomal analysis are usually covered if the attending physician can demonstrate the medical necessity of testing for the patient, such as a family history of specific genetic defects, or advanced maternal age (greater than 35 years). The use of these tests to determine fetal sex alone is not covered by most plans.

3. *In utero* **fetal surgery** is surgery that is performed on a fetus while it is in the mother's womb. It is also possible to remove the fetus from the womb, perform surgery, and return it to the womb, allowing the pregnancy to continue to term. If the surgery is covered, it is often covered as the mother's expense as a complication of pregnancy.

4. *In vitro* **fertilization** is the fertilization of the ovum outside the body (i.e., within a test tube or a petri dish).

Charges for *in vitro* fertilization may be covered. Refer to the plan for verification.

5. **Abortion** is the premature expulsion of an embryo or nonviable fetus. There are three different types of abortions:

   a. A spontaneous abortion occurring naturally.
   b. A therapeutic abortion intentionally induced because the life of the mother would be endangered if the pregnancy were allowed to continue to term.
   c. An elective abortion intentionally induced to terminate an unwanted pregnancy.

   Coverage for abortions varies greatly from plan to plan. Spontaneous and therapeutic abortions are covered by most plans; however, elective abortions are often excluded. In addition, some plans may pay for certain services, including abortion, for spouses but not for dependent children. Therefore, read the plan document carefully before you process these types of expenses.

ACTIVITY #2

Maternity Billing

Directions: Answer the following questions without looking back at the material just covered. Write your answers in the space provided.

1. Why might maternity charges not be combined and lumped together under a single appropriate code?

   _____

   _____

2. List the four common maternity billing procedures.

   a. _____

   b. _____

   c. _____

   d. _____

Delivery with Tubal Ligation

Sterilization is a surgical method to achieve permanent infertility. Sterilization procedures include tubal ligations for females and vasectomies for males. It is becoming more common for health plans to cover sterilization procedures.

When the plan provides coverage for sterilization procedures and a tubal ligation is performed during the same operative session as a vaginal delivery, the UCR fee (or the actual charge, whichever is less) for the delivery is allowed at 100% and the sterilization fee is reduced to 50% of the UCR charge.

When a sterilization procedure is performed during the same hospitalization as that for a vaginal delivery but not in the same operative session, 100% of the fee or UCR is allowed for each procedure.

When a tubal ligation is performed during the same operative session as a cesarean section or intraabdominal surgery, the C-section should be processed under the appropriate CPT/RVS code and the tubal should be processed under CPT code 58611. The UCR for both the C-section and the tubal ligation should be allowed at 100%, as the relative value for 58611 has already been reduced.

Vaginal delivery

| With tubal ligation | 59400–100% |
| During same operative session | 58605–50% |

Vaginal delivery

| With tubal ligation | 59400–100% |
| Not during same operative session | 58605–100% |

C-section delivery

| With tubal ligation | 59510–100% |
| During same operative session | 58611–50% |

C-section delivery

| With tubal ligation | 59510–100% |
| Not during same operative session | 58605–100% |

If a plan does not cover sterilization, the expense for a tubal ligation, regardless of when it is performed, would be denied as an expense that is not covered.

Cosmetic Surgery

Cosmetic surgery is a surgical procedure that is performed solely to improve appearance and is usually not covered by benefit plans.

To properly handle possible cosmetic claims, you must become familiar with the terminology. The following are some of the more common cosmetic procedures and they are not usually covered. However, you should investigate each claim and evaluate it on an individual basis. Establish the primary intent of each procedure to determine whether the procedure is cosmetic or reconstructive.

Although some procedures are cosmetic in nature, they may also be performed for functional reasons. For instance, a blepharoplasty is the removal of excessive skin and fat from the eyelids. Certainly, removal of excessive skin and fat improves the person's appearance. However, it can also be a procedure with medical value. Most plans will cover blepharoplasty when the skin overhang is so extensive that it interferes with the patient's peripheral vision.

When the restorative or cosmetic nature of the procedure is not obvious, you must investigate the claim by carefully reviewing the following documents:

- Hospital admission history and physical
- Operative report
- Pathology report
- Preoperative and postoperative photographs
- A narrative report from a referring physician, if available.

Preoperative and Postoperative Photographs

Providers routinely take preoperative and postoperative photographs. These photos are sometimes needed to determine whether a surgery was solely cosmetic in nature.

To request photographs, use a standard request for additional information form letter. You should request the operative report for the procedure at the same time.

When you receive the operative report and photographs, compare them with the claim to determine the reason for the surgery. If the surgery appears to be cosmetic in nature, forward the claim, along with the photographs and any reports, to a consultant for review.

Possible Cosmetic Procedures

Following is a list of common surgical procedures that may be considered cosmetic in nature. Keep in mind that numerous other procedures and services fall under a cosmetic heading. This sample list is for training purposes only, and you should consult the individual plan guidelines prior to processing a surgery claim.

PRACTICE PITFALLS

Following are three general guidelines regarding cosmetic surgeries:

1. Cosmetic surgery performed purely for cosmetic reasons is not covered. However, cosmetic surgery after an accident, injury, or surgical procedure may be covered (e.g., breast reconstruction after a mastectomy).
2. When there is an underlying condition, the surgery is not considered cosmetic, regardless of the nature of the surgery (e.g., removal of a scar if there is an underlying disease).
3. When you are processing a surgical claim, determine the primary reason for the surgical procedure. If the treatment is due to injury or disease, the surgery is not considered cosmetic.

Blepharoplasty Surgical repair of drooping eyelids. This condition may impair peripheral vision. The surgery may be done on the upper lid only, the lower lid only, or both upper and lower lids. Surgery of both lids requires the use of modifier -50.

When blepharoplasty is performed on the upper lid, the removal of the fat decreases the bulging lid, relieving the patient of a perpetual "tired look" about the eyes and thus imparting a more youthful appearance. The diagnosis most often listed on the claim is blepharochalasis, acquired atrophy of the skin of the upper eyelid, which occurs naturally in aging. Blepharoplasty may also be performed for ptosis, which is an abnormal downward displacement of the eyelid due to muscle weakness, eyelid trauma, facial nerve paralysis, or loss of innervation. As this condition worsens, the tissue obstructs the pupil and progressively impairs the patient's vision. The operative report for treatment of functional blepharoptosis will describe structural rearrangement such as palpebral muscle shortening; resection of part of the upper lid, including the tarsal plate; nerve and muscle transplantation; and facial sling.

Vision impairment is the only condition for which an upper-lid blepharoplasty would not be considered cosmetic.

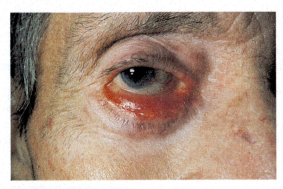

FIGURE 7-4   An ectropion
Source: Dr. P. Marazzi/Science Source

The documentation required to assess visual impairment includes at least one of the following:

- Results of a tangent screen examination.
- Results of a confrontation test.
- Results of perimeter testing.

The latter tests measure the patient's peripheral vision and support the medical record and preoperative photos in establishing the functional need for surgery.

Claims received for lower-lid blepharoplasty are usually purely cosmetic. The surgery consists of removing the herniated fat pads in the lower lid and excising the redundant skin. Three conditions in which a blepharoplasty of the lower lid may be indicated and not considered cosmetic are

1. *Ectropion*—A condition in which the margin of the upper or lower eyelid turns outward, as in Figure 7-4 ●. When the lower lid is involved, involuntary tearing often constitutes the most annoying symptom. Surgery consists of removing a portion of the inside of the lid to cause the eyelid to turn inward. This is a functional correction.
2. *Entropion*—A condition in which the margin of the upper or lower eyelid turns in, causing the eyelashes to rub against and irritate the eyeball. If a secondary infection occurs, scarring of the cornea may ensue with subsequent loss of vision. Therefore, it is important to correct the condition in the early stages of development. Surgery consists of cutting away a portion of the inside of the eyelid in a way that causes the eyelid to turn outward. This is a functional correction.
3. *Lid Lesions*—A condition in which a cyst-like mass called a chalazion, meibomian, or tarsal cyst results in chronic inflammation of the meibomian gland in the eyelid. Another type of lesion is a hordeolum or sty, which is an infection of the eyelash that is associated with whitish pus under the skin. When medical treatment fails to alleviate the condition, surgery may be performed to remove the affected area. Tumors constitute the third type of lesion that might require surgical care.

In a blepharoplasty, the surgeon removes the pockets of fat in the upper and lower lids beneath the skin. The ellipse of skin must be cut off to elevate the drooping eyebrow. The surgeon sews the margins together with the final suture line lying with the eyebrow's upper hairline. The redundant skin of the lower lid is undermined, and the excess fat is removed along with the redundant skin. The wound is then sutured with fine silk.

The structure line in the upper eyelid partially coincides with the old one; the one in the lower lid is disguised by the eyelashes. The rest of the two sutures coincide with the natural creases about the eye.

Breast Augmentation   Surgical enlargement of the breast by use of implants. Implants come in various types but are most often gel- or fluid-filled sacs.

Breast Prosthesis   An artificial sac implanted in the chest muscles to replace or enlarge the breast. Many types of prostheses are available.

Breast Reconstruction   A procedure in which an implant is placed under the skin or muscle of the chest wall to restore the contour of a missing breast. This procedure is usually covered when it is used to restore the appearance of a patient who has had a mastectomy due to cancer, fibroadenoma, or fibrocystic breast disease. Claims submitted for breast reconstruction should include the diagnosis of the underlying disease and the date of the previously performed mastectomy. In the case of breast cancer, only charges submitted for reconstruction for the removed breast are considered covered expenses. Charges submitted for reduction mammoplasty on the unaffected side (to make the unaffected breast appear similar in size and shape to the reconstructed breast) are considered cosmetic and are usually not covered.

Asymmetry is a condition in which the breasts are grossly dissimilar in size, shape, or arrangement on the chest wall. As a slight discrepancy between the breasts is normal, the condition must be severe to be considered functional.

Breast Reduction   Surgical procedure to reduce the size of the breast. This surgery may be covered in extreme cases (usually when over one pound of fat is removed on each side).

Cheiloplasty   Surgery for the lips. Like the skin and mucous membranes of other parts of the body, the lips are subject to precancerous and cancerous lesions. These lesions most often occur in fair-skinned persons who have a long history of exposure to sunlight.

In *hyperkeratosis*, a common precancerous condition, the mucosa of the lip becomes paler, thinner, and more fragile with numerous cracks and fissures. Gradually, ulcerations appear which repeatedly break down and heal. Treatment consists of removing the entire involved lip surface and advancing the inner lining of the lip to cover the defect. This procedure is called *lip stripping and resurfacing* and is considered medically necessary.

A cheiloplasty can also be done to make the lips narrower, to enlarge them, or to create a "cupid's bow" (the dip in the edge line of the upper lip). When it is done for these reasons, cheiloplasty is considered cosmetic.

Chemical Peel or Chemical Abrasion   A procedure with the same effect as dermabrasion, except that caustic chemicals such as phenol or trichloracetic acid are used. The technique creates a superficial chemical burn. After the skin has healed, fine wrinkles appear flattened and the skin is tightened. This procedure is considered purely cosmetic.

Cleft Lip and Palate Repair Correction of a birth defect in which the two sides of the face fail to unite properly in the early stage of prenatal development, resulting in a fissure or split in the lip and/or palate (roof) of the mouth. A cleft lip may occur unilaterally or bilaterally. An incomplete cleft lip occurs when a bridge of skin connects the cleft and noncleft sides. If a skin bridge does not exist, the cleft is complete. Deformity of the nose usually accompanies a cleft lip in the form of distortion and displacement of the lower lateral nasal cartilage.

Surgery to correct a cleft lip or palate should be scheduled when a child is old enough to tolerate the procedure safely, usually at about 10 weeks of age with a weight of about 10 pounds and a hemoglobin of 10 g/dL. By that time, the tissues are large enough that they may be accurately repaired. Further correction of the nasal deformity, often with simultaneous revision of minor lip irregularities, may be done when the child is older, and final surgery may be delayed until adolescence to allow for full maturity of the facial features. Services to correct this congenital defect are considered functional.

However, claims for services related to cleft lip (and possibly palate) repair in persons who are older than adolescent age should be reviewed, as they may be purely cosmetic repairs and not functional repairs of a defect.

Collagen or Zyderm Injections Injection into the skin of Zyderm, a medical grade of collagen (taken from cows). When it is injected into fine lines or small defects in the skin, it temporarily plumps up the indented areas, making them appear less pronounced. Usually, supplemental injections must be performed about every six to nine months. Collagen injections are strictly cosmetic.

Congenital Anomaly Repair Surgical correction of a birth defect. Depending on the defect, a congenital abnormality may or may not be covered by a plan.

Dermabrasion A procedure using abrasive materials (sandpaper, emery paper, or wire brushes) to remove acne scars, birthmarks, fine wrinkles, or other skin defects. When the skin grows back, the surface irregularities have been smoothed away. Although dermabrasion is usually considered a cosmetic procedure, check the plan guidelines; it may be covered to restore the skin to the appearance of a presickness state or to treat cases of severe acne.

Electrolysis Epilation Removal of hair by destruction of the hair follicle (root) with an electric current. In women, the usual diagnosis submitted is hirsutism, which is a condition of adult male hair growth in a female. Electrolysis does not treat the underlying condition, which is a hormonal imbalance, and it is therefore considered purely cosmetic.

Gynecomastia Correction Surgery to correct a swelling of the breast tissue in the male. If an underlying hormonal disease has been ruled out, the condition is treated by removing a small section of the breast tissue, which may be covered by some plans.

Hair Transplantation Moving healthy hair follicles from one location on the body to another location, usually the head. Alopecia areata is a condition in which patchy areas of baldness occur. Male pattern baldness (androgenic alopecia), loss of hair from the crown of the head, occurs in about 30% of adult males. A few medications have been shown to promote the regrowth of hair in some instances. Transplantation treats the symptoms but not the condition; therefore, it is usually considered cosmetic.

Hypertrophied Breast/Macromastia Surgery Surgery to correct abnormal enlargement of the female breasts caused by hormonal factors or obesity. The condition may require a mastectomy when the weight of the breast tissue causes physical complaints. Among the symptoms are shoulder, neck, and back pain; numbness of the hand and arm caused by the bra straps compressing the brachial plexus (the group of nerves in the area between the neck and the shoulder that innervate the arm); and chronic inflammation of the skin of the opposed surfaces (intertrigo). Documentation to substantiate the functional nature of this procedure includes preoperative and postoperative photos, admission history, and physical examination information that includes the patient's height and weight, discharge summary, operative report, and pathology report.

Each administrator has their own guidelines. Therefore, you should research all claims involving hypertrophied breasts before making a payment, to verify the applicable guidelines.

Keloid Removal Surgical removal of a keloid, a thick scar resulting from excessive growth of fibroid tissue. Any open wound can develop keloid scarring. Therefore, this scarring may occur following surgery. Keloid scar surgery is not usually considered cosmetic.

Lipectomy The surgical removal of fatty tissue. The removal of this fatty tissue may be accomplished by standard surgical techniques (incisional approach) or by liposuction, which consists of "sucking" out the fatty tissue through a vacuum tube that is inserted through small incisions. Regardless of the method used, the surgical removal of the redundant fatty tissue is considered cosmetic.

Mammoplasty Surgery to reduce (reduction mammoplasty) or enlarge (augmentation mammoplasty) the size of the breast. Augmentation mammoplasty is performed for the conditions of amastia and hypomastia. *Amastia* is defined as the congenital absence of mammary tissue in an adult female. Amastia can be unilateral (one-sided) or bilateral (two-sided). *Hypomastia* is defined as abnormal smallness of the mammary gland and, like amastia, it can affect one or both breasts. In cases in which one breast is normal and the other is markedly small or absent, hypomastia causes asymmetry.

Mastectomy Excision or amputation of the breast, usually required as a result of a malignant disease. This procedure is not the same as a reduction mammoplasty. There are three types of mastectomies:

1. *Radical mastectomy* is the removal of the breast tissue (mammary gland), pectoral muscles, axillary lymph nodes, and associated skin and subcutaneous tissue. This procedure is used to treat cancer but may result in the partial loss of arm movement. Usually, radical mastectomy is followed by reconstructive surgery to restore the appearance of the remaining tissue.

2. *Modified radical mastectomy* is the same as the radical procedure except that the pectoral muscles are left intact. This procedure can usually be performed during the earlier stages of cancer (stage I or II). Modified radical mastectomy is usually also followed by reconstructive procedures.

3. *Subcutaneous mastectomy* is a technique in which most of the breast tissue is removed but the skin and areola are preserved. Unlike the other two methods, immediate reconstruction can usually be done by inserting a Silastic prosthesis into the subcutaneous pocket left by the excision of the breast tissue or under the pectoralis major muscle. Subcutaneous mastectomy and reconstruction for multipathology breasts (e.g., in patients with fibrocystic disease or fibroadenoma) consists of removing the mammary tissue and inserting a prosthesis (implant) under the remaining skin to maintain the breast contour. The surgery is used to treat chronic mastitis in patients who experience incapacitating breast pain or those who have repeated breast biopsies of the cystic nodules to rule out cancer.

To show the medical necessity of a mastectomy, the documentation requested from the physician should include a history of removal of lumps or repeated aspirations of the cysts, as well as the laboratory results of the previous biopsies.

Mentoplasty/Genioplasty   Surgery to change the size and shape of the chin with an implant. This procedure is done for a small (microgenic) or moderately receding chin when there is no underlying defect in the jaw itself. The surgeon makes a small incision under the chin and inserts a silicone implant, giving increased prominence to the chin.

Otoplasty   Plastic surgery to change the position or configuration of the ear or ears. The most common deformities that require an otoplasty are

- *Protruding or Lop Ears*—Protruding ears are set at a greater than 25-degree angle from the skull. They may protrude due to cartilage deformities to such an extent that they form a right angle on the side of the head. In the case of a lop ear, the ear is bent upon itself. Prominent ears are usually caused by lack of definition of the antihelical fold. This defect is described in the diagnosis and operative report.

  The best age to perform corrective surgery for these conditions is about 13 to 14 years, when the ear has attained almost maximum growth. However, because these conditions can cause serious emotional and psychological problems, surgery may be done before the child reaches school age. This surgery is usually considered cosmetic.

- *Microtia*—A congenital defect characterized by a small, malformed, malpositioned ear remnant. Affected children almost always have a hearing deficit. Repair begins at age five or six years and is performed in a series of surgeries. The surgery is considered reconstructive.

Palatoplasty   Plastic surgery of the palate, usually to correct a cleft palate.

Panniculectomy   Removal of a sheet or layer of fatty tissue. This procedure is most often done to remove excess fatty tissue from the abdomen.

"-Plasty"   The surgical suffix that means to mold or shape.

Rhinoplasty   Cosmetic repair of the external part of the nose to change its size or shape. This procedure does not involve the internal functioning of the nose, although it is performed entirely within the nose to prevent scarring.

A rhinoplasty consists of five major steps:

1. Elevating the skin from the bony and cartilaginous dorsum.
2. Removing the hump or lowering a prominent dorsum.
3. Narrowing the nasal pyramid to compensate for the flatness caused by the hump removal.
4. Shortening the nose if necessary.
5. Modeling the tip or lower cartilaginous complex to proportions that are consistent with the previous steps.

Key words to look for in determining whether surgery on the nose is cosmetic are "modifications of alar cartilages" and "lowering the dorsum." It is never necessary to modify the alar cartilages or lower the dorsum other than for cosmetic reasons. It is also never necessary to do alar base excisions for functional reasons. In fact, this procedure constricts the airway and does the opposite of improving air flow.

Rhinoplasties are often combined with a septoplasty or submucous resection. Therefore, it is essential to properly investigate these claims to determine whether and what part of the nasal procedure is necessary to correct a functional defect versus what part has been done purely for cosmetic purposes.

The test used to document airway obstruction is called *rhinomanometry*. It is the measurement of the airflow and pressure within the nose during respiration, and it calculates the resistance or obstruction. Unfortunately, this test is not often performed.

The structures of the nose responsible for airway obstruction are the septum and the nasal turbinates. The septum is made up of the downward projection of the ethmoid bone at the back, the vomer bone at the bottom, and the triangular-shaped septal cartilage, which divides the nasal cavity (internal nose) into two wedge-shaped cavities. An accident can displace the septal cartilage where it meets the vomer or ethmoid bones, causing one side of the nasal cavity to become narrower and to obstruct the airway.

Rhytidectomy   Surgical removal of wrinkles. This procedure is usually cosmetic unless it interferes with the normal function of a body part.

Rhytidoplasty (facelift)   Removal of facial wrinkles. Wrinkles result from the absorption of subcutaneous fat, a decrease in the thickness and elasticity of the skin, and the skin's failure to adhere to the deeper tissues—all processes that are part of the normal physiology of aging. This procedure is possibly one of the most graphic examples of a purely cosmetic procedure.

Senile Ptosis of the Eyelids Repair   Surgical correction of a condition in which the skin of the eyelids sags or droops, sometimes causing vision impairment. Ptosis in general refers to a drooping or sagging organ part.

Septoplasty   Surgical correction of a deviated nasal septum, the dividing wall between the two nasal cavities. In this condition, the dividing wall between the two nasal cavities is deflected (turned) away from the center of the nose. The surgery involves only the internal functioning of the nose and is usually covered. Septoplasty or submucous resection of the septum involves undermining the mucous membrane that covers the septum. This procedure is also referred to as "raising the mucoperichondrial and mucoperiosteal flaps." The surgeon then cuts into the cartilage at its base, allowing it to be moved over and straightened.

Submental Lipectomy   Removal of fat deposits under the chin. The region under the chin (submental region) and the neck often requires special attention. A submental lipectomy through a separate incision may be required to remove the fat deposits beneath the chin, thus correcting the appearance of double chins. Suturing and repositioning of the neck muscle (platysma) is done to obliterate jowls. This procedure is usually considered cosmetic.

Submucous Resection   Removal of a portion of the nasal septum.

Tattoo Removal   This procedure is always considered cosmetic.

Temporomandibular Joint Surgery   Osteoplastic surgery of the jaw for prognathism (projection of the jaw(s) beyond the projection of the forehead), micrognathism (abnormal smallness of jaws), and other variations may be cosmetic or functional, depending on the degree of malocclusion.

Turbinates Repair   Resection of the **bony** projections from the side walls of the internal nose. The purpose of the turbinates is to warm and moisten air. They divide each nasal cavity into three passageways. A submucous resection of the turbinates consists of undermining the mucous membrane that covers them and removing a portion of the bone, thereby enlarging the nasal passageway. A submucous resection is a functional correction and is therefore an eligible expense.

Wart and Mole Removal   Warts and m**o**les are discolorations of the skin that protrude above the normal skin elevation. Often they are associated with other diseases and conditions, especially cancer. Therefore, many plans will cover the removal of warts and moles.

ACTIVITY #3

Billing Restorative and Cosmetic Procedures

Directions: Answer the following questions without looking back at the material just covered. Write your answers in the space provided.

1. List the documents that must be reviewed during a claim investigation when the restorative or cosmetic nature of the procedure is not obvious.

   a. _____

   b. _____

   c. _____

   d. _____

   e. _____

2. Why do providers take preoperative and postoperative photographs of a patient? _____

   _____

   _____

3. What is the procedure for requesting and using preoperative and postoperative photographs to process a claim? _____

   _____

   _____

   _____

Obesity Surgery

Exogenous obesity is caused by overeating. Treatment for this condition is not considered treatment of a disease and is usually not covered by most plans until the level of obesity reaches a life-threatening point. Most administrators have defined this level as being 100 pounds or 30% over the weight that is considered optimal for a person of a particular height and bone frame.

Endogenous obesity is obesity caused by an internal malfunction, usually hormonal (e.g., thyroid disorder). Treatment for this type of obesity or for the underlying cause is considered treatment of a disease and is eligible under most plans. This is a comparatively rare condition.

Most administrators require the following documentation to be submitted for review before the scheduled treatment:

- Current weight and height
- Frame type (small, medium, large)
- History of weight loss in the past (e.g., what diets have been tried, what level of success)
- Concurrent medical complications such as high blood pressure or diabetes
- Family history of obesity or other health problems.

The following three procedures are the most common ones that have been used to combat exogenous obesity:

1. *Gastric Balloon/Garren Gastric Bubble*—A procedure in which a balloon is inserted into the stomach, thus giving the person the impression of being "full." Because many overweight people eat not because they are hungry but because of habit or compulsion, this has not been an effective method. In addition, many complications, including death, have resulted from this procedure. Therefore, it is no longer considered an accepted medical practice.

2. *Gastric Bypass*—A procedure in which the stomach is bypassed, allowing food to empty directly into the large intestine. The theory behind this procedure is that the food, nutrients, and fats are not thoroughly broken down and digested if they do not go through the stomach. When fewer calories are accessible to the body for storage, the individual loses weight. This procedure is usually considered to be a permanent one, although it can be reversed. See CPT code 43846.

3. *Gastric Stapling*—A procedure in which a portion of the stomach is stapled off to reduce the size of the stomach. This procedure decreases the amount of food that may be eaten at a single meal. See CPT code 43843.

Most procedures for obesity surgery have side effects. Some of the side effects may be so severe for some people that the procedure will need to be reversed. Therefore, only the severely obese should consider any of these methods of treatment.

The alternatives to surgery include the following services that are usually not covered under benefit plans:

- Special diets and dietary supplements
- HCG (human chorionic gonadotropin) and vitamin injections
- Acupuncture
- Appetite suppressants
- Biofeedback
- Hypnosis
- Hospital confinement for weight reduction
- Exercise programs
- Health centers, weight loss centers, or other similar programs
- Diet books and instructions

PRACTICE **PITFALLS**

Many insurance companies wait until they receive the surgeon's billing before they pay any assistant surgeon or anesthesiologist bill. This practice reduces errors because the primary surgeon usually has a better understanding of the actual surgical procedures performed. Furthermore, it allows the medical biller to ensure that the assistant surgeon and anesthesiologist have billed properly.

If a surgeon is a PPO provider but the assistant surgeon or anesthesiologist is not, some insurance carriers will not penalize the patient for not using a PPO assistant surgeon or anesthesiologist, because the patient does not normally select the assistant surgeon or anesthesiologist.

Cosurgeons

Under some circumstances, two surgeons, usually with similar skills, may operate simultaneously as primary surgeons performing distinct, separate parts of a total surgical service. They are referred to as **cosurgeons**. For example, two surgeons may simultaneously apply skin grafts to different parts of the body, or two surgeons may repair different fractures of the same patient.

When you are coding a claim for cosurgeons, use the following modifiers:

- Modifier -80, assistant at surgery. This modifier includes M.D., D.O., and Doctor of Podiatric Medicine (D.P.M.) provider types and describes an assistant surgeon providing full assist to the primary surgeon.
- Modifier -81, minimal assistant at surgery. This modifier includes M.D., D.O., and D.P.M. provider types and describes an assistant surgeon providing minimal assistance to the primary surgeon. This modifier may be used when more than one assistant is involved or if one person assists during a portion of the surgery. This modifier is not intended for use by nonphysician assistants such as registered nurses (RNs) or physician assistants (PAs).

- Modifier -82, assistant at surgery when a qualified resident surgeon is not available to assist the primary surgeon. This modifier includes M.D., D.O., and D.P.M. provider types. When you receive a claim for cosurgeons, you should refer to the plan guidelines or administrative guidelines before processing. Usually, cosurgeon procedures are referred to a consultant, supervisor, or Medical Review Department before processing.

Assistant Surgeons

Complex surgeries may require a primary surgeon and an assistant surgeon. The job of the **assistant surgeon** is to assist the primary surgeon as required. The assistant surgeon may close the operative wound, perform hemostasis of the wound edges, and suture the vessels. As the assistant surgeon is not the physician primarily responsible for the patient, the UCR allowance is considerably less than that for the surgeon.

In order for a plan to cover an assistant surgeon, the complexity of the surgical procedure must medically require an assistant. (See Appendix C for Assistant Surgeon Procedures.) Obviously, an assistant surgeon would not be covered for minor surgery (e.g., acne surgery).

As a rule, you may use the following guidelines to determine whether an assistant is required:

1. The place of service is either a hospital (inpatient or outpatient), or a surgi-center. Seldom are major surgeries performed in an office.
2. Followup days are listed in the *RVS* for each procedure. Services without followup days are usually not complex enough to require an assistant.

The allowance for an assistant surgeon is 20% of the surgery allowance (UCR). Modifier -80 is used to designate the assistant surgeon's fee.

EXAMPLE:

Procedure 15570 has a unit value of 10.0. The conversion factor is $38.50. Therefore,

10 units × $38.50 = $385. 20% of $385 = $77.

Using the previously stated guidelines, $77 is the UCR fee for an assistant surgeon for this procedure.

Some procedures do not require the expertise of an M.D. assistant, but they do require technical help. For these procedures, PAs are often used. When these professionals are used in lieu of an M.D. assistant, modifier -81 is used. The allowed amount is usually calculated at 10%–15% of the surgeon's allowance, depending on the insurance carrier's practice and plan definition. The most common percentage used is 10%.

EXAMPLE:

Procedure 15570 has a unit value of 10 units. The conversion factor for surgery is $38.50. Therefore,

10 units × $138.50 = $385. $385 × 10% = $38.50,

and the allowable amount for the PA is $38.50.

Although an assistant surgeon is considered medically necessary when a C-section is performed, you should still review the physician's coding. The assistant is entitled to 20% (or 10% if he or she is a P.A.) of the delivery only and his or her assistance should not be submitted under the global code that includes the antepartum and postpartum care.

If more than one procedure is performed, the multiple/bilateral guidelines apply. The reasoning is that the assistant surgeon allowable is 20% of the surgeon's allowable. Thus, the first procedure would be calculated at 20% of the allowed amount and the subsequent procedures would be calculated at the allowed amount × 50% × 20%.

Podiatry

Podiatry provides services for the feet. The services are usually provided by a podiatrist with the professional designation D.P.M.

The joints of the feet are very complex. When surgery is performed, the medical biller must review the claim for accuracy before sending it to the claims examiner. The claims examiner must review the claim carefully too, as it will also be complex. In this chapter we will discuss some of the procedures performed on the foot and some guidelines that have been established regarding payment of podiatry claims.

ACTIVITY #4

Billing for Surgical Procedures

1. What are therapeutic procedures? _____

2. What is the difference between a cosmetic procedure and a reconstructive procedure? _____

3. Define lump sum billing in relation to maternity charges. _____

4. When would charges for amniocentesis or chromosomal analysis usually be covered? _____

5. Are collagen injections a cosmetic procedure? ____

6. What is the name of the surgical procedure for excision or amputation of the breast? _____

7. What is a deviated nasal septum? _____

8. Modifier _____ is used to designate the assistant surgeon's fee.

9. The allowance for an assistant surgeon is _____ of the surgery allowance.

10. Would an assistant surgeon be required for acne surgery? _____

PRACTICE PITFALLS

Because of the complexity of podiatry claims, most administrators have special handling guidelines for podiatric care and surgery. Many plans have provisions that place a UCR limitation and a daily maximum on podiatric claims. In addition, most of these claims may also be referred to a consultant for review, prior to payment.

The UCR fee allowance for podiatric surgery is determined the same way as any other surgical procedure. The most common problem in determining the correct UCR allowance is the excessive detail in which the surgery is sometimes described. At times, the podiatrist describes and bills each procedure independently, even though some procedures are incidental to the major operation performed.

Refer to the Surgery section in this chapter for further information on multiple, bilateral, and incidental surgeries. The following four handling procedures may help you identify the correct breakdown of the surgeries performed:

1. Separate the procedures performed on each foot. The foot that has the most or major surgery is identified as the primary foot.

2. List the independent procedures and identify the metatarsal or phalange by digit (e.g., great toe #1, second toe #2).

3. Determine whether more than one procedure has been performed on one joint, one toe, or adjacent parts of the foot. No additional allowance is made for secondary procedures because all such procedures are considered incidental (part of the major procedure).

4. After you have identified all the independent procedures for both the primary and secondary foot, you may locate the correct CPT surgical procedure code.

Surgical Coding for Podiatry

To select the correct CPT code, identify the diagnosis and the required procedures that are necessary to correct the medical problem. For example, a bill with a diagnosis of "hammertoe" may list service for an arthroplasty, a capsulotomy, and a tenotomy with a separate charge for each procedure. In this case, you should allow the benefit for repair of hammertoe (CPT code 28285). The separate procedures are included in the hammertoe repair CPT code.

Here are eight rules that you should consider when determining the correct surgical codes:

1. Only one bunion surgery is allowable per foot.
2. Only one bone operation is allowable per toe.
3. Only one capsulotomy/tenotomy is allowable per metatarsal.
4. No increase is allowable for K wires (stabilizing wires placed in the foot). These wires are considered a necessary part of the procedure and do not warrant an extra benefit.
5. Generally, one operation is allowable per incision.
6. Taylor's bunion is not a bunion.

7. Unna's boot (gauze soaked in zinc oxide) is considered part of the surgery itself and does not warrant an additional allowance. When the boot is used for treatment of leg ulcers, additional benefits may be allowed.

8. Flexible casts are nothing more than a tape or bandage and do not warrant a casting benefit.

Remember that these are general guidelines only. The actual administration of podiatry claims varies greatly among companies. Therefore, you should refer to the benefit plan summary prior to processing the claim payment.

Conditions of the Foot and Treatment Procedures

Foot surgeries usually involve some incision of the skin and, in some cases, of the bone. Skin heals in phases. In the first phase, skin grows together, after which stitches may be removed. The scar may look slightly inflamed. Some redness and swelling are normal. After about six months, the scar blends with the surrounding skin. Scarring varies according to the individual.

Bone also heals in phases. A bonelike "cement" forms first, bridging the affected bone and enabling it to bear some weight. Later, this extra bone dissolves. The healing process varies from person to person and also depends on the health and age of the person.

Ligaments are flexible bands of fiber joining bone to bone. **Joints** are the locations where two bones meet. The foot is flexible because it contains 33 complex joints. (See Figure 7-5 ●.)

Bunions

A **bunion** is an enlargement of a bone in a joint at the base of the big toe. Bunions are most often inherited. Contrary to what many people believe, bunions are not caused by wearing tight shoes, although tight-fitting shoes can aggravate them. The simplest bunion procedure is the Silver procedure, which does not involve any surgery in the first metatarsal interspace; all other bunion procedures do.

In the McBride procedure, the surgeon removes the bump on the outside of the first metatarsal, removes the sesamoid, and severs the abductor and short tendon. If tenotomies are not performed, the procedure is a Silver.

Reverdin or Reverdin and Green bunionectomy involves the removal of the bunion on the outside of the first metatarsal and a wedge osteotomy of the first metatarsal to bring the toe into proper alignment.

The Austin, Reverdin, Peabody, Mitchell, Wilson, and Rue bunionectomies all involve some kind of osteotomy in the head of the metatarsal and all have the same CPT code of 28296. A metatarsal base osteotomy is a valid second procedure (28306).

The Akin osteotomy involves the removal of a cylindrical wedge of the proximal phalanx of the great toe, after which the gap is closed with a screw, wire, or pin. This cylindrical wedge can be taken from either the distal or proximal end of the phalanx. If this procedure is performed along with the Akin bunionectomy, the CPT code is 28298. When the Akin osteotomy and bunionectomy are performed at the same time, the claim should reflect one surgery per foot.

The Keller bunionectomy with Silastic implant involves the removal of a bunion from the first metatarsal, excision of the head of the proximal phalanx, and insertion of the Silastic head into the end of the phalanx so that it forms a new gliding joint.

POSITIONAL BUNIONS. A **positional bunion** develops when a bony growth on the side of the metatarsal bone enlarges the joint, forcing the joint capsule to stretch over it. As this growth pushes the big toe toward the others, the tendons on the inside tighten and force the big toe further out of alignment. The bunion presses against the shoe, irritating the skin and causing increased pain.

To treat a positional bunion, the bump is removed (positional bunionectomy). The surgeon may also remove a wedge

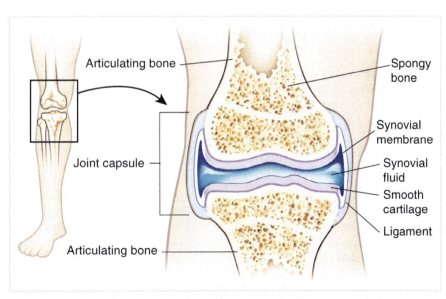

FIGURE 7-5 A typical joint

of the joint capsule to reposition it and may release tight tendons. The patient may have to wear a special wooden shoe or splint for about three weeks postoperatively.

STRUCTURAL BUNIONS. A **structural bunion** occurs when the angle between the first and second metatarsal bones increases to a point at which it is greater than normal. The increased angle of the metatarsal makes the big toe bow toward the other toes. This is usually an inherited tendency. Treatment of a structural bunion (structural bunionectomy) involves repositioning the bone. The patient may have to wear a splint or a special shoe for about six weeks postoperatively.

A structural bunion becomes severe when the angle between the metatarsal bones of the first and second toes exceeds the angle of a mild structural bunion. The big toe bows toward the others, sometimes causing the second and third toes to buckle.

To correct a severe structural bunion, a surgeon may perform a base osteotomy to remove a wedge of bone so that the metatarsal can be repositioned. Tiny K wires or screws may be used to stabilize the bone. The foot and ankle may be immobilized with a cast; no weight should be placed on the foot for several weeks.

DEGENERATIVE DISEASE. Degenerative disease is not a bunion, but it is often associated with bunions. This is because an untreated bunion can increase wear and tear on the joint of the big toe, break down the cartilage, and pave the way for degenerative diseases such as arthritis, osteoarthritis, and rheumatoid arthritis.

Treatment of degenerative conditions involves removal of all bunions and replacement of the degenerated joint with a silastic (plastic) implant. The patient may wear a splint or a special shoe for several weeks. However, he or she may regain the ability to walk within one or two days after surgery.

TAYLOR'S BUNIONECTOMY. Taylor's procedure is not a bunion operation; rather, it is the removal of a small bone portion of the fifth metatarsal. It is often done with an osteotomy. The procedure may accompany an incidental removal of the outside of the first phalanx.

Hammertoes

Hammertoes are inherited muscle imbalances or abnormal bone lengths that can make the toes buckle under, causing their joints to contract. Subsequently, the tendons shorten. A flexible hammertoe is one in which the buckled joint can be straightened manually with the hand. It may progress and become rigid over time. Rigid hammertoes are fixed and cannot be manually straightened. Corns, irritation, pain, and loss of function are common symptoms and may be more severe in rigid than in flexible hammertoes.

SURGICAL REPAIR. There are two different types of hammertoe repair: simple and radical. Regardless of the procedure, only one hammertoe operation is allowable per toe. Some of the more common hammertoe repair procedures are tenotomy, capsulotomy, osteotomy, arthroplasty, and arthrodesis.

Tenotomy and **capsulotomy** are performed to release the buckling and the top and bottom tendons. The joint capsules may also have to be cut. When a tenotomy and capsulotomy are performed on the same joint, only one operation is allowable per joint.

When an osteotomy is performed in conjunction with a tenotomy and capsulotomy, the additional procedure is incidental.

In an **arthroplasty**, the surgeon removes a portion of the joint and straightens the toe. The resulting gap will fill in with fibrous tissue. Removal of the joint and fusion of the bones constitute an alternative treatment.

The fifth (little) toe may curl inward beneath the fourth toe so that the nail faces outward. This inherited problem results in corns and pain. A derotation arthroplasty is performed to remove a wedge of skin and bone to uncurl (derotate) the toe. The patient may have to use a bandage, splint, and sometimes a surgical shoe for several weeks following surgery.

Plantar Calluses

A **metatarsal plantar callus** occurs when the metatarsal bone is longer or lower than the others so that it hits the ground first at every step with more force than it is equipped to handle. As a result, the skin under this bone thickens and becomes hardened into a callus. The callus causes irritation and pain. The treatment is a V osteotomy in which the surgeon cuts the metatarsal bone in a V shape, then lifts the end of the bone and aligns it with the other bones. The V shape holds the bone in its new position, preventing it from rocking to the left or the right.

A fifth metatarsal plantar callus is caused by walking improperly on the outside of the foot. The extra pressure may cause the skin under the bone to thicken, causing irritation and pain.

A **dorsal osteotomy** is performed by removing a small wedge of bone from the top (dorsal) side of the base of the fifth metatarsal bone. This elevates the bone and relieves pressure on the callus. The bone is then fixed with tiny wires or screws.

Dwyer Osteotomy Surgical Procedure

The **Dwyer procedure** is the treatment for a deformity of the calcaneus or large heel bone. It consists of a wedge resection of a portion of the calcaneus bone, closed with a staple, pin, or screw fixation.

Bone Spurs

A **bone spur** is a bony overgrowth on the bone. Bone spurs have a variety of causes and usually result in pain, interfere with the use of the foot, and detract from its appearance.

A **heel spur** is an overgrowth of bone on the heel. It may be stimulated by muscles that pull from the heel bone along the bottom of the foot. High-arched feet are especially apt to have excessively tight muscles in this area.

Treatment of bone spurs involves releasing the band of tight muscles to relieve the stress, then surgically removing the bone spur. The patient may need to use crutches for up to two weeks after surgery to avoid bearing weight on the foot.

A bone spur may occur alone or with a hammertoe, usually resulting in pain and interfering with the use of the foot. An overgrowth under the toenail can press up into the tissue underneath the growth plate, deforming the nail above. This condition is especially painful when shoes are worn.

COMMON SURGICAL PROCEDURES. The most common exostosis (bony growth) on the foot is the heel spur. In most cases, surgery is the most effective way to treat a heel spur. A plantar fasciotomy performed at the same time as a surgery for heel spurs is an incidental procedure, as a fasciotomy must be done to cut through the area before the surgeon can locate the heel spur. In many cases, the use of **orthosis** (an orthopedic appliance) is as effective as surgery.

Treatment for subungual exostosis smooths down the spur with a tiny rasp. The rasp resembles a dental burr and is inserted through a small incision.

Ingrown Toenails

An **ingrown toenail** is a nail in which one or both corners or sides of the nail grow into the skin of the toe. Irritation, redness, an uncomfortable sensation of warmth, swelling, pain, and infection can result.

SURGICAL PROCEDURES. Removal of a nail margin can be done with or without excising the root or matrix. To allow surgical benefits for the total excision of the nail and matrix, the claim documentation must be indicated that the root and matrix are being permanently removed. Excision of subungual exostosis is sometimes used to describe the removal of one or two margins. This is not a separate procedure.

On a partial ingrown toenail, only one or two sides grow into the skin. The treatment is a partial matrixectomy in which a wedge of the nail and the underlying nail bed are removed. The nail portion can be surgically removed with a scalpel or by chemical means. This is a simple and brief procedure.

In severe cases of ingrown toenails, the entire nail grows into the skin on both sides. This is called a completely ingrown toenail. Usually, significant pain is present. Treatment is a total **matrixectomy** that removes the nail and growth plate, either surgically or chemically. The body then produces a "**false nail**," that is, tough skin that mimics a real nail. This false nail usually grows in within a few months after the surgery.

Warts

Warts are caused by a virus and are contagious. They often grow in groups and spread to the fingers and other areas of the body. Warts occurring on the soles of the feet are called plantar warts, are painful, and may affect walking. Usually, these warts grow on the soles, but they may occur on the toes or on the top of the foot. Treatment entails scooping out the wart with a curette, a spoon-shaped surgical instrument. The base is then cauterized (burned either electrically or chemically) to discourage regrowth.

Neuromas

A **neuroma** is a tumor arising from the connective tissue of the nerves. There are four interspaces between the toes of the

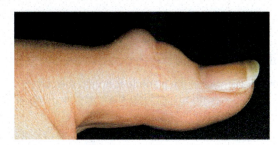

FIGURE 7-6   A ganglion
Source: Dr. P. Marazzi/Science Source

foot, and neuromas most often occur in the second interspace. Neuromas are commonly bilateral, but rarely does more than one occur on the same foot or in the first interspace.

If any other surgical procedure is performed on the first toe or on the metacarpophalangeal M-P joint of the second, third, fourth, or fifth toes, no additional allowance is available for removal of neuromas from the adjacent interspace. This procedure should not call for any increased allowance for microsurgery.

When a nerve is pinched between two metatarsal bones (usually the third and fourth metatarsals), the nerve may become enlarged. Abnormal bone structure contributes to the cause, but too-tight shoes can aggravate the condition. The treatment is to remove a small portion of the nerve. As a result, this area is permanently numbed.

Ganglions

Ganglions are fluid-filled sacs that may grow on a joint capsule or tendon, as in Figure 7-6 ●. The location and size of ganglions vary and the cause is unknown. Ganglions cause irritation, swelling, and pain when they press against nerves. Treatment involves excising the ganglion by separating it from the surrounding tissues. If it is not removed completely, a ganglion may grow back.

Miscellaneous Issues

High-arched feet (pes cavus) are caused by an imbalance of muscles and nerves and are often inherited. High arches can cause various problems such as calluses and foot, heel, ankle, or tendon pain. Treatment depends on the specific problems caused by the high arches. Usually, surgery or orthoses are prescribed.

Flat feet (pes planus) are also hereditary and are caused by a muscle imbalance. Feet with low, relaxed arches may create problems such as hammertoes and bunions; arch, foot, and leg fatigue; calf pain, and an overly tight heel cord (which makes the foot even flatter). Loose joints may move too freely, causing pain and instability. Surgery and orthoses may also be used to treat this condition. **Orthotic devices** are prescribed custom-made arch supports that fit inside most shoes and "bring the floor up to your feet." To make this support, a podiatrist takes a plaster impression of the feet. The orthotic device is made of leather, plastic, or other material, depending on the particular foot problem.

ACTIVITY #5

Billing of Podiatry Procedures

Directions: Fill in the blank spaces with the correct word without looking back at the material just covered.

1. A _____ is an enlargement of a bone in a joint at the base of the big toe. They are most often inherited.

2. _____ are also hereditary and are caused by a muscle imbalance.

3. _____ are inherited muscle imbalances or abnormal bone lengths that can make the toes buckle under, causing their joints to contract. Subsequently, the tendons shorten.

4. _____ are caused by an imbalance of muscles and nerves and are often inherited.

5. An _____ occurs when one or both corners or sides of the nail grow into the skin of the toe.

6. A _____ occurs when the metatarsal bone is longer or lower than the others so that it hits the ground first at every step with more force than it is equipped to handle. As a result, the skin under this bone thickens and becomes hardened into a callus.

7. A _____ is a tumor arising from the connective tissue of the nerves.

8. A _____ is a bony overgrowth on the bone.

9. _____ are caused by a virus and are contagious. They often grow in groups and spread to the fingers and other areas of the body.

Assistant Surgeon for Podiatry

Because of the complexity of the bones, joints, and tendons in the foot, many podiatric surgeries that are performed on an inpatient basis require an assistant surgeon. Some of these surgeries also require an assistant surgeon when they are performed in a doctor's office.

PRACTICE PITFALLS

Because it is difficult to determine the allowable expense and the correct surgical allowance for podiatry claims, you should refer questionable claim situations to a supervisor, review department, or consultant. Here are some guidelines or situations that may warrant a consultant's review:

1. Charges for the insertion or removal of K wire

2. Microsurgical repair of nerves

3. Serial surgery. **Serial surgery** is surgery on several individual toes or joints in which only one surgical procedure is performed in each operative visit. For example, surgery on one toe is followed by surgery on another toe one week later, followed by still other surgeries after that. Or, surgery is performed on one joint, followed by surgery on a different joint of the same toe at a later date. This process can last days, weeks, or even months.

4. Fragmented fees billed at 100% for each procedure. This situation may also include misrepresented CPT codes.

5. Vascular studies (e.g., temperature gradient studies, Doppler studies, or plethysmography). These tests can be considered medically necessary in certain situations or for certain conditions (e.g., diabetes, peripheral vascular disease). You will need test results and the patient's history for review.

6. Possibly unnecessary services or procedures:
   - Use of nitrous oxide anesthesia
   - Operating room charge for office surgery
   - Preoperative sedatives
   - Use of steroid injections, arthrocentesis, or power equipment on the day of surgery
   - Rental of TENS unit
   - More than two postoperative X-rays. The exception is major bone surgery and delayed bunion surgery.

It is generally accepted medical practice to allow an assistant surgeon to work on soft tissue surgeries, with the exception of surgery for ingrown toenails. Multiple or bilateral procedures may also require an assistant surgeon. Single-toe procedures for excision of dome and simple hammertoe procedures usually do not warrant the use of an assistant surgeon.

When they are allowed, the assistant surgeon's benefits are paid according to the standard policy provisions for assistant surgeons.

Before referring a claim for review, the claims examiner should request all necessary documentation, including the operating report and the patient diagnosis and history. In addition, diagnostic tests, before and after photos, X-rays, and the physician's daily office notes may also be necessary for review on some claims. The medical biller must code according to the documentation to avoid the need for these claim reviews.

If a claim is sent for referral, the claims examiner should first make a determination and pay any and all services that are not being questioned. The examiner should send written notification to the provider with the payment regarding which services are pending a consultant's review.

When the consultant returns his or her review, some services may be allowed and others denied. The claims examiner should verify the plan guidelines and benefits and make a payment determination on the claim.

The consultant's report and the name, address, and phone number of the consultant are the property of the company and should never be given to the claimant. This information should be retained as part of the claim file.

Surgery Modifiers

Following are some examples of modifiers that are frequently used with surgery procedures.

-22 Increased Procedural Services

-32 Mandated Services

-47 Anesthesia by Surgeon

-50 Bilateral Procedure

-51 Multiple Procedures

-52 Reduced Services

-54 Surgical Care Only

-55 Postoperative Management Only

-56 Preoperative Management Only

-57 Decision for Surgery

-62 Two Surgeons

-66 Surgical Team

-80 Assistant Surgeon

-81 Minimum Assistant Surgeon.

Anesthesia

Anesthesia is the artificially induced loss of feeling and sensation, with or without loss of consciousness. The anesthesiologist providing the service bills for his or her services. The four kinds of anesthesia administration are

1. General anesthesia.
2. Regional anesthesia.
3. Intravenous (IV) sedation.
4. Acupuncture.

General Anesthesia

General anesthesia produces a state of unconsciousness. It may be brought about by inhalation of gases such as ether, nitrous oxide, and ethylene or by drugs administered intravenously, such as sodium pentothal. General anesthesia produces preliminary excitement, replaced by a loss of voluntary control. Loss of consciousness occurs when the anesthetic reaches the brain, with hearing being the last sense to be lost. Most major operations, particularly on the upper abdomen, chest, head, and neck, are performed under general anesthesia. A number of side effects may accompany general anesthesia, many of which cannot be controlled or predicted. General anesthesia is considered more dangerous than other forms of anesthesia. Therefore, anesthesiologists have one of the highest malpractice insurance rates.

Prior to surgery requiring general anesthesia, the anesthesiologist usually meets with the patient to assess his or her general health and record age, weight, concurrent medical problems, family history, and other pertinent data. Anesthesiologists are reluctant to administer general anesthesia to patients who are extremely obese or who have blood pressure or respiratory problems because they have the highest risk factors.

General anesthesia can be used in outpatient surgery. However, it requires a prolonged postoperative recovery period (usually two to four hours), and therefore it is commonly reserved for use in a facility setting (outpatient hospital, surgicenter). The administration of general anesthesia in a doctor's or dentist's office is considered very dangerous, although some specialists do so routinely.

Regional Anesthesia

Regional anesthesia is the loss of sensation of a part of the body due to the interruption of nerve conduction. While regional anesthesia is in effect, the patient remains conscious. This method is adequate for many operations and is considerably less dangerous than general anesthesia. Regional anesthesia can be safely performed on an outpatient basis. The three types of regional anesthesia are topical, local, and nerve block.

Topical anesthesia is applied directly to the surface of the area to be anesthetized. The conjunctiva and mucous membranes of the mouth, throat, urethra, and bladder are areas that are most effectively anesthetized by a topical application.

Local anesthesia affects only a localized area. The drug is directly introduced by injection into the skin and subcutaneous tissues. The anesthesia injection wears off very quickly; therefore, only short procedures can be performed painlessly. Superficial biopsies, mole excisions, and suturing of lacerations are the most common procedures performed with local anesthesia.

For **nerve block anesthesia**, a drug is injected close to the nerve so that the nerve impulses are interrupted, thereby producing a loss of sensation.

Spinal anesthesia is a specialized type of nerve block. The spinal nerves are blocked in either the subarachnoid or the epidural space. The term **spinal anesthesia** generally refers to nerves blocked in the subarachnoid space. **Epidural anesthesia** refers to the nerves blocked in the epidural space. Epidural anesthesia is frequently used for maternity claims.

According to the American Society of Anesthesiologists guidelines, the anesthesia value for maternity claims is base units + time units. Because the epidural is administered throughout labor and the physician is not in constant attendance, many insurance carriers and PPOs have developed special guidelines for maternity anesthesia. To process these claims accurately, be sure to develop a full understanding of the office procedures.

Another type of spinal anesthetic is a **saddle block**, named because the injection produces a loss of feeling in the region of the body that corresponds to the area that makes contact with a riding saddle (buttocks, perineum, and thighs). Spinal anesthesia was formerly used frequently for normal deliveries. Now, it is mainly used on operations within the peritoneal cavity and on the lower extremities.

Intravenous Sedation

IV sedation is a medication composed of a sedative and a painkiller administered intravenously to produce a semiconscious state. A common mixture is meperidine (Demerol) and diazepam (Valium). This type of anesthesia is often used in dental surgical procedures and in many diagnostic procedures, such as bronchoscopy and esophagogastroduodenoscopy, in which the surgical invasion is obtained through an existing orifice. This type of anesthesia is commonly referred to as "twilight sleep."

Acupuncture

Acupuncture can be used as another form of anesthesia. There are more than 1000 acupuncture locations on the body, and each location or combination of locations produces a different physiological effect. Sometimes, only one needle is necessary to achieve the desired result; other times many needles are required. The patient remains awake and can talk during the procedure. Acupuncture works similarly to the way nerve block anesthesia works. Although this type of anesthesia is most popular in China, it is also used in the United States.

Hypnosis

Hypnosis is the creation of a state in which the subconscious mind is allowed to take over and the conscious mind is more or less inactive. Some patients choose hypnosis rather than conventional forms of anesthesia.

Most plans do not cover hypnosis services, though a few may cover hypnosis when it is used in lieu of covered anesthesia.

Anesthesia CPT Coding

The coding for anesthesia services depends on the area of the body on which the surgeon is operating. Anesthesia CPT codes, shown in Table 7-2 ●, range from 00100 to

TABLE 7-2 Anesthesia CPT® Codes

Head	00100-002222
Neck	00300-00352
Thorax	00400-00474
Intrathoracic	00500-00580
Spine and Spinal Cord	00600-00670
Upper Abdomen	00700-00797
Lower Abdomen	00800-00882
Perineum	00902-00952
Pelvis (except hip)	01112-01190
Upper leg (except knee)	01200-01274
Knee and Popliteal Area	01320-01444
Lower Leg (below knee, includes ankle and foot)	01462-01522
Shoulder and Axilla	01610-01682
Upper Arm and Elbow	01710-01782
Forearm, Wrist and Hand	01810-01860
Radiological Procedures	01916-01936
Burns, Excisions or Debridement	01951-01953
Obstetric	01958-01969
Other Procedures	01990-01999

01999. As specific surgeries usually are not included in these codes, there are no special circumstances for any given body area. For that reason we will list the subsections without further comment.

Anesthesia Handling Procedures

An anesthesiologist may be classified as either a **hospital staff anesthesiologist** (employed by the hospital) or an **independent anesthesiologist** (self-employed or not employed by the hospital). Charges made by a hospital for the services of a staff anesthesiologist are usually covered as a hospital ancillary expense. Charges by an outside anesthesiologist vary according to plan provision, but they are usually covered under either a separate Basic anesthesia benefit or under a Major Medical benefit. When you are processing claims, do not confuse the professional anesthesia expense with the charges that may appear on a hospital bill. The anesthesia charges on a hospital bill are for the actual anesthesia drug, the anesthesia machine, and other associated supplies.

Anesthesia may be administered by any of the following individuals:

Medical doctor (M.D.)

Anesthesiologist (Anes.)

Certified Registered Nurse Anesthetist (CRNA)

Anesthetic Assistant (AA)

RVS Ground Rules

The American Society of Anesthesiologists developed a coding system which has been adopted by the CPT. The CPT code range for anesthesia is 00100–01999. The *RVS* uses 00100–01999 or 10000–69999 (same as surgery) for coding anesthetic services. Anesthesia unit values are listed in the *RVS* for procedures that require anesthesia to be administered by an anesthesiologist. Remember that local anesthesia is never allowable separately. Therefore, anesthesia benefits are those that are allowed on procedures which require more than a local anesthesia.

These units (for all schedules) are used when

* The anesthesia is personally administered by a licensed physician, and
* The physician remains in constant attendance during the procedure for the sole purpose of administering and monitoring the anesthesia service.

Basic/Base Units

The basic or base anesthesia units are designed to allow for the usual preoperative and postoperative care, the administration of anesthesia, and the administration of fluids or blood incident to the anesthesia or surgery. Usually, monitoring services such as ECG, blood pressure oximetry, capnography, mass spectrometry, and monitoring of blood gases are also included in the basic value and should not be billed separately.

Remember that the surgical unit values include surgery, local infiltration, and digital block or topical anesthesia.

Time Units

The length of time that a person is under anesthesia determines the amount of money that will be considered allowable for the procedure. Anesthesia time begins when the anesthesiologist starts to physically prepare the patient for the induction of anesthesia in the operating room area (or its equivalent). The time ends when the anesthesiologist is no longer in constant attendance, usually when the patient is ready for postoperative supervision.

There are two ways of calculating the anesthesia time, depending on individual payer guidelines:

1. Actual time
2. Block time.

ACTUAL TIME. Some carriers allow one time unit for each 15 minutes, regardless of the amount of time that a patient is under anesthesia. Any fractional portions of a 15-minute block (e.g., one minute, five minutes) are calculated to the nearest tenth of a unit. Thus, each 1.5 minutes is worth 0.1 units.

BLOCK TIME. For the first four hours, time units are computed by allowing 1.0 time unit for each 15 minutes or fraction thereof. After four hours, 1.0 unit is allowed for each 10 minutes. If the time is less than 10 minutes, 1.0 unit is allowed for spans between five and 10 minutes. The reason for this is that the risks of injury or adverse effects significantly increase with time. Therefore, extra compensation is provided for extended anesthesia time.

For example, if the anesthesia time were 50 minutes, a total of 4.0 time units would be allowed (1.0 unit for every 15 minutes = 3.0 units, plus 1.0 unit for the additional five minutes). Therefore, the same number of units would be allowed for a 50-minute procedure, a 55-minute procedure, or a one-hour procedure. Table 7-3 ● provides an example of anesthesia Block Time units.

Many anesthesiologists bill time according to a military clock, that is, by a 24-hour standard. When you are using military time, do not worry about converting the time to a regular clock. The regular time is unimportant. Instead, concentrate on determining the time units involved. Consider the following example:

1. Total time: 13:15 to 14:25
   13:15 to 14:15 = 1 hour = 4.0 units
   14:15 to 14:25 = 10 min = 1.0 unit
                   1 hour 10 min = 5.0 units
2. Total time: 15:20 to 18:25
   15:20 to 18:20 = 3 hours = 12.0 units
   18:20 to 18:25 = 5 min = 1.0 unit
                   3 hour 5 min = 13.0 units

EXCEPTIONS. Time units are usually not allowed for the following procedures/situations:

- Daily management of epidural of subarachnoid drug administration (01996)

TABLE 7-3 Example of Anesthesia Block Time Units

Anesthesia Time	Units of Occurrence
5 min – 19 min	1 unit
20 – 34 min	2 units
35 min – 49 min	3 units
50 min – 1 hr 04 min	4 units
1 hr 5 min – 1 hr 19 min	5 units
1 hr 20 min – 1 hr 34 min	6 units
1 hr 35 min – 1 hr 49 min	7 units
1 hr 50 min – 2 hr 4 min	8 units
2 hr 5 min – 2 hr 19 min	9 units
2 hr 20 min – 2 hr 34 min	10 units
2 hr 35 min – 2 hr 49 min	11 units
2 hr 50 min – 3 hr 4 min	12 units
3 hr 5 min – 3 hr 19 min	13 units
3 hr 20 min – 3 hr 34 min	14 units
3 hr 35 min – 3 hr 49 min	15 units
3 hr 50 min – 4 hr 4 min	16 units
4 hr 5 min – 4 hr 14 min	17 units
4 hr 15 min – 4 hr 24 min	18 units
4 hr 25 min – 4 hr 34 min	19 units
4 hr 35 min – 4 hr 44 min	20 units
4 hr 45 min – 4 hr 54 min	21 units
4 hr 55 min – 5 hr 4 min	22 units

- Administration of epidural anesthesia for maternal delivery (62282)
- Anesthesia for patient of extreme age, under one year or over 70 years (99100)
- Anesthesia complicated by use of total body hypothermia (99116)
- Anesthesia complicated by use of controlled hypotension (99135)
- Anesthesia complicated by emergency conditions (99140).

These codes are normally paid according to the base units multiplied by the conversion factor. No allowance is made for time units.

ACTIVITY #6

Anesthesia Billing

Directions: Answer the following questions without looking back at the material just covered. Write your answers in the space provided.

1. What are the anesthesia charges on a hospital bill for? _____

_____

_____

_____

(Continued)

2. What four types of individuals are qualified to administer anesthesia?

a. _____

b. _____

c. _____

d. _____

3. When does anesthesia time begin and end? _____

_____

_____

Calculating Anesthesia

The anesthesia allowance is calculated by adding the basic units to the time units and multiplying that amount by the conversion factor. This procedure applies to all schedules.

Basic Unit Value for the procedure
+ Time Unit Value
+ Modifier Unit Value (if applicable)
Total Anesthesia Value

Total Anesthesia Value × plan/Basic Conversion Factor = Anesthesia basic allowance or plan UCR

Multiple Procedures

For anesthesia claims with multiple procedures, the basic units for the major procedure (the procedure with the greatest number of basic units) are the only basic units allowed. The basic units for the secondary procedure are not taken into account. The additional expense is accommodated by allowing the extra time units that are necessary to complete the multiple procedures.

Network Anesthesia

Carriers that pay different percentages for network and non-network providers will often pay the anesthesiologist at the network rate if the chosen surgeon is a network provider, regardless of whether the anesthesiologist is a part of their network. The reason for this policy is that the surgeon usually chooses the anesthesiologist. Thus, the patient is not penalized for a choice that he or she was not allowed to make.

Modifiers

In addition to the modifiers listed previously which denote who performed the services, some carriers use additional modifiers for anesthesia services.

Physical status modifiers are represented by the initial P, followed by a single digit from 1 to 6.

P1: A normal healthy patient

P2: A patient with mild systemic disease

P3: A patient with severe systemic disease

P4: A patient with severe systemic disease that is a constant threat to life

P5: A moribund patient who is not expected to survive without the operation

P6: A patient who has been declared brain-dead and whose organs are being removed for donation.

Optional modifiers denote special conditions. The following are the valid anesthesia two-digit modifier codes. (For additional information, consult your CPT.)

-22: Increased procedural services

-23: Unusual anesthesia

-32: Mandated services

-51: Multiple procedures, but not bilateral.

Some carriers require that a modifier be used to identify who performed the anesthesia service, and what type of service it was. These modifiers are HCPCS Level II modifiers. The following modifier codes are used for this purpose:

AA: Anesthesia services performed by an anesthesiologist

AD: Anesthesia was medically supervised by a physician for more than four concurrent procedures

QK: Medically directed by a physician; two through four concurrent procedures

QX: Anesthesia administered by a CRNA with medical direction by a physician

QY: Medical direction on one CRNA by an anesthesiologist

QZ: Anesthesia administered by a CRNA without medical direction by a physician.

Unusual Circumstances

Occasionally, the use of modifier -22 or -23 will indicate that unusual procedures were performed. This modifier is often used to explain why the amount of time shown on an anesthesia claim is greater than usual. **Unusual services** are services that are rarely provided, unusual, or variable and that may warrant an additional anesthesia fee. These situations can include

- Severe or multiple injuries.
- Procedures in the head, neck, or shoulder region which can disrupt the administration of anesthesia.
- Unusual or lengthy monitoring.
- Procedures where care must be taken to avoid certain areas of the body.
- Procedures or situations where the patient must be placed in an unusual position (e.g., sitting).

Coding these claims can be difficult; the medical biller must ensure that the coding matches the documentation. When these claims are processed, the examiner should request a copy of the operative report, the hospital medical records, detailed records from the anesthesiologist regarding the services performed, and the length of time the patient was under anesthesia. This information will allow you to determine whether the anesthesiologist billed the correct code or whether there were additional complications that could increase the amount of time the anesthesiologist attended the patient.

Some insurance carriers will allow an additional percentage for unusual services claims (e.g., an additional 25% benefit), and some will allow a specific amount of units (e.g., an additional three units is not uncommon). There are a number of other carriers who do not allow any additional benefit. The rationale for not allowing more is that the additional time involved in the procedure is enough to compensate the anesthesiologist for the unusual services. Be sure to consult plan guidelines prior to processing claims with unusual services modifiers. You may need to refer many of these claims for medical review.

Qualifying Circumstances

Many anesthesia services are provided under particularly difficult circumstances, which include extraordinary conditions of the patient, notable operative conditions, and unusual risk factors. This section includes a list of important qualifying circumstances that make a significant impact on the character of the anesthesia service provided. These procedures would not be reported alone but as additional procedures qualifying an anesthesia procedure or service. The claim may include more than one.

99100   Anesthesia for patient of extreme age, under one year or over 70 years

99116   Anesthesia complicated by use of total body hypothermia

99135   Anesthesia complicated by use of controlled hypotension

99140   Anesthesia complicated by emergency conditions. Most plans require the emergency conditions to be specified. Treatment is considered emergency treatment when its delay would lead to a significant increase in the threat to life or body part.

Many providers will allow additional units for qualifying circumstances.

EXAMPLE:

99100 – 1 additional unit

99116 – 5 additional units

99135 – 5 additional units

99140 – 2 additional units

Examining Tips

Many insurance carriers will allow additional units for some modifiers.

EXAMPLE:

P1 – No additional value

P2 – No additional value

P3 – 1 additional unit

P4 – 2 additional units

P5 – 3 additional units

P6 – No additional units

Monitored Anesthesia Care

Monitored anesthesia care (MAC) is the monitoring of a patient's vital signs during an operation in anticipation of the need for general anesthesia. There are several reasons that this monitoring may be necessary:

- The patient may have an adverse physiological reaction to the procedure.
- The patients may have a low pain threshold or may experience intense pain.
- It may become necessary to expand the operative field (e.g., a mass may be biopsied under a local anesthetic; however, if the surgeon locates additional tumors, more radical surgery would be done during the same operative session).
- The patient may be combative.
- The patient may be a neonate or pediatric patient who may become frightened or combative.
- The patient may be mentally impaired and may become uncooperative due to his or her impairment.
- It may become necessary to administer drugs which are required to be administered by an anesthesiologist, even though they may not produce unconsciousness in a patient.

In order for an anesthesiologist to be reimbursed for MAC, the following services are required:

- Preoperative visit and evaluation, including medical history, anesthesia history, taking of medication information, and physical exam.
- Preoperative evaluation of all available pertinent reports (e.g., lab, X-ray).
- Patient discussion and signing of informed consent.
- Monitoring of vital signs during the operative procedure, including oxygenation, ventilation, circulation, temperature, and maintenance of the patient's airway.
- Diagnosis and treatment of any clinical problems which occur during the procedure.
- Administration of medications or other agents to ensure patient safety and comfort during the procedure.
- Postoperative patient management, including evaluation of the patient, time-based record of vital signs and level of consciousness, and reporting of any complications, adverse reactions, or unusual events.
- Postanesthesia visits (as needed).
- A complete record of all drugs used and amounts.

In order for MAC to be reimbursed, the anesthesiologist must be present during the entire operative procedure. If all the preceding requirements are met, a MAC anesthesiologist is reimbursed at the same amount as routine anesthesiology, as the same level of attention and care is required.

The modifier -QS on the claim denotes that the claim is for MAC services.

Medical Direction of Anesthesiology

At times, the actual monitoring of the patient will be performed by an AA or a CRNA under the direction of a physician. In such cases, the physician is responsible for

- Conducting the preoperative evaluation of the patient.
- Ordering the drugs.
- Determining the anesthesia treatment plan.
- Handling or participating in the most demanding anesthesia procedures, including induction and emergence.
- Monitoring the course of anesthesia and the patient's situation at frequent intervals.
- Handling any emergency situations.
- Providing all postanesthesia care.

The AA or CRNA is responsible for

- Understanding the anesthesia plan.
- Providing the continuous administration of the anesthesia.
- Monitoring the patient's vitals.
- Remaining in contact with the physician and summoning him or her if needed.

This division of labor allows a directing physician to handle anesthesia for several patients at the same time. However, most payers limit the number of patients a physician may direct at one time to four or fewer.

In such cases, most carriers will split the anesthesiologist allowance, allowing 50% for the directing physician and 50% for the AA or CRNA, provided that the directing physician is not directing the care of more than four patients concurrently. If the physician is directing the care of more than four patients at a time, some payers will set reimbursement at 25% for the directing physician and 75% for the AA or CRNA. Others will consider the anesthesiologist's services to be supervisory. In other words, in their view the anesthesiologist is simply overseeing the work of the AA or CRNA, not directing the specifics of the work. Reimbursement for supervisory anesthesiologists is often calculated at three base units per procedure. No time units are allowed, unless an anesthesiologist can document that he or she was present and attending during the induction of the anesthesia, in which case one time unit is allowed.

Anesthesiologists are required to certify the number of patients for whom concurrent care was handled at any given time during the operative session.

Pain Control

Occasionally, an anesthesiologist may be called on to perform services to ease intractable or chronic pain. **Intractable pain** is hard to manage and is often severe enough to limit a patient's movement or abilities. In such cases, relief may be obtained through an injection or intravenous infusion of pain medication.

Many insurance carriers will allow payment for these services if the following conditions are met:

- The pain cannot be managed through other means (e.g., oral or traditional pain medications).
- The pain is severe enough that it interferes with daily living.
- A complete medical evaluation has been performed to assess the source of the pain.
- All other reasonable medical treatments (including psychological approaches) were considered or tried and found to be unsuccessful or potentially harmful.
- Transcutaneous electrical nerve stimulation (TENS) was unsuccessful.
- Pharmacological or physical therapy programs were found to be unsuccessful or potentially harmful.

Often block treatments for intractable pain are limited to three per year. You should request medical records to evaluate the success of the treatment. These cases will often need to be referred for review.

Patient-Controlled Anesthesia

Some conditions allow the patient to administer their own pain medication (or anesthetic). This is often done using an **infusion pump**, a machine which contains medication and administers a small dose when the patient presses a button. The machine is attached to the outside of the body and the medication flows through a line running into a vein (for intravenous medications) or under the skin (for subcutaneous medications). Safeguards on the machine prevent an overdose from occurring and prevent a second dose from being administered before the first dose has had a chance to take effect.

Infusion pumps have been shown to provide equal or better pain relief than other methods and have a lower overall dosage level.

Many carriers will allow benefits for the placement and use of an infusion pump if all of the following criteria are met:

- The unit and pain medication are prescribed by a licensed physician.
- The medical condition being treated is a covered expense.
- The medical condition being treated requires long-term pain control.
- The pain is manageable by pharmacological means and no other pain control (or very limited additional pain control) is necessary.
- The unit is used in a hospital setting, or, if it is used in a home setting, the use is monitored by an RN on a regular basis.

As with many other new forms of anesthesia, plan guidelines vary widely. Be sure to check contract provisions before processing infusion pump claims. If the plan does allow for payment, there will often be separate charges for the infusion pump, professional charges for the placement of the infusion pump, and charges for the medications that are placed in the infusion pump.

● **ONLINE INFORMATION:** Find a website that describes and discusses an infusion pump. Research how the pump works and learn some advantages and disadvantages of its use.

Miscellaneous

Epidural anesthesia is often provided during labor for normal deliveries. Time of administration tends to run four or more hours. Some administrators provide their own rules, and some plans do not cover anesthesia during labor at all. Therefore, verify the guidelines that apply to the plan you are processing.

General anesthesia is usually administered when shock therapy is provided. Many plans do not cover anesthesia for this purpose or may have special handling guidelines. Verify the guidelines before processing these claims.

A standby anesthesiologist may be asked to be available while diagnostic procedures are performed on a patient who may require emergency surgery. If the anesthesiologist is not rendering treatment, administering anesthesia, or monitoring vital signs, but is charging merely for being available, the charge is usually not a covered expense. However, verify first before processing the claim.

If surgery is cancelled for medical reasons prior to the surgery, the anesthesiologist may be reimbursed for conducting evaluation and management. In such cases, the claim should use an evaluation and management code and should provide full documentation of the reason for the cancellation of surgery.

CHAPTER REVIEW

Summary

- Surgery charges may be the most complicated charges you will encounter. That is why there are so many guidelines covering surgery, multiple surgery, assistant surgery, and cosmetic surgery. If for any reason you are unsure how to process a claim, request the medical opinion of a senior coder or examiner, as appropriate for your position.
- The use of an assistant surgeon always depends on the medical necessity of the procedure performed.
- The charges for podiatry services vary from simple to complex.
- Because podiatry surgery guidelines vary from company to company, check with the administrator before processing these types of claims.
- Anesthesia plays an important role in patient care.
- The guidelines we have just covered will enable you to process anesthesia charges, no matter what method or type of anesthesia is administered.
- There is almost always an anesthesia charge when major surgery is performed, and you as the claims examiner are responsible for processing these charges. The medical biller from the surgeon, the anesthesiologist, and the facility where surgery was performed will all submit bills.
- Use the preceding guidelines to calculate anesthesia time and to identify the provider of services (anesthesiologist, nurse anesthetist, or surgeon).

Review Questions

Directions: Answer the following questions without looking back at the material just covered. Write your answers in the space provided.

1. Define surgery. _____

2. Are cosmetic surgical procedures usually covered by benefit plans? _____

3. What are the four types of surgical procedures? (List them and indicate under what circumstances each type of procedure would be used.)

   a. _____

   b. _____

   c. _____

   d. _____

4. What does the physician's charge for surgery performed in the office generally include? _____

5. Identify two situations that would warrant separate payment for preoperative care.

6. What does the surgical unit value include? _____

7. When can the follow-up care be billed separately? _____

8. What are cosurgeons? _____

9. What are By Report procedures and what other term may be used to indicate these procedures? _____

10. What services are normally provided in maternity cases?

11. What is podiatric surgery? _____

_____

12. Define ligaments. _____

_____

13. How many complex joints are in the foot? _____

14. How many bunion surgeries are normally allowed per foot? _____

15. What is an orthotic device? _____

_____

16. What are the four methods of anesthesia administration?

a. _____

b. _____

c. _____

d. _____

17. What is the American Society of Anesthesiologists code range for anesthesia? _____

18. What is the *RVS* code range for anesthesia? _____

19. The total anesthesia unit values consist of _____ and _____ units.

20. True or False: Most plans cover anesthesia for shock therapy. _____

If you were unable to answer any of these questions, refer back to that section and then fill in the answers.

ACTIVITY #7

Find the Terms

Directions: Find and circle the words listed here. Words can appear horizontally, vertically, diagonally, forward, or backward.

```
Y  V  M  N  R  O  P  V  V  J  P  E  R  K  N  S  I  S  Q  T  O  H
P  M  K  U  I  E  C  M  C  I  J  Q  C  I  T  C  E  X  S  O  T  Y
L  G  O  W  L  H  C  R  U  J  D  O  W  R  F  C  P  E  Q  P  P  P
A  N  L  T  W  T  U  O  O  P  L  S  U  I  I  X  R  U  T  I  N  N
N  I  U  T  O  A  I  K  N  B  N  C  G  V  P  I  Z  W  X  C  I  O
T  Q  D  F  Z  E  Q  P  E  S  T  O  R  X  A  U  R  B  C  A  A  S
A  C  M  Z  L  Q  T  L  L  U  T  E  I  L  C  R  M  W  X  L  P  I
R  Y  L  P  X  K  D  S  R  E  S  R  S  S  V  H  L  I  W  A  E  S
C  D  L  D  H  D  U  A  O  L  P  U  U  P  U  Z  A  O  I  N  L  E
A  U  Y  Z  A  R  L  Y  A  L  R  R  M  C  N  F  N  M  L  E  B  R
L  T  X  S  G  B  P  U  K  G  A  P  O  S  T  W  N  Y  L  S  A  U
L  C  E  E  U  T  S  X  E  F  T  S  N  C  B  I  O  I  O  T  T  T
U  V  R  N  G  U  X  R  X  A  L  F  R  B  E  K  O  K  U  H  C  C
S  Y  I  Y  N  I  Y  Q  J  N  W  J  K  O  Y  D  E  N  Z  E  A  N
A  O  M  U  H  A  M  M  E  R  T  O  E  S  D  R  U  W  H  S  R  U
N  S  E  R  U  D  E  C  O  R  P  K  C  O  L  B  E  R  E  I  T  P
S  Y  A  D  P  U  W  O  L  L  O  F  F  Q  H  P  A  P  E  A  N  U
B  S  H  E  C  L  C  F  Y  F  X  L  M  B  C  V  S  P  O  S  I  C
E  Z  M  T  N  P  P  U  V  Z  Y  K  D  W  F  H  T  M  L  R  U  A
Y  W  E  V  I  Q  R  D  X  M  N  S  B  N  F  O  F  M  I  A  T  K
N  E  R  V  E  B  L  O  C  K  A  N  E  S  T  H  E  S  I  A  R  M
G  L  O  B  A  L  A  P  P  R  O  A  C  H  X  G  Z  E  K  H  L  J
```

1. Block Procedures
2. By Report
3. Dorsal Osteotomy
4. Followup Days
5. Global Approach
6. Hammertoes
7. Hypnosis
8. Infusion Pump
9. Intractable Pain
10. Multiple Procedures
11. Nerve Block Anesthesia
12. Plantar Callus
13. Reconstruction
14. Saddle Block
15. Serial Surgery
16. Structural Bunion
17. Surgery
18. Topical Anesthesia
19. Unusual Services

ACTIVITY #8

Matching

Directions: Match the following terms with the proper definition by writing the letter of the correct definition in the space next to the term.

1. ___U___ Assistant Surgeon
2. ___N___ Chromosomal Analysis
3. ___R___ Cosurgeons
4. ___I___ Diagnostic Procedures
5. ___K___ Endogenous Obesity
6. ___Q___ Epidural Anesthesia
7. ___A___ Exogenous Obesity
8. ___P___ False Nail
9. ___M___ General Anesthesia
10. ___O___ Hospital Staff Anesthesiologist
11. ___V___ In Vitro Fertilization
12. ___T___ Independent Anesthesiologist
13. ___H___ Ingrown Toenail
14. ___S___ IV Sedation
15. ___J___ In Utero Fetal Surgery
16. ___G___ Metatarsal Plantar Callus
17. ___I___ Monitored Anesthesia Care
18. ___F___ Physical Status Modifiers
19. ___E___ Positional Bunion
20. ___C___ Regional Anesthesia
21. ___D___ Spinal Anesthesia
22. ___B___ Therapeutic Procedures

a. Obesity caused by overeating.

b. Procedures performed to remove or correct the functioning of a body part that is diseased or injured.

c. Anesthesia that produces the loss of sensation of a part of the body due to the interruption of nerve conduction.

d. A specialized type of nerve block in which the spinal nerves are blocked in either the subarachnoid or the epidural space.

e. A bony growth on the side of the metatarsal bone that enlarges the joint, forcing the joint capsule to stretch over it.

f. Modifiers that are used to indicate various physical conditions and that are represented by the initial P, followed by a single digit from 1 to 6.

g. A condition that occurs when the metatarsal bone is longer or lower than the others so that it hits the ground first at every step with more force than it is equipped to handle.

h. A nail in which one or both corners or sides of the nail grow into the skin of the toe.

i. The monitoring of a patient's vital signs during an operation in anticipation of the need for a general anesthesia.

j. Surgery on a fetus while it is in the mother's womb, or removal of the fetus from the womb, performance of surgery, and return of the fetus back to the womb, with the pregnancy continuing to term.

k. Obesity caused by an internal malfunction, usually hormonal (e.g., thyroid disorder).

l. Procedures performed to determine the presence of disease or the cause of the patient's symptoms.

m. Anesthesia that produces a state of unconsciousness.

n. A diagnostic study performed on the amniotic fluid to determine whether any abnormalities in the number or structure of the fetal chromosomes are present.

o. An anesthesiologist employed by the hospital.

p. A tough section of skin that mimics a real nail.

q. Anesthesia which blocks the nerves in the epidural space.

r. Two surgeons, usually with similar skills, operating simultaneously as primary surgeons and performing distinct, separate parts of a total surgical service.

s. A medication composed of a sedative and a painkiller administered intravenously to produce a semiconscious state.

t. An anesthesiologist who is self-employed or not employed by the hospital.

u. A surgeon who assists a primary surgeon. He or she may close the operative wound, ensure hemostasis of the wound edges, and suture vessels.

v. The fertilization of the ovum within a test tube.

Keywords and concepts you will learn in this chapter:

Balance Billing

Benefit Period

Carriers

Deficit Reduction Act of 1984 (DEFRA)

Diagnosis-Related Group (DRG)

Electronic Remittance Notice (ERN)

End-Stage Renal Disease (ESRD)

Intermediaries

Limiting Charge (LC)

Maintenance of Benefits

Medicaid

Medicare

Medicare Allowance

Medicare Remittance Advice

Medicare Summary Notice (MSN)

Medicare Supplements

Nonparticipating Physicians

Outliers

Part A

Part B

After completing this chapter, you will be able to:

- Explain the impact of TEFRA and DEFRA on health insurance plans.

- State the eligibility requirements for Medicare.

- List the types of nonparticipating facilities that Medicare will not cover.

- Describe the types of Medicare coverage and the benefits for each.

- Explain what reasonable charges are and how they affect Medicare payments to providers.

- Describe what acceptance of assignment is and how it affects Medicare payments to the provider.

- List the claims that require acceptance of assignment.

- Explain how the limiting charge rule affects the payment of claims.

- Discuss how to estimate Medicare benefits.

Part C
Part D
Participating Physicians
Railroad Retirement
Reasonable Charges
Social Security Disability
Tax Equity and Fiscal Responsibility
Act of 1982 (TEFRA)

- Explain and describe DRG billing.

- Show how a DRG benefit is calculated with a given scenario.

- Describe the purpose of the Medicaid program.

- List Medicaid eligibility requirements.

Medicare is a federally funded program that allows many people to obtain services who may not be able to afford coverage or qualify for it otherwise. Its official title is the Federal Health Insurance Benefit Plan for the Aged and Disabled, Title XVIII of Public Law 89-97 of the Social Security Act of 1965. This program provides health insurance for people 65 years of age or older and certain persons who are totally disabled or have a diagnosis of end-stage renal disease (ESRD). The Medicare program is overseen by the CMS. (See Figure 8-1 ●.)

Social Security Administration offices throughout the United States take applications for Medicare, determine eligibility, and provide general information about the program. The actual processing of the claims is administered by many different insurance companies, usually one or two within each state. Consequently, as a medical biller or claims examiner you will see diversity in the application or denial of benefits and in the Medicare Remittance Notice (MRN) forms. The **Medicare Remittance Advice** is used to convey payments to providers who accept assignment for Medicare claims. The **Electronic Remittance Notice (ERN)** is the electronic version of the MRN. The **Medicare Summary Notice (MSN)** is an explanation of benefits sent to the Medicare beneficiary, detailing the processing of claims submitted for payment.

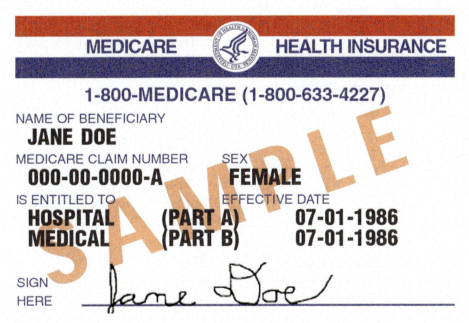

FIGURE 8-1   Sample Medicare Insurance Card
Source: Medicare.gov

TEFRA/DEFRA

The **Tax Equity and Fiscal Responsibility Act of 1982 (TEFRA)** and the **Deficit Reduction Act of 1984 (DEFRA)**—and their amendments—have redirected the financial responsibility for medical coverage of active employees aged 65 years and older and their spouses aged 65 years and older. When this federal program was introduced, it selected Medicare as the primary payer for persons who have reached their 65th birthday, regardless of their employment status.

Initially, TEFRA regulations did not apply to the spouses over age 65 of active employees who were under 65 years of age. DEFRA became effective on January 1, 1985, and amended TEFRA so that now spouses who are 65 years and older of active employees who are under age 65 can elect their primary coverage as either Medicare or the private group plan.

The employers affected by these Acts are those who regularly employ 20 or more workers for each working day in at least 20 weeks of the current or preceding calendar year. Employees of such employers must be offered coverage under the group plan on the same basis as other employees. Each employee who is or who becomes affected must complete and sign an election form choosing the primary plan.

If the employee chooses coverage under the employer's group plan, the group plan will be the primary payer on all medical services and Medicare will be the secondary payer. If the employee rejects coverage under the group plan and chooses Medicare, the employee and spouse by law can be covered only by Medicare. The group plan will not provide secondary coverage.

Employers with fewer than 20 employees are exempt from the TEFRA/DEFRA regulations, and Medicare is the primary carrier for their active employees and spouses aged 65 years or older. Medicare is also the primary carrier for all retired employees and for active employees and their spouses under age 65 who are totally disabled with conditions including ESRD.

After you have determined that the group plan is subject to TEFRA/DEFRA (because the employer has 20 or more employees), next you must determine whether the individual is eligible for Medicare.

Medicare Eligibility

Medicare eligibility is provided on the basis of one of these three principles:

1. Age
2. Disability
3. ESRD.

An individual is eligible for Medicare coverage on the first day of the month in which he or she reaches age 65. Persons who are born on the first day of the month are eligible on the first day of the month preceding their birthday.

EXAMPLE:

Birthday June 15, eligible for Medicare on June 1.

Birthday June 1, eligible for Medicare on May 1.

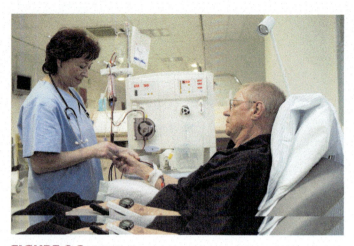

FIGURE 8-2 Dialysis
Source: Olaf Doering/Alamy

No premium is charged if the person or the person's spouse has worked 10 years in Medicare-covered employment.

Medicare coverage for totally disabled persons begins on the first of the 25th month from the date approved for **Social Security Disability** or **Railroad Retirement** benefits. The covered individuals include disabled workers of any age, disabled widows between the ages of 50 and 65, disabled beneficiaries age 18 and over who receive Social Security benefits because of disability incurred before age 22, blind individuals, and railroad retirement annuitants.

ESRD is a condition in which a person's kidneys fail to function. As a result, the patient needs dialysis treatments. (Refer to the Physician's, Clinical, and Hospital Services Claims chapter for a review of this type of service.) Because of the many problems associated with ESRD, patients are considered to be totally disabled, even though some persons with this disease continue to work. As a result, the following special rules apply to ESRD patients.

The employer's group health plan is the primary payer for the first 30 months after a patient (under age 65) with ESRD becomes eligible for Medicare. This 30-month period begins on the earlier of

- The month in which a regular course of renal dialysis, as shown in Figure 8-2 ●, is initiated.
- The month in which the patient is hospitalized for a kidney transplant.

Medicare is the secondary payer during this 30-month period but will revert to the primary status beginning with the 31st month. As a general rule, all services provided under a dialysis program are assigned to Medicare.

Providers of Service

Providers of services and medical equipment suppliers under Medicare must meet all licensing requirements of the state in which they are located. To be a participating provider under the Medicare program and receive payments for services, a provider must meet additional Medicare requirements. All providers must bill Medicare for a patient who has Medicare benefits, regardless of whether the provider participates in the

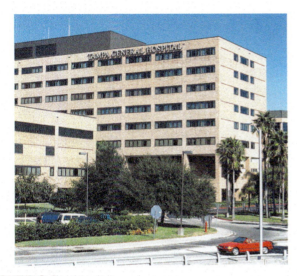

FIGURE 8-3 Hospital
Source: Michal Heron/Pearson Education/PH College

program. Medicare does not pay for the following care received in nonparticipating facilities:

- Hospital care (see Figure 8-3 ●)
- Skilled nursing facility (SNF)
- Home health agency
- Hospice
- Outpatient rehabilitation
- Dialysis facilities
- Ambulatory surgical centers
- Independent physical therapists
- Independent occupational therapists
- Clinical laboratories
- Portable X-ray suppliers
- Rural health clinics

The Parts of Medicare

There are four parts to the Medicare program: Part A, Part B, Part C, and Part D.

1. **Part A** is considered the basic plan or hospital insurance. This part covers facility charges for acute inpatient hospital care, skilled nursing, home healthcare, and hospice care.
2. **Part B** is the medical (supplementary, voluntary) insurance that covers physician services, outpatient hospital services, home healthcare, outpatient speech and physical therapy, and durable medical equipment.
3. **Part C** is the Medicare advantage portion that includes coverage in an HMO, PPO, and so on.
4. **Part D** is the prescription drug component (effective 2006) introduced by the Medicare Prescription Drug, Improvement, and Modernization Act of 2003.

Part A

Part A, the hospital coverage portion of Medicare, automatically applies for the following individuals when they enroll in Medicare:

- All people age 65 and over, if they are entitled to either monthly Social Security benefits or pensions under the Railroad Retirement Act. (See Figure 8-4 ●.)

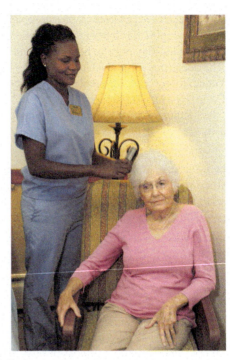

FIGURE 8-4 Retired Elder on Medicare
Source: Pat Watson/Pearson Education/PH College

- Some spouses who receive Medicare benefits derived strictly from their eligible spouse's work credits. The eligible spouse's social security number followed by the appropriate letter indicates that benefits are based on the eligible spouse.

Effective July 1, 1973, all people aged 65 years and older who are not otherwise eligible for Part A may enroll by paying the full cost of such coverage, provided they also enroll in Part B. Part A claims are processed by private insurance companies called **intermediaries** or Part A Medicare Administrative Contractors (MACs).

BENEFITS. A Part A deductible amount is taken from the first inpatient hospital admission. The use of Medicare benefits for an inpatient is measured by benefit periods. A **benefit period** begins with the first day of admission to the hospital. A benefit period ends after the patient has been discharged from the hospital or SNF for a period of 60 consecutive days (including the day of discharge). If the patient is then readmitted, a new benefit period begins and another inpatient deductible is taken.

If a member remains in the hospital for an extended period of time, additional copayments may be required. Medicare deducts the copay amount from the billed amount and then pays the amount that exceeds the copay.

The inpatient hospital copayments are calculated as follows:

- First day–60th day = Patient pays deductible only, no additional copayment.
- 61st day–90th day = Patient pays additional copayment per day.
- 91st day–150th day = Patient pays higher additional copayment per day.

These days are known as the 60-day Lifetime Reserve. These copayments are not renewable.

For SNFs, there is a separate copayment schedule and requirement. To be eligible for this benefit, the patient must have a three-night qualifying stay prior to being admitted to the SNF. In addition, the doctor must certify that the patient needs skilled nursing and rehabilitative care on a daily basis. Custodial care is not covered, nor is it available for occasional rehabilitative care. In addition, the Medicare intermediary must approve the stay.

Here is an example of SNF copayments:

- First day–20th day = Patient has no copayment. Because patients are usually admitted from an acute care facility, where they paid a deductible, Medicare generally pays 100% of the allowable copayment for the SNF.
- 21st day–100th day = Patient pays a set copayment per day.

A patient may be admitted multiple times during a calendar year. However, the maximum number of allowable days is 100 per benefit period.

Part B

Part B is the supplementary medical insurance, which covers physician and outpatient hospital services. It is considered a supplemental plan because each participant must pay a stipulated amount each month for the benefits. Private insurance companies, called **carriers** or Part B MACs, process Part B claims. (See Figure 8-5 ●.)

The rules, limits, and maximums under this coverage are subject to change annually.

> ● **ONLINE INFORMATION:** Visit the www.medicare.gov website to find the current premium and coverage for Medicare B.

BENEFITS. The Part B deductible is a per-calendar-year charge. After the deductible has been satisfied, generally 80% of the approved charge will be paid.

Beginning January 1, 2006, the Medicare Part B deductible will be indexed to the increase in the average cost of Part B services for Medicare beneficiaries. In other words, the amount charged for the Part B deductible will depend on the amount spent by Medicare for payments for services.

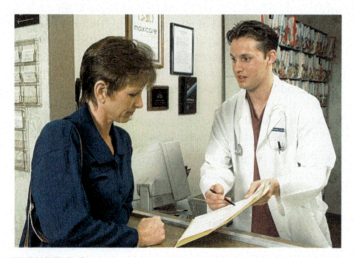

FIGURE 8-5 Part B pays for Physician Office Services
Source: Michal Heron/Pearson Education/PH College

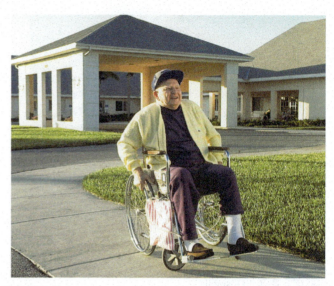

FIGURE 8-6 Long-Term Care Services are not covered by Medicare
Source: Michal Heron/Pearson Education/PH College

Services That Are Not Covered under Medicare Part A or Part B

Medicare does not cover everything. Here is a partial list of the items and services that are not covered:

- Acupuncture
- Deductibles, coinsurance, or copayments for healthcare services
- Dental care and dentures (with only a few exceptions)
- Cosmetic surgery
- Custodial care (help with bathing, dressing, using the bathroom, and eating) at home, in a nursing home, or in another long-term care facility like the one shown in Figure 8-6 ●
- Eye refractions
- Healthcare received during travel outside the United States
- Hearing aids and hearing exams for the purpose of fitting a hearing aid
- Hearing tests (other than for fitting a hearing aid) that have not been ordered by one's doctor
- Long-term care, such as custodial care in a nursing home
- Orthopedic shoes (with only a few exceptions)
- Routine foot care such as cutting of corns or calluses (with only a few exceptions)
- Routine eye care and most eyeglasses
- Nonpreventative screening tests and screening laboratory tests (with some exceptions)
- Shots (vaccinations) (with some exceptions)
- Some diabetic supplies (such as syringes or insulin, unless the insulin is used with an insulin pump or the patient joins a Medicare Prescription Drug Plan).

Part C

Medicare beneficiaries may choose to receive covered items and services from a Medicare Health Maintenance Organization, which is a private insurance company that charges a premium and copays. If a Medicare beneficiary selects this coverage, he or she must receive services according to the selected carrier's arrangements. When patients are enrolled in a Medicare HMO, these patients must submit claims to the HMO. Senior citizens with these plans cannot bill the remaining amounts or copays to Medicare.

Part D

In an effort to provide better health coverage for Medicare beneficiaries, the Medicare Prescription Drug, Improvement, and Modernization Act of 2003 authorized limited coverage of prescription drug benefits for Medicare beneficiaries. This coverage started in 2006. The beneficiary must enroll in a plan and must pay premiums or copayments for certain medications for some plans. The beneficiary would be wise to consult a pharmacy regarding which plan would best cover his or her particular medications. These plans are provided through private insurance companies.

> ● **ONLINE INFORMATION:** Pretend you have coverage through Medicare and want to know which Medicare D program to choose. Find the Internet tools to check medications you take and determine which Part D program is best for you.

ACTIVITY #1

Parts of Medicare

Directions: Answer the following questions after reviewing the material just covered. Write your answers in the space provided.

1. What is the difference between Medicare Part A and Part B? _____

   _____

   _____

2. List five services that are not covered under Medicare Part A or Part B.

   a. _____

   b. _____

   c. _____

   d. _____

   e. _____

3. Medicare Part A claims are processed by private companies called _____

4. How does one find the Medicare A deductible for inpatient hospitalization? _____

5. How does one enroll in Part B benefits? _____

Approved or Reasonable Charges

Medicare payments are based on **reasonable charges**, which are the amounts approved by the Medicare carrier according to what is considered reasonable for the geographic area in which the doctor practices. Because of the way that the approved amounts are determined and because of high rates of inflation in medical care prices, the approved amounts are often significantly less than the actual charges billed by providers. The charge approved by the carrier is the lower of either the charge

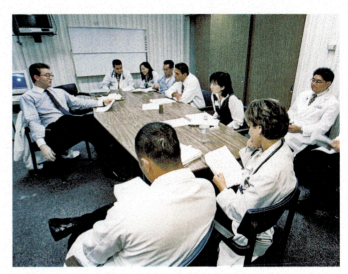

FIGURE 8-7 Doctors discussing financial decisions
Source: Jonathan Nourok/PhotoEdit

billed by the provider or the prevailing charge (which is based on all the customary charges in the locality for each type of service), as determined by Medicare.

The participating provider must write off the amounts that are more than the Medicare-approved amount. (See Figure 8-7 ●.) Unfortunately, the Medicare members, who often are on a fixed income, are held responsible for a large portion of the bill if they see a nonparticipating provider.

> ▶ **CRITICAL THINKING QUESTION:** Where would you advise a patient who requires medical services and has Medicare insurance to seek medical care?

Medicare Assignment of Benefits

A participating provider must agree to accept assignment on all Medicare claims. If this is done, the payment goes directly to the provider for all claims, rather than to the member. In addition, the provider has agreed to accept the amount approved by the Medicare carrier as payment in full for the covered services. The patient is not responsible for any amount over the Medicare-approved amount. In such a case, the secondary carrier is also not responsible for the amount in excess of the Medicare-approved amount.

Physicians Who Accept Medicare Assignment

When a physician agrees to accept Medicare assignment for a bill, Medicare pays the physician directly for that bill. The physician may bill the patient only for any deductibles or coinsurance that Medicare has deducted from the assigned bill. As a result, the total fee that a physician may receive from Medicare and from beneficiaries for an assigned bill is limited by what Medicare deems an appropriate fee for the particular service or procedure (the **Medicare allowance**).

To encourage physicians to accept assignment, Medicare has set a higher allowance for physicians who agree to accept assignment for all bills for Medicare-eligible persons. These physicians are called **participating physicians**. Participating physicians agree not to practice **balance billing**, which is charging patients the excess not covered by the Medicare allowance.

The phrase "participating physician" can be confusing because physicians who sign these agreements are not the only ones who treat Medicare patients. Physicians who treat Medicare-eligible patients but who decide whether to accept assignment on a case-by-case basis are called **nonparticipating physicians**. In exchange for the freedom to make this choice for each patient, nonparticipating physicians receive only 95% of the allowed amount that Medicare participating physicians receive. When they are setting their physician fees, they cannot charge more than 115% of the Medicare-allowed amount for nonparticipating providers.

Mandatory Assignment

Providers may or may not accept Medicare assignment. However, there are some services for which they are required to accept assignment:

- Clinical diagnostic laboratory services
- Medicare patients who also are eligible for Medicaid
- Ambulatory surgery centers
- Method II home dialysis supplies and equipment

EXAMPLE 1:

Participating provider; accepts assignment.

Billed Charge	Medicare Approved Amount	Medicare Pays	Member Pays
$42	$35	(Part B deductible $124)	$35 (ded)
$90	$75	$75 to ded = $0 paid	$75 (ded)
$480	$400	$400 − $14 to ded = $386 × 80% = $308.80 paid	$14 (ded) + $77.20 (20%) = $91.20

EXAMPLE 2:

Nonparticipating provider; does not accept assignment.

Billed Charge	Medicare Approved Amount	Medicare Pays	Member Pays
$42	$33.25 ($35 × 95%)	$33.25 to ded = $0 paid	$33.25 (ded) + 4.99 (LC 15%) = $38.24
$90	$71.25 ($75 × 95%)	$71.25 to ded = $0 paid	$71.25 (ded) + 10.69 (LC 15%) = $81.94
$480	$380.00 ($400 × 95%)	$380.00 − $19.50 = $360.50 × 80% = $288.40	$19.50 (ded) + $72.10 (20%) + $57.00 (LC 15%) = $148.60

Some nonparticipating providers routinely write off any amounts that are not covered by Medicare. This practice is prohibited by law. It means that Medicare covers 100% of the bill, so there is no monetary incentive to the patient not to overuse services.

Coordination of Benefits with Medicare

There are a variety of ways in which group health plans coordinate their payments with Medicare when Medicare is primary and the group plan is secondary. The most common methods in use include the following:

- Nonduplication of Medicare
- Maintenance of benefits

- Physician's assistant, nurse midwife, nurse specialist, nonphysician anesthetist, clinical psychologist, and clinical social worker services

In addition, a all physicians, nonphysician practitioners, and suppliers must take assignment on all claims for drugs and biologicals furnished to any patient enrolled in Medicare Part B.

Limiting Charges

A **limiting charge (LC)** is the maximum amount that the federal government allows nonparticipating physicians to charge Medicare patients for a given service. The LC applies to services that are billed on a nonassigned basis. The LC for these services is 115% of the nonparticipating fee schedule amount.

Balance billing by nonparticipating physicians is strictly limited to this amount. Participating physicians are not affected because they are not allowed to balance bill Medicare patients for any services. The LC applies only to physicians' services. Ambulance companies and other nonphysician providers are not subject to LC regulations.

Following are two examples of how this rule affects the payment of claims.

- Coordination of benefits
- Medicare supplemental coverage.

Nonduplication of Medicare Benefits

Calculation of benefits under the nonduplication approach is the same as with COB except that allowable expenses are those that are listed as covered expenses under the group plan. To compute benefits under this approach, use the following guidelines:

1. Compute regular group benefits. Apply all eligibility requirements, deductibles, limitations, and maximums. This is the plan's normal liability (NL).
2. If the claim is Medicare assigned, the Medicare-approved amount is used as the base. This will give you the balance amount.

PRACTICE **PITFALLS**

The following are additional examples of LC s for balance billing by nonparticipating providers.

EXAMPLE 1:
Participating provider; accepts assignment.

Billed Charge	Medicare-Approved Amount	Medicare Pays	Member Pays
$182	$135	$135 – $124 to ded = $11 × 80% = $8.80 paid (Part B deductible $124)	$124 (ded) + 2.20 (20%) = $126.20

EXAMPLE 2:
Nonparticipating provider; does not accept assignment.

Billed Charge	Medicare Approved Amount	Member Pays	Medicare Pays
$182	$ 128.25 ($135 × 95%)	$128.25 – $124 to ded = $4.25 × 80% = $3.40 paid (Part B deductible $124)	$124 (ded) + .85 (20%) + 19.24 (LC 15%) = $144.09

PRACTICE **PITFALLS**

Following are two examples of calculation of benefits using the nonduplication of Medicare benefits approach.

EXAMPLE 1:
Plan benefits: $150 deductible; no charges have been applied toward the deductible amount 80% payable for all expenses, participating provider; Medicare-assigned.

Billed Charges	Plan-Allowed Charges	Plan Normal Liability (NL)	Medicare-Allowed Amount	Medicare Payment	Payment
$175.00 Office Visit	$125.00	$0.00 ($125 applied to ded)	$125.00	$.80 ($125 – $124 ded = $1 × 80%)	$260.00 Lesser of Plan or Medicare-allowed Amount – $108.80 Medicare/Primary Payer Payment $151.20 Balance Due **$124.80 Payment Made by Plan**
$165.00 Lab	$150.00	$100.00 ($150 – $25 ded = $125 × 80%)	$135.00	$108 ($135 × 80%)	The plan pays the lesser of the NL ($124.80) or the Balance Due ($151.20).
$31.00 Meds	$31.00	24.80 ($31 × 80%)	$0.00	$0.00 (Not Covered)	The patient's out-of-pocket amount is $26.40 ($151.20 – $124.80).
Totals $371.00	**$306.00**	**$124.80**	**$260.00**	**$108.80**	

EXAMPLE 2:
Same plan benefits as in Example 1, nonparticipating provider; not Medicare assigned.

Billed Charges	Plan-Allowed Charges	Plan Normal Liability (NL)	Medicare-Allowed Amount	Medicare Payment	Payment
$175.00 Office Visit	$125.00	$0.00 ($125 applied to ded)	$118.75	$0.00 ($118.75 applied to ded)	$284.05 Lesser of Plan Allowed or Medicare Balance Billable Amount ($247 × 115% = $284.05) –$98.40 Medicare/Primary Payer Payment $185.65 Balance Due **$124.80 Payment Made by Plan**
$165.00 Lab	$150.00	$100.00 ($150 – $25 ded = $125 × 80%)	$128.25	$98.40 ($128.25 – $5.25 ded = $123.00 × 80%)	The plan pays the lesser of the NL ($124.80) or the Balance Due ($185.65).
$31.00 Meds	$31.00	24.80 ($31 × 80%)	$0.00	$0.00 (Not Covered)	The patient's out-of-pocket amount is $60.85 ($185.65 – $124.80).
Totals $371.00	**$306.00**	**$124.80**	**$247.00**	**$98.40**	

a. Subtract the amount paid by Medicare from the Medicare-approved amount.

b. Compare the balance with the plan's normal liability (the amount determined in the first step).

    1. If the normal liability amount is equal to or greater than the balance amount, the balance amount is paid by the plan.

    2. If the normal liability amount is less than the balance amount, the normal liability amount is paid.

3. If the claim is not Medicare-assigned, the base is the lesser of the plan's eligible expense.

a. Subtract the amount paid by Medicare from the plan's approval amount (calculated in the first step).

b. Compare the balance with the plan's normal liability (the amount determined in number two)

    1. If the normal liability amount is equal to or greater than the balance amount, the balance is paid by the plan.

    2. If the normal liability (NL) amount is less than the balance, the normal liability amount is paid.

4. The credit reserve is calculated based on the difference between the plan's liability (calculated in number one) and the amount actually paid by the plan.

Maintenance of Benefits

Maintenance of benefits refers to a provision in many group health plans that allows the person who has Medicare to "maintain" the same group benefits as members who do not have Medicare. Benefit credits are not established. To determine the benefits payable under this provision, use the following guidelines:

1. Compute the normal liability (NL), both Basic or Major Medical benefits, that would be payable in the absence of Medicare (perform a line-for-line calculation). Apply all eligibility requirements, deductibles, limitations, and contractual maximums.

2. Determine the amount the provider is allowed to collect. This will be the Medicare-allowed amount if the claim is assigned, or the Medicare balance billable amount (MBBA) if the claim is not assigned.

3. Use the lesser of number one or number two as the base.

4. Compare the amount paid by Medicare to the base.

5. If the amount paid by Medicare is greater than the base, no payment will be issued by the plan. The insured has received at least the same in benefits as he would have received under the plan.

6. If the base is greater than the amount paid by Medicare, pay the difference. The insured will now have received the amount they would have received if there was no Medicare coverage, up to the amount of the Medicare-allowed amount or the balance billing limit.

Under maintenance of benefits, when a group plan and Medicare are both providing benefits on the same expenses, the total benefits provided should equal what the benefit would have been under the group plan alone as if the member did not have Medicare. However, since most plans exclude any amount for which there would be no charge in the absence of the insurance, the Medicare allowed amount (on assigned claims) or Medicare balance billable amount (on nonassigned claims) must be taken into consideration.

Regular group benefits are provided for charges covered by the group plan but not covered at all by Medicare.

Standard Coordination of Benefits

Standard COB with Medicare is calculated as with any other COB claim. Allowable expenses are based on the amount approved by Medicare on an assigned claim; or the amount approved by the plan or Medicare, whichever is greater, on a nonassigned claim. However, payment is only made up to the Medicare-allowable amount on assigned claims, and up to the MBBA amount on nonassigned claims. If the plan's normal liability is greater than the payment made, the difference between the plan's normal liability and the payment is reserved for future claims payments. Also, as with other COB claims, allowable expenses are considered those payable in whole or part by one or both plans. Benefit credit reserve is established and used to cover allowable expenses. (See Figure 8-8 ● for Medicare Secondary Payer rules.)

Medicare Secondary Payer

If the patient...	And this condition exists...	Then the program pays first...	And this program pays second...
Is age 65 or older, and is covered by a group health plan through a current employer or spouse's current employer...	The employer has fewer than 20 employees...	**Medicare**	group health plan
	The employer has 20 or more employees, or at least one employer is a multi-employer group that employs 20 or more individuals...	group health plan	**Medicare**
Has an employer retirement plan and is age 65 or older or is disabled and age 65 or older...	The patient is entitled to Medicare...	**Medicare**	Retiree coverage
Is disabled and covered by a large group health plan from work, or is covered by a family member who is working...	The employer has fewer than 100 employees...	**Medicare**	large group health plan
	The employer has 100 or more employees, or at least one employer is a multi-employer group that employs 100 or more individuals...	large group health plan	**Medicare**
Has end-stage renal disease and group health plan coverage...	Is in the first 30 months of eligibility or entitlement to Medicare...	group health plan	**Medicare**
	After 30 months...	**Medicare**	group health plan
Has end-stage renal disease and COBRA coverage...	Is in the first 30 months of eligibility or entitlement to Medicare...	COBRA	Medicare
	After 30 months...	**Medicare**	COBRA
Is covered under Workers' Compensation because of job-related illness or injury...	The patient is entitled to Medicare...	Workers' Compensation (for health care items or services related to job-related illness or injury)	**Medicare**
Has black lung disease and is covered under the Federal Black Lung Program...	The patient is eligible for the Federal Black Lung Program...	Federal Black Lung Program (for health care services related to black lung disease)	**Medicare**
Has been in an auto accident where no-fault or liability insurance is involved...	The patient is entitled to Medicare...	No-fault or liability insurance (for accident-related health care services)	**Medicare**
Is age 65 or older OR is disabled and covered by Medicare and COBRA...	The patient is entitled to Medicare...	**Medicare**	COBRA
Has Veterans Health Administration (VHA) benefits...	Receives VHA authorized health care services at a non-VHA facility...	VHA	Medicare may pay when the services provided are Medicare-covered services and are not covered by the VHA

FIGURE 8-8 Medicare Secondary Payer Rules

PRACTICE **PITFALLS**

The following are two examples of calculation of benefits using the maintenance of benefits approach.

EXAMPLE 1:

Plan benefits: $150 deductible; no charges have been applied toward the deductible amount; 80% payable for all expenses; Participating provider; Medicare assigned.

Billed Charges	Plan Allowed Charges	Plan Normal Liability (NL)	Medicare Allowed Amount	Medicare Payment	Payment
$175.00 Office Visit	$125.00	$0.00 ($125 applied to ded)	$125.00	$.80 ($125 − $124 ded = $1 × 80%)	$124.80 Base −$108.80 Medicare/Primary Payer Payment **$16.00 Payment Made by Plan**
$165.00 Lab	$150.00	$100.00 ($150 − $25 ded = $125 × 80%)	$135.00	$108 ($135 × 80%)	$260.00 Lesser of the Plan or Medicare Allowed
$31.00 Meds	$31.00	24.80 ($31 × 80%)	$0.00	$0.00 (Not Covered)	The patient's out-of pocket amount is $135.20 ($260.00 − $108.80 − $16.00)
Totals $371.00	$306.00	$124.80	$260.00	$108.80	

EXAMPLE 2:

Same plan benefits as in Example 1, nonparticipating provider; not Medicare assigned.

Billed Charges	Plan Allowed Charges	Plan Normal Liability (NL)	Medicare Allowed Amount	Medicare Payment	Payment
$175.00 Office Visit	$125.00	$0.00 ($125 applied to ded)	$118.75	$0.00 ($118.75 applied to ded)	$124.80 Base −$98.40 Medicare/Primary Payer Payment
$165.00 Lab	$150.00	$100.00 ($150 − $25 ded = $125 × 80%)	$128.25	$98.40 ($128.25 − $5.25 ded = $123.00 × 80%)	**$26.40 Payment Made by Plan** $284.05 Lesser of Plan Allowed or Medicare Balance Billable Amount ($247 × 115%)
$31.00 Meds	$31.00	24.80 ($31 × 80%)	$0.00	$0.00 (Not Covered).	The patient's out-of-pocket amount is $159.25
Totals $371.00	$306.00	$124.80	$247.00	$98.40	($284.05 − $98.40 − $26.40)

PRACTICE **PITFALLS**

The following are examples or calculation of benefits using standard COB.

EXAMPLE 1:
Plan benefits: $150 deductible; no charges have been applied toward the deductible amount; participating provider; Medicare assigned.

Billed Charges	Plan Allowed Charges	Plan Normal Liability (NL)	Medicare-Allowed Amount	Medicare Payment	Payment
$175.00 Office Visit	$125.00	$0.00 ($125 applied to ded)	$125.00	$.80 ($125 – $124 ded = $1 × 80%)	$260.00 Medicare-Allowed Amount –$108.80 Medicare/Primary Payer Payment $151.20 Balance Due **$124.80 Payment Made by Plan**
$165.00 Lab	$150.00	$100.00 ($150 – $25 ded = $125 × 80%)	$135.00	$108 ($135 × 80%)	The plan pays the lesser of the NL ($124.80) or the difference; up to the Medicare-allowed amount.
$31.00 Meds	$31.00	24.80 ($31 × 80%)	$0.00	$0.00 (Not Covered)	The patient's out-of-pocket amount is $26.40 ($151.20 – $124.80).
Totals $371.00	$306.00	$124.80	$260.00	$108.80	

EXAMPLE 2:
Same plan benefits as in #1, nonparticipating provider; not Medicare assigned.

Billed Charges	Plan-Allowed Charges	Plan Normal Liability (NL)	Medicare-Allowed Amount	Medicare Payment	Payment
$175.00 Office Visit	$125.00	$0.00 ($125 applied to ded)	$118.75	$0.00 ($118.75 applied to ded)	$284.05 (Medicare Balance Billable Amount) ($247 × 115%) –$98.40 Medicare/Primary Payer Payment $185.65 Balance Due **$124.80 Payment Made by Plan**
$165.00 Lab	$150.00	$100.00 ($150 – $25 ded = $125 × 80%)	$128.25	$98.40 ($128.25 – $5.25 ded = $123.00 × 80%)	Plan pays the lesser of the NL ($124.80) or the Balance Due ($185.65), up to the balance billing limit.
$31.00 Meds	$31.00	$24.80 ($31 × 80%)	$0.00	$0.00 (Not Covered)	The patient's out-of-pocket amount is $60.85 ($185.65 – $124.80).
Totals $371.00	$306.00	$124.80	$247.00	$98.40	

EXAMPLE 3:
Benefits payable at 85% of PPO schedule. Deductible $150, deductible satisfied; participating provider; Medicare assigned.

Billed Charges	Plan-Allowed Charges	Plan Normal Liability (NL)	Medicare-Allowed Amount	Medicare Payment	Payment
$5,000.00 Inpatient Hospital Charges	$2,200.00 PPO Contract Rate	$1,870.00 (PPO Allowance $2,200 × 85%)	$4,000.00	$2,438.40 ($4,000.00 – $952 (2006 inpatient ded) = $3048.00 × 80%)	**$1,561.60 Payment Made by Plan** The payment includes the inpatient deductible amount ($952.00) + $609.60 (20% copayment).

In Example 3, the PPO provider has a contractual obligation to provide care on this claim for $2,200. This requirement is due to a contract between the provider and the PPO. Amounts over $2,200 are not usually collectible.

Until early 1999, the insurance carrier had no liability in this example because Medicare paid more than the normal liability and because the provider is part of the plan network and contractually has to write off charges over $2,200. This would leave no patient responsibility and no insurance liability.

However, providers claimed that insurance carriers and PPOs were in violation of the Social Security Act Anti-Kickback Clause. This section of the Act basically states that an insurance company or PPO cannot make a provider write off the Medicare patient responsibility amount. Therefore, the patient responsibility amount is payable by the insurance carrier up to the plan's normal liability in the absence of Medicare. In this example, the plan must pay the $1,561.60 patient responsibility amount on this claim, as their normal liability is higher than this amount.

Medicare Supplements

Medicare supplements (also called Medigap) are private insurance separate plans written exclusively for Medicare participants. These plans charge the participants a fee. They may offer the policyholder a supplement plan with optional benefits. Common options are as follows:

- Physician's services—Covers Part B deductible and 20% coinsurance for reasonable charges. Reasonable charges means that amounts reduced by Medicare because of prevailing fees are not covered under the plan, even though the plan's prevailing fee may be higher than the Medicare fee when the bill is assigned. If the bill is not assigned, the plan's UCR or Medicare's UCR is the amount allowable, whichever is greater.
- Hospital services—Covers Part A deductible and may or may not cover the various copays not covered by Medicare.

In response to the changes in Medicare, supplemental plans have become more flexible. Therefore, the benefits can be complex and comprehensive or very basic. Read plan provisions carefully to determine which items are covered and which are not. As the purpose of a Medicare supplement plan is to cover the patient's responsibility, many charges that are covered are paid at 100%.

ACTIVITY #2

Computing Benefits

Directions: Answer the following questions after reviewing the material just covered. Write your answers in the space provided.

1. Explain how you would compute benefits under each method for payment.

   a. _____ Nonduplication of Medicare

   _____

   _____

   b. Maintenance of benefits _____

   _____

   c. Coordination of benefits _____

   _____

   d. Medicare supplemental coverage _____

   _____

2. Why is there such variability in benefits for Medicare supplemental plans, ranging from basic benefits to complex and comprehensive benefits? _____

   _____

Estimating Medicare Coverage

Sometimes a member is entitled to Medicare coverage but has not enrolled. Many policies specify that the group plan will estimate what Medicare would have paid if the person had been enrolled properly. Other policies specify that benefits may be reduced only when the member is actually enrolled in Medicare. In the latter situation, the plan will provide its regular benefits and the Medicare payment will not be estimated.

To estimate a Medicare payment, use the following guidelines:

Hospital: Part A

1. Provide full benefits toward the Medicare deductible and coinsurance amounts.
2. Provide regular group benefits for services or items covered by the group plan but not covered by Medicare.

Professional: Part B

1. Determine the plan's UCR for the billed charges. The UCR amount is considered the estimated Medicare-approved amount.
2. Multiply 80% of the estimated approved amount (#1). This is your estimated Medicare payment.
3. After you have estimated Medicare's payment, you can proceed with calculating the COB (as shown).

Diagnosis-Related Group Billing

In the early 1980s, Medicare instituted **diagnosis-related group (DRG)** payments for inpatient hospital claims. Under the DRG system, Medicare makes a flat-rate payment on the basis of the patient's diagnosis rather than the hospital's itemized billing. If the hospital can treat the patient for less than Medicare's estimate, the hospital keeps the savings. If treatment costs more, the hospital must absorb the loss. Neither Medicare nor the patient is responsible for the excess amount. Examples of DRGs include treatment of a hip fracture, cancer treatment, initiation of dialysis, and other common short-stay procedures.

Exceptions

Provisions have been made for cases that are atypically expensive (based on the diagnosis) because of complications or an abnormally long confinement. Known as **outliers**, these cases will be reimbursed on an itemized or cost-percentage basis rather than by using DRG. The bill from the hospital must indicate that the case is an outlier.

Exclusions

Excluded from DRG payments are long-term custodial care, children's care, and psychiatric and rehabilitative hospital care. Some states have obtained waivers from DRG, so you should consult your state department of insurance to determine whether it is excluded.

Benefit Payment Calculations

As shown in the following examples, the maximum liability under a plan consists of only the following expenses:

- Expenses that are covered by the plan.
- Expenses that the insured is legally obligated to pay.

PRACTICE PITFALLS

EXAMPLE 1:
Itemized hospital bill exceeds Medicare DRG allowance.

Hospital Bill	$8,700
DRG Allowance	$7,000
Medicare Payment	$6,048
	(DRG Allowance − $952)
Member's Responsibility	$ 952
Hospital Write-off	$1,700

Although the Medicare DRG allowance is less than the itemized hospital bill, the insured is legally obligated to pay only the $952 Part A deductible. Therefore, the difference between the itemized hospital bill amount and the DRG allowance is excluded as not covered. The plan's benefits would be based on the DRG allowance of $7,000, and the $1,700 is not covered because it may exceed the DRG allowance.

EXAMPLE 2:
Medicare DRG allowance exceeds itemized billed amount.

Hospital Bill	$ 8,700
DRG Allowance	$10,000
Medicare Payment	$ 9,048
	(DRG Allowance − $952)
Member's Responsibility	$ 952

Although the Medicare payment exceeds the itemized hospital bill, the insured is legally obligated to pay the $952 Part A deductible. Handling of this type of billing also varies. Check the payer guidelines before processing the claim.

Medicaid

The Medicaid program was established under Title XIX of the Social Security Act of 1965. **Medicaid** is a jointly funded federal–state entitlement program, designed to provide healthcare services to certain low-income and medically needy people. It covers children, the aged, blind or disabled people, and people who are eligible to receive federally assisted income maintenance payments. The purpose of this program is to provide financially and medically needy people with access to medical care. The Medicaid program is overseen by the CMS.

Medicaid is the largest program providing medical and health-related services to America's neediest people. Within broad national guidelines which the federal government provides, each state

1. Establishes its own eligibility standards.
2. Determines the type, amount, duration, and scope of services.
3. Sets the rate of payment for services.
4. Administers its own program.

Thus, the Medicaid program varies considerably from state to state.

By law, Medicaid is always secondary to private group healthcare plans. If Medicaid inadvertently pays as the primary plan, it can exercise its right of recovery and seek reimbursement from the private plan. The private plan is required by law to process Medicaid's request for reimbursement and pay back to Medicaid the monies that Medicaid paid the provider.

Medicaid Eligibility

The regulations governing eligibility under the Medicaid program are complex. Individuals may be entitled to coverage due to medical, family, or financial situations. Having private insurance does not preclude an individual from being eligible for Medicaid benefits.

The Medicaid program does not process its own claims. Medicaid contracts with other organizations who act as the fiscal intermediary, similar to Medicare. The intermediary processes the claims according to specifications set forth by the Medicaid program.

The rates under Medicaid are based on the results of reimbursement studies conducted by the CMS. Reimbursement for hospital inpatient services is based on each facility's reasonable cost of services as determined from audit cost reports and annual limitations on reimbursable increases in cost.

If the patient is covered by private insurance in addition to Medicaid, the provider may bill the patient's private insurance. There is a three-year statute of limitations from the date of service for recovering payment. In addition, there is a three-year subrogation right. Medicaid is the last plan to pay.

In order for a claimant's services to be covered under Medicaid, the claimant must be a Medicaid beneficiary and the provider must be an approved Medicaid provider. To be an approved provider, the provider of services must agree to accept Medicaid's determination of approved amounts as binding. This is similar to Medicare's approved amount on assigned claims, in which the provider is not allowed to bill the patient for any amount not approved by Medicaid. In recent years, many providers have dropped out of the Medicaid program because Medicaid's allowances and payments were extremely low. Some were even lower than those provided by Medicare.

> ● **ONLINE INFORMATION:** Go to your state government website and research the Medicaid eligibility requirements for your state.

CHAPTER REVIEW

Summary

- Medicare is administered through the CMS.
- Each year, it establishes rules and guidelines for payment and covered charges.
- Medical billers and claims examiners must stay informed of the changes in the Medicare system. You can do this by subscribing to the Medicare bulletin that is usually published by the fiscal intermediary for Medicare in the local area.
- By using the Medicare bulletins and applying the guidelines we have covered in this chapter, medical billers or claims examiners will establish a consistent approach to processing Medicare claims, which will result in competent and accurate claim decisions.
- Medicaid guidelines vary from state to state.
- Medicaid bulletins are produced to assist you in interpreting the rules for coverage and to determine which charges Medicaid covers.
- These bulletins are available to Medicaid providers and are primarily used by billers; however, they may be helpful to claims examiners too. Contact your Medicaid intermediary for copies of the bulletins.

Review Questions

Directions: Answer the following questions after reviewing the material just covered. Write your answers in the space provided.

1. What is Medicare? _____
_____
_____

2. What are the three Medicare eligibility programs?

   a. _____
   b. _____
   c. _____

3. Medicare _____ is considered the basic plan or hospital insurance.

4. Medicare _____ is the medical insurance that covers doctors' services, outpatient services, and so on.

5. What does it mean when a provider accepts assignment of benefits in relation to Medicare?
_____
_____

6. What is the purpose of the Medicaid program? _____
_____

7. True or False: By law, Medicaid is always primary to private group health insurance plans. _____

8. In what situation are providers allowed to bill or submit a claim to the Medicaid beneficiary?
_____

9. The _____ is a bill that lists the healthcare services paid by the Medicaid program on behalf of a person who has indicated that he or she has other healthcare coverage benefits available.

10. In order for a claimant's services to be covered under Medicaid, the claimant must be a _____ and the provider must be an _____.

If you were unable to answer any of these questions, refer back to that section and then fill in the answers.

Coordination of Benefits Practice

Directions: Using the Medicare Remittance Notice that follows, compute the COB payment amount for the claims that are listed on the notice. Use the COB Worksheet provided in Appendix B.

MEDICARE REMITTANCE NOTICE

DATE: FEBRUARY 27, CCYY
CHECK SEQUENCE NO.: 2AF-01241351-2
PAGE 1 OF 1

BENEFICIARY NAME	SVC FR MO-DY	TO DY-YR	PLACE TYPE	PROCEDURE DESCRIPTION	AMOUNT BILLED	AMOUNT APPROVED	SEE NOTE	DEDUCTIBLE	COINSURANCE	MEDICARE PAYMENT	SECONDARY CARRIER UCR	SECONDARY CARRIER LIABILITY	PAYMENT AMOUNT
HELGA HEARTACHE	02-06	02-06	23	93000	340.00	297.18	56						
	02-06	02-06	23	93545	770.00	699.23	56						
	02-06	02-06	23	85025	40.00	21.21	56						
	02-06	02-06	23	86901	45.00	27.34	56						
	02-06	02-06	23	85610	30.00	19.57	56						
Accepts assignment	CLAIM NOTE			TOTALS	1,225.00	1,064.53	442	124.00	188.11	752.42	846.32	507.79	_____
BARRY BROKEN	01-26	01-26	23	992885	882.00	699.00	56						
Accepts assignment	CLAIM NOTE			TOTALS	882.00	699.00	442	124.00	115.00	460.00	882.00	433.80	_____
HELGA HEARTACHE	02-09	02-09	21	33217	245.00	189.46	56						
	02-09	02-09	21	33225	500.00	167.38	56						
	02-09	02-09	21	33240	295.00	295.00							
Accepts assignment	CLAIM NOTE			TOTALS	1,040.00	651.84	442	0.00	130.37	521.47	895.63	716.51	_____
ALMA ALVAREZ	02-02	02-02	11	99213	330.00	227.56	56						
Does not accept assignment	CLAIM NOTE			TOTALS	330.00	227.56	442	124.00	20.71	82.85	289.44	145.06	_____
ALMA ALVAREZ	02-02	02-02	11	76092	165.00	127.57	56						
Accepts assignment	CLAIM NOTE			TOTALS	165.00	127.57	442	0.00	25.51	102.06	124.07	105.56	_____
BARRY BROKEN	01-26	01-26	21	70260-27	70.00	61.12	56						
	01-26	01-26	21	71020-27	55.00	43.21	56						
	01-26	01-26	21	735502-7	80.00	70.88	56						
	01-26	01-26	21	73590-27	100.00	83.83	56						
	01-26	01-26	21	70450-27	325.00	180.67	56						
	01-26	01-26	21	73718-27	770.00	622.39	56						
Accepts assignment	CLAIM NOTE			TOTALS	1,400.00	1,062.10	442	0.00	212.42	849.68	1,203.30	1,082.97	_____
HELGA HEARTACHE	02-06	02-06	23	99285	1,600.00	1,306.70	56						
	02-06	02-06	23	99285	420.00	383.13	56						
Does not accept assignment	CLAIM NOTE			TOTALS	2,020.00	1,689.83	442	0.00	337.97	1,351.86	1,595.78	1,156.62	_____
BARRY BROKEN	01-26		21	21800	560.00	499.99	56						
	01-26		21	27758	215.00	116.32	56						
	01-26	01-26	21	27784	200.00	159.56	56						
	01-26	01-26	21	62000	150.00	130.99							
Accepts assignment	CLAIM NOTE			TOTALS	1,125.00	906.86	442	0.00	181.37	725.49	975.80	878.22	_____

56 - Medicare limits payment to this amount.
442 - Total for these charges.

HELGA HEARTACHE - Ninja
BARRY BROKEN - ABC
ALMA ALVAREZ - XYZ

(Continued)

Instructions for COB Worksheet

Place the patient's name and the year that services were rendered in the box on the top of the COB calculation sheet.

1. The total allowable amount of this claim is the higher of either the primary plan's allowable amount or the secondary plan's allowable amount.

2. Add up the primary insurance carrier payment for this claim. (If the carrier is Medicare, this is the allowable amount minus the amount paid by Medicare.)

3. Subtract Line 2 from Line 1.

4. Find the secondary insurance carrier's NL for this claim.

5. Find the lesser of Line 3 or Line 4.

This is the actual amount of the secondary insurance payer on this claim.

To Calculate Credit Reserve:

6. Find the NL amount for the secondary insurance carrier for this claim (from Line 4).

7. Find the actual payment for the secondary insurance carrier for this claim (from Line 5).

8. Subtract Line 7 from Line 6. This is the amount of money the secondary carrier has saved by paying secondary on this claim. This amount becomes part of the credit reserve.

9. Enter the credit reserve amount for all previous claims for this patient.

10. Add Line 8 and Line 9. This is the total credit reserve for this patient.

ACTIVITY #4

Word Search

Directions: Find and circle the words listed. Words can appear horizontally, vertically, diagonally, forward, or backward.

```
C  B  L  U  E  C  G  E  A  S  M  R  R  P  T  M  T  M  B  K  G  K  N  C  M
L  E  D  Q  X  N  U  N  P  P  H  F  U  W  D  A  E  U  U  V  Y  F  E  D  E
U  O  W  W  H  F  D  O  I  U  G  G  X  K  W  D  F  V  F  T  V  L  E  Y  D
O  R  J  U  V  P  T  S  I  L  F  S  Y  Q  I  Z  O  E  S  R  U  T  M  E  I
C  O  A  W  S  A  A  A  T  A  L  Z  S  C  P  N  C  T  E  U  P  P  C  C  C
U  V  Z  W  M  D  K  R  Y  A  F  I  A  W  J  W  B  A  I  W  K  B  J  U  A
Q  J  K  Y  T  R  R  Q  O  D  G  R  B  D  B  E  T  B  J  A  B  A  B  F  R
Y  K  O  C  M  K  Z  U  S  V  E  E  H  E  G  D  N  V  I  N  Z  S  V  O  E
H  S  F  K  B  V  B  P  T  A  I  C  R  C  C  J  A  M  X  H  S  F  K  E  S
F  S  M  L  Y  Y  P  W  L  Q  N  E  G  E  M  N  H  F  Q  E  U  E  Q  U  U
L  E  Y  Z  P  K  E  L  S  E  Q  A  W  C  N  G  A  L  F  L  G  K  U  R  P
U  N  M  W  S  H  O  O  R  N  K  V  D  L  G  A  A  L  W  U  T  Z  P  T  P
N  V  V  E  E  W  P  U  R  T  U  Q  D  T  T  W  L  G  A  E  M  D  M  S  L
S  E  G  R  A  H  C  E  L  B  A  N  O  S  A  E  R  D  O  B  B  D  K  P  E
Q  V  Q  N  O  J  A  V  P  I  B  F  E  V  F  B  D  V  I  A  R  J  E  B  M
L  M  C  N  U  E  Z  F  O  R  H  J  G  M  L  L  S  D  T  S  A  S  H  Y  E
N  E  C  M  I  R  F  W  H  S  L  G  D  I  F  N  D  K  A  C  E  Q  K  X  N
Y  P  A  R  T  I  C  I  P  A  T  I  N  G  P  H  Y  S  I  C  I  A  N  S  T
R  R  C  N  U  G  W  A  Y  T  R  F  X  O  N  B  P  J  S  T  Y  W  S  O  S
I  A  P  T  X  C  G  O  S  H  A  N  E  G  M  J  C  G  K  E  K  L  X  E  V
H  C  B  D  L  Q  P  H  S  R  B  F  H  F  Y  L  I  I  E  H  R  C  Y  D  V
J  X  E  K  C  N  W  L  W  N  E  Z  D  C  F  O  G  F  S  T  X  T  V  O  K
Z  O  N  J  V  T  Q  C  R  K  P  V  W  A  G  I  B  Q  H  Y  J  P  E  O  B
X  H  F  I  U  P  L  K  M  D  L  V  B  A  C  C  X  T  I  L  D  N  U  X  K
A  T  S  S  E  I  R  A  I  D  E  M  R  E  T  N  I  Z  M  D  P  L  Z  V  G
```

1. Balance Billing
2. End-Stage Renal Disease
3. Intermediaries
4. Medicare Allowance
5. Medicare Supplements
6. Participating Physicians
7. Reasonable Charges

ACTIVITY #5

Matching

Directions: Match the following terms with the proper definition by writing the letter of the correct definition in the space next to the term.

1. _____ Deficit Reduction Act of 1984
2. _____ Diagnosis-Related Group
3. _____ Maintenance of Benefits
4. _____ Medicare Remittance Notice
5. _____ Medicare Summary Notice
6. _____ Nonparticipating Physicians
7. _____ Tax Equity and Fiscal Responsibility Act of 1982

a. A federal act that redirected the financial responsibility for medical coverage of active employees age 65 years and older and their spouses aged 65 years and older to Medicare.

b. Physicians who treat Medicare-eligible patients but who decide whether to accept assignment on a case-by-case basis.

c. A flat-rate payment is made according to the patient's diagnosis rather than the hospital's itemized billing.

d. The Act that amended TEFRA so that spouses aged 65 years and older of active employees who are under age 65 can elect their primary coverage as either Medicare or the private group plan.

e. A COB provision in many group health plans that allows the person who has Medicare to "maintain" the same group benefits as members who do not have Medicare.

f. A document used to convey payments to providers who accept assignment for Medicare claims.

g. An explanation of benefits sent to the Medicare beneficiary, detailing the processing of claims submitted for payment.

Workers' Compensation

Keywords and concepts you will learn in this chapter:

Adjudicated

Company Activities

Death Benefits

Doctor's First Report of Occupational Injury
or Illness (First Report)

Job-Related Injuries

Lien

Nondisability Claims

Occupational Illnesses

Permanent and Stationary

Permanent Disability

Physician's Final Report

Rehabilitation Benefit

Reexamination Report

Subjective Findings

Temporary Disability

Vocational Rehabilitation

Work Hardening

Workers' Compensation (WC)

After completing this chapter, you will be able to:

- Describe the eligibility requirements and basic benefits of Workers' Compensation (WC).

- List situations or places that would be covered by WC if an accident were to occur.

- List the type of claims for which WC provides coverage.

- Describe the three disability levels for WC claims.

- Describe the benefits provided by WC coverage.

- Describe the Doctor's First Report and how it is used.

- State the information that should be included in a Doctor's First Report and Subsequent Progress Reports.

- List the factors that may delay the close of a WC case.

- List signs to look for that may indicate fraud or abuse in a WC case.

- Properly complete lien documents.

Workers' Compensation (WC) is a separate medical and disability reimbursement program which provides 100% coverage for job-related injuries, illnesses, or conditions arising out of and in the course of employment. The employer, by law, is responsible for paying the benefits due to an injured employee for work-related injuries and illnesses. WC insurance includes benefits for medical care expenses, disability income, and death benefits.

When you receive a claim for treatment of an accident, it is important to obtain a statement of exactly what happened so that you can determine whether the claim is covered by WC or by the patient's regular insurance. **Job-related injuries** include any injuries that happen during the performance of work-related duties, as shown in Figure 9-1 ●, whether they occur in or out of the office.

Occupational illnesses are any disorders, illnesses, or conditions which arise at work or from exposure to factors at work. Occupational illnesses may be caused by inhaling, directly contacting, absorbing, or ingesting a hazardous agent. Some occupational illnesses may take years to develop or may remain latent for a number of years before flaring up. For this reason, some states have WC laws which cover employees for years after they cease active employment in a field. For example, construction employees who dealt repeatedly with asbestos may develop asbestosis years after exposure. (See Figure 9-2 ●.)

Federal WC programs cover federal employees, coal miners (under the black lung program), longshoremen, and harbor workers. State WC laws cover everyone else. States set up their own guidelines, and the federal government mandates a minimum level of benefits.

Each state's WC Appeals Board has the sole authority to oversee the rights and benefits of an injured or ill employee. It is through this Appeals Board that an applicant (employee) will file their WC application.

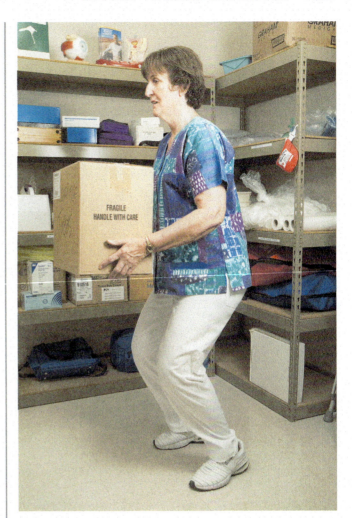

FIGURE 9-1   Lifting injuries are common Workers' Compensation claims
Source: Michal Heron/Pearson Education/PH College

As a general limitation, most health insurance plans specify that the claimant will not be entitled to payment for "bodily injury or disease resulting from and arising out of any employment or occupation for compensation or profit."

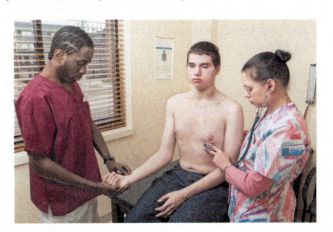

FIGURE 9-2   Worker being tested for lung related injuries
Source: Michal Heron/Pearson Education/PH College

Most health insurance plans will investigate a claim and then provide benefits for medical care if they suspect that a claim is work-related. Because the resolution of a WC case usually takes one to two years, private plans are obligated to pay the benefits for which the member is entitled. Then they file a **lien** with the member and the WC Board to recover plan losses when the case is settled. (Liens are explained in more detail later in this chapter.)

After the WC carrier has accepted liability for the claim, the plan will discontinue providing benefits for medical care. At that point, the plan would deny the claim on the basis that it is work-related.

> • **ONLINE INFORMATION:** Locate your state WC Appeals Board on the Internet. What services are available via the website? It will be helpful for you to know this information when you are processing WC claims.

Employee Activities

The following section contains some general guidelines for what the WC Board in most states recognizes as an injury or illness, according to the type of activity, not the type of injury.

Company Activities

Company activities can be defined as the following:

1. An injury sustained while attending an activity sponsored by an employer for the purpose of obtaining some business gain (e.g., company party for morale purposes; sporting activity to which the employee is transported, at which the company may gain advertisement by having the employee wear a shirt with a company logo).
2. An injury sustained during an activity for which the company provides remuneration.
3. An injury sustained by an employee who was pursuing his or her occupation.

Use of Company Vehicles

Most WC laws provide coverage for an injury sustained while driving or riding as an authorized passenger in a company vehicle. This is true whether the injury is incurred in the course of the person's occupation, or whether the vehicle is provided as a part of the employee's benefits to use to and from work.

The law's interpretation of "in the course of employment" is very different from most laymen's interpretation. For instance, a person who is injured while eating lunch at a company-sponsored event may be covered by WC. Therefore, always do an investigation and let the claims specialist handle the final determination.

Business Trips

Most WC laws provide coverage for a person who is on a business trip. This coverage is applicable as long as the person is engaged in employment duties. For example, an employee might be eating dinner on a business trip when he is cut by the jagged edge of a table. Because dinner is not part of the employee's duties, any injury during that time will not be considered a WC issue. Of course, there are always exceptions to this rule.

Company Parking Lot

Most WC laws provide that if an employee is injured in a parking lot which is owned by or maintained by the person's employer and furnished to the person free of charge, the employee may be covered under WC. In addition, coverage would extend, in some instances, to an injury sustained by the employee while on neutral ground between the parking lot and the place of employment. An exception would be if such incidents were specifically excluded in the WC law, or if the injuries were sustained from willful or negligent actions on the part of the employee.

Usually, WC is not liable for injuries sustained in a parking lot which is owned by the employer and where the employee pays a rental fee for the parking space. In such instances, the employee has a free choice to park elsewhere, which would relieve the employer of any and all responsibility.

> ▶ **CRITICAL THINKING QUESTION:** How would an employer notify employees about parking lot safety to prevent WC injuries?

Occupational Disease

Most of the time, coverage will extend to employees who contract a disease that develops due to working within a certain industry.

LUNG CONDITIONS. For instance, most states provide compensation for individuals who worked with asbestos material over a period of years who later develop asbestosis or silicosis. Other lung diseases, such as mesothelioma and lung cancer, are common WC claims.

SKIN CONDITIONS. Likewise, individuals can develop dermatitis from working with certain chemicals, such as those found in the exterminating, painting, or cleaning industries, or any job that involves working with latex. Rashes, welts, and itching can all be signs of a reaction to a chemical. Even if an employee has been working around the chemicals for a long period of time, new reactions can appear. At the first sign of skin irritation or difficulty breathing when exposed to chemicals, the employee should report the symptoms to the WC representative or physician.

REPETITIVE MOVEMENT CONDITIONS. Another common type of disorder developed on the job is repetitive movement injuries such as carpal tunnel syndrome due to typing or hammering in the same manner on a daily basis. It is difficult to prove that the condition is a result of work, and the employee must show that he or she is using any ergonomically provided equipment and still developed the condition.

Infectious or Communicable Diseases. In the healthcare industry, it is common to contract an infectious or communicable disease at some point in one's career. However, it is debatable whether these are WC issues. For example, if an employee contracts the norovirus from caring for patients who also have the virus, some employers would allow WC to obtain antiviral medication. If the physician provides time off for the employee to recover so that he or she can return to work without being contagious to others, the employee may have the right to collect payment for lost wages. Some situations are clear-cut WC issues, such as a situation in which a nurse contracts hepatitis or HIV from an accidental needle stick. The nurse would be covered and treated under WC insurance.

Sometimes a claimant submits a claim for an occupational illness to the WC Board and also has a concurrent nonoccupational illness for which he or she may be reimbursed under the plan. In such instances, the provider should complete a separate billing indicating the charges that were solely for the treatment of the nonoccupational disability.

Noncovered Activities

Usually, employees need to be on the clock to be considered "working." If an employee punches out, then continues to work and is injured, the injury may not be covered by WC. If an employee visits the workplace during nonworking hours, an injury during this time would not be covered. Certain other conditions will negate WC benefits as well. Examples include being under the influence of drugs or alcohol when the employee sustains the injury or performing a task without proper safety equipment.

Types of Claims

WC provides benefits for

1. **Medical expenses**, including medical services, hospital treatment, surgery, medications, prosthetics or appliances, and durable medical equipment. (See Figure 9-3 ●.)
2. **Temporary disability**, allowing payments to continue to the employee even though he or she is not currently working. Payments are based on the employee's salary and the length of the disability. Payments are usually not taxable as income.
3. **Permanent disability**, in the form of weekly or monthly payments or as a lump sum distribution.
4. **Death benefit**, to compensate spouses and dependents for the loss of an employee. Some states also provide a burial benefit to help cover the cost of funeral services.
5. **Vocational rehabilitation**, to cover rehabilitation services or vocational retraining for permanently disabled employees who are unable to continue in their present position.

There are three types of WC claims. They are nondisability claims, temporary disability claims, and permanent disability claims.

Nondisability Claims

Nondisability claims are for minor injuries that do not prevent the patient from continuing to work. In this case, the patient is able to continue working throughout the extent of the injury. On the first visit to the physician, the physician completes a **Doctor's First Report of Occupational Injury or Illness (First Report)**. The physician submits this form and a copy of the bill to the WC carrier. If you receive a claim with an attached First Report, consult company guidelines to determine whether the claim should be pended for a WC determination or paid with a lien attached.

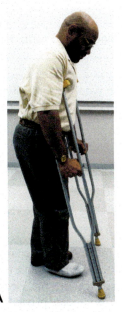 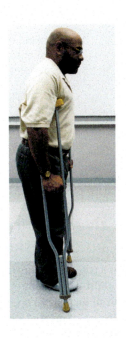 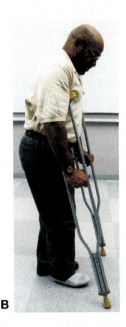 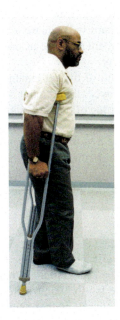

A

B

FIGURE 9-3   Rehabilitation

Source: Pat Watson/Pearson Education/PH College

Temporary Disability Claims

Temporary disability claims are submitted when the patient is not able to perform her job requirements until she recovers from the injury involved. When a physician sees a patient in this situation, the physician submits a First Report. Then he or she issues ongoing reports every two to three weeks until the patient is discharged to return to work.

Each state has a waiting period before temporary disability becomes effective, usually three to seven days (except in the Virgin Islands, where the waiting period is one day). During temporary disability, the employee is paid a portion of his or her salary as a tax-free benefit. Temporary disability ends when the patient is able to return to work, even if he or she has limitations or must return to a different department, or when the patient's condition ceases to improve and the patient is left with a permanent disability. Most healthcare plans do not have a disability benefit (for either temporary or permanent disability) or death benefits. Therefore, the medical biller should check the health insurance before submitting such a claim. The health claims examiner should not receive a disability claim unless the insurance plan has a provision for one. If a claims examiner does receive a disability claim, he or she should deny it as not a covered benefit.

> ● **ONLINE INFORMATION:** Research your state's waiting period by accessing the state WC website.

Permanent Disability Claims

Permanent disability usually commences after a temporary disability when it is determined that the patient will not be able to return to work. The physician prepares a discharge report stating that the patient is **permanent and stationary**. Unfortunately, this report means that the patient is expected to have the disability for the rest of his or her life. The WC Board will review the case and, if the disability is determined to be permanent, the Board will release a *"Compromise and Release."* This is a settlement from the insurance carrier for a payment to the injured party.

The amount of the settlement is based on the age of the disabled employee, the amount of money that he or she was earning at the time of the injury, and the severity of the injury. The older an employee is, the higher the disability rating. This is because a younger patient is believed to have a better chance of finding other employment or of being retrained for another job than an older employee would. In addition, the patient may be eligible to receive death benefits and rehabilitation benefits.

Death Benefit

A **death benefit** compensates the family of a deceased employee for the loss of income that the employee would have provided to the family. Some states also provide a burial benefit to assist the family with the funeral and burial expenses for the employee.

Rehabilitation Benefit

If an employee is found to have a permanent disability, some states allow for a **rehabilitation benefit**. This benefit is used to retrain the employee in a physical ability which will help him or her to seek future employment (e.g., proper use of a wheelchair; use of the left hand if the person has lost his or her right hand.)

Some states participate in a "**work hardening**" program, wherein an employee is assigned therapy similar to his or her work in an attempt to strengthen the employee and build up his or her endurance toward a full day's work. Often employees in such a program return to work on a limited or restricted basis. Physicians, therapists, employers, insurance carriers, and all others concerned with the employee's case must keep in constant communication to ensure that the patient does not return to work either sooner or later than optimal.

Many states also allow for vocational rehabilitation or retraining in a different job field when the employee is unable to return to his or her former position. Vocational training can include courses in colleges and vocational schools or on-the-job training programs. Often employees are paid a weekly allowance (as in the case of temporary disability) while they are attending school and for a limited time after graduation while they are searching for a job. After this time expires, the employee is considered to be off temporary disability and expected to have returned to work. Vocational rehabilitation can also include job guidance, resume preparation, and placement services.

> ## ACTIVITY #1
>
> ### Types of Claims
>
> **Directions:**   Answer the following questions after reviewing the material just covered. Write your answers in the space provided.
>
> 1. What kind of claim would be filed if, after an injury, the patient is no longer able to perform his or her job requirements? _____
> _____
>
> 2. What kind of claim would be filed if the patient is able to continue working throughout the injury? ____
> _____
>
> 3. What is the "work hardening" program? _____
> _____

Privacy in Processing Workers' Compensation Claims

If a patient is being treated for a work-related injury, all records relating to the injury and treatment should be kept separate from the patient's regular medical records. Because employers are covering the costs of treatment, privacy guidelines are somewhat different from the normal privacy agreement

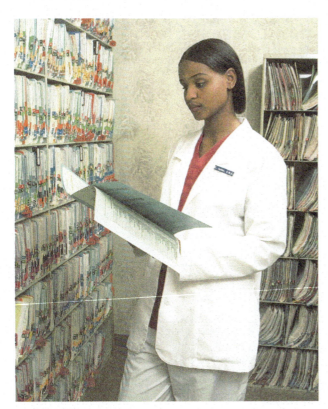

FIGURE 9-4   Medical Assistant making sure to file WC information appropriately
Source: Michal Heron/Pearson Education/PH College

between the insured party and the provider. In WC cases, the agreement is actually between the medical provider and the employer, not the provider and the patient (employee). The employer may request to see records regarding the injury, and these records may be subpoenaed. No information pertaining to the employee's nonwork-related treatment should be made a part of this file, so that confidentiality between the provider and the patient is not breached for nonwork-related treatments and conditions. (See Figure 9-4 ●.)

A medical biller will need the following information to submit a claim; the claims examiner will need a copy of the following reports to process a claim properly:

• Doctor's First Report
• Subsequent Progress Reports
• Physician's Final Report.

Adjudication means that the claim or benefit case has been closed. Delay of adjudication can occur due to unresolved factors affecting the case.

Doctor's First Report

Regardless of the type of claim or benefits, the doctor must file a First Report of Injury, shown in Figure 9-5 ●. This form may have a different name, depending on the state; however, nearly all states require the completion of a similar form. This form requests basic information regarding the date, time, and location of the injury or illness and the treatment, the patient's subjective complaints and objective findings,

the diagnosis, and the treatment needed. **Subjective findings** are those that cannot be discerned by anyone other than the patient (e.g., pain, discomfort). The physician is likely to give an opinion on the extent of pain, a description of activities that produce pain, notes on any other findings, and a treatment plan.

Physicians must report injury, disability, or death within a specified time period. This period varies from immediately on knowledge of the incident to within 30 days. Different states set different time limits and different requirements for reporting. There may also be different levels of injury (e.g., injury, disability, death).

This report is considered a legal document and it should be signed in ink by the physician. All information should be typed or printed clearly. The original copy of the form should be sent to the insurance carrier. One copy is retained in the patient's records, and many providers also send a copy to the employer.

If the physician chooses to send a narrative report along with the standard report, he or she includes the following information:

• A history of the accident, injury or illness
• The diagnosis
• Any connection between the primary injury and any subsequent injuries, especially if the interrelating factors between the primary and secondary injuries are not immediately discernable
• Subjective and objective findings, including the treatment plan and when the employee might return to work. (See Figure 9-6 ●.)

Progress Reports

Following the First Report, the physician follows up with progress reports (sometimes called supplemental reports) every two weeks or each time the patient is seen by the doctor. (See Figure 9-7 ●.) Although many states have forms for progress reports, they may allow a narrative report to be filed instead of the specified form. Progress reports are always sent at the end of a hospitalization, even if the patient is expected to be readmitted later. They often serve as both a report on the patient's condition and as a bill.

If the patient's condition changes significantly, a **Reexamination Report**, or a detailed progress report, should be filed with the insurance carrier.

Physician's Final Report

The medical biller may be asked to compile the physician's final report for the claims examiner. By obtaining a copy of this report, the claims examiner can monitor a patient's progress. Then, if claims are received at a later time, it is easier to determine whether subsequent treatment is related to the original WC injury. If the injury is determined to be related to the WC injury, the claim should be denied and the patient should submit the claim to the WC insurance carrier.

The WC carrier may wait until the physician indicates that the patient's condition is permanent and stationary before

STATE OF CONFUSION

DOCTOR'S FIRST REPORT OF OCCUPATIONAL INJURY OR ILLNESS

Within five days of your initial examination, for every occupational injury or illness, send two copies of this report to the employer's workers' compensation insurance carrier or the insured employer. Failure to file a timely doctor's report may result in assessment of a civil penalty. In the case of diagnosed or suspected pesticide poisoning, send a copy of the report to Division of Labor Statistics and Research, P.O. Box 555555, Anytown, USA 12345-6789, and notify your local health officer by telephone within 24 hours.

	PLEASE DO NOT USE THIS COLUMN
1. INSURER NAME AND ADDRESS	
2. EMPLOYER NAME	Case No.
3. Address: No. and Street City Zip	Industry
4. Nature of business (e.g., food manufacturing, building construction, retailer of women's clothes.)	County
5. PATIENT NAME (first name, middle initial, last name) 6. Sex ☐Male ☐ Female 7. Date of Mo. Day Yr. Birth:	Age
8. Address: No. and Street City Zip 9. Telephone number ( )	Hazard
10. Occupation (Specific job title) 11. Social Security Number	Disease
12. Injured at: No. and Street City County	Hospitalization
13. Date and hour of injury Mo. Day Yr. Hour ___ a.m. ___ p.m. or onset of illness 14. Date last worked Mo. Day Yr.	Occupation
15. Date and hour of first Mo. Day Yr. Hour ___ a.m. ___ p.m. examination or treatment 16. Have you (or your office) previously treated patient? ☐Yes ☐No	Return Date/Code

Patient please complete this portion, if able to do so. Otherwise, doctor please complete immediately, inability or failure of a patient to complete this portion shall not affect his/her rights to workers' compensation under the California Labor Code.

17. **DESCRIBE HOW THE ACCIDENT OR EXPOSURE HAPPENED.** (Give specific object, machinery or chemical. Use reverse side if more space is required.)

18. **SUBJECTIVE COMPLAINTS** (Describe fully. Use reverse side if more space is required.)

19. **OBJECTIVE FINDINGS** (Use reverse side if more space is required.)
A. Physical examination

B. X-ray and laboratory results (State if none or pending.)

20. **DIAGNOSIS** (if occupational illness specify etiologic agent and duration of exposure.) Chemical or toxic compounds involved? ☐Yes ☐ No
ICD-9cm Code ___ ___ ___ - ___ ___

21. Are your findings and diagnosis consistent with patient's account of injury or onset of illness?   ☐Yes ☐No   If "no", please explain.

22. Is there any other current condition that will impede or delay patient's recovery?   ☐Yes ☐No   If "yes", please explain.

23. **TREATMENT RENDERED** (Use reverse side if more space is required.)

24. If further treatment required, specify treatment plan/estimated duration.

25. If hospitalized as inpatient, give hospital name and location   Date   Mo.   Day   Yr.   Estimated stay
admitted

26. WORK STATUS -- Is patient able to perform usual work?   ☐Yes   ☐No
If "no", date when patient can return to: Regular work ___/___/___
Modified work ___/___/___   Specify restrictions _____

Doctor's Signature _____   License Number _____
Doctor Name and Degree (please type) _____   IRS Number _____
Address _____   Telephone Number _____

FORM 5021 (Rev. 4)

Any person who makes or causes to be made any knowingly false or fraudulent material statement or material representation for the purpose of obtaining or denying workers' compensation benefits or payments is guilty of a felony.

FIGURE 9-5   Example of a Doctor's First Report

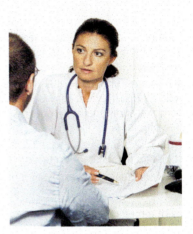

FIGURE 9-6   Worker being interviewed for Doctor's First Report
Source: Lisa S./Shutterstock

finalizing a claim. The physician then notifies the WC carrier that no further treatment is needed (or that no further treatment will significantly alter the patient's condition) and that the patient has been discharged. This is called the **Physician's Final Report**. Some states require the final report to be submitted on a specified form, and some states use the same form for both subsequent and final reports. The Physician's Final Report indicates that the patient has been discharged; gives the level of the patient's permanent disability, if any; and states the balance due on the patient's account (usually provided as a patient's statement showing services, dates of service, charges, and any payments rendered). After this information has been received, the WC carrier will establish the level of permanent disability (if any), medical and other expenses will be paid, and the case will be closed.

Delay of Adjudication

When a patient is released to work, all benefits have been paid, and the case is closed, the claim is said to have been **adjudicated**. Often adjudication occurs within two to eight weeks after the physician submits the report stating that the patient has been discharged and is able to return to work. Meanwhile, the medical

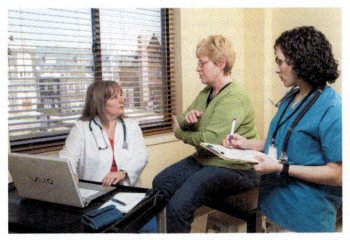

FIGURE 9-7   Worker talking to Doctor and Nurse
Source: Michal Heron/Pearson Education/PH College

biller may bill the health insurance, and after the case is determined to be WC, the WC money will go to the insurance company.

If the patient suffers a permanent disability, adjudication can take much longer, especially if the level of permanent disability is contested and a lawsuit ensues. The following additional factors may delay the close of a case:

1. Confusion or questions on any of the reports submitted by the employer, employee, or physician. This can include conflicting information from one or more parties, vague or ambiguous terminology (especially by the physician), or illegible items.
2. Omitted information on a report, including incomplete forms, boxes that are not filled in, or missing signatures.
3. Incorrect billing or questions on the billing provided by the physician.
4. Insufficient progress reports to update the insurance carrier on the status of the patient.

ACTIVITY #2

Claims Processing

Directions: Answer the following questions after reviewing the material just covered. Write your answers in the space provided.

1. Why is a member's records about a work-related injury and treatment be kept separate from the patient's regular medical records? _____
_____

2. When is a patient's claim considered adjudicated? ___
_____

3. Answer the following three-part question about the WC process.
   a. Which report is considered a legal document? ___
   _____
   b. Should it be typed/printed or handwritten? _____
   _____
   c. How should it be signed? _____

Fraud and Abuse

Unfortunately, fraud and abuse occur frequently in the WC system. Many employees, employers, providers, and insurance carriers find it easy to defraud the system and reap significant financial awards. WC insurance agencies have even had to hire detectives to watch the behavior of employees who are suspected of participating in an illegal claim.

In the past, there have been few deterrents to abusing the system. It was frequently possible to find a doctor who was willing to testify that injuries were more serious than was first thought. Likewise, numerous lawyers stepped in and set up relationships with doctors to produce claims where no actual injury or illness existed. This is especially true when work-related stress became a popular diagnosis for any one of a number of ailments.

PRACTICE PITFALLS

Although most claims are legitimate, the medical biller and the health claims examiner should recognize what constitutes fraud. The following lists detail some signs of fraud or abuse. Be suspicious if an injured employee

- cannot clearly describe the pain or injury, or changes the description each time he or she relates details of the incident.
- is overly dramatic regarding the injury. (See Figure 9-8 ●.)
- complains of an injury which cannot be substantiated by medical evidence (e.g., soft tissue injuries which cannot be seen on an X-ray; continued insistence that there is a serious injury, even when there is medical evidence to the contrary).
- delays the reporting of an injury, especially an injury that is reported on a Monday when the employee claims it happened on Friday.

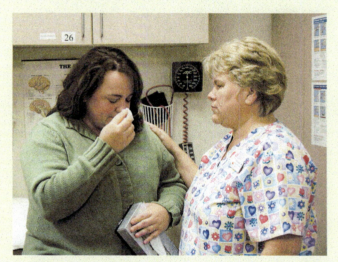

FIGURE 9-8   Patient overly emotional to get doctor to extend WC disability
Source: Dylan Malone/Pearson Education/PH College

- reports the injury to an attorney or regulatory agency prior to reporting the injury to his or her employer.
- changes physicians frequently, or shows up for a first treatment but seems unhappy with the diagnosis and changes physicians (the patient may be seeking a physician who will grant additional time off or will testify to a greater degree of injury).
- is a short-term employee, or was scheduled to terminate employment just after the injury occurred.
- has a history of unusual or an excessive number of WC claims.

Be suspicious of a medical provider who

- orders or performs unnecessary procedures or tests.
- inflates the severity of the injury to qualify for higher reimbursement (e.g., lists a fracture as open rather than closed, bills for a high-complexity exam rather than a moderate-complexity exam).
- charges for services that were never performed, or adds additional procedures onto existing claims.
- makes multiple referrals to a lab, clinic, or hospital and receives a referral fee from these organizations.
- states that an injury exists and needs treatment when no injury is actually present.
- sends in duplicate billings with information changed (e.g., dates) to make it appear that services were performed more than once.
- files many claims with subjective injuries (e.g., pain, strain, emotional disturbance, inability to perform certain functions).
- files claims for several employees of the same company that show similar injuries (i.e., injuries for which reports or X-rays may be duplicated).

Be suspicious of an attorney who

- pressures an insurer to process and pay a claim immediately.

These instances suggest that medical billers and claims examiners should be alert to possible fraud or abuse. If you suspect fraud, report it to the appropriate authority immediately. If anyone becomes aware of fraud by any means, note it in the claim file and refer the information to a supervisor. A medical biller or claims examiner can be guilty of fraud if they knew about the fraud and did nothing to prevent it. This is true even if the person receives no money from the fraud.

Liens

Because it can take months or even years for a WC claim to be paid by the WC insurance carrier, many health insurance carriers will pay these claims, then place a lien to recoup the money when the claim is settled. A lien is a legal document that expresses claim on the property of another for payment of a debt. (See Figure 9-9 ●.) A lien is completed and submitted to the attorney representing the injured party to be paid at the time of monetary settlement of the WC claim.

A lien should be sent along with copies of the EOBs. Whenever additional payments are made, submit a copy of the EOB to the attorney so that all payments will be included in the lien. All services must be for the care of the injury covered under the WC claim.

Many states have a special lien form for WC purposes. These forms can be obtained through the local Division of Industrial Accidents. (See Figure 9-10 ● for a sample copy of a state lien form.) The insurance claims examiner completes the lien form and sends copies to the WC appeals board, the patient's attorney, the patient, and the WC insurance carrier. A copy should also be kept for the claims files.

TO: Attorney _____

_____

_____, Confusion

RE: Medical Reports and Insurance Carrier Lien

FOR_____

    I do hereby authorize the above insurance carrier to furnish you, my attorney, with a full report of any records and resultant payments of myself in regard to the accident in which I was involved.

    I hereby authorize and direct you, my attorney, to pay directly to said insurance carrier such sums as may be due and owed for payment of medical services rendered me or the provider of services both by reason of this accident and by reason of any other bills that are due, and to withhold such sums from any settlement, judgment or verdict as may be necessary to adequately protect said insurance carrier. And I hereby further give a lien on my case to said insurance carrier against any and all proceeds of any settlement, judgment or verdict which may be paid to you, my attorney, or myself as the result of the injuries for which I have been treated or injuries in connection therewith.

    I fully understand that I am directly and fully responsible for reimbursement of any payments for all medical bills submitted for services rendered and that this agreement is made solely for said insurance carrier's additional protection and in consideration of its awaiting payment. And I further understand that such payment is not contingent on any settlement, judgment or verdict by which I may eventually recover said fee.

Dated: _____   Patient's Signature: _____

    The undersigned being attorney of record for the above patient does hereby agree to observe all the terms of the above and agrees to withhold such sums from any settlement, judgment or verdict as may be necessary to adequately protect said insurance carrier named above.

Dated: _____   Attorney's Signature: _____
Mr./Ms. Attorney: Please sign, date, and return one copy to our office at once.

Keep one copy for your records.

FIGURE 9-9   Example of a Lien filed by an insurance company

WORKERS' COMPENSATION APPEALS BOARD

STATE OF CONFUSION

CASE NO. _____

NOTICE AND REQUEST FOR ALLOWANCE OF LIEN

_____

LIEN CLAIMANT   ADDRESS

VS.

_____

INJURED WORKER   ADDRESS

_____

EMPLOYER   ADDRESS

_____

INSURANCE CARRIER   ADDRESS

The undersigned hereby requests the Workers' Compensation Appeals Board to determine and allow as a lien the sum of
_____ dollars ($_____) against
any amount now due or which may hereafter become payable as compensation to _____
                                                                                    INJURED WORKER
on account of injury sustained by him/ her on _____.
                                                          DATE

This request and claim for lien is for: (Mark appropriate box)
- ❑   The reasonable expense incurred by or on behalf of said injured worker for medical treatment to cure or relieve from the effects of said injury; or
- ❑   The reasonable medical expense incurred to prove a contested claim; or
- ❑   The reasonable value of living expenses of said injured worker or of his dependents, subsequent to the injury, or
- ❑   The reasonable living expenses of the wife or minor children, or both, of said injured worker, subsequent to the date of injury, where such injured worker has deserted or is neglecting his family; or
- ❑   The reasonable fee for interpreter's services performed on _____.
                                                                      DATE

NOTE: ITEMIZED STATEMENTS MUST BE ATTACHED
The undersigned declares that he delivered or mailed a copy of this lien claim to each of the above-named parties on

_____
ATTORNEY FOR LIEN CLAIMANT   DATE

_____
ADDRESS OF ATTORNEY FOR LIEN CLAIMANT   LIEN CLAIMANT

INJURED WORKER'S CONSENT TO ALLOWANCE OF LIEN

I consent to the requested allowance of a lien against my compensation.

_____
ATTORNEY FOR INJURED WORKER   INJURED WORKER

DEPARTMENT OF INDUSTRIAL RELATIONS
DIVISION OF INDUSTRIAL ACCIDENTS

FIGURE 9-10   Example of a State Required Lien form

If a lien is not filed, all monies recovered at the close of the case technically belong to the member. It is then the member's responsibility to cover the medical expenses. If any liens are filed, the member must first pay the liens, and then pay any other resultant expenses. Therefore, if the lawyer files a lien and his fees exhaust most of the money, there will be little or no money left for other expenses. If at all possible, members should be persuaded to pay for medical services prior to settlement of the claim.

If a lien is filed, the examiner should have the copy of the lien letter signed by the patient and his or her attorney. This makes the attorney responsible for payment of the physician's bills. If the attorney does not remit the necessary funds from the member's settlement, the attorney must cover the payments for medical services.

A lien should have a specified time limit on it, often a period of one year. If settlement has not been reached by that time, or if there are ongoing charges on the member's account relating to the WC injury, an amended lien should be filed. The subsequent lien should state the balance of the patient's account and should have the word AMENDED stamped across the top or below the Appeals Board Case Number.

The examiner should place all files with liens in a special section and hold them until the cases have been settled. It is illegal to continually bill or harass the member when a lien agreement has been signed. (See Figure 9-11 ●.) In effect, the lien acknowledges the insurance carrier's agreement to wait for reimbursement until the case has been settled. The examiner should contact the member's attorney at least once every three months for an update on the case and to determine when settlement is expected to occur. You should also contact the attorney within two weeks after the date settlement is expected to find out the results of the case and to ask when reimbursement will be provided to pay the claim.

In some states, the law provides that the insurance carrier will be paid before the attorney or member collect any monies from the settlement. Check the statutes in your state. If your state has such a provision, attorneys may not collect their fee and then state that insufficient funds were recovered

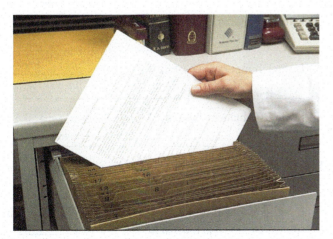

FIGURE 9-11   File to keep unprocessed lien claims
Source: Michal Heron/Pearson Education/PH College

to cover the outstanding medical expenses. Some states also allow the insurance carrier to bill the member for any funds which were not received from the settlement. Once again, check the laws of your state to determine whether members can be billed or whether any amounts not collected should be written off.

Liens are an inexpensive way of ensuring that the insurance carrier will be reimbursed for payments made. The cost is much less than suing the member and assures that payment will be received when the dispute between the member and the WC insurance carrier is settled. A lien is a legal document that will be recognized by the court and will provide protection in the event of litigation.

> ▶ **CRITICAL THINKING QUESTION:** If you are not sure that the patient is going to receive WC benefits for an injury, who should you bill for the physician fees?

Reversals

Occasionally, an accident which was thought to be WC will turn out to be the responsibility of the injured. This can happen when a patient hides or omits facts regarding when and how the accident occurred. It can also be discovered that there is a nonindustrial, underlying condition which caused the accident.

Preexisting Medical Conditions

If an employee has a medical condition that causes an event and as a result of that event the employee is injured, the WC coverage could be compromised. For example, a patient may have epilepsy and suffer a seizure at work. Any injuries that the employee directly received on the job site could be considered WC; however, the treatment of the underlying epileptic condition would not be WC. Another example would be if an employee has multiple sclerosis and falls down the stairs due to difficulty with depth perception; this accident could be attributed to the multiple sclerosis rather than being a workplace injury.

Employee Negligence

In some cases, the employee may be found to be negligent in their actions, or willfully disregarding established workplace rules. In such cases, injuries sustained as the result of the employee's negligence may not be considered industrial accidents. For example, if an employee is told that she must refrain from wearing hoop earrings, but she chose to wear them anyway, she may be considered liable for her medical costs if the earrings are caught on machinery and ripped from her ear, resulting in an injury.

Other examples include use of equipment without using the safety equipment that was also provided. The Occupational Safety Hazard Association provides guidelines for various industries on what personal protective equipment must be provided for employees' use in hazardous areas or using hazardous equipment. For example, a prep cook would be expected to use the protective shield on a meat slicer to avoid cutting his or her fingers or hands in the slicer. If the cook disregarded this safety precaution and removed the shield, he or she might not be covered by WC for any injuries sustained. Similarly, a welder who chose not to use the heat-protective gloves and mask might not be covered by WC.

> ● ONLINE INFORMATION: To check out various industrial safety guidelines, visit www.osha.gov.

Inattention to Workers' Compensation Treatment

If an employee is injured and then does not follow through on the treatment indicated, he or she is risking noncoverage by WC. For example, an employee slips in a water spill and sprains his wrist catching himself. The employee goes to the WC clinic for treatment. The physician completes her initial report and prescribes a wrist brace and physical therapy to aid the wrist in healing properly. If the employee does not wear the wrist brace or does not follow through with physical therapy until the physician releases him, he is at risk of noncoverage of further injuries to his wrist.

In all of these scenarios, the WC Board could deny payment on the claim. All claims for treatment should then be submitted to the employee's regular insurance carrier. In these cases, the claims and subsequent payments would become part of the patient's regular file.

CHAPTER REVIEW

Summary

- WC insurance is a separate medical insurance program that covers work-related injuries, disabilities, and death. A wide range of activities may be covered under WC laws.
- WC provides nondisability claims, temporary disability claims, permanent disability claims, death benefits, and rehabilitation benefits to injured employees.
- Vocational rehabilitation or training in a different job field is part of WC in many states.
- The Doctor's First Report of Occupational Injury or Illness is a major factor in the employer's or insurance company's decision to accept or contest the WC claim. The basic information requested on the form are the date, time, and location of the injury or illness and treatment rendered.
- The Physician's Final Report is usually the last report and states that the patient has been discharged.
- The physician must notify the WC carrier that no further treatment is needed.
- The claim is said to be adjudicated when all the benefits have been paid and the patient is released to work.
- Some factors that may delay the close of a case are confusion or questions on any of the reports, omitted information on a report, incorrect billing or questions on the billing, and insufficient progress reports.

Review Questions

Directions: Answer the following questions without looking back at the material just covered. Write your answers in the space provided.

1. What is Workers' Compensation? _____

_____

2. What items are likely to cause a delay in adjudication of a case? _____

_____

_____

_____

3. What do you do if a patient says he has a WC injury but he has nothing from the employer to prove it? _____

_____

_____

4. What is a lien? _____

_____

5. Why should you file a lien? _____

_____

6. What signatures should you get on a lien? _____

_____

7. Define Temporary Disability. _____

_____

8. Define Permanent Disability. _____

_____

9. What is a nondisability claim? _____

_____

10. If an employee is injured while he or she is at a company-sponsored game, is it considered a WC case? _____

_____

If you were unable to answer any of these questions, refer back to that section and then fill in the answers.

ACTIVITY #3

Word Search

Directions: Find and circle the words listed here. Words can appear horizontally, vertically, diagonally, forward, or backward.

```
Z  S  E  S  C  N  U  E  V  H  T  U  Q  Z  F  A  L  G  N  T  M  W  V
T  C  H  Z  M  O  L  B  X  C  M  X  N  D  D  W  Y  U  J  X  E  Q  M
S  I  N  B  P  I  M  G  F  V  Z  F  G  F  N  U  E  T  J  E  T  A  P
N  W  R  D  R  T  A  P  D  S  R  G  F  F  X  Q  G  A  C  N  I  V  W
S  L  Q  E  X  A  T  L  A  F  N  C  T  W  Q  T  D  T  A  U  P  Y  E
K  V  E  R  G  S  F  Q  C  N  Y  Y  D  Z  Q  U  D  U  A  P  Y  Y  C
B  V  R  D  H  N  N  B  R  Y  Y  Z  Q  K  O  T  M  R  Q  D  O  D  M
T  I  F  E  N  E  B  N  O  I  T  A  T  I  L  I  B  A  H  E  R  Y  K
V  V  E  F  E  P  R  D  C  P  M  I  C  U  C  V  N  P  D  T  T  B  N
L  O  G  I  I  M  F  V  K  U  Z  A  L  T  H  Y  G  H  R  P  C  M  W
O  T  L  U  B  O  W  H  T  S  K  Q  E  I  I  H  K  O  V  F  I  B  V
X  K  R  S  P  C  M  G  T  K  U  J  K  N  B  V  I  M  K  U  C  R  O
K  B  M  I  A  S  Y  B  D  W  K  R  N  M  Q  A  I  D  X  F  X  W  N
Q  A  V  Z  N  R  U  P  Z  B  B  R  J  C  I  O  S  T  P  B  Z  M  V
W  J  D  O  O  E  S  A  K  Y  Y  K  B  O  T  I  N  I  I  W  B  A  S
R  R  H  E  Z  K  A  P  C  S  O  Y  P  D  Y  I  F  D  D  E  R  D  S
Z  F  J  A  L  R  V  B  Q  Q  D  J  A  W  V  N  H  B  I  N  S  C  N
U  E  S  S  P  O  F  T  K  F  J  N  O  M  M  O  L  E  N  D  O  X  J
U  G  X  O  V  W  N  T  A  R  Y  F  A  X  S  Q  X  A  F  S  Z  N  G
J  O  B  R  E  L  A  T  E  D  I  N  J  U  R  I  E  S  P  T  N  Q  J
S  C  U  U  I  U  J  K  P  X  N  T  M  W  Z  J  W  K  T  C  R  W  W
R  O  V  M  H  H  D  I  U  Y  W  C  W  B  X  I  O  Z  J  P  C  Q  R
S  V  Q  Q  I  M  D  V  W  U  Q  F  L  F  L  C  G  U  T  D  G  Q  W
```

1. Company Activities
2. Job-Related Injuries
3. Nondisability Claims
4. Rehabilitation Benefit
5. Workers' Compensation

ACTIVITY #4

Matching

Directions: Match the following terms with the proper definition by writing the letter of the correct definition in the space next to the term.

1. _____ Doctor's First Report of Occupational Injury or Illness
2. _____ Occupational Illnesses
3. _____ Permanent and Stationary
4. _____ Temporary Disability
5. _____ Vocational Rehabilitation

a. Retraining in a different job field when the employee is unable to return to his or her former position.

b. Claims for the time during which the patient is not able to perform his or her job requirements until he or she recovers from the injury involved.

c. Any disorders, illnesses, or conditions that arise at work or from exposure to factors at work.

d. A term meaning that nothing more can be done and the patient will have the disability for the rest of his or her life.

e. The report completed by a physician at a WC patient's first visit.

CHAPTER 10

Managed Care Claims

Keywords and concepts you will learn in this chapter:

Capitation

Eligibility Roster

Group Model

Independent Physician Associations (IPAs)

Individual Practice Organizations (IPOs)

Medical Groups

Network Model

Preventive Coverage

Primary Care Provider (PCP)

Staff Model

Stop-loss

Treatment Authorization Request (TAR)

Withhold

After completing this chapter, you will be able to:

- Describe the main types of managed care organizations and how they work.
- List the common managed care benefits.
- Describe the various types of health maintenance organizations and how they work.
- Explain the differences and similarities between HMOs and PPOs.
- Describe Preferred provider organizations and how they work.
- Describe how risk for expenses is shared between Groups or independent physician associations and managed care plans.
- Explain how providers are reimbursed in a capitation agreement.
- Explain how fee-for-services procedures are usually billed.
- Discuss the information on a Treatment Authorization Request Form.
- Describe how a specialist referral is obtained.
- Identify the steps required to obtain a second opinion.
- Describe limitations that may exist with prescription coverage.

- Outline the steps to processing an MCP claim.

- Demonstrate the ability to perform calculations when processing a claim.

- Properly complete a denial notice.

- Define stop-loss.

The health insurance industry has been transformed in recent years with the rise of managed care networks and HMOs. Managed care is a system for organizing the delivery of health services so that the cost of care is reduced and the quality of care is maintained or improved. Managed care plans (MCPs) were created in an attempt to bring healthcare costs under control by having providers share some of the financial risks of healthcare with patients and insurance carriers. Managed care techniques are most often practiced by organizations and professionals who assume part or all of the risk associated with providing the medical care for a defined population of patients. Managed care is best described as a multifaceted system for providing healthcare while maintaining reasonable costs.

There are many different types of managed care organizations, including HMOs, PPOs, gatekeeper PPOs, exclusive provider organizations, physician hospital organizations, and management service organizations. Several of these types of care were previously discussed in the Introduction chapter under "Types of Insurance." In this chapter, we will focus on processing claims in an HMO setting.

Health Maintenance Organizations

Under an HMO arrangement, members pay a set amount every month, and the HMO agrees to provide all their care or to pay for the covered care that they cannot provide. The HMO hires physicians and sets up hospitals (or contracts with existing physicians and hospitals). The member chooses a specific provider for his or her care called a **primary care provider or primary care physician (PCP)**. Members sign up for HMO coverage through their employer or through an individual policy.

Many HMOs require a copayment amount from the member for each visit, usually a nominal amount of $10 to $50. This is the entire amount the patient must pay. As a result of the Affordable Care Act, members receive preventive benefits that previously were not covered by most indemnity plans. These benefits include annual physicals, mammograms, and Pap smears (shown in Figure 10-1 ●). Another benefit of belonging to an HMO is the lack of paperwork for the patient; the provider completes any paperwork for reimbursement.

Members of an HMO are locked into visiting their PCPs, rather than going to any in-network physician, although they may switch PCPs at any time throughout the plan year and may receive referrals from the PCP to specialists. If the member wishes to see a provider other than their PCP, he or she must usually seek preapproval from the HMO or must cover the costs out of pocket.

The most common types of HMO organizations are

- **Staff model.** This is the original concept of HMO services. A physician or provider is hired to work at the HMO's own facility. The physician is usually paid a salary and may receive additional bonuses. He or she works only for the HMO and sees no outside patients.
- **Group model.** The HMO contracts with providers or provider Groups to provide services. These practitioners agree to see only HMO members, but they do so at their own facilities.

Staff Model HMOs

In a staff HMO, the HMO owns the facility and hires the staff. When a patient comes for an appointment, the HMO collects the copayment amount. The HMO keeps this money and adds it to premiums to cover its costs of doing business.

The practitioners on staff, whether they are physicians, nurses, or specialists (e.g., X-ray technicians, cardiac specialists) are paid a standard salary based on the work they do and

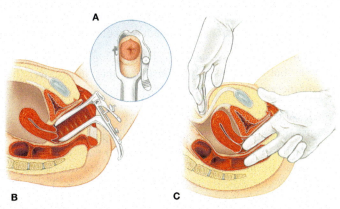

FIGURE 10-1 Preventative services such as yearly pap smears are covered under HMO plans.

the hours they spend at work. The amount remains the same regardless of the number of patients they see or the number of procedures they perform.

The HMO covers all costs, including the costs of the facilities, equipment, supplies, and personnel (including doctors, nurses, specialists, accountants, and any other personnel who are needed to keep the company running).

Patients often make appointments through the HMO, rather than through the provider. This arrangement allows the HMO to monitor the number of patients the provider sees and keep track of the services performed. If the patient needs additional services (e.g., a referral to a specialist, lab tests, X-rays), the staff provider will write an order for the services, letting the HMO know that these services are needed.

Because providers are not reimbursed per procedure, they have no incentive to perform or order services that the patient does not need.

If an HMO feels that a provider is referring too many patients for additional services, the HMO will limit the number of referrals that the provider may make or may insist on additional documentation to justify the services.

In this model, there are no claims to process because the HMO handles all costs and services.

Group Model HMOs

In a Group HMO, a medical facility or Group bands together to provide services for HMO patients at their own facilities. It is similar to the staff model HMO in that the providers receive salaries based on their qualifications and working hours. However, rather than receiving payment directly from the HMO, they receive their salaries from the Group. The Group itself receives a capitation amount from the HMO to cover a wide range of services.

EXAMPLE:

The HMO has 10,000 members who each pay an average premium of $150 per month. The HMO contracts with a Group to provide all provider visits, outpatient X-ray and DXL charges, and outpatient or minor surgery charges for 1,000 of these patients. (Other Groups will handle the remaining patients.) In exchange for these services, the HMO will pay a capitated payment of $50 per member for these 1,000 members. Thus, the Group receives $50,000 per month to cover these services. The Group then hires or contracts with providers to work for them for a salary. The providers are paid a set amount each month from this pool of money.

If there are any services which the Group is contracted to provide, but cannot supply themselves, they must cover the cost of these services.

EXAMPLE:

The Group contract requires the Group to provide chiropractic services for those patients who need it. However, there are not enough of these patients for the Group to keep a chiropractor on staff on a regular basis. Thus, the Group makes an arrangement with a chiropractor to provide these services at a reduced fee (say, $50 per visit). When patients need chiropractic services, they are referred

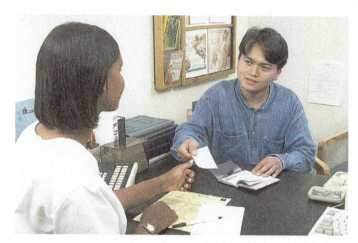

FIGURE 10-2   Collecting payments at each visit
Source: Michal Heron/Pearson Education/PH College

to this contracted chiropractor. The chiropractor collects the copayment amount from the patient (say, $20), and the Group pays the remaining $30 for the visit to the chiropractor.

If the patient needs services which are not covered by the provider Group (i.e., hospital services), the Group refers the patient back to the HMO. The HMO will then provide these services at one of its facilities. These facilities may either be wholly owned by the HMO and thus paid as a staff model, or they may be another Group that has contracted with the HMO to provide all inpatient hospital treatment. If the hospital is a staff arrangement, the HMO covers all costs. If it is a Group arrangement, they receive a capitated amount (e.g., $75 per person per month). Any amount remaining from the premiums after all Groups have been paid their capitated amounts is used to cover the costs of services that they are contractually obligated to cover, but for which there is no provider under contract (e.g., prescriptions).

In a Group model, patients may see different doctors in the Group each time they visit the Group offices. The Group collects the copayment amount for each visit, as shown in Figure 10-2 ●, and uses it to cover the costs of staff, facilities and supplies.

Rather than building their own facilities, some HMOs contract with hospitals to take over a specified number of beds or a wing of an existing hospital. This arrangement developed due to the increased costs of building a new hospital facility and the decreased utilization of hospitals. HMOs encourage doctors to shorten the length of time that patients stay at hospitals. Thus, some hospitals have only 40% to 50% of their beds filled at any given time. Sharing a facility with an HMO can be a good way to provide the HMO with the resources and treatment options that it needs while at the same time increasing the revenues of the hospital. HMO personnel usually care for patients at these facilities.

Individual Practice Organizations

Individual Practice Organizations (IPOs) (sometimes called Independent Practice Associations) are legal entities composed of a network of private physicians who have organized to negotiate contracts with insurance companies and HMOs.

There are two arms to this type of organization. The HMO arm acts as an insurer, oversees the program, enrolls members, collects premiums, and handles the claims. The medical Group arm organizes physicians and contracts with the HMO for discounted rates on services. The medical Group as a whole is paid a capitation amount for each member, and the Group oversees the care of the members and attempts to control costs.

The individual physicians (who are members of the medical Groups) agree to see HMO patients in their own offices along with their regular fee-for-service clients. These providers are able to easily gather a large number of patients by joining the IPO. At the same time, they retain their autonomy and freedom, unlike traditional HMO doctors who are hired by the HMO and placed on salary.

This type of arrangement allows the HMO to add numerous doctors, giving patients a wider freedom of choice. As doctors are paid a capitation amount according to the number of members they see, there is no additional cost to the HMO for adding more doctors.

In a **network model**, the HMO contracts with several providers in a locale, allowing some overlap of geographic area. This arrangement gives subscribers a wider choice and allows an HMO to increase its subscriber base without worrying about unduly overloading a single provider. In the network model, providers see not only the HMO members, but their regular fee-for-service patients as well.

There are two payment types within HMOs: those that utilize capitation, and those that pay according to services provided. Capitation pays a provider a set amount per month for the treatment of a patient. The provider is paid each month, regardless of whether the patient visits the provider. The savings of being paid for patients who do not visit is usually offset by patients who require more treatment than the average member.

Most HMOs require the Group or IPO to have a certain number of physicians in varying specialties. For example, the list must often include a general practitioner or internist, a pediatrician (see Figure 10-3 ●), an obstetrician/gynecologist, a cardiologist, etc. This arrangement allows the Group to treat all aspects of the patient's care and to provide appropriate services to all members who choose that Group/IPO as their PCP.

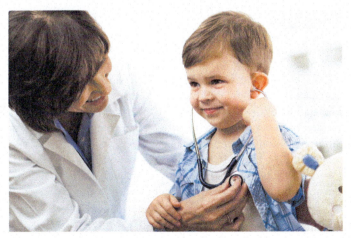

FIGURE 10-3   A pediatrician with a child
Source: StockLite/Shutterstock

> ▶ **CRITICAL THINKING QUESTION:** What are some advantages and disadvantages of each HMO model? Why might an individual patient select one model over another?

HMO Coverage

Often HMOs offer a higher level of coverage than traditional indemnity plans.

Physician Visits

HMOs cover physician visits, necessary testing, and also treatment by a specialist (when the patient is referred by his or her PCP). The patient usually has to pay a copayment for each physician visit at the time of service. In addition, the patient usually pays a copayment to the specialist at the time of service. The specialist copays are generally higher than those for PCP visits.

Specialty Care

HMOs tend to cover prenatal care, emergency care, home healthcare, skilled nursing care, drug and alcohol abuse treatment, physical therapy, allergy treatment, and inhalation therapy, often to a higher degree than coverage provided by indemnity plans. Each type of service will likely have an associated copay. Mental health treatments often require a higher copayment than physician visits and are often limited to short-term care. There also are usually limits on the number of visits. Beginning in 2014, as a result of the Affordable Care Act, mental health and substance treatment became part of the essential benefits package, a set of healthcare services that must be covered by certain plans.

Physical therapy is sometimes covered only for a brief period of time and only if significant improvement is expected for the patient. The American Physical Therapy Association is attempting to establish physical therapy as an essential service under the Affordable Care Act.

Controversial or experimental procedures (e.g., laser surgery, gastric stapling) often are not covered. Cosmetic procedures are almost never covered.

Hospitalization

Most HMO plans cover hospitalization in full. However, many plans require a per-day inpatient copayment, and if a patient is seen in the ER, he or she often must pay a copayment for the ER visit as well.

Preventive Services

Even before healthcare reform, HMOs covered preventive services. **Preventive coverage** provides for services such as an annual physical, cancer screening (e.g., Pap smears, mammograms), flu shots, immunizations, and well-baby care. With funding from the Affordable Care Act, HMO plans also cover health education, cessation of smoking classes, nutrition counseling (especially for diabetics and those who need weight control), or exercise classes.

Vision Services

Eye exams for both children and adults are covered by most HMOs; however, additional vision services (e.g., glasses,

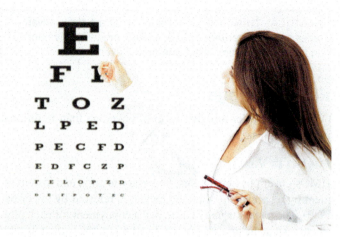

FIGURE 10-4   Eye exams are typically covered by HMOs
Source: Andresr/Shutterstock

contacts) may not be covered. In some cases, additional coverage for these items is available. (See Figure 10-4 ●.)

Prescription Drugs

Plans that cover prescription drugs often require a copayment from the member for each prescription. Prescriptions are often limited to a 30-day supply, but some HMOs do not limit the number of prescriptions that may be filled in a month. Some HMOs may offer a discounted rate for a three-month supply of medication.

Required Provisions

HMOs that are federally qualified must provide the following essential health benefits:

1. Preventive and wellness services and chronic disease management.
2. Hospitalization.
3. Rehabilitative services and devices.
4. Mental health and substance use disorder services.
5. Emergency and ambulatory patient services.
6. Maternity and newborn care.

> ● **ONLINE INFORMATION:** Search online for the Affordable Care Act of 2010 for an overview of the healthcare law. Find the timeline for the elements of the Laws enactments. Take note of the changes that will come about as a result of the Act. Consider which changes will have the most effect on you, your family, and your job responsibilities.

Preferred Provider Organization

A **Preferred Provider Organization (PPO)** is a popular alternative to HMOs. The PPO plan is very similar to HMO plans; however, the PPO allows a patient to see any physician or specialist within the network without a referral. This saves the patient time because he or she does not need to go through the PCP to get referrals to see specialists. PPOs may have copayments or coinsurance that is the responsibility of the patient. The PPO plan is usually more expensive than an HMO plan.

Groups/Independent Physician Associations

Medical groups are groups of physicians who are signed under or work for the same company. **Independent Physician Associations (IPAs)** are groups of providers who have banded together for the sole purpose of signing a contract with an MCP.

Most MCPs require the Group or IPA to have a certain number of physicians in varying specialties. For example, they often must have a general practitioner or internist, a pediatrician, an obstetrician, a gynecologist, a cardiologist, or any combination of specialties. This rule allows the Group to treat all aspects of the patient's care and to provide appropriate services to all members who choose that Group/IPA as their PCP.

MCP to Group/IPA Risk

MCPs often use existing providers to deliver care to their patients by signing the providers to contracts. They introduce a mechanism for financial risk-sharing by providing cost incentives to providers in order to contain their expenditures (i.e., the provider is paid a set amount, regardless of the services that he or she provides to the patient).

In many MCP situations, the risk for patient services is shared between the Group/IPA and the MCP. The contract between the Group/IPA and the MCP outlines who is responsible for what services and what conditions or limitations apply to those services.

Risk determinations may be

- *No risk*—The MCP collects and keeps the monthly capitation amount and merely pays providers on a fee-for-service basis for the treatment rendered to members. This is similar to a regular insurance carrier setup, except that the member pays only the copay amount, not deductibles or copayment percentage. This arrangement is almost never seen.
- *Partial risk*—The MCP is responsible for most services; however, the capitation covers basic services.
- *Shared risk*—The MCP and the Group/IPA share the responsibility for services. A contract designates which services or treatments are covered by the MCP and which are covered by the provider.
- *Full risk*—The Group/IPA is responsible for most, if not all of the services. The MCP is just in the business of selling policies and writing contracts with Groups/IPAs.

Most MCP contracts with providers are on a shared-risk basis. The MCP provides a list to the Group/IPA of all possible services (often indicated by CPT® codes and descriptions), and an indication of who is responsible for those services. (See Figure 10-5 ●.) A letter code often designates who is responsible for payment for that service (e.g., G = Group/IPA responsibility, H = MCP/HMO responsibility).

This document also lists any services that are denied and the appropriate copayment amount for many of these services.

Group/IPA to Physician Risk

In addition to the MCP transferring all or part of the risk to the Group/IPA, the Group/IPA may transfer some or all of their

Covered Services	MEDICARE		COMMERCIAL						
	Standard	Medi-Medi	AMG	Rocky	CAT	MIPC	CAIT	SBA	RICE
Abortion - Elective (CPT 59840 - 59841) Note: Refer to Super Panel contracts for financial responsibility for specific procedures	G/P[1]	G/P[2]	G/P[2]	G/P[1]	G/P[2]	G/P[2,3]	G/P[4]	G/P[4]	G/P[4]
Abortion - Therapeutic (CPT 59812 - 59857) If the life of the mother could be endangered if the fetus is carried to term, or in cases of fetal genetic defect.	-	G	G	G	G	G	G	G	G
Acupuncture	-	-	-	-	-	-	-	-	G
Acute Care • Facility Component	P	P	P	P	P	P	P	P	P
• Hospital Based Physicians, including clinical and anatomical pathologist (CPT 80002 - 83999), radiologist (CPT 70010 - 76499), anesthesiologist (CPT 00100 - 01999, 99100 - 99140)	P	P	P	P	P	P	P	P	P
• Professional Component, including consultations and follow up care visits (CPT 99217 - 99239, 99251 - 99275)	G	G	G	G	G	G	G	G	G
• Closed panel physicians under contract with a hospital for test reading (e.g. EKG)[5]	P	P	P	P	P	P	P	P	P
• Special services and reports, miscellaneous (CPT 99000 - 99090, 99175 - 99199)	G	G	G	G	G	G	G	G	G

[1] Not covered except in cases of rape or incest, or when the life of the mother would be endangered if the fetus were brought to term.
[2] Covered for the first thirteen (13) weeks of pregnancy only.
[3] Copay for HIPC is the same as for in-patient hospitalization.
[4] Covered through the second trimester (24 weeks) of pregnancy only.
[5] Plan to confirm closed panel status.

Legend: G = Medical Group Responsibility; P = Plan/HMO Responsibility; G/P = Shared Responsibility; -- = Not Covered

This chart shows a sampling of CPT codes and the party that bears responsibility for covering costs for each procedure under numerous different plans. It is important to check the correct column for the plan being processed to determine if services are covered or not.

FIGURE 10-5 Distribution of Responsibility

risk to an individual capitated provider as well. The levels of risk transferred to the capitated provider include

- *No risk*—The Group/IPA keeps the entire capitation payment and providers are paid on a fee-for-service basis. There are usually no withholds or bonuses as part of the provider's contract. (A **withhold** is a portion of the monthly capitation amount that is retained by the MCP; these will be covered later in the chapter.) However, the contract agreement often incorporates a fee schedule, so the amount that the provider receives for services will be determined by the fee schedule.

- *No referral risk transferred*—All or part of the payment to the provider involves risk, but the risk is not tied to referrals. Only the capitation amount, bonuses, and withholds are at risk (e.g., the provider may perform more services than the capitation, withholds, and bonuses cover). Under this arrangement, referral means any service that is not provided by the provider. Essentially, it is expected that the capitation, withholds, and bonuses are the only payments for any and all care that the provider renders to the member. The provider is not responsible for paying for referrals, and the amount of money paid to the provider is not affected by the provider's decision to make referrals to other providers.

- *Referral risk is transferred, but is not substantial*—Part of the payment to the provider depends on the decisions the provider makes to refer patients to other providers. However, that part of the payment is not substantial (i.e., it is under 25%). Therefore, if this type of provider makes too many patient referrals to other providers, up to 25% of his or her capitation amount may be withheld.

- *Substantial risk for referrals is transferred, but stop-loss protection is in place*—If more than 25% of total payments to the provider are at risk for referrals, the medical Group/IPA must have aggregate or per-patient stop-loss protection in place. Stop-loss protection means that if the costs to the provider exceed a specified amount, the provider will be reimbursed by the group/IPA for at least 90% of expenditures over that amount.

In general, the higher the risk that is transferred to the provider, the higher the capitation amount. If less risk is transferred to the provider, the Group/IPA keeps a higher percentage of the capitation amount to cover its expenses.

ACTIVITY #1

HMOs

Directions: Fill in the blank spaces with the correct word, after reviewing the material just covered.

1. Most HMO contracts with providers are on a _____ _____ basis.

2. In addition to the _____ transferring all or part of the risk to the Group/IPA, the Group/IPA may turn around and transfer some or all of their risk to an individual _____.

3. In general, the _____ the risk that is transferred to the provider, the _____ the capitation amount.

Capitation Payments

Capitation is the practice of paying a provider a set amount per month to treat MCP members and provide other administrative duties. When an MCP and a provider sign a contract, they make an agreement regarding a capitated fee. This fee often depends on the type of plan under which the patient is covered. It may be affected by varying factors, such as the gender, age, and overall health of the patient. The provider and MCP will also agree which services are covered by the capitation amount.

Often, capitation amounts pay for all the basic treatment the patient needs during the month. If the patient does not see the physician that month, the physician keeps the fee. If the patient becomes ill and requires treatment, the physician is expected to provide the necessary services without receiving additional compensation from the MCP. Usually, the amount saved and the extra amount spent balance out. With this type of arrangement, the physician has an incentive to minimize lab tests and keep treatment costs to a minimum.

The capitation amount for each provider is determined by the number of patients who are included on either the active or new member roster. The PCP usually receives capitation payments for the previous month. The amount of the capitation payment varies according to the coverages or plans that have been selected. Additional amounts may be provided for patients who have entered a hospice or skilled nursing care facility, as well as those who have been diagnosed with specific diseases (e.g., HIV, ESRD).

The MCP may retain a portion of the monthly capitation amount, called a withhold, to protect the HMO from inadequate patient care or financial management by the PCP. They also may withhold a portion to ensure the quality of care given to patients and promptness of payments to outside providers. This amount is outlined in the contract signed by the group and the MCP.

PRACTICE **PITFALLS**

The 123 MCP withholds 3% of the capitation amount to cover financial insolvency and unpaid claims by the Group/IPA. If all obligations have been met, this amount will be returned when the group terminates its contract with the MCP. In addition, the 123 MCP will withhold 5% of the capitation for its Medical Management Incentive Program. This program stipulates that the 5% will be reimbursed to the Group/IPA if the following guidelines are met:

- 25% of the withheld amount will be reimbursed if the provider/Group/IPA has submitted less than their budgeted amount of hospital expenses that are covered by the HMO.

- 10% of the amount will be reimbursed for above-average customer satisfaction. The MCP will randomly survey patients to determine their satisfaction with the provider and the services rendered. If the provider receives above-average scores in customer satisfaction, he or she will receive this amount.

- 10% of the withheld amount will be reimbursed for low disenrollment. If the provider/Group maintains less than 2% disenrollment (patients terminating MCP coverage or transferring to another provider), then they will receive this amount.
- 40% of the withheld amount will be reimbursed for high quality of care. The level of care will be determined by a review of medical records by the MCP. If the Medical Review Panel agrees with the treatment given at least 80% of the time, the provider will receive this amount.
- 15% of the withheld amount will be reimbursed for protocol compliance. This is calculated as follows:

    - 5% for compliance with all facility requirements, as determined by an audit of the facility.
    - 5% for timeliness of claim payments.
    - 5% for timeliness of submission of all contractually required statements to the MCP.

If the provider meets all the stipulations outlined here, he or she will keep the 5% quality care amount.

Billing for Services

Although the monthly capitation amount covers most services, some services will be reimbursed on a fee-for-service basis. This means that the provider will bill the MCP for these services at the time of service. Most agreements between a provider and an MCP list the services that are covered by the capitation amount or those that are on a fee-for-service basis. Fee-for-service procedures are usually billed on a CMS-1500 form, the same as non-MCP services, or they may be electronically billed if required. (See Figure 10-6 ●.)

Authorizations, Referrals, and Second Opinions

In an effort to contain their costs, MCPs often require preauthorizations for treatment that is their financial responsibility. They may also require a SSO Consultation regarding the proposed treatment.

Preauthorization

Most MCPs require the provider or member to obtain preauthorization for services which are the financial responsibility of the MCP. This request is often made using a **Treatment Authorization Request (TAR)** form. The provider lists the diagnosis and proposed treatment plan, along with any needed followup care.

The provider submits the TAR to the MCP for approval. Then the MCP evaluates the proposed treatment and informs the provider and member whether or not they will cover the services. If the MCP decides that the services are not necessary, they will deny payment. The provider and member must then decide whether they will abandon the treatment, seek authorization for an alternate treatment, or go ahead with the treatment with the understanding that the patient is completely responsible for the charges.

The MCP may decide that an SSO Consultation is needed before they make a determination. In such a case, the member must have the SSO performed prior to the services and with enough time for the MCP to evaluate the second surgeon's response to determine whether they will cover the services.

Often a TAR approval is valid for a limited time, usually 30 days. If services are not performed within that time, the provider will need to complete an additional TAR and obtain another preauthorization. In the case of ongoing treatments (e.g., chemotherapy, dialysis), the provider may need to obtain monthly authorization of services covered by the MCP, as shown in Figure 10-7 ●.

All routine followup care and/or hospital stays should be included in the one authorization.

If the TAR lists a specific date of surgery and the surgery is approved, the surgery should be performed on the date indicated on the TAR. If there is no date listed, TARs are often good for 30 days from the date of approval. Services must be performed within that time period in order for the TAR approval to be valid. If a TAR was approved but services were not performed within the required time period, and no additional TAR was submitted, the Group/IPA may be responsible for payment of services, not the MCP.

The TAR approval will also indicate the number of days that the patient may remain in the hospital (if it is an inpatient stay). Any days beyond this number are not covered by the MCP unless an additional TAR is submitted and approved, verifying the need for additional services.

Different rules may apply for inpatient admission for psychiatric care or chemical dependency.

EMERGENCY TREATMENT AUTHORIZATION REQUESTS. Many MCPs have an emergency request procedure which allows a physician to fax the TAR and receive overnight approval for treatment.

If a member is unable to wait the 24 hours for treatment, he or she should seek assistance in the ER of the nearest hospital. The hospital will then contact the MCP for an emergency treatment request. Many MCPs require the member to seek emergency treatment at an MCP facility if possible. Only if the emergency is threatening to life or limb should the member go to a non-MCP facility.

SAMPLE

(1500)

HEALTH INSURANCE CLAIM FORM
APPROVED BY NATIONAL UNIFORM CLAIM COMMITTEE 08/05

☐☐☐ PICA   PICA ☐☐☐

1. MEDICARE   MEDICAID   TRICARE   CHAMPVA   GROUP   FECA   OTHER   1a. INSURED'S I.D. NUMBER   (For Program in Item 1)
CHAMPUS   HEALTH PLAN   BLK LUNG
☐(Medicare #) ☐(Medicaid #) ☐(Sponsor's SSN) ☐(Member ID#) ☐(SSN or ID) ☐(SSN) ☐(ID)

2. PATIENT'S NAME (Last Name, First Name, Middle Initial)   3. PATIENT'S BIRTH DATE   SEX   4. INSURED'S NAME (Last Name, First Name, Middle Initial)
MM DD YY   M☐ F☐

5. PATIENT'S ADDRESS (No, Street)   6. PATIENT RELATIONSHIP TO INSURED   7. INSURED'S ADDRESS (No, Street)
Self☐ Spouse☐ Child☐ Other☐

CITY   STATE   8. PATIENT STATUS   CITY   STATE
Single☐ Married☐ Other☐

ZIP CODE   TELEPHONE (Include Area Code)   Full-Time Part-Time   ZIP CODE   TELEPHONE (Include Area Code)
Employed☐ Student☐ Student☐

9. OTHER INSURED'S NAME (Last Name, First Name, Middle Initial)   10. IS PATIENT'S CONDITION RELATED TO: 11. INSURED'S POLICY GROUP OR FECA NUMBER

a. OTHER INSURED'S POLICY OR GROUP NUMBER   a. EMPLOYMENT? (Current or Previous)   a. INSURED'S DATE OF BIRTH   SEX
☐YES ☐NO   MM DD YY   M☐ F☐

b. OTHER INSURED'S DATE OF BIRTH   SEX   b. AUTO ACCIDENT?   PLACE (State)   b. EMPLOYER'S NAME OR SCHOOL NAME
MM DD YY   M☐ F☐   ☐YES ☐NO

c. EMPLOYER'S NAME OR SCHOOL NAME   c. OTHER ACCIDENT?   c. INSURANCE PLAN NAME OR PROGRAM NAME
☐YES ☐NO

d. INSURANCE PLAN NAME OR PROGRAM NAME   10d. RESERVED FOR LOCAL USE   d. IS THERE ANOTHER HEALTH BENEFIT PLAN?
☐YES ☐NO   If yes, return to and complete item 9 a-d

READ BACK OF FORM BEFORE COMPLETING & SIGNING THIS FORM.
12. PATIENT'S OR AUTHORIZED PERSON'S SIGNATURE I authorize the release of any medical or other information necessary to process this claim. I also request payment of government benefits either to myself or to the party who accepts assignment below.

SIGNED _____   DATE _____

13. INSURED'S OR AUTHORIZED PERSON'S SIGNATURE I authorize payment of medical benefits to the undersigned physician or supplier for services described below.

SIGNED _____

14. DATE OF CURRENT   ILLNESS (First symptom) OR INJURY (Accident) OR PREGNANCY (LMP)   15. IF PATIENT HAS HAD SAME OR SIMILAR ILLNESS, GIVE FIRST DATE MM DD YY   16. DATES PATIENT UNABLE TO WORK IN CURRENT OCCUPATION
MM DD YY   FROM MM DD YY   TO MM DD YY

17. NAME OF REFERRING PHYSICIAN OR OTHER SOURCE   17a.   18. HOSPITALIZATION DATES RELATED TO CURRENT SERVICES
17b. NPI   FROM MM DD YY   TO MM DD YY

19. RESERVED FOR LOCAL USE   20. OUTSIDE LAB? $ CHARGES
☐YES ☐NO

21. DIAGNOSIS OR NATURE OF ILLNESS OR INJURY (Relate Items 1,2,3 or 4 to Item 24E by Line)   22. MEDICAID RESUBMISSION
1. |___.___   3. |___.___   CODE ___   ORIGINAL REF. NO.
2. |___.___   4. |___.___   23. PRIOR AUTHORIZATION NUMBER

24. A. DATE(S) OF SERVICE			B. PLACE OF SERVICE	C. EMG	D. PROCEDURES, SERVICES, OR SUPPLIES (Explain Unusual Circumstances)		E. DIAGNOSIS POINTER	F. $ CHARGES	G. DAYS OR UNITS	H. EPSDT Family Plan	I. ID. QUAL.	J. RENDERING PROVIDER ID. #
From MM DD YY	To MM DD YY				CPT/HCPCS	MODIFIER						
1											NPI	
2											NPI	
3											NPI	
4											NPI	
5											NPI	
6											NPI	

25. FEDERAL TAX ID NUMBER   SSN EIN ☐☐   26. PATIENT'S ACCOUNT NO.   27. ACCEPT ASSIGNMENT? (For govt. claims, see back) ☐YES ☐NO   28. TOTAL CHARGE $ 29. AMOUNT PAID $ 30. BALANCE DUE $

31. SIGNATURE OF PHYSICIAN OR SUPPLIER INCLUDING DEGREES OR CREDENTIALS (I certify that the statements on the reverse apply to this bill and are made a part thereof)   32. SERVICE FACILITY LOCATION INFORMATION   33. BILLING PROVIDER INFO & PH. #

SIGNED _____   DATE _____   a.   b.   a.   b.

NUCC Instruction Manual available at: www.nucc.org   PLEASE PRINT OR TYPE   APPROVED OMB 0938-0999 FORM CMS-1500 (08/05)

CARRIER

PATIENT AND INSURED INFORMATION

PHYSICIAN OR SUPPLIER INFORMATION

FIGURE 10-6   CMS-1500

Verbal Control No. *1	Type of Service Requested *2 ☐ ☐ Drug Other	Is Request Retroactive? ☐ ☐ YES NO *3	Is Patient Medicare Eligible? ☐ ☐*4 YES NO	Provider Phone No. *5	Patient's Authorized Representative (IF ANY) Enter name and address: *6

Provider Name and Address *7 | **Provider Number** *8 | **FOR STATE USE** Provider, your request is: *9
☐ Approved as Requested
☐ Approved as Modified (items marked below as authorized may be claimed)
☐ Denied
☐ Deferred
By: _____ Medi-Cal Consultant
Comments/Explanation

Name and Address of Patient Patient Name (Last, First, MI) *10 | **Medicaid Identification Number** *11

Street Address | **Sex** *12 **Age** *13 | **Date of Birth** | *14 |

City, State, Zip Code | **Patient Status** *15 ☐ Home ☐ Board & Care

Phone Number *16 | ☐ SNF/ICF ☐ Acute

Diagnosis Description *17 | **ICD-9 CM *18 Diagnosis Code**

Medical Justification *19

*20

Line No.	Authorized Yes | No	Approved Units	Specific Services Requested	Units of Service	NDC/UPC or Procedure Code	Quantity	Charges
1	☐ ☐	*21	*22	*23	*24	*25	*26
2	☐ ☐						
3	☐ ☐						
4	☐ ☐						
5	☐ ☐						
6	☐ ☐						

To the best of my knowledge, the above information is true, accurate and complete and the requested services are medically indicated and necessary to the health of the patient.

*27

Signature of Physician or Provider   Title   Date

Authorization is valid for services provided *28
From Date   To   Date
| | | |

Office | **Sequence Number** *29

FIGURE 10-7   State Treatment Authorization Request Form

In such cases, the hospital is required to provide life-saving measures. Any measures not required to sustain life must be approved by the MCP before they are rendered. Many hospitals are aware of this situation and will immediately call the MCP before treating an MCP member who has sought treatment at their facility.

The MCP will do an immediate review of the patient's situation and authorize individual services. However, each service will need to be authorized prior to being rendered, unless it is necessary to sustain the life of the patient.

If the patient is stable, the MCP will often have the patient transferred to their own facility for treatment.

PRACTICE PITFALLS

EXAMPLE:
June Jenkins was involved in a diving accident. When she was pulled from the water, she was not breathing and it appeared her neck was broken. At the ER, the doctors were able to perform life-saving measures (i.e., CPR and insertion of a breathing tube). However, before they could do a spinal X-ray or MRI, they needed authorization from the MCP. Only after the MCP authorized these procedures was the hospital assured of payment on the services they provided to determine the extent of June's injury. If the hospital had performed these services prior to receiving authorization, June would have been responsible for full payment of the unauthorized procedures.

If the Group/IPA is financially responsible for ER services, then they are responsible for managing the member's utilization of ER services and for paying the cost of these services. The group must provide written information to its members on how to access these services. The Group/IPA must have procedures for the authorization of these services. They may not deny payment on the basis of lack of notification or lack of authorization for these services.

Under the Affordable Care Act, health plans are prohibited from requiring patients to get prior approval before seeking emergency services from an out-of-network provider or hospital. Health plans also are prevented from requiring higher copayments or coinsurance for out-of-network ER services.

Utilization Review

Many insurance carriers began creating utilization review (UR) departments in an effort to control costs and avoid unnecessary procedures. Although this process was started among traditional insurance carriers, managed care carriers have taken the concept a step further, creating complete UR departments and reviewing every outside procedure that may require additional costs.

Furthermore, UR committees are becoming more selective in the items and providers they choose to review. Procedures that are nearly always allowed, such as cystourethroscopy, are being automatically allowed, whereas more questionable procedures, such as MRI of the knee, are being reviewed. In addition, some insurers are tracking the records of providers. Providers who are known to order tests or procedures that are nearly always necessary are less closely watched than those who have a history of ordering questionable procedures.

● **ONLINE INFORMATION:** Perform online research on UR programs. What is the utilization process? What are some circumstances that might trigger a UR?

Specialist Referrals

If a member wishes to see a specialist, the member must discuss the request with his or her PCP. If the PCP denies the request, he or she must follow the procedures for denial of services, including sending a denial letter to the member.

If the PCP agrees with the member's request or recommends the member to see a specialist, he or she should complete an appropriate referral form and approve it by the Group/IPA. The decision to refer or not to refer a member is a medical judgment that should be made by the PCP and the Group/IPA, especially as the financial responsibility for these visits often falls with the PCP or Group/IPA. Of course, if the member wishes to have a referral to a specialist for a service that is the financial responsibility of the MCP, he or she must obtain preauthorization.

If the referral authorization is approved, the member will receive a written notice listing the name, address, and phone number of the specialist and either an appointment time or information about how to schedule an appointment.

The Group/IPA is required to have contracts with its specialists. They must maintain contracts with a sufficient number of specialists so that members are not inconvenienced by excessive waiting times for appointments.

Second Opinions

If a member requests a specific treatment and the MCP determines that this treatment or service is not medically necessary, would be detrimental to the patient, or would provide no medical benefit to the member, they may deny the service (i.e., refuse to cover the treatment). The denial letter should contain a statement regarding why services are denied.

Many MCPs have a second-opinion policy that is designed to resolve differences of opinion regarding proposed treatment among PCPs, members, specialists, and the managed care program. Second opinions are often provided in the following situations:

- At the request of the member before a surgical or other invasive procedure
- If the PCP's opinion is contrary to the member's expressed expectations, even after the physician has counseled the member
- If the opinion of the PCP differs substantially from the recommended treatment plan of the specialist on the case
- At the request of the MCP.

There are several steps in the second-opinion process:

1. A request is made by the PCP, member, consultant, or MCP for a second opinion. This request may be either verbal or in writing.
2. The patient's chart is documented with the request.
3. An internal review is done. This is a second opinion performed by another physician who is affiliated with the same Group/IPA as the PCP.
4. If the member is still dissatisfied or if the two opinions differ substantially, the member may contact the MCP to request an external review. This is an opinion provided by a physician who is not affiliated with the Group/IPA to which the member belongs. After receiving the request for the external review, the MCP reviews the records. If they deem it necessary to have an external review, they will inform the PCP and the member. The MCP may send the member to a physician of their choosing.

5. All records are forwarded to the MCP's Chief Medical Officer, who determines the proper course of treatment. The PCP will then be informed of the decision, and it is his or her responsibility to carry out the proposed treatment plan. This may mean treating the patient themselves or referring the member to a specialist for treatment.

Financial responsibility for second opinions is usually split among the Group/IPA and the MCP as follows:

1. The Group/IPA is responsible for the internal review.
2. The MCP is responsible for the external review unless the Group/IPA failed to document the internal review, did not properly complete a TAR and obtain authorization before sending the member for an external review, or reached a decision that differs substantially from the opinion of the external review physician.

All activities regarding the second-opinion process must be thoroughly documented in the patient's record. Anytime the MCP must bear financial responsibility for any services, including the external review, a TAR must be completed and the treatment must be preauthorized. (See Figure 10-8 ●.)

Because there may be substantial delays in receiving authorizations and/or referrals, causing member complaints, some MCPs are now allowing members to refer themselves for a second opinion. However, they are limited to obtaining a second opinion from another provider who is affiliated with the same MCP, and the number of times they may refer themselves for a second opinion is limited (e.g., once every six months).

Denials of Service after a Second Opinion

After the member has exhausted the second-opinion process or chooses not to proceed with the process (i.e., accepts the decision of the internal review), the Group/IPA must send a denial letter to the member. A copy of this letter must also be sent to the MCP with any supporting documentation.

This letter must state the patient's name, the date that services were requested, the services that were requested, and the reason for the denial of services.

The MCP often keeps a log of these denials. If they feel that a Group/IPA is denying too many treatments, they may ask for a review of the record to monitor the quality of care given to the patients.

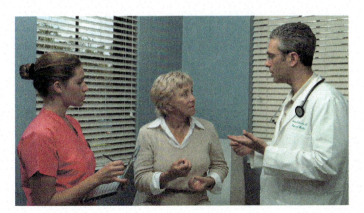

FIGURE 10-8   MCPs have second opinion policies
Source: Michal Heron/Pearson Education/PH College

Miscellaneous Services

Certain rules may apply to select types of service under an MCP agreement. These services can include outpatient surgery, ER services, durable medical equipment, and prescriptions.

Outpatient Surgery

Some MCPs provide a list of surgeries that must be performed in an outpatient setting. This is most often done in a shared-risk contract when the Group/IPA is financially responsible for outpatient services and the MCP is responsible for inpatient services.

It is important to know which surgeries must be performed on an outpatient basis. If physicians do not follow these guidelines, the Group/IPA may be financially responsible for all inpatient costs in relation to the surgery.

The medical biller and examiner should be aware of this list and keep it handy. If a provider submits a claim for inpatient surgery that should have been performed on an outpatient basis, the claim should be denied and returned to the provider.

If the provider feels that the surgery should have been performed inpatient due to complications or other circumstances, he or she should have submitted a TAR and waited for approval prior to surgery.

ACTIVITY #2

Authorizations, Referrals, and Second Opinions

Directions: Answer the following questions after you review the material just covered. Write your answers in the space provided.

1. What form is usually submitted for a member to obtain preauthorization for services which are the financial responsibility of the MCP? _____

2. Who is financially responsible for second opinions? ____
_____

3. What is utilization review? _____
_____

Prescription Coverage

When an MCP offers prescription coverage to a member, there are often limitations:

1. The member must purchase the drugs from an MCP-contracted facility. If the member obtains prescriptions from a noncontracted pharmacy, he or she will bear the cost of the pharmacy services. There may be exceptions to this rule for emergency situations, situations in which the patient is outside the service area, or times when the prescription is not available from a contracted pharmacy.
2. The MCP may limit drugs and medications to a 30-day supply.
3. The MCP will usually only cover prescription drugs, not over-the-counter medications.

4. The MCP may only include oral and topical drugs. Injectable drugs are often not covered under the pharmacy benefit, but they may be covered under the medical benefit. This is especially common for injectable medications which the patient needs for survival (e.g., insulin for a diabetic).

5. The MCP may limit coverage to the generic equivalent of a drug if it is available. If there is no generic equivalent, the MCP will often cover the brand name at the standard copayment amount. However, if there is a generic equivalent, the MCP may only cover the cost of the generic equivalent. Thus, the member will be charged the standard copay, plus the difference between the generic and the brand-name medication.

Some generic drugs are not the same as their brand-name counterparts. They may have a similar yet different active ingredient, or they may be provided in a different dosage amount from the brand-name drug. In such cases, they are not considered to be therapeutically equivalent. When a patient wants a brand-name drug that does not have a therapeutically equivalent generic version, the MCP may require the physician to prescribe the generic drug, or the plan may allow the full benefit for the brand-name drug.

Claim Payments

Now that you understand some of the basic rules regarding eligibility, preauthorizations, referrals, and second opinions, we will discuss the steps for a medical biller to process an MCP claim. After the following brief overview of the process, each item will be discussed in more detail.

1. Check the member's eligibility, determine which contract covers the member, and find the person's PCP (if applicable).
2. Check the member's contract to determine whether the services are covered and what the copayment or other amounts are.
3. Determine who is financially responsible for payment on the claim by using the Distribution of Responsibility chart.
4. Check whether the proper referrals, preauthorizations, or second opinions were done.
5. If the referrals, preauthorizations, or second opinions were done, send in the claim.

Claims examiners follow a similar process to the medical biller, verifying the details of the insurance policy, after which they follow these steps:

1. Determine the allowed amount for the procedure.
2. Determine whether there should be a reduction of benefits due to improper referrals, incomplete authorizations, or other limitations.
3. Subtract the amount of any copayment given by the member.
4. Pay the remaining amount.

Check Member Eligibility

When you are processing MCP claims, as with other types of claims, eligibility is the first item to consider. Check the **eligibility**

roster to determine the effective dates of the patient's coverage, find the contract that covers the patient, and find his or her PCP (the Group/IPA responsible for the person's primary care).

The MCP's providers often have three eligibility rosters to consider:

1. The **active member roster** lists those whose coverage has continued into the next month. This usually means the insured; if they receive benefits through their employer, the employer has paid the monthly premium to continue coverage for another month.
2. The **new member roster** shows those patients who have signed up for MCP coverage and have chosen the provider as their PCP. The new member roster also shows those patients who have recently chosen this provider as their PCP.
3. The **terminated member roster** shows those members whose coverage has been terminated.

The claims examiner will often have a computerized eligibility roster which shows not only the dates that the member was eligible, but also the plan under which they are covered and the name of their PCP. The plan under which the patient is covered will not only determine the covered services, but will also determine who is responsible for payment of each individual service.

Check the Member's Contract

After you have determined the plan, go through the member's contract. Like other contracts, this one will list the items covered, the amount of copayments, and any excluded items. Any amounts that are excluded would be automatically denied.

Determine Financial Responsibility

For items that are covered, you will need to determine who is responsible for payment of the item. When Groups or providers sign up with an MCP, they agree to cover certain services in exchange for a capitation amount. When providers signs up, they will sign up for certain plans. They may be providers on some plans, but not on others.

Refer to the Distribution of Responsibility chart shown in Figure 10-1. This chart (often many pages long) shows who is responsible for the payment on each plan. The responsible party will be either the provider (regardless of whether it is a Group or individual provider), or the MCP. On some items, the responsibility may be shared. In these cases you will need to refer to the specific contract, which will explain in greater detail who has financial responsibility for the services.

Items are often listed on the Distribution of Responsibility chart by CPT number. If a chart lists items alphabetically, you may have to look up the procedure code in the CPT to determine what the service is. In addition, many Distribution of Responsibility charts that are listed alphabetically may have an indexed listing by CPT code in the back.

After you have located the proper procedure code, follow the line across until you are under the plan name for the plan that covers the member. Determine whether the responsibility lies with the provider or the MCP. Be sure to check if there are any provisions regarding coverage. These provisions will often be referenced by a small number with a more detailed explanation at the bottom of the page (e.g., see abortion in Figure 10-1).

If the provider is responsible for payment of the services, these items are considered covered by the capitation amount and no further payment is due on those services. Check the provider that is listed on the claim. If the provider submitting the claim was the member's PCP, then charges should be denied as being covered by the capitation amount. If the provider on the claim is not the PCP, the claim should be forwarded to the PCP for payment.

If there are services for which the PCP is responsible and services for which the MCP is responsible on the same claim, process the claim and pay the items for which the MCP is responsible. Deny the items for which the PCP is responsible and forward the claim to the PCP for further processing, if needed.

> ▶ CRITICAL THINKING QUESTION: Identity theft is a growing concern in healthcare. How would you advise a medical clinic to correctly identify patients and prevent identity theft?

Check Referrals, Preauthorizations, or Second Opinions

The services that are the financial responsibility of the MCP should have been preceded by referrals or preauthorizations. In some cases, a second opinion may also have been required. Check to be sure that all the proper paperwork was done.

If the paperwork was not done, check the contract to determine the impact on the coverage of those services.

The preauthorization often is accessible by computer, so the claims examiner should be able to check it quickly and easily. Often a preauthorization number will be included on the claim. (See block 23 on the CMS-1500, Figure 10-6.) If a preauthorization number is not included, you must check the system for the preauthorization. Not having a preauthorization number on the claim is often not considered a valid reason for denying payment on a service, as the claims examiner has access to that information.

If the referrals, preauthorizations, or second opinions were done, process the claim.

If they were not done, deny or reduce benefits accordingly and process the claim.

Patient Encounter Forms

The Group/IPA must report all patient encounters (i.e., visits) to the MCP, regardless of whether the visit occurs at the Group/IPA or at one of its contracted providers. This information is often reported on an encounter form. If the Group/IPA does not have data regarding an encounter (which may happen if they are not contractually obligated to cover the services), but they receive information regarding the encounter, they should report what they know about the encounter to the MCP.

The MCP may specify the use of a designated form for reporting encounters, or they may use the CMS-1500. Generally, the medical biller will start with the encounter form and then complete the claim form (CMS-1500).

Encounters for consultation, second opinions, and other outside visits should be reported prior to adjudication and/or payment of the claim.

Some MCPs have their providers or Group/IPAs report patient encounters on a CMS-1500. The only difference between this form and a routine CMS-1500 is block 24F, charges. If the charges are covered by a capitation amount, then there is no charge for these services. Therefore, the indicated charges will be $0. The total charges and the balance due will likewise be $0.

If services are rendered by a provider and are not covered by the normal capitation amount, the amount for these charges should be placed in block 24F. Some MCPs may have providers or Group/IPAs submit charges that are the MCP's responsibility on a separate claim form from those that are covered under capitation. Thus, there may be two claim forms for the same provider, patient, and dates of service.

ACTIVITY #3

Managed Care

Directions: Answer the following questions after you review the material just covered. Write your answers in the space provided.

1. List the four things a claims examiner needs to check before a claim can be processed, denied, or reduced.

   a. _____

   b. _____

   c. _____

   d. _____

2. Under what circumstances would a payment be covered by the capitation amount? _____

   _____

3. Under what circumstances would a payment be denied as being covered by the capitation amount? _____

   _____

Processing the Claim

You are now ready to begin the actual calculations to process the claim. When claims are submitted, they often are accompanied by a Claim Transmittal Form, shown in Figure 10-9 ●. This form will indicate the type of claim being submitted and the authorization number for these claims.

Determine the Allowed Amount

Start by determining the allowed amount for the procedure. Most MCPs will have a fee schedule which will list each CPT code and the allowed amount for that code. Some MCPs that cover a wide area may have an *RVS* and Conversion Factor Report. In these cases, calculate the allowed amount using these factors in the same way you would calculate indemnity.

If there is a contracted amount for services, the processing of the claim should adhere to the terms in the contract. Usually

```
                                                    Provider Network Services
                                                   CLAIMS TRANSMITTAL FORM

         Date:

         To:    Claims Services

         From: _____ , Administrator for _____

         The attached claims are the responsibility of [the MCP].

         Authorization Number

         _____Inpatient Hospital (IP) Charges

         _____Outpatient Surgery (OPS) Facility Charges

         _____Anesthesia for approved IP or OPS

         _____Radiology for approved IP, OPS or SNF

         _____Pathology for approved IP, OPS or SNF

         _____Emergency services which resulted in admission to Inpatient status

         _____Ambulance

         _____Durable Medical Equipment

         _____Dialysis Facility Charges

         _____Radiation Therapy

         _____Member not on roster for date of service.  Include relevant roster page(s).


         NOTE: Use a separate form for each type of Plan expense.  Multiple providers
         may be grouped if the authorization number is the same.

                [The MCP] will not send denial notices for services which are the
         responsibility of the Group/IPA.

                Refer to the Medical Services Agreement for questions of coverage and
         financial responsibility.
```

FIGURE 10-9 Claim Transmittal Form

a fee schedule will accompany contracted terms. This fee schedule may be different for each provider with which the Group/IPA contracts. Pull the proper contract and determine the correct allowed amount.

Calculate Any Reduced Benefits

If the member or PCP did not obtain the proper referrals, preauthorizations, or second opinions, determine the impact on the payment. This effect is often stated in either the contract with the member (if it was the member's responsibility to obtain the proper paperwork) or the MCP's contract with the Group/IPA.

   If the benefits are reduced, calculate the impact of the reduction (e.g., if benefits are reduced to 50% if preauthorization is not obtained, multiply the allowed amount by 50%).

Be sure that you look at all paperwork carefully. If the preauthorization allowed three days of inpatient care and the member spent four days in the hospital, services for the last day may not be covered or may be reduced. In such a case, you may need to request an itemized billing to determine the dates that services were provided so you can determine which services should be denied.

Subtract the Copayment

Check the member's contract. Each item should list a copayment amount if a copayment is required from the member. Be sure you are checking the proper category. Often there are different copayment amounts for different types of services.

Rover Insurers, Inc.
5931 Rolling Road
Ronson, CO 81369

December 15, CCYY
Claim For: Abby Addison
Claim Number: 478-78-4
Group Policy Number: 41935
Member's ID Number: 001-00-RED

Dear Ms. Addison:

We received a claim for you. The following details the benefits that were paid on this claim. Please save this form for your tax records. If you have any questions, please contact the customer service office.

DATE OF SERVICE	PROCEDURE	BILLED AMOUNT	ALLOWED AMOUNT	% OF PAYMENT	PAYMENT AMOUNT	DENIED AMOUNT	REASON CODE
11/06/CCYY	HOSP CONSULT	$200.00	$140.00	90%	$ 36.00**	$ 60.00	55
11/07-08/CCYY	HOSP VISIT	$150.00	$100.00	90%	$ 90.00	$ 50.00	55
11/09/CCYY	HOSP D/C	$100.00	$ 75.00	90%	$ 67.50	$ 25.00	55
TOTAL		$450.00	$315.00		$193.50	$135.00	

55 Denied amount exceeds the amount covered under your plan.
** $100 applied to deductible.

FIGURE 10-10   Sample EOB

The amount of the member's copayment is always subtracted from the allowed amount. If the provider neglected to collect this amount at the time services were rendered, the provider is responsible for contacting the patient and collecting it. Thus, even if the claim states that no money was collected from the member, the copayment amount should always be subtracted from the allowed amount.

Pay the Remaining Amount

After you have calculated any reduced benefits and subtracted the copayment amount, pay the remaining amount. As the member is always responsible for the copayment, and usually only the copayment, any resulting benefits are generally due to the provider. The member should not have paid more than the copayment amount. If the member did pay more than the copayment amount, the provider is responsible for reimbursing the member for any amounts that he or she overpaid.

An EOB should accompany all claim payments, showing the calculation of the benefits and providing an explanation for why any services were denied or reduced. A notice should also accompany the EOB, stating that this is the contracted amount for this service and no amounts other than the copayment may be collected from the member. (A sample EOB is shown in Figure 10-10 ●.)

Of course, if you are working for a staff-model HMO, there is no payment due for the services that were rendered by the HMO-owned facility. This is because the providers in this type of facility are paid a salary, regardless of the number of members they see or the services they provide.

Denial of a Claim or Service

If you deny a claim or service, you must include a denial letter with the EOB, indicating the reason for the denial. The denial notice must also include a statement that the provider has the right to appeal the denial within 60 days and must provide the address where the member can file an appeal. If it appears that services were not medically necessary or were not true emergency services, then you must send the claim through a medical review process. The medical review should use the presenting diagnosis, rather than the discharge diagnosis, as the basis for their decision making and must consider the member's understanding of the medical circumstances which led to the emergency service.

All denial notices must contain an explicit reason, in layman's terms, of why the claim is being denied. If the MCP provides a list of denial reasons, then you should write the appropriate denial reason on the denial letter. You may not use a code unless you indicate the meaning of that code on the denial letter.

In addition, all denial letters must meet the following criteria:

1. The decision to deny must be correct and based on approved medical practices.
2. The denial reason must be clear to the member and CMS-approved denial reasons must be used.
3. The denial letter must include mandated appeals language and the correct health plan address.
4. The denial letter must be sent to the appropriate parties (the provider, the member, or both).
5. The denial notice must be issued within the required time frame.

Excess Risk Limit Cost Summary

I. Group Name: _____   Enrollee Name: _____   II.

    Address: _____   Enrollee PF#: _____

    _____   Date of Elegibility: _____

    Contact Person: _____   Contract Year: _____

    Phone Number: _____   For HIV/AIDS cases, list qualifying hospital stays:

    Date Submitted: _____

Type of submission	
__ Original	__ Medicare
__ Supplemental	__ Commercial
__ Resubmittal	__ OO Care
__ AIDS/HIV	__ CCC

III.

Provider of Service / Provider #	Date of Service	CPT, RVS, or SMA code	Units	Billed Amount	Amount Paid	For HMO use only
					TOTAL THIS PAGE:	

FIGURE 10-11   Excess Risk (Stoploss) Form

Appeals

Under the Affordable Care Act, patients have the right to appeal health insurance plan decisions. When it issues the first denial of payment, the plan must notify the patient of (1) the reason for denial, (2) the patient's right to file an appeal, (3) the patient's right to request an external review if the internal review was unsuccessful, and (4) the availability of the state's Consumer Assistance Program. The plan must respond to the appeal within 72 hours for denial of a claim for urgent care, within 30 days for denial of claims for nonurgent care, and within 60 days for denial of a claim for services already received.

If a member or provider appeals a denied claim, the MCP will review the claim and determine whether to uphold or reverse the denial. If the MCP determines that the services should have been covered and that the services were the financial responsibility of the Group/IPA, it will inform the Group/IPA of its decision and will instruct the Group/IPA to pay the claim.

Reinsurance/Stop-loss

Stop-loss is an attempt to limit payments by an insured person or a Group/IPA in the case of a catastrophic illness or injury to a member.

Many MCPs include a stop-loss or reinsurance clause. This clause may state that the Group/IPA will be financially responsible for the first set amount (e.g., $7,000) in expenses for each member in a contract year. After those expenses have been paid, the MCP will reimburse the Group/IPA for verified expenses which exceed the set amount.

If the provider's contract has a stop-loss clause, it is important that the claims examiner be aware of the amount. Any services which exceed that set amount should be covered by the MCP. Often the MCP will require that a claim for reimbursement be submitted on specific forms. An example of a stop-loss form is shown in Figure 10-11 ●.

CHAPTER REVIEW

Summary

- Managed care contracts were created in an attempt to bring healthcare costs under control by having doctors share some of the financial risks of healthcare with the patient and the insurance carrier.
- HMOs are the most common type of managed care model.
- A written contract dictates those services which the provider will cover and those which the MCP will cover.

- A provider submits a claim to the MCP for those services that are the plan's financial responsibility. The claim must be processed and paid or denied in a timely manner.
- The rules governing payment of MCP claims vary from those of indemnity claims.
- As you process a claim for an MCP, you must consider where the financial responsibility lies, along with whether or not preauthorizations, referrals, or second opinions were handled properly.

Review Questions

Directions: Answer the following questions after reviewing the material just covered. Write your answers in the space provided.

1. What is an HMO? _____
   _____

2. In a _____, a facility or Group bands together to provide services for HMO patients at their own facilities.

3. What is a capitation payment? _____
   _____

4. What is a TAR and what is its purpose? _____
   _____

5. What is stop-loss? _____
   _____

If you were unable to answer any of the questions, refer back to that section and then fill in the answers.

ACTIVITY #4

Find the Terms

Directions: Find and circle the words listed here. Words can appear horizontally, vertically, diagonally, forward, or backward.

```
A C K H Z Q Q G M D I E V C Q Z N W V F
W H S K W S O X R L Y F I Q M K I B A N
X T B M L D U S P O I N T V Q Z V S F Z
Q A I O O Q J X E C U O C R S O P W W C
P I L L R U B Q D P H P D J D I E J W M
F H L Q E I W B H H L E M J T I F P C S
N E T W O R K M O D E L C O V C N G L C
K W W O N N B P M L I C G E D T Y V S T
X G S D A P A M C V W J R P K E L S C F
Q Z F Z W Q E P S C Y N X I F G L T N E
R V B D L Z G W Y P O P J S X Y U O L C
Q E X S U X O Q I I M B Y T K B N P I E
R J C H M P M X T T N P K S U B L L Q E
J A K K L D N A Z F H R W X P Z T O C U
I B H Y Z B Z S X O Y H N C T Y N S K Y
B G X O J I H G N U H Q O V J F Q S B J
O R U T L U G I I N P Z U L Y S T M U U
U O D I B G Y E V K X Y U C D N K G E J
H V T G V B F A Z I M O V Z E L K R G E
O U Q I F R N B Z U C W M Y C X O Q S G
```

1. Group Model
2. Network Model
3. Stop-loss
4. Withhold

ACTIVITY #5

Matching

Directions: Match the following terms with the proper definition by writing the letter of the correct definition in the space next to the term.

1. _____ Eligibility Roster
2. _____ Independent Physician Associations
3. _____ Individual Practice Organizations
4. _____ Primary Care Provider
5. _____ Treatment Authorization Request

a. A legal entity composed of a network of private physicians who have organized to negotiate contracts with insurance companies and HMOs.

b. The provider chosen by a member, who is responsible for all the member's healthcare needs.

c. A form used to request authorization for services that are the financial responsibility of the HMO.

d. A listing which shows the effective dates of the patient's coverage, the contract under which they are covered, and their primary care provider.

e. Groups of providers who have banded together for the sole purpose of signing a contract with an MCP.

CHAPTER 11
Claims Auditing

CHAPTER 12
Processing Non-Medicare Claims

CHAPTER 13
Processing Medicare Claims

CHAPTER 14
Processing Workers' Compensation Claims

Keywords and concepts you will learn in this chapter:

Audit

Audit Analysis Report

Audit of Findings

Audit Scope

Billing Integrity

Certificate of Compliance Agreement (CCA)

Compliance Planning

Corporate Integrity Agreement (CIA)

Corrective Action

Medicaid Fraud Control Unit (MFCU)

Office of Inspector General (OIG)

Open Letters

Recovery Audit Contractors (RAC)

Self-Disclosure Protocol (SDP)

Statistical Sampling

Zone Program Integrity Contractor (ZPIC)

After completing this chapter, you will be able to:

- Describe the responsiblities of the Office of Inspector General.

- List the requirements under Corporate Integrity Agreements (CIAs).

- Identify the types of audits performed on claims.

- Describe the phases of an audit.

- Explain the components that must be included in post audit compliance education.

- List the items included in a self-disclosure protocol.

As healthcare needs increase and federal and state funding amounts remain tentative, Medicare and Medicaid programs must be vigilant in recovering funds paid for fraudulent claims and overpayments, and must ensure that providers are providing the service for which they are billing. In this chapter, we will explore the work of the **Office of Inspector General (OIG)** to monitor these programs through auditing. Internal auditing programs are of the utmost importance and are required by the Patient Protection and Affordable Care Act of 2010.

Office of Inspector General

The OIG was created by the Inspector General Act of 1978. (See Figure 11-1 ●.) The responsibilities have changed to include oversight over programs funded through the American Recovery and Reinvestment Act of 2009 (ARRA). The OIG assesses whether the Department of Health and Human Services (HHS) is using funds from the ARRA in accordance with legal and administrative requirements. The OIG is involved with the CMS in conducting audits of the Medicare and Medicaid programs.

Recovery and Reinvestment Act Responsibilities

The OIG is responsible for the following duties as assigned through the ARRA:

- Review agency spending plans prepared by HHS management.
- Outline steps that HHS management should take to obtain meaningful audit coverage.
- Conduct risk assessments of programs receiving funding, including health information technology and other non-Medicaid programs.
- Assess recipients' capability to manage and account for funds in accordance with federal regulations.

Corporate Integrity Agreements

- Healthcare providers who are found guilty under any of the civil false claims statues need a **Corporate Integrity Agreement (CIA)**. The OIG is responsible for negotiating these settlements after federal healthcare program investigations have been completed. CIAs typically involve completion of five or more years of monitored compliance.
- Use of a compliance officer and committee.

- Development of compliance standards and policies, including a confidential disclosure program.
- Implementation of an employee training program about compliance standards and policies.
- Completion of external independent annual reviews of compliance.
- Restriction of employment of ineligible persons.
- Reporting of overpayments, reportable events, and investigations or legal proceedings.
- Annual reporting to the OIG of compliance efforts.

OIG Reviews

The OIG completes an ongoing review related to the ARRA including a review of state Medicaid agency compliance with ARRA requirements and other HHS programs that are not covered in this text.

Open Letters

The OIG makes efforts to educate the healthcare industry about regulations and standards that must be met. One avenue that the OIG uses is **open letters** to notify the industry of changes or OIG initiatives to prevent fraud and abuse in the Medicare and Medicaid System. An example of such a letter is shown in Figure 11-2 ●. This letter refers to the self-disclosure program in which the OIG agrees to collaborate with individuals or agencies that find potential fraud and self-report it to the OIG.

ACTIVITY #1

The OIG

Directions: List five things you have learned about the OIG.

1. _____
2. _____
3. _____
4. _____
5. _____
   _____

● **ONLINE INFORMATION:** By visiting oig.hhs.gov/compliance/open-letters/, you can view all of the open letters from the OIG over the past decade.

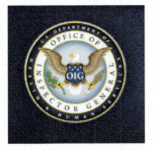

FIGURE 11-1 Office of Inspector General Banner
Source: Courtesy of the Office of Inspector General

DEPARTMENT OF HEALTH & HUMAN SERVICES

Office of Inspector General

Washington, D.C. 20201

An Open Letter to Health Care Providers

March 24, 2009

This Open Letter refines the OIG's Self-Disclosure Protocol (SDP) to build upon the initiative announced in my April 24, 2006, Open Letter. The 2006 Open Letter promoted the use of the SDP to resolve matters giving rise to civil monetary penalty (CMP) liability under both the anti-kickback statute and the physician self-referral ("Stark") law. As part of our ongoing efforts to evaluate and prioritize our work, these refinements aim to focus our resources on kickbacks intended to induce or reward a physician's referrals. Kickbacks pose a serious risk to the integrity of the health care system, and deterring kickbacks remains a high priority for OIG.

To more effectively fulfill our mission and allocate our resources, we are narrowing the SDP's scope regarding the physician self-referral law. OIG will no longer accept disclosure of a matter that involves only liability under the physician self-referral law in the absence of a colorable anti-kickback statute violation. We will continue to accept providers into the SDP when the disclosed conduct involves colorable violations of the anti-kickback statute, whether or not it also involves colorable violations of the physician self-referral law. Although we are narrowing the scope of the SDP for resources purposes, we urge providers not to draw any inferences about the Government's approach to enforcement of the physician self-referral law.

To better allocate provider and OIG resources in addressing kickback issues through the SDP, we are also establishing a minimum settlement amount. For kickback-related submissions accepted into the SDP following the date of this letter, we will require a minimum $50,000 settlement amount to resolve the matter. This minimum settlement amount is consistent with OIG's statutory authority to impose a penalty of up to $50,000 for each kickback and an assessment of up to three times the total remuneration. See 42 U.S.C. § 1320a-7a(a)(7). We will continue to analyze the facts and circumstances of each disclosure to determine the appropriate settlement amount consistent with our practice, stated in the 2006 Open Letter, of generally resolving the matter near the lower end of the damages continuum, i.e., a multiplier of the value of the financial benefit conferred.

These refinements to OIG's SDP are part of our ongoing efforts to develop the SDP as an efficient and fair mechanism for providers to work with OIG collaboratively. Further information about our SDP can be found at: http://oig.hhs.gov/fraud/selfdisclosure.asp. I look forward to continuing our joint efforts to promote compliance and protect the Federal health care programs and their beneficiaries.

Sincerely,

/Daniel R. Levinson/

Daniel R. Levinson
Inspector General

FIGURE 11-2 Example Open Letter from the OIG

Requirement	Explanation
Single, identifiable entity	Professional staff are required to work full-time on MFCU duties only
State Administered	Federal government pays matching funds up to 75% after the first three years of paying 90% matching funds
Interdisciplinary Model	A team of investigators, auditors, and attorneys must be available in the MFCU
Authority	MFCUs must have statewide authority to prosecute cases or have ability to refer suspected criminal violation to appropriate authority
Expanded Authority	MFCU's investigate Medicaid funded facilities, board and care facilities and in some cases Medicare or other government program run facilities.

FIGURE 11-3   MFCU Requirements

Auditing

Many type of audits have been used over the years to eliminate fraud and/or abuse of Medicare and Medicaid programs. An **audit** is a formal examination or systematic check of a program. Audits are conducted on claims for Medicare and Medicaid. The most recent types of auditors are described here.

Recovery Audit Contractors

Recovery Audit Contractors (RACs) are government-contracted auditors whose task is to find and stop Medicare fraud. RACs are assigned by CMS nationwide to audit hospitals, medical practices, rehabilitative centers, and long-term care providers' claims for potential fraud or overpayment. One of the most common errors that must be corrected by repayment is lack of medical necessity. Thus, a major focus of claims management is reviewing claims for justification of medical necessity. Medical necessity is defined by CMS through evidence-based research that certain procedures or treatments are necessary for the patients' health.

Zone Program Integrity Contractor

Zone Program Integrity Contractor (ZPIC) is the latest auditing program paid by CMS and designed to look at billing trends and patterns of Medicare billing. The purpose of the ZPIC program is to prevent waste, fraud, and abuse in the Medicare system. Providers who have higher than average Medicare billings in their community are the first to receive these **billing integrity** audits.

The ZPIC program provides higher authorization to contractors than the RAC program. ZPICs have CMS-set performance standards and have the goal of identifying cases of suspected fraud, investigating them, and acting immediately on the findings. Penalties to be given at the ZPIC program's discretion include suspension of payments, denial of payments, and recoupment of overpaid claims. The worst-case scenario for providers is referral to the OIG for criminal or civil prosecution.

Medicaid Fraud Control Units

Medicaid Fraud Control Units (MFCUs) investigate and prosecute Medicaid fraud as well as patient abuse and neglect in healthcare facilities. The OIG hires, certifies, and annually recertifies each MFCU. MFCUs must be compliant with OIG statues, regulations, and policies to be recertified.

MFCUs are independent state-level organizations that audit for performance standards and make recommendations to programs for improvement. The OIG MFCU requirements are listed in Figure 11-3 ●.

ACTIVITY #2

Types of Audits

Directions: Describe the differences among the three audits discussed in this chapter.

_____

_____

_____

_____

_____

Audit Findings

To understand audit findings, you must first understand how an audit is conducted. Sometimes the organization is notified that an audit will be conducted on certain days and the organization is given a list of records that will be reviewed so the facility can be ready for the auditor. Other times, there is no notification until the auditors walk in the door. Many audits are conducted offsite and auditors only request copies of portions of the records. (See Figure 11-4 ●.)

Phases of an Audit

Depending on the type of audit, or **audit scope**, the auditor reviews a random sampling or a specific sample of claims. The

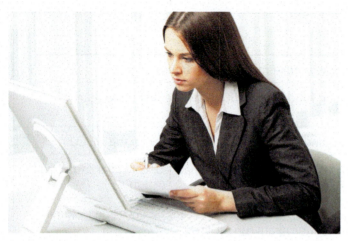

FIGURE 11-4 Completing an audit report
Source: Konstantin Chagin/Shutterstock

audit scope details what is being investigated, who will conduct the audit, and when the process will occur. During this initial phase, the auditor chooses a **statistical sampling** of records. Statistical sampling is a method in which the auditor selects enough claims to be considered statistically valid rather than reviewing every claim. The method that is used to determine what is statistically valid has to do with the size of the client population, the type of services billed, and the number of claims submitted. A computer program called RAT-STATS is the primary statistical tool for OIG's Office of Audit Services.

> ▶ CRITICAL THINKING QUESTION: If you are notified of an upcoming audit and the records that will be needed for the audit, what should you do prior to the auditor's arrival?

The next phase is data gathering. The auditor will gather all the data from the claim, the medical record, the billing policies and procedures, and so on from the organization. These data are entered into a system. Most likely it is the RAT-STATS program, although that program was created in the 1970s and auditing organizations may use different data collection systems. There may or may not be a period during which the organization is allowed to provide missing data.

After the audit, the audit information is analyzed and put into a report that includes recommendations for corrective action and a compliance plan. This report is called an **audit analysis report**. The report will detail the findings and the immediate conditions for continuation in the Medicare and/or Medicaid program.

Most companies conduct an **audit of the findings**. The purpose of auditing the findings is to validate the audit results by answering the following questions:

1. Are the findings valid?
2. Is there any missing information that can be provided to clarify the audit?
3. Are there similar problems in nonaudited claims?
4. What systemic problems may be the cause of the errors?

After these questions have been answered, a compliance plan is created.

Certificate of Compliance Agreement

Although there are immediate **corrective actions** that may be given under the auditor's authority, there will be further corrective actions if the provider does not attain compliance. After the compliance plan is complete, the organization will receive a **certificate of compliance agreement**. This certificate is only applicable as long as the organization continues to follow the compliance plan.

Compliance Planning

The OIG provides a series of materials that give guidance on compliance. One of the programs relates to preventing compliance issues (in voluntary compliance programs). Another is used to create a **compliance plan** to rectify issues that were found during the audit. The educational materials supplied by the OIG are directed at specific venues in the healthcare industry, such as hospitals, nursing homes, third-party billers, and durable medical equipment suppliers. The OIG provides these materials to encourage the providers to develop and use internal controls to monitor adherence to statutes, regulations, and program requirements. Some companies go so far as to use the same RAT-STATS software to fulfill the claims review requirements for corporate integrity agreements.

Compliance Education

Postaudit compliance education must include the findings of the audit, the identified systemic problems, a corrective plan, and measures to prevent fraud and abuse of the Medicare and Medicaid program. This education is required for all employees and is a part of the new-hire orientation process, as shown in Figure 11-5 ●. Figure 11-6 ● shows an agenda provided by the OIG for educating employees about compliance. The OIG website oig.hhs.gov/compliance/provider-compliance-training/ contains accompanying materials to provide training materials.

> ▶ CRITICAL THINKING QUESTION: How would you handle a suspicion of fraud or healthcare abuse by a coworker?

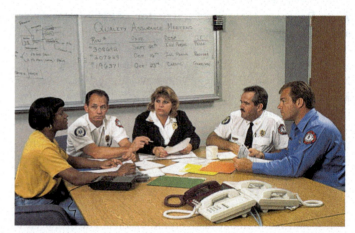

FIGURE 11-5 Teaching compliance in new-hire orientation
Source: Michal Heron/Pearson Education/PH College

PROVIDER COMPLIANCE TRAINING
TAKE THE INITIATIVE.
Cultivate a Culture of Compliance With Health Care Laws

HEAT

AGENDA

8:00 – 8:30	Attendee Registration
8:30 – 8:35	Welcome Remarks *Meredith Williams and Amanda Walker* Industry Guidance Branch, Senior Counsel OIG/HHS
8:35 – 8:40	Overview of OIG *Sheri Denkensohn*, Special Assistant to the Inspector General OIG/HHS
8:40 – 9:00	Keynote Speech *Inspector General Daniel Levinson* OIG/HHS
9:00 – 10:05	Session 1: <u>Cultivating a Culture of Compliance</u> Navigating the Fraud and Abuse Laws *Meredith Williams* Compliance Program Basics *Amanda Walker* Operating an Effective Compliance Program *Tony Maida*, Administrative & Civil Remedies Branch, Deputy Branch Chief OIG/HHS Understanding Program Exclusions *Geeta Kaveti*, Administrative & Civil Remedies Branch, Associate Counsel OIG/HHS
10:05 – 10:25	Break

HEALTH CARE FRAUD PREVENTION AND ENFORCEMENT ACTION TEAM (HEAT)
OFFICE OF INSPECTOR GENERAL (OIG)

FIGURE 11-6   Example Compliance Education Agenda

HEAT PROVIDER COMPLIANCE TRAINING
TAKE THE INITIATIVE.
Cultivate a Culture of Compliance With Health Care Laws

10:25– 11:30	Session 2: Know Where to Go When a Compliance Issue Arises

Navigating the Government
James Cannatti, Industry Guidance Branch, Senior Counsel
OIG/HHS

Overview of Centers for Medicare and Medicaid Services
Nancy O'Connor, Regional Administrator
CMS/HHS

Importance of Documentation
Dr. Julie Taitsman, Chief Medical Officer
OIG/HHS

OIG Subpoenas, Audits, Surveys, and Self-Disclosure Protocol
Tony Maida

11:30 – 11:50	Break
11:50 – 12:50	Session 3: Understanding the Consequences of Health Care Fraud

Health Care Fraud Enforcement Panel
Spencer Turnbull, HEAT Initiative Administrator
OIG/HHS

Dr. Peter Budetti, Center for Program Integrity, Deputy Administrator
CMS/HHS

Nick DiGiulio, Office of Investigations, Special Agent in Charge
OIG/HHS

John Pease, Assistant United States Attorney
Eastern District of Pennsylvania

Jacqueline Franklin, Supervisory Criminal Investigator
Medicaid Fraud Control Unit of Washington, D.C.

12:50 – 12:55	Adjournment

HEALTH CARE FRAUD PREVENTION AND ENFORCEMENT ACTION TEAM (HEAT)
OFFICE OF INSPECTOR GENERAL (OIG)

FIGURE 11-6 *(Continued)*

Self-Disclosure Protocol

Part of any compliance plan is the education of employees on **self-disclosure protocol**. Essentially, they must be told that it is important for them to report fraudulent or abusive practices. Providers who wish to voluntarily disclose self-discovered evidence of potential fraud to OIG may do so under the Provider Self-Disclosure Protocol (SDP). Self-disclosure gives providers an opportunity to avoid the costs and disruptions associated with an OIG-directed investigation or audit.

The OIG endeavors to work cooperatively with providers who are forthcoming, thorough, and transparent in their disclosures in resolving these matters. The *Federal Register* related to self-disclosure (Volume 63, Number 210) reads in part,

> While no written agreement setting out the terms of the self-assessment will be required, the OIG expects the commitment of the health care provider to disclose specific information and engage in specific self-evaluation steps relating to the disclosed matter. In contrast to the pilot disclosure program, the fact that a disclosing health care provider is already subject to Government inquiry (including investigations, audits or routine oversight activities) will not automatically preclude a disclosure.

Submission of a Self-Disclosure

A voluntary disclosure statement must be submitted in writing to the OIG office and should contain the following elements:

1. Name, address, provider number, and position of the disclosing party
2. Knowledge of any current government investigations or audits into the organizations practices
3. Full description of matter being reported
4. Description of parties involved in the potentially fraudulent activity
5. The reason that the disclosing party believes the activity is a violation of federal law
6. A certifying statement that the statements provided in the self-disclosure are truthful and made in good faith.

● **ONLINE INFORMATION:** To view the entire Federal Register notice related to self-disclosure, visit oig.hhs.gov/compliance/self-disclosure-info.

ACTIVITY #3

Self-Disclosure Letter

Directions: Assume that you have seen a coworker upcoding claims to get better reimbursement. Using the preceding list of required items, compose a hypothetical self-disclosure letter.

PRACTICE PITFALLS

Internal auditing or reviews that check claims prior to processing are the safest way for a company to prevent fraud and abuse. It is helpful to create an interdepartmental committee that reviews claims for errors. Committee members should not review portions of a claim in which they have input. For example, a physical therapist who records minutes spent with a patient for claims should not review rehabilitation minutes for appropriateness during these committee reviews. Instead, a biller could review the minutes, and the physical therapist could review the biller's entries on the claim form. This practice of committee reviews is in itself a safety check for individuals who attempt fraud during the billing practice.

Other preventative measures are training employees in compliance and conducting background checks on employees for abuse, fraud investigations, or convictions in the past. One way to conduct a search of potential employees' background related to healthcare fraud is to search for their names in the exclusions website exclusions.oig.hhs.gov/. The site lists anyone who is excluded from working in a capacity that is funded by Medicare or Medicaid monies.

CHAPTER REVIEW

Summary

- The OIG is the governing agency that monitors for Medicare and Medicaid fraud or abuse.
- The types of audits used by the OIG include Recovery Audit Contractors (RACs), Zone Program Integrity Contractors (ZPICs) and the Medicaid Fraud Control Units (MFCUs).
- Corporate Integrity Agreements and Certified Compliance Agreements are part of OIG's relationship-building process with providers of healthcare.
- Auditing involves phases of sample identification, data collection, data analysis, and data reporting.
- Audit findings are examined to ensure validity and to determine a compliance plan.
- Organizations can voluntarily create a compliance plan, self-report potential fraudulent activities, or be audited and face potential corrective action.
- Compliance plans include educating employees about the corporate compliance plan and teaching them how to disclose potentially fraudulent activities.

Review Questions

Directions: Choose the best answer to each question.

1. Which agency monitors Medicare and Medicaid practices for fraud and abuse?

    a. DEA

    b. OIG

    c. CMS

    d. FDA

2. Which of the following audits has most recently been added to Medicare and Medicaid audits?

    a. RACs

    b. MFCUs

    c. ZPICs

    d. None of the above

3. Which of the following is not a requirement to be a MFCU?

    a. Be solely state funded

    b. Be an independent agency

    c. Have state-wide authority

    d. Be composed of an interdisciplinary team

4. Which of the following terms is a negotiated agreement between the OIG and an organization that has been found guilty of fraud?

    a. Certificate of Corporate Agreement

    b. Certified Integrity Agreement

    c. Corporate Integrity Agreement

    d. Certificate of Corporate Compliance

5. Which of the following is not a part of a compliance plan?

    a. Compliance education plan

    b. Self-disclosure education

    c. Agreement to follow corrective actions

    d. Payments for the cost of auditing

Directions: Indicate whether the statement is true or false.

6. Self-disclosure of potential fraudulent activities to the OIG guarantees that the person disclosing will not be prosecuted.

7. Voluntarily creating a compliance plan is a sign of guilt.

8. Educating employees about compliance with Medicare and Medicaid regulations is a good idea that moves the company toward achieving compliance.

9. Organizations choose which records will be reviewed by auditors.

10. Auditors will always notify the organization of their planned dates for auditing.

ACTIVITY #4

Matching

Directions: Match the key word to its definition.

1. Audit
2. Recovery Audit Contractors
3. Medicaid Fraud Control Units
4. Audit Scope
5. Audit Analysis Report
6. Corrective Action
7. Zone Program Integrity Contractors
8. Statistical Sampling
9. Audit of Findings
10. Self-Disclosure Protocol

a. Auditing program paid by CMS and designed to look at billing trends and patterns of Medicare billing.

b. A formal examination or systematic check of a program.

c. A method in which enough claims are chosen to be considered statistically valid.

d. Investigate and prosecute Medicaid fraud as well as patient abuse and neglect in healthcare facilities.

e. Government-contracted auditors whose task is to find and stop Medicare fraud.

f. A type of audit.

g. A report detailing the findings and the immediate conditions for continuation in the Medicare and/or Medicaid program.

h. Validating the audit results.

i. OIG collaboration to gather information on potential fraudulent actions.

j. Remedies imposed after an audit.

Processing Non-Medicare Claims

12

After completing this chapter, you will be able to:

Choose key information from insurance contracts to complete a claim.

Set up a file to track claims that require more information.

Organize family files for tracking aggregate deductibles.

Review a claim for accuracy.

Find appropriate documentation in a medical record when more information is required.

Complete a team audit for claim appropriateness.

Identify whether a claim should be approved, whether it requires more information, or whether it should be denied.

275

The next three chapters provide practice for the medical biller and health claims examiner. As the work that people with these job titles do can take different forms, we will explore both the provider billing side and claims processing side of situations. In this chapter, the activities will focus on billing for services rendered, reviewing those claims prior to sending them for payment, and handling claims examining at the processing end of the spectrum. As described in earlier chapters, these functions are the primary responsibilities of medical billers and health claims examiners.

> ● **ONLINE INFORMATION:** There are several organizations associated with medical billing and claims examining. The American Academy of Professional Coders (AAPC) (www.aapc.com), American Health Information Management Association (AHIMA) (www.ahima.org), and Medical Association of Billers (MAB) (physicianswebsites.com/) are a few worth investigating.

Billing for Services Rendered

It is the responsibility of the medical biller to gather the necessary information for submitting a health insurance claim and to be a part of the final review before the claim is sent to the insurance for payment. It is essential to be proficient in accurately performing these tasks, both to promote the success of the medical practice and to ensure that payments are received on time.

In this section, we will study how to select key information from an insurance contract, use it to complete a claim, and set up a tracking system for claims on families with aggregate deductibles or coinsurance.

Use the following scenario to complete the activities in this section. The Lang family has four members participating in the Ball Insurance Company Plan found in Appendix A. You work for the provider, Dr. Annette Adams, whom they all visit for primary care. Your medical office is comprehensive, providing X-rays and most lab work on-site. Assume that the Lang family has not filed any previous claims and that the activities are additive.

ACTIVITY #1

Jonny Lang Breaks a Leg

Directions: Complete CMS-1500 claim forms for the listed events and supplemental bills for the patient on the example patient bill form. Find the CMS-1500 and Patient Bill forms in Appendix B.

1. On March 3, CCYY, eight-year-old Jonny Lang fell out of a tree and broke his tibia. His parents brought him to the office, where he received the following services:
   a. Complex office visit of an established patient ($50.00)
   b. X-ray of the affected tibia ($120.00)
   c. Closed conscious sedation for setting of the tibia bone ($320.00)
   d. Casting of the leg ($120.00)
   e. Second X-ray of leg to assure proper casting ($120.00)
   f. Administration of a tetanus shot ($25.00)
2. On April 15, CCYY, Jonny returned to have his cast removed, incurring the following charges:
   a. Office visit of established patient, 40 minutes ($65.00)
   b. Cast removal ($100.00)

ACTIVITY #2

Sani Lang Has a Fainting Episode

Directions: Complete the CMS-1500 insurance claim for the following services. Also complete a Family Deductible Tracking Form to track the family aggregate deductible and coinsurance and create a bill for the patient. Find these forms in Appendix B.

1. On May 1, CCYY, Sani Lang got dizzy and fainted. The family insisted that she go to the doctor to get checked out. At the doctor's office, she incurred the following charges:
   a. Office visit of established patient ($50.00)
   b. Blood draw for labs (complete blood count, CBC) ($40.00)
2. On May 6, CCYY, Sani had a followup appointment to review her laboratory results. Here are the charges incurred:
   a. Office visit with counseling and teaching about blood pressure ($60.00)
   b. Automated blood pressure cup ($75.00)

ACTIVITY #3

Angie Lang Has a Sports Physical

Directions: Complete the CMS-1500 insurance claim for the following services. Also continue the family tracking form and create a bill for the patient. These forms can be found in Appendix B.

1. On June 20, CCYY, Angie Lang had a physical that was required for her to play summer sports in a local community center. The following charges were incurred:
   a. Sports physical of established patient ($65.00)
   b. Administration of MMR immunizations ($25.00)
   c. Administration of tetanus shot ($25.00)

> ▶ **CRITICAL THINKING QUESTION:** What is different about a sports physical? Is there a specific code for a sports physical?

ACTIVITY #4

Sani Lang Has a Car Accident

Directions: Utilizing the list of charges provided in Figure 12-1 ●, create claim forms for the following situations. For patients with more than one visit, it is appropriate to bill for both visits on one claim form. (Note: You are only charging for the services of your medical practice.) Assume that all deductibles and out-of-pocket maximums have been met.

1. On November 16, CCYY, Sani was taken to the emergency room after a car accident, where she was evaluated for a broken arm. This accident was a one-car accident, and therefore, the medical bills should be billed to the medical insurance company. When the emergency room doctor discovered that she had a hairline fracture in her arm, she was sent home with a brace with instructions to follow up with her physician in two weeks when the swelling has gone down.

2. On November 30, CCYY, Sani went to your office and had an X-ray, had her arm put in a cast, and had a followup X-ray after the casting.

3. On November 16, CCYY, Jonny was taken to your office with a cut on his head from the car accident. He required 21 stitches with a local anesthetic. He also had an X-ray of his head to make sure there was no internal injury, which there was not.

4. On November 22, CCYY, Jonny returned to the office to have his stitches removed.

5. On November 16, CCYY, Hui Lang came to the office with a sore ankle after being in the car accident. Hui had an X-ray of his right ankle and was fitted with a soft boot for stabilization of the sprained ankle.

6. On January 2, CCNY, Sani returned to the office to have her cast removed. Because she was previously diagnosed with osteoporosis, a follow-up X-ray was taken of the arm to ensure proper healing. The X-ray was negative for abnormality.

7. On December 3, CCYY, Hui returned to the office for a followup to his sprained ankle. The ankle did not appear

Item	Fee
Cast removal	$100.00
Casting of an arm, wrist or hand	$120.00
Cleaning and stitching of wound <25 stitches	$200.00
Irrigation and drainage of a wound	$250.00
Local anesthetic for stitches	$ 75.00
Office visit complex 45 min	$ 50.00
Office visit minor 25 min	$ 25.00
Office visit moderate 26-44 min	$ 45.00
Removal of sutures	$ 25.00
Single x-ray	$120.00
Splint for ankle	$ 75.00

FIGURE 12-1 Partial pricing list for physician fee services

to be healing, so a follow-up X-ray was taken and he was referred to an orthopedist for further evaluation.

8. On December 24, CCYY, Jonny returned to the office with redness, swelling, and tenderness at the site where he previously had stitches. The doctor determined that the area was infected, provided irrigation and drainage of the area, and restitched his head with a local anesthetic.

9. On January 2, CCNY, Jonny returned to the office to have his stitches removed.

Committee Review of Claims

As discussed in Chapter 11, one important role of the medical biller to be a part of a team audit for claim appropriateness. This review will increase the likelihood of submitting clean claims and provide checks and balances against insurance fraud or abuse.

In this section you will review three completed claims as if you were on a committee and were assigned to verify that medical necessity has been established. The reason for this particular review

is that medical necessity is the number one reason for denial of claims; thus, it makes sense that this would be a major part of a final review of claims prior to sending them for insurance payment.

● **ONLINE INFORMATION:** Several automobile insurance companies have websites that help a medical biller determine whether to bill the automobile insurance or the patient's healthcare insurance policy. Conduct a search on the differences and add it to your resource file.

ACTIVITY #5

Medical Necessity

Directions: In the figures that follow (Figure 12-2 ●, Figure 12-3 ●, and Figure 12-4 ●), you will find three claims that have errors. You are reviewing the diagnosis codes and procedure codes for medical necessity. Review and correct the claims to be clean.

(1500)

HEALTH INSURANCE CLAIM FORM
APPROVED BY NATIONAL UNIFORM CLAIM COMMITTEE 08/05

☐☐ PICA

PICA ☐☐

1. MEDICARE MEDICAID TRICARE CHAMPVA GROUP FECA OTHER	1a. INSURED'S I.D. NUMBER (For Program in Item 1)
☐(Medicare #) ☐(Medicaid #) ☐(Sponsor's SSN) ☐(Member ID#) ☑(SSN or ID) ☐(SSN) ☐(ID)	32156743

CHAMPUS / HEALTH PLAN / BLK LUNG

2. PATIENT'S NAME (Last Name, First Name, Middle Initial)	3. PATIENT'S BIRTH DATE SEX	4. INSURED'S NAME (Last Name, First Name, Middle Initial)
DOE, JOE F.	MM DD YY M☐ F☐	DOE, JOE F.

5. PATIENT'S ADDRESS (No, Street)	6. PATIENT RELATIONSHIP TO INSURED	7. INSURED'S ADDRESS (No, Street)
1432 SYCHAMORE ST	Self☐ Spouse☐ Child☐ Other☐	1432 SYCHAMORE ST

CITY	STATE	8. PATIENT STATUS	CITY	STATE
LAS VEGAS	NV	Single☐ Married☐ Other☐	LAS VEGAS	NV

ZIP CODE	TELEPHONE (Include Area Code)		ZIP CODE	TELEPHONE (Include Area Code)
84312	(502)4316714	Full-Time Part-Time Employed☐ Student☐ Student☐	84312	(502)4316714

9. OTHER INSURED'S NAME (Last Name, First Name, Middle Initial)	10. IS PATIENT'S CONDITION RELATED TO:	11. INSURED'S POLICY GROUP OR FECA NUMBER
a. OTHER INSURED'S POLICY OR GROUP NUMBER	a. EMPLOYMENT? (Current or Previous) ☐YES ☒NO	a. INSURED'S DATE OF BIRTH SEX MM DD YY 03 04 1941 M☒ F☐
b. OTHER INSURED'S DATE OF BIRTH SEX MM DD YY M☐ F☐	b. AUTO ACCIDENT? PLACE (State) ☐YES ☒NO	b. EMPLOYER'S NAME OR SCHOOL NAME BLUE CORP
c. EMPLOYER'S NAME OR SCHOOL NAME	c. OTHER ACCIDENT? ☐YES ☒NO	c. INSURANCE PLAN NAME OR PROGRAM NAME BLUE INS
d. INSURANCE PLAN NAME OR PROGRAM NAME	10d. RESERVED FOR LOCAL USE	d. IS THERE ANOTHER HEALTH BENEFIT PLAN? ☐YES ☒NO If yes, return to and complete item 9 a-d

READ BACK OF FORM BEFORE COMPLETING & SIGNING THIS FORM.

12. PATIENT'S OR AUTHORIZED PERSON'S SIGNATURE I authorize the release of any medical or other information necessary to process this claim. I also request payment of government benefits either to myself or to the party who accepts assignment below.	13. INSURED'S OR AUTHORIZED PERSON'S SIGNATURE I authorize payment of medical benefits to the undersigned physician or supplier for services described below.
SIGNED *SIGN ON FILE* DATE_ 4/10/CCYY	SIGNED *SIGN ON FILE*

14. DATE OF CURRENT MM DD YY 04 09 CCYY ILLNESS (First symptom) OR INJURY (Accident) OR PREGNANCY (LMP)	15. IF PATIENT HAS HAD SAME OR SIMILAR ILLNESS, GIVE FIRST DATE MM DD YY	16. DATES PATIENT UNABLE TO WORK IN CURRENT OCCUPATION MM DD YY MM DD YY FROM TO
17. NAME OF REFERRING PHYSICIAN OR OTHER SOURCE	17a. / 17b. NPI	18. HOSPITALIZATION DATES RELATED TO CURRENT SERVICES MM DD YY MM DD YY FROM TO
19. RESERVED FOR LOCAL USE		20. OUTSIDE LAB? $ CHARGES ☐YES ☒NO

21. DIAGNOSIS OR NATURE OF ILLNESS OR INJURY (Relate Items 1,2,3 or 4 to Item 24E by Line)	22. MEDICAID RESUBMISSION CODE ORIGINAL REF. NO.
1. │ 205 . 00 3. │	
2. │ 4. │	23. PRIOR AUTHORIZATION NUMBER

24. A. DATE(S) OF SERVICE		B. PLACE OF SERVICE	C. EMG	D. PROCEDURES, SERVICES, OR SUPPLIES (Explain Unusual Circumstances) CPT/HCPCS MODIFIER	E. DIAGNOSIS POINTER	F. $ CHARGES	G. DAYS OR UNITS	H. EPSDT Family Plan	I. ID. QUAL.	J. RENDERING PROVIDER ID. #
From MM DD YY	To MM DD YY									
1	04 09 CCYY	04 09 CCYY	11		9 9 2 0 3	1	0	1		NPI	ANNETTE SMITH 20142014
2					8 0 0 6 9	1	0	1		NPI	
3					8 0 0 4 7	1	0	1		NPI	
4										NPI	
5										NPI	
6										NPI	

25. FEDERAL TAX ID NUMBER SSN EIN	26. PATIENT'S ACCOUNT NO.	27. ACCEPT ASSIGNMENT? (For govt. claims, see back)	28. TOTAL CHARGE	29. AMOUNT PAID	30. BALANCE DUE
341-56-2143 ☐☒	54164	☒ YES ☐ NO	$ 0 00	$ 0 00	$ 0 00

31. SIGNATURE OF PHYSICIAN OR SUPPLIER INCLUDING DEGREES OR CREDENTIALS (I certify that the statements on the reverse apply to this bill and are made a part thereof) SIGNED *SIGN ON FILE* DATE	32. SERVICE FACILITY LOCATION INFORMATION 4216 CENTER ST HOLLYWOOD, CA a. b.	33. BILLING PROVIDER INFO & PH. # (461)3215612 ANNETTE SMITH a. b. 20142014

NUCC Instruction Manual available at: www.nucc.org   PLEASE PRINT **OR** TYPE   APPROVED OMB 0938-0999 FORM CMS-1500 (08/05)

CARRIER / PATIENT AND INSURED INFORMATION / PHYSICIAN OR SUPPLIER INFORMATION

FIGURE 12-2 Find the error in this claim form

1500

HEALTH INSURANCE CLAIM FORM
APPROVED BY NATIONAL UNIFORM CLAIM COMMITTEE 08/05

PICA | | | PICA

1. MEDICARE   MEDICAID   TRICARE   CHAMPVA   GROUP   FECA   OTHER
CHAMPUS   HEALTH PLAN   BLK LUNG
☐(Medicare #) ☐(Medicaid #) ☐(Sponsor's SSN) ☐(Member ID#) ☑(SSN or ID) ☐(SSN) ☐(ID)

1a. INSURED'S I.D. NUMBER   (For Program in Item 1)
X3Y4111

2. PATIENT'S NAME (Last Name, First Name, Middle Initial)
JONES, DAWN F.

3. PATIENT'S BIRTH DATE   SEX
MM 10 | DD 26 | YY 1955   M☐   F☑

4. INSURED'S NAME (Last Name, First Name, Middle Initial)
JONES, DAWN F.

5. PATIENT'S ADDRESS (No, Street)
1356 QUAKER ST

6. PATIENT RELATIONSHIP TO INSURED
Self ☑   Spouse ☐   Child ☐   Other ☐

7. INSURED'S ADDRESS (No, Street)
1356 QUAKER ST

CITY OATVILLE   STATE AL

8. PATIENT STATUS
Single ☑   Married ☐   Other ☐

CITY OATVILLE   STATE AL

ZIP CODE 92314   TELEPHONE (Include Area Code) (505)106-1066

Full-Time ☐   Part-Time ☐
Employed ☐   Student ☐   Student ☐

ZIP CODE 92314   TELEPHONE (Include Area Code) (505)106-1066

9. OTHER INSURED'S NAME (Last Name, First Name, Middle Initial)

10. IS PATIENT'S CONDITION RELATED TO:

11. INSURED'S POLICY GROUP OR FECA NUMBER
1026543

a. OTHER INSURED'S POLICY OR GROUP NUMBER

a. EMPLOYMENT? (Current or Previous)
☐ YES   ☑ NO

a. INSURED'S DATE OF BIRTH   SEX
MM 10 | DD 26 | YY 1955   M☐   F☑

b. OTHER INSURED'S DATE OF BIRTH   SEX
MM | DD | YY   M☐   F☐

b. AUTO ACCIDENT?   PLACE (State)
☐ YES   ☑ NO

b. EMPLOYER'S NAME OR SCHOOL NAME
GENERAL OAT CO

c. EMPLOYER'S NAME OR SCHOOL NAME

c. OTHER ACCIDENT?
☐ YES   ☑ NO

c. INSURANCE PLAN NAME OR PROGRAM NAME
PLANS FOR LIFE

d. INSURANCE PLAN NAME OR PROGRAM NAME

10d. RESERVED FOR LOCAL USE

d. IS THERE ANOTHER HEALTH BENEFIT PLAN?
☐ YES   ☑ NO   If yes, return to and complete item 9 a-d

READ BACK OF FORM BEFORE COMPLETING & SIGNING THIS FORM.
12. PATIENT'S OR AUTHORIZED PERSON'S SIGNATURE I authorize the release of any medical or other information necessary to process this claim. I also request payment of government benefits either to myself or to the party who accepts assignment below.

SIGNED *SIGN ON FILE*   DATE

13. INSURED'S OR AUTHORIZED PERSON'S SIGNATURE I authorize payment of medical benefits to the undersigned physician or supplier for services described below.

SIGNED *SIGN ON FILE*

14. DATE OF CURRENT   ILLNESS (First symptom) OR INJURY (Accident) OR PREGNANCY (LMP)
MM 03 | DD 04 | YY CCYY

15. IF PATIENT HAS HAD SAME OR SIMILAR ILLNESS, GIVE FIRST DATE   MM | DD | YY

16. DATES PATIENT UNABLE TO WORK IN CURRENT OCCUPATION
FROM MM | DD | YY   TO MM | DD | YY

17. NAME OF REFERRING PHYSICIAN OR OTHER SOURCE

17a.
17b. NPI

18. HOSPITALIZATION DATES RELATED TO CURRENT SERVICES
FROM MM | DD | YY   TO MM | DD | YY

19. RESERVED FOR LOCAL USE

20. OUTSIDE LAB? $ CHARGES
☐ YES   ☒ NO

21. DIAGNOSIS OR NATURE OF ILLNESS OR INJURY (Relate Items 1,2,3 or 4 to Item 24E by Line)
1. 748.00
2.
3.
4.

22. MEDICAID RESUBMISSION
CODE   ORIGINAL REF. NO.

23. PRIOR AUTHORIZATION NUMBER

24. A. DATE(S) OF SERVICE From MM DD YY	To MM DD YY	B. PLACE OF SERVICE	C. EMG	D. PROCEDURES, SERVICES, OR SUPPLIES (Explain Unusual Circumstances) CPT/HCPCS	MODIFIER	E. DIAGNOSIS POINTER	F. $ CHARGES	G. DAYS OR UNITS	H. EPSDT Family Plan	I. ID. QUAL.	J. RENDERING PROVIDER ID. #
1	03 04 CCYY	03 04 CCYY	11		99213		1	0			NPI	5614311067
2					88048		1	0			NPI	5614311067
3											NPI	
4											NPI	
5											NPI	
6											NPI	

25. FEDERAL TAX ID NUMBER   SSN EIN
98-51634   ☐ ☑

26. PATIENT'S ACCOUNT NO.
143651

27. ACCEPT ASSIGNMENT? (For govt. claims, see back)
☑ YES   ☐ NO

28. TOTAL CHARGE $ 0

29. AMOUNT PAID $ 0

30. BALANCE DUE $ 0

31. SIGNATURE OF PHYSICIAN OR SUPPLIER INCLUDING DEGREES OR CREDENTIALS (I certify that the statements on the reverse apply to this bill and are made a part thereof)

SIGNED *SIGN ON FILE*   DATE

32. SERVICE FACILITY LOCATION INFORMATION
a.
b.

33. BILLING PROVIDER INFO & PH. # (505)555-5555
ANY PROVIDER
1356 MEMBERS
OATVILLE, AL 92314
a.   b. 5614311067

NUCC Instruction Manual available at: www.nucc.org   PLEASE PRINT OR TYPE   APPROVED OMB 0938-0999 FORM CMS-1500 (08/05)

CARRIER   PATIENT AND INSURED INFORMATION   PHYSICIAN OR SUPPLIER INFORMATION

FIGURE 12-3   Find the error in this claim form

FIGURE 12-4 Find the error in this claim form

Examining Claims

The claims examiner has an important role in validating whether claims are payable. The insurance industry would not survive if insurance companies paid invalid claims or overpaid claims that were incorrectly billed. Validating claims is an important step that is often accomplished by an intermediary or claims examiner. This person is hired by the insurance company to determine whether claims are valid for payment, require more information, or should be denied.

The examiner determines the status of each claim. The claims that are cleared for payment are sent for payment process-ing. The claims that need more information are sent back to the provider with a request for further information in order to process the claim. The claims that are denied are also sent back to the provider and patient with an explanation of denial. The most common reasons for denials are lapse in insurance coverage, use of a nonparticipating provider, and lack of medical necessity.

> ▶ **CRITICAL THINKING QUESTION:** Are there ethical issues involved in being a claims examiner? How would you ensure that you are being fair and impartial as you determine what claims to approve?

ACTIVITY #6

Claims Examination

The following claims (Figure 12-5 ●, Figure 12-6 ●, and Figure 12-7 ●) have been submitted to the Rover Insurance Company. Your responsibility is to review the following claims and determine whether all claims are fine as is or whether any of the claims requires further information. If any of the claims does require more information, select form(s) from Appendix B and complete.

(1500)

HEALTH INSURANCE CLAIM FORM
APPROVED BY NATIONAL UNIFORM CLAIM COMMITTEE 08/05

☐☐☐ PICA   PICA ☐☐☐

1. MEDICARE	MEDICAID	TRICARE CHAMPUS	CHAMPVA	GROUP HEALTH PLAN	FECA BLK LUNG	OTHER	1a. INSURED'S I.D. NUMBER (For Program in Item 1)
☐ (Medicare #)	☐ (Medicaid #)	☐ (Sponsor's SSN)	☐ (Member ID#)	☒ (SSN or ID)	☐ (SSN)	☐ (ID)	564321

2. PATIENT'S NAME (Last Name, First Name, Middle Initial)
WASH MARTHA T.

3. PATIENT'S BIRTH DATE   MM 09 DD 10 YY 1947   SEX M☐ F☒

4. INSURED'S NAME (Last Name, First Name, Middle Initial)

5. PATIENT'S ADDRESS (No, Street)
1001 WHITE HOUSE DR

6. PATIENT RELATIONSHIP TO INSURED
Self ☒ Spouse ☐ Child ☐ Other ☐

7. INSURED'S ADDRESS (No, Street)

CITY   WASHINGTON   STATE DC

8. PATIENT STATUS
Single ☒ Married ☐ Other ☐

CITY   STATE

ZIP CODE 00001   TELEPHONE (Include Area Code) (202)111-1111

Full-Time Part-Time
Employed ☒ Student ☐ Student ☐

ZIP CODE   TELEPHONE (Include Area Code) ( )

9. OTHER INSURED'S NAME (Last Name, First Name, Middle Initial)

10. IS PATIENT'S CONDITION RELATED TO:

11. INSURED'S POLICY GROUP OR FECA NUMBER
10514321

a. OTHER INSURED'S POLICY OR GROUP NUMBER

a. EMPLOYMENT? (Current or Previous)
☐ YES ☒ NO

a. INSURED'S DATE OF BIRTH   MM DD YY   SEX M☐ F☐

b. OTHER INSURED'S DATE OF BIRTH   MM DD YY   SEX M☐ F☐

b. AUTO ACCIDENT?   PLACE (State)
☒ YES ☐ NO CO

b. EMPLOYER'S NAME OR SCHOOL NAME
GEORGE COMPANY

c. EMPLOYER'S NAME OR SCHOOL NAME

c. OTHER ACCIDENT?
☐ YES ☒ NO

c. INSURANCE PLAN NAME OR PROGRAM NAME
FLAG INSURANCE

d. INSURANCE PLAN NAME OR PROGRAM NAME

10d. RESERVED FOR LOCAL USE

d. IS THERE ANOTHER HEALTH BENEFIT PLAN?
☐ YES ☒ NO   If yes, return to and complete item 9 a-d

READ BACK OF FORM BEFORE COMPLETING & SIGNING THIS FORM.
12. PATIENT'S OR AUTHORIZED PERSON'S SIGNATURE I authorize the release of any medical or other information necessary to process this claim. I also request payment of government benefits either to myself or to the party who accepts assignment below.

SIGNED SIGN ON FILE   DATE

13. INSURED'S OR AUTHORIZED PERSON'S SIGNATURE I authorize payment of medical benefits to the undersigned physician or supplier for services described below.

SIGNED SIGN ON FILE

| 14. DATE OF CURRENT   MM 04 DD 11 YY CCYY   ◀ ILLNESS (First symptom) OR INJURY (Accident) OR PREGNANCY (LMP) | 15. IF PATIENT HAS HAD SAME OR SIMILAR ILLNESS, GIVE FIRST DATE MM DD YY | 16. DATES PATIENT UNABLE TO WORK IN CURRENT OCCUPATION   FROM MM 04 DD 11 YY CCYY   TO MM 08 DD 11 YY CCYY |

17. NAME OF REFERRING PHYSICIAN OR OTHER SOURCE

17a.
17b. NPI

18. HOSPITALIZATION DATES RELATED TO CURRENT SERVICES
FROM MM DD YY   TO MM DD YY

19. RESERVED FOR LOCAL USE

20. OUTSIDE LAB?   ☐ YES ☐ NO $ CHARGES

21. DIAGNOSIS OR NATURE OF ILLNESS OR INJURY (Relate Items 1,2,3 or 4 to Item 24E by Line)
1. 814.00
2.
3.
4.

22. MEDICAID RESUBMISSION
CODE   ORIGINAL REF. NO.

23. PRIOR AUTHORIZATION NUMBER

24. A. DATE(S) OF SERVICE From MM DD YY	To MM DD YY	B. PLACE OF SERVICE	C. EMG	D. PROCEDURES, SERVICES, OR SUPPLIES (Explain Unusual Circumstances) CPT/HCPCS	MODIFIER	E. DIAGNOSIS POINTER	F. $ CHARGES	G. DAYS OR UNITS	H. EPSDT Family Plan	I. ID. QUAL.	J. RENDERING PROVIDER ID. #
1	04 11 CCYY	04 11 CCYY	11		73580		1	50 00	2		NPI	521212212
2					27825		1	250 00			NPI	
3					29345		1	100 00			NPI	
4											NPI	
5											NPI	
6											NPI	

25. FEDERAL TAX ID NUMBER   SSN EIN ☐☐

26. PATIENT'S ACCOUNT NO. 511111

27. ACCEPT ASSIGNMENT? (For govt. claims, see back) ☒ YES ☐ NO

28. TOTAL CHARGE $ 400 00

29. AMOUNT PAID $ 0

30. BALANCE DUE $ 400 00

31. SIGNATURE OF PHYSICIAN OR SUPPLIER INCLUDING DEGREES OR CREDENTIALS (I certify that the statements on the reverse apply to this bill and are made a part thereof)

SIGNED SIGN ON FILE   DATE

32. SERVICE FACILITY LOCATION INFORMATION
1001 WALL STREET
WASHINGTON DC 00212

a.   b.

33. BILLING PROVIDER INFO & PH. # (513)6662222
ANY PROVIDER

a.   b. 521222212

NUCC Instruction Manual available at: www.nucc.org   PLEASE PRINT OR TYPE   APPROVED OMB 0938-0999 FORM CMS-1500 (08/05)

FIGURE 12-5   Received CMS-1500 Form

```
(1500)
HEALTH INSURANCE CLAIM FORM
APPROVED BY NATIONAL UNIFORM CLAIM COMMITTEE 08/05
```

PICA		PICA

1. MEDICARE   MEDICAID   TRICARE   CHAMPVA   GROUP   FECA   OTHER
CHAMPUS   HEALTH PLAN   BLK LUNG
☑(Medicare #) ☐(Medicaid #) ☐(Sponsor's SSN) ☐(Member ID#) ☑(SSN or ID) ☐(SSN) ☐(ID)

1a. INSURED'S I.D. NUMBER   (For Program in Item 1)

2. PATIENT'S NAME (Last Name, First Name, Middle Initial)
SANCHEL FARTH T.

3. PATIENT'S BIRTH DATE   SEX
MM DD YY
01 01 1945   M☒ F☐

4. INSURED'S NAME (Last Name, First Name, Middle Initial)

5. PATIENT'S ADDRESS (No, Street)
2121 TUNNEL ST

6. PATIENT RELATIONSHIP TO INSURED
Self ☒ Spouse ☐ Child ☐ Other ☐

7. INSURED'S ADDRESS (No, Street)

CITY ALBUMIUM   **STATE** AL

8. PATIENT STATUS
Single ☐ Married ☒ Other ☐

CITY   **STATE**

ZIP CODE 21343   **TELEPHONE (Include Area Code)** (213)4312121

Full-Time Part-Time
Employed ☒ Student ☐ Student ☐

ZIP CODE   **TELEPHONE (Include Area Code)** ( )

9. OTHER INSURED'S NAME (Last Name, First Name, Middle Initial)
SANCHEL FARTH

10. IS PATIENT'S CONDITION RELATED TO:

11. INSURED'S POLICY GROUP OR FECA NUMBER
561324735

a. OTHER INSURED'S POLICY OR GROUP NUMBER
62134

a. EMPLOYMENT? (Current or Previous)
☐YES ☒NO

a. INSURED'S DATE OF BIRTH   SEX
MM DD YY
01 01 1945   M☒ F☐

b. OTHER INSURED'S DATE OF BIRTH   SEX
MM DD YY
01 01 1945   M☒ F☐

b. AUTO ACCIDENT?   PLACE (State)
☐YES ☒NO

b. EMPLOYER'S NAME OR SCHOOL NAME
RAILROAD PACIFIC

c. EMPLOYER'S NAME OR SCHOOL NAME
RAILROAD PACIFIC

c. OTHER ACCIDENT?
☐YES ☑NO

c. INSURANCE PLAN NAME OR PROGRAM NAME
MEDICARE

d. INSURANCE PLAN NAME OR PROGRAM NAME
RAILWAY HEALTH

10d. RESERVED FOR LOCAL USE

d. IS THERE ANOTHER HEALTH BENEFIT PLAN?
☒ YES ☐NO   If yes, return to and complete item 9 a-d

READ BACK OF FORM BEFORE COMPLETING & SIGNING THIS FORM.
12. PATIENT'S OR AUTHORIZED PERSON'S SIGNATURE I authorize the release of any medical or other information necessary to process this claim. I also request payment of government benefits either to myself or to the party who accepts assignment below.

SIGNED SIGN ON FILE   DATE

13. INSURED'S OR AUTHORIZED PERSON'S SIGNATURE I authorize payment of medical benefits to the undersigned physician or supplier for services described below.

SIGNED SIGN ON FILE

14. DATE OF CURRENT
MM DD YY
10 21 CCYY
ILLNESS (First symptom) OR
INJURY (Accident) OR
PREGNANCY (LMP)

15. IF PATIENT HAS HAD SAME OR SIMILAR ILLNESS, GIVE FIRST DATE MM DD YY

16. DATES PATIENT UNABLE TO WORK IN CURRENT OCCUPATION
MM DD YY   MM DD YY
FROM   TO

17. NAME OF REFERRING PHYSICIAN OR OTHER SOURCE

17a.
17b. NPI

18. HOSPITALIZATION DATES RELATED TO CURRENT SERVICES
MM DD YY   MM DD YY
FROM   TO

19. RESERVED FOR LOCAL USE

20. OUTSIDE LAB? $ CHARGES
☐YES ☐NO

21. DIAGNOSIS OR NATURE OF ILLNESS OR INJURY (Relate Items 1,2,3 or 4 to Item 24E by Line)
1. 250 . 00   3.
2.   4.

22. MEDICAID RESUBMISSION
CODE   ORIGINAL REF. NO.

23. PRIOR AUTHORIZATION NUMBER

24. A. DATE(S) OF SERVICE						B. PLACE OF SERVICE	C. EMG	D. PROCEDURES, SERVICES, OR SUPPLIES (Explain Unusual Circumstances) CPT/HCPCS MODIFIER	E. DIAGNOSIS POINTER	F. $ CHARGES	G. DAYS OR UNITS	H. EPSDT Family Plan	I. ID. QUAL.	J. RENDERING PROVIDER ID. #
From			To											
MM	DD	YY	MM	DD	YY									
1 10	21	CCYY	10	21	CCYY	11		90211	1	50 00	1		NPI	321456125
2													NPI	
3													NPI	
4													NPI	
5													NPI	
6													NPI	

25. FEDERAL TAX ID NUMBER   SSN EIN
☐☐

26. PATIENT'S ACCOUNT NO.
5613421

27. ACCEPT ASSIGNMENT?
(For govt. claims, see back)
☐YES ☐NO

28. TOTAL CHARGE
$ 50 00

29. AMOUNT PAID
$ 50 00

30. BALANCE DUE
$ 00 00

31. SIGNATURE OF PHYSICIAN OR SUPPLIER INCLUDING DEGREES OR CREDENTIALS
(I certify that the statements on the reverse apply to this bill and are made a part thereof)

SIGNED SIGN ON FILE   DATE

32. SERVICE FACILITY LOCATION INFORMATION
TEMPLE AVE 2041E.
ALBUMIUM, AL 21343

a.   b.

33. BILLING PROVIDER INFO & PH. # (313)4445555
TED DOCTOR

a.   b. 321456125

```
NUCC Instruction Manual available at: www.nucc.org    PLEASE PRINT OR TYPE    APPROVED OMB 0938-0999 FORM CMS-1500 (08/05)
```

FIGURE 12-6   Received UB-04 Form

1500

HEALTH INSURANCE CLAIM FORM
APPROVED BY NATIONAL UNIFORM CLAIM COMMITTEE 08/05

☐☐☐PICA   PICA ☐☐☐

1. MEDICARE	MEDICAID	TRICARE CHAMPUS	CHAMPVA	GROUP HEALTH PLAN	FECA BLK LUNG	OTHER	1a. INSURED'S I.D. NUMBER	(For Program in Item 1)
☐(Medicare #)	☐(Medicaid #)	☐(Sponsor's SSN)	☐(Member ID#)	☑(SSN or ID)	☐(SSN)	☐(ID)	561111111	

2. PATIENT'S NAME (Last Name, First Name, Middle Initial)	3. PATIENT'S BIRTH DATE	SEX	4. INSURED'S NAME (Last Name, First Name, Middle Initial)
JONES JACK P.	MM 04 DD 09 YY 1986	M☒ F☐	

5. PATIENT'S ADDRESS (No, Street)	6. PATIENT RELATIONSHIP TO INSURED	7. INSURED'S ADDRESS (No, Street)
PARSON ROAD N 2001	Self ☒ Spouse ☐ Child ☐ Other ☐	

CITY PARSON VILLE	STATE TN	8. PATIENT STATUS	CITY	STATE
		Single ☒ Married ☐ Other ☐		

ZIP CODE 92167	TELEPHONE (Include Area Code) (921)6169216	Employed ☐ Full-Time Student ☐ Part-Time Student ☐	ZIP CODE	TELEPHONE (Include Area Code) ( )

9. OTHER INSURED'S NAME (Last Name, First Name, Middle Initial)	10. IS PATIENT'S CONDITION RELATED TO:	11. INSURED'S POLICY GROUP OR FECA NUMBER 134-21-6514

a. OTHER INSURED'S POLICY OR GROUP NUMBER	a. EMPLOYMENT? (Current or Previous) ☒ YES ☐ NO	a. INSURED'S DATE OF BIRTH MM DD YY SEX M☐ F☐

b. OTHER INSURED'S DATE OF BIRTH MM DD YY SEX M☐ F☐	b. AUTO ACCIDENT? PLACE (State) ☐ YES ☒ NO	b. EMPLOYER'S NAME OR SCHOOL NAME CONSTRUCT HOMES

c. EMPLOYER'S NAME OR SCHOOL NAME	c. OTHER ACCIDENT? ☐ YES ☒ NO	c. INSURANCE PLAN NAME OR PROGRAM NAME CONSTRUCT PLAN

d. INSURANCE PLAN NAME OR PROGRAM NAME	10d. RESERVED FOR LOCAL USE	d. IS THERE ANOTHER HEALTH BENEFIT PLAN? ☐YES ☒ NO If yes, return to and complete item 9 a-d

READ BACK OF FORM BEFORE COMPLETING & SIGNING THIS FORM.

12. PATIENT'S OR AUTHORIZED PERSON'S SIGNATURE I authorize the release of any medical or other information necessary to process this claim. I also request payment of government benefits either to myself or to the party who accepts assignment below. SIGNED _SIGN ON FILE_ DATE_____	13. INSURED'S OR AUTHORIZED PERSON'S SIGNATURE I authorize payment of medical benefits to the undersigned physician or supplier for services described below. SIGNED _SIGN ON FILE_

14. DATE OF CURRENT MM DD YY 10 20 CCYY ILLNESS (First symptom) OR INJURY (Accident) OR PREGNANCY (LMP)	15. IF PATIENT HAS HAD SAME OR SIMILAR ILLNESS, GIVE FIRST DATE MM DD YY 08 11 CCYY	16. DATES PATIENT UNABLE TO WORK IN CURRENT OCCUPATION MM DD YY MM DD YY FROM TO

17. NAME OF REFERRING PHYSICIAN OR OTHER SOURCE	17a.	18. HOSPITALIZATION DATES RELATED TO CURRENT SERVICES MM DD YY MM DD YY
	17b. NPI	FROM TO

19. RESERVED FOR LOCAL USE	20. OUTSIDE LAB? $ CHARGES ☐YES ☐NO

21. DIAGNOSIS OR NATURE OF ILLNESS OR INJURY (Relate Items 1,2,3 or 4 to Item 24E by Line)

1. | 847 . 30   3. |
2. | 4. |

22. MEDICAID RESUBMISSION CODE   ORIGINAL REF. NO.
23. PRIOR AUTHORIZATION NUMBER

24. A. DATE(S) OF SERVICE		B. PLACE OF SERVICE	C. EMG	D. PROCEDURES, SERVICES, OR SUPPLIES (Explain Unusual Circumstances)		E. DIAGNOSIS POINTER	F. $ CHARGES	G. DAYS OR UNITS	H. EPSDT Family Plan	I. ID. QUAL.	J. RENDERING PROVIDER ID. #
From MM DD YY	To MM DD YY			CPT/HCPCS	MODIFIER						
10 20 CCYY	10 20 CCYY	11		90211			50 00			NPI	521664444
										NPI	
										NPI	
										NPI	
										NPI	
										NPI	

25. FEDERAL TAX ID NUMBER SSN EIN ☐☐	26. PATIENT'S ACCOUNT NO. 51362	27. ACCEPT ASSIGNMENT? (For govt. claims, see back) ☒ YES ☐ NO	28. TOTAL CHARGE $ 50 00	29. AMOUNT PAID $ 0	30. BALANCE DUE $ 50 00

31. SIGNATURE OF PHYSICIAN OR SUPPLIER INCLUDING DEGREES OR CREDENTIALS (I certify that the statements on the reverse apply to this bill and are made a part thereof) SIGNED _SIGN ON FILE_ DATE____	32. SERVICE FACILITY LOCATION INFORMATION 1050 PARSON LANE PARSON, TN 43261	33. BILLING PROVIDER INFO & PH. # (313)333-2122 PROVIDER T.D.W.
	a. b.	a. b. 521664444

NUCC Instruction Manual available at: www.nucc.org   PLEASE PRINT OR TYPE   APPROVED OMB 0938-0999 FORM CMS-1500 (08/05)

● **FIGURE 12-7**   Received CMS-1500 Form

CHAPTER REVIEW

Summary

- The medical biller is responsible for choosing key information from insurance contracts to complete a claim correctly. The key information includes diagnosis and justifications for medical necessity.
- Use tracking forms that indicate which claims were sent back to providers for more information, so that you can ensure none of the claims are lost in a mail shuffle.
- When a family is covered by the same insurance company and an aggregate deductible applies, track the aggregation.
- Reviewing claims for accuracy is one of the responsibilities of a medical biller or claims examiner. This task includes verifying that the coding is correct, the information regarding patient identification is accurate, and the fees are appropriately assessed.
- The medical biller should prioritize claims that are returned for further information. It is important to identify and relay information for insurance claims to be paid. Some insurance companies have time limits for turnaround.
- Performing a final audit of claims prior to sending them to the insurance company for payment can save time in gathering requested information for returned claims and ensure timely payment. These audits are often completed by a team of people who review various parts of the claim for accuracy.
- The claims examiner reviews claims for approval of payment, determines which claims require more information (and requests such information), and identifies those that are to be denied.

Review Questions

Directions: Using the information you have learned in this chapter, answer the following questions.

Multiple Choice

1. Which of the following job titles is most likely to perform the task of completing a health insurance claim?

   a. medical examiner

   b. medical biller

   c. claims examiner

   d. receptionist

2. What is the most common reason for denial of a claim?

   a. wrong address of insured

   b. wrong insurance group number

   c. lack of diagnosis supporting medical necessity

   d. lack of information related to the cause of an injury

3. What does it mean when a family has an aggregate deductible?

   a. A certain number of family members must meet the individual deductible before the aggregate deductible is met.

   b. The individual deductibles do not matter; if anyone in the family meets the family deductible, it is considered met for everyone in the family.

   c. The individual deductibles must be met first, and then the family deductible has to be met.

   d. As soon as one person meets the individual deductible, the money that person has paid goes toward other family members' individual deductibles.

4. Why is it important for the medical biller to return requested information to insurance companies in a timely manner?

   a. There are deadlines that stop an insurance company from ever paying on a claim after a certain length of time.

   b. The claim will not be processed without the necessary information.

   c. The claim may affect deductibles and coinsurance for future claims.

   d. For the sake of efficiency, the most urgent matters should be completed first.

5. What technique can prevent claims from being denied or returned for lack of information?

   a. doing an internal committee audit before sending the claims for processing

   b. supervisory review of claims

   c. external intermediary review of claims

   d. keeping a log of returned claims to avoid making the same mistakes on future claims

True/False

6. Medical necessity is only important for Medicare claims.

7. Deductibles are the amount a patient pays for office visits.

8. When there are injuries in an automobile accident, the patient is responsible for filing a claim to the automobile insurance company.

9. Medical necessity is determined by having the diagnosis and procedure codes match accordingly.

10. A medical biller and a claims examiner may have similar job tasks.

Processing Medicare Claims

After completing this chapter, you will be able to:

- Determine the appropriate E/M codes to enter on a Medicare claim.

- Identify why a Medicare audit downcoded a service.

- Choose key information from the medical record to complete a claim.

- Review a Medicare claim for accuracy and medical necessity.

- Find appropriate documentation in a medical record when more information is required.

- Complete a team audit for claim appropriateness.

Continuing our exploration of health claims examining, this chapter discusses the necessity of auditing Medicare claims for accuracy to avoid Medicare audits and overpayment claims. We will focus on coding Medicare claims from medical records and/or encounter forms, determining the appropriate E/M code and diagnosis codes from information in the medical record, and auditing Medicare claims for submission readiness. In addition, we will analyze a postaudit review, which will reveal why the Medicare auditor downcoded a claim. Clarifying the results of the audit can help us create a plan of action to ensure that improved documentation is provided as required.

Evaluation and Management Coding for Medicare Claims

The key to Medicare E/M coding is verifying that the code used is deemed medically necessary for the patient, given the information in the medical record. As presented in earlier chapters, the key ingredients of an E/M code are

- Extent of history taken at this encounter.
- Examination time and technicality.
- Level of medical decision making necessary.
- Counseling at this encounter.
- Coordination of care conducted at this encounter.
- Nature of presenting problem for this encounter.
- Overall time spent with the patient for this encounter.

The first three items on this list are the primary basis for choosing an E/M code. After determining the history, examination, and medical decision-making level, the medical biller selects an E/M code based on how many of the three categories meet or exceed the description of the E/M code.

New Patient, Initial Observation, Initial Hospital, or Emergency Room Care

For the categories of new patient, initial observation, initial hospital care, or emergency room care, the E/M stated criteria must meet all three of the key components. For example, if all three components meet or exceed the description for 99204 (New patient office visit with comprehensive history, comprehensive exam, and moderate medical decision-making complexity), then this is the correct code. If only two of the categories match this description, then the code 99203 is correct instead. It is important only to code the level that documentation for medical necessity of the encounter supports.

Established Patient and Subsequent Care Visits

For established patient visits or subsequent care visits to the hospital or other care facility, only two of the three criteria must be met in order to use the indicated E/M code. For example, if a patient is in the hospital and the code 99225 is selected for a subsequent observation care (expanded problem-focused interval history, expanded problem-focused examination, and medical decision making of moderate complexity), only two of these criteria need apply. Therefore, if the medical decision-making was low complexity but the other two criteria were expanded problem focused, it is still appropriate to use the 99225 code. This information is clearly outlined in the CPT® manual and should be reviewed to verify coding accuracy.

Time

Time spent with the patient, with patient representatives, or on coordination of care only counts when it takes 50% or more of the time for the total visit. Therefore, the time category would be considered in instances where the medical record clearly reflects that the time of the session spent on counseling or consultation encompassed more than 50% of the total visit time.

> ● **ONLINE INFORMATION:** For a current fact sheet and resource guide to using E/M codes, download www.cms.gov/Outreach-and-Education/Medicare-Learning-Network-MLN/MLNProducts/Downloads/Evaluation_Management_Fact_Sheet_ICN905363.pdf.

ACTIVITY #1

E/M Coding

Directions: Match the E/M code for physician office visit to the description of the three key components.

Criterion	E/M Code
1. History—problem focused of new patient Examination—problem focused Decision Making—straightforward	a. 99204
2. History—comprehensive of new patient Examination—comprehensive Decision Making—high complexity	b. 99214
3. History—detailed of new patient Examination—detailed Decision Making—low complexity	c. 99201
4. History—detailed of established patient Examination—expanded problem focused Decision Making—low complexity	d. 99203
5. History—detailed of established/patient Examination—detailed Decision Making—low complexity	e. 99213

ACTIVITY #2

Determining Medical Complexity

Directions: Use Table 13-1 ● (the criteria found in the CPT manual) to determine the medical complexity of the case presented.

Case 1: Mary Stanza is an established patient with a history of high cholesterol, hypertension, and obesity. She is seeing the doctor today for chest pain. What is the probable level of decision making for this patient? _____

Explain your reasoning: _____

_____

_____

Case 2: Jonny Boiler is an established pediatric patient who is brought in by his mother with red spots all over his body. He has a fever, the spots itch, and his school has reported several cases of chicken pox. What level of decision making is involved in this case? _____

Explain your reasoning: _____

_____

_____

Case 3: Mark Lapooze is an established adult patient who is presenting with low back pain. After examination, the physician determines that as Mr. Lapooze's symptoms do not reflect a definitive diagnosis, she will need to rule out kidney stones, back injury, or other inflammation of organs in that area. She orders labs and X-rays first and then sends Mr. Lapooze to have a scan for kidney stones. What level of decision making is involved in this case? _____

Explain your reasoning: _____

_____

_____

TABLE 13-1 CPT Criteria for Determining Medical Decision Making

Number of Diagnoses or Management Options	Amount and/or Complexity of Data to Be Reviewed	Risk of Complications and/or Morbidity or Mortality	Level of Decision Making
Minimal	0 or minimal	Minimal	**Straightforward**
Limited	Limited	Low	**Low complexity**
Multiple	Moderate	Moderate	**Moderate complexity**
Extensive	Extensive	High	**High complexity**

Note: Only 2 of the three categories have to be met to qualify for that level of decision making.

Use of Encounter Forms

Providers often use an encounter form to communicate common diagnostic and procedural codes to the medical biller. It is sometimes called the superbill because it serves as documentation of the visit, payment collected, and coding for billing purposes. Encounter forms can be a useful tool when you are coding a Medicare claim; however, they cannot be the only tool you use. The medical record documentation must justify the encounter coding and, in the end, justify the Medicare claim submitted.

> ● **ONLINE INFORMATION:** Search the Internet for encounter forms or superbill examples so that you can compare providers of similar services.

ACTIVITY #3

Encounter Forms

Directions: The following scenarios provide an encounter form and the corresponding medical note. Use the CPT and *International Classification of Diseases* (ICD) manuals to provide the codes for a Medicare claim.

For case #1, see Figure 13-1 ● and Figure 13-2 ●. List the codes for the Medicare claim here:

_____

For Case #2, see Figure 13-3 ● and Figure 13-4 ●. List the codes for the Medicare claim here:

_____

For Case #3, see Figure 13-5 ● and Figure 13-6 ●. List the codes for the Medicare claim here:

_____

Patient Name **Mary Stanza**

Capital City Medical
123 Unknown Boulevard, Capital City, NY 12345-2222

Date of Service
MM/DD/CCYY

New Patient			Arthrocentesis/Aspiration/Injection		Laboratory	
Problem Focused	99201		Arthrocentesis/Aspiration/Injection		Amylase	82150
Expanded Problem, Focused	99202		Small Joint	20600	B12	82607
Detailed	99203		Interm Joint	20605	CBC & Diff	85025
Comprehensive	99204		Major Joint	20610	Comp Metabolic Panel	(80053)
Comprehensive/High Complex	99205		**Other Invasive/Noninvasive**		Chlamydia Screen	87110
Well Exam Infant (up to 12 mos.)	99381		Audiometry	92552	Cholesterol	82465
Well Exam 1–4 yrs.	99382		Cast Application		Digoxin	80162
Well Exam 5–11 yrs.	99383		Location Long Short		Electrolytes	80051
Well Exam 12–17 yrs.	99384		Catheterization	51701	Ferritin	82728
Well Exam 18–39 yrs.	99385		Circumcision	54150	Folate	82746
Well Exam 40–64 yrs.	99386		Colposcopy	57452	GC Screen	87070
			Colposcopy w/Biopsy	57454	Glucose	82947
			Cryosurgery Premalignant Lesion		Glucose 1 HR	82950
			Location (s):		Glycosylated HGB A1C	83036
Established Patient			Cryosurgery Warts		HCT	85014
Post-Op Follow Up Visit	99024		Location (s):		HDL	83718
Minimum	99211		Curetement Lesion		Hep BSAG	87340
Problem Focused	99212		Single	11055	Hepatitis panel, acute	80074
Expanded Problem Focused	99213		2–4	11056	HGB	85018
Detailed	(99214)		>4	11057	HIV	86703
Comprehensive/High Complex	99215		Diaphragm Fitting	57170	Iron & TIBC	83550
Well Exam Infant (up to 12 mos.)	99391		Ear Irrigation	69210	Kidney Profile	80069
Well exam 1–4 yrs.	99392		ECG	93000	Lead	83655
Well Exam 5–11 yrs.	99393		Endometrial Biopsy	58100	Liver Profile	80076
Well Exam 12–17 yrs.	99394		Exc. Lesion Malignant		Mono Test	86308
Well Exam 18–39 yrs.	99395		Benign		Pap Smear	88155
Well Exam 40–64 yrs.	99396		Location		Pregnancy Test	84703
Obstetrics			Exc. Skin Taqs (1–15)	11200	Obstetric Panel	80055
Total OB Care	59400		Each Additional 10	11201	Pro Time	85610
Injections			Fracture Treatment		PSA	84153
Administration Sub. / IM	90772		Loc		RPR	86592
Drug			w/Reduc w/o Reduc		Sed. Rate	85651
Dosage			I & D Abscess Single/Simple	10060	Stool Culture	87045
Allergy	95115		Multiple or Comp	10061	Stool O & P	87177
Cocci Skin Test	86490		I & D Pilonidal Cyst Simple	10080	Strep Screen	87880
DPT	90701		Pilonidal Cyst Complex	10081	Theophylline	80198
Hemophilus	90646		IV Therapy—To One Hour	90760	Thyroid Uptake	84479
Influenza	90658		Each Additional Hour	90761	TSH	84443
MMR	90707		Laceration Repair		Urinalysis	81000
OPV	90712		Location Size Simp/Comp		Urine Culture	87088
Pneumovax	90732		Laryngoscopy	31505	Drawing Fee	36415
TB Skin Test	86580		Oximetry	94760	Specimen Collection	99000
TD	90718		Punch Biopsy		**Other:**	
Unlisted Immun	90749		Rhythm Strip	93040	**EKG**	
Tetanus Toxoid	90703		Treadmill	93015	**Chest X-Ray**	
Vaccine/Toxoid Admin <8 Yr Old w/ Counseling	90465		Trigger Point or Tendon Sheath Inj.	20550		
Vaccine/Toxoid Administration for Adult	90471		Tympanometry	92567		
Diagnosis/ICD-9: **Chest Pain**			**HTN, Obesity,**			
			Hyperlipidemia			

I acknowledge receipt of medical services and authorize the release of any
medical information necessary to process this claim for healthcare payment only. I do authorize payment to the provider.

Patient Signature *Mary Stanza*

Total Estimated Charges: _____

Payment Amount: _____

Next Appointment: _____

FIGURE 13-1 Encounter Form #1

Physician Note:

S: Established patient Mary Stanza age 45 presents with chest pain, "tight, heavy, constant." This pain is acute and has lasted, "3-4 hours." Ms. Stanza reports she has been resting to see if the pain would cease and when it didn't she came to the office.

O: Blood pressure is elevated at 160/95; No Temp, Pulse is 80, Respirations 20; Pulse OX on room air is 93%; Denies GI, Neuro, and other physical symptoms. 25 minutes spent examining patient.

A: Chest pain of unknown origin, chronic HTN, Obesity, and Hyperlipidemia.

P: Sent to Emergency room for chest x-ray, labs, and EKG.

Patient: Mary Stanza   **Medical Record Number:** 201456

FIGURE 13-2   Physician Note #1

Patient Name **Jonny Boiler**

Capital City Medical
123 Unknown Boulevard, Capital City, NY 12345-2222

Date of Service
MM/DD/CCYY

New Patient		Arthrocentesis/Aspiration/Injection		Laboratory	
Problem Focused	99201	Arthrocentesis/Aspiration/Injection		Amylase	82150
Expanded Problem, Focused	99202	Small Joint	20600	B12	82607
Detailed	99203	Interm Joint	20605	CBC & Diff	85025
Comprehensive	99204	Major Joint	20610	Comp Metabolic Panel	80053
Comprehensive/High Complex	99205	**Other Invasive/Noninvasive**		Chlamydia Screen	87110
Well Exam Infant (up to 12 mos.)	99381	Audiometry	92552	Cholesterol	82465
Well Exam 1–4 yrs.	99382	Cast Application		Digoxin	80162
Well Exam 5–11 yrs.	99383	Location Long Short		Electrolytes	80051
Well Exam 12–17 yrs.	99384	Catheterization	51701	Ferritin	82728
Well Exam 18–39 yrs.	99385	Circumcision	54150	Folate	82746
Well Exam 40–64 yrs.	99386	Colposcopy	57452	GC Screen	87070
		Colposcopy w/Biopsy	57454	Glucose	82947
		Cryosurgery Premalignant Lesion		Glucose 1 HR	82950
		Location (s):		Glycosylated HGB A1C	83036
Established Patient		Cryosurgery Warts		HCT	85014
Post-Op Follow Up Visit	99024	Location (s):		HDL	83718
Minimum	99211	Curettement Lesion		Hep BSAG	87340
Problem Focused	(99212)	Single	11055	Hepatitis panel, acute	80074
Expanded Problem Focused	99213	2–4	11056	HGB	85018
Detailed	99214	>4	11057	HIV	86703
Comprehensive/High Complex	99215	Diaphragm Fitting	57170	Iron & TIBC	83550
Well Exam Infant (up to 12 mos.)	99391	Ear Irrigation	69210	Kidney Profile	80069
Well exam 1–4 yrs.	99392	ECG	93000	Lead	83655
Well Exam 5–11 yrs.	99393	Endometrial Biopsy	58100	Liver Profile	80076
Well Exam 12–17 yrs.	99394	Exc. Lesion Malignant		Mono Test	86308
Well Exam 18–39 yrs.	99395	Benign		Pap Smear	88155
Well Exam 40–64 yrs.	99396	Location		Pregnancy Test	84703
Obstetrics		Exc. Skin Tags (1–15)	11200	Obstetric Panel	80055
Total OB Care	59400	Each Additional 10	11201	Pro Time	85610
Injections		Fracture Treatment		PSA	84153
Administration Sub. / IM	90772	Loc		RPR	86592
Drug		w/Reduc w/o Reduc		Sed. Rate	85651
Dosage		I & D Abscess Single/Simple	10060	Stool Culture	87045
Allergy	95115	Multiple or Comp	10061	Stool O & P	87177
Cocci Skin Test	86490	I & D Pilonidal Cyst Simple	10080	Strep Screen	87880
DPT	90701	Pilonidal Cyst Complex	10081	Theophylline	80198
Hemophilus	90646	IV Therapy—To One Hour	90760	Thyroid Uptake	84479
Influenza	90658	Each Additional Hour	90761	TSH	84443
MMR	90707	Laceration Repair		Urinalysis	81000
OPV	90712	Location Size Simp/Comp		Urine Culture	87088
Pneumovax	90732	Laryngoscopy	31505	Drawing Fee	36415
TB Skin Test	86580	Oximetry	94760	Specimen Collection	99000
TD	90718	Punch Biopsy		**Other:**	
Unlisted Immun	90749	Rhythm Strip	93040		
Tetanus Toxoid	90703	Treadmill	93015		
Vaccine/Toxoid Admin <8 Yr Old w/ Counseling	90465	Trigger Point or Tendon Sheath Inj.	20550		
Vaccine/Toxoid Administration for Adult	90471	Tympanometry	92567		
Diagnosis/ICD-9: **Exposure to Chicken Pox**		**Fever, Rash**			

I acknowledge receipt of medical services and authorize the release of any medical information necessary to process this claim for healthcare payment only. I do authorize payment to the provider.

Patient Signature *Jonny Boiler*

Total Estimated Charges: _____

Payment Amount: _____

Next Appointment: _____

FIGURE 13-3   Encounter Form #2

Physician Note:

S: Established patient Jonny Boiler presents with exposure to chicken pox at his school, fever, and rash that itches.

O: Jonny has fever of 101.2; apparent red rash (looks similar to chicken pox); had vaccine as a young child. No other dermatological instigators suspected.

A: Probable Chicken pox, fever, rash.

P: Stay away from others until sores are scabbed over; drink plenty of fluids, Tylenol for the fever and over the counter anti-itch medications. Recheck in 2 weeks if not resolved will do chicken pox titer.

Patient: Jonny Boiler   **Medical Record Number:** 201556

FIGURE 13-4   Physician Note #2

Patient Name **Mark Lapooze**

Capital City Medical
123 Unknown Boulevard, Capital City, NY 12345-2222

Date of Service
MM/DD/CCYY

New Patient			Arthrocentesis/Aspiration/Injection		Laboratory	
Problem Focused	99201		Arthrocentesis/Aspiration/Injection		Amylase	82150
Expanded Problem, Focused	99202		Small Joint	20600	B12	82607
Detailed	99203		Interm Joint	20605	CBC & Diff	85025
Comprehensive	99204		Major Joint	20610	Comp Metabolic Panel	80053
Comprehensive/High Complex	99205		**Other Invasive/Noninvasive**		Chlamydia Screen	87110
Well Exam Infant (up to 12 mos.)	99381		Audiometry	92552	Cholesterol	82465
Well Exam 1–4 yrs.	99382		Cast Application		Digoxin	80162
Well Exam 5–11 yrs.	99383		Location Long Short		Electrolytes	80051
Well Exam 12–17 yrs.	99384		Catheterization	51701	Ferritin	82728
Well Exam 18–39 yrs.	99385		Circumcision	54150	Folate	82746
Well Exam 40–64 yrs.	99386		Colposcopy	57452	GC Screen	87070
			Colposcopy w/Biopsy	57454	Glucose	82947
			Cryosurgery Premalignant Lesion		Glucose 1 HR	82950
			Location (s):		Glycosylated HGB A1C	83036
Established Patient			Cryosurgery Warts		HCT	85014
Post-Op Follow Up Visit	99024		Location (s):		HDL	83718
Minimum	99211		Curettement Lesion		Hep BSAG	87340
Problem Focused	99212		Single	11055	Hepatitis panel, acute	80074
Expanded Problem Focused	99213		2–4	11056	HGB	85018
Detailed	(99214)		>4	11057	HIV	86703
Comprehensive/High Complex	99215		Diaphragm Fitting	57170	Iron & TIBC	83550
Well Exam Infant (up to 12 mos.)	99391		Ear Irrigation	69210	Kidney Profile	80069
Well exam 1–4 yrs.	99392		ECG	93000	Lead	83655
Well Exam 5–11 yrs.	99393		Endometrial Biopsy	58100	Liver Profile	80076
Well Exam 12–17 yrs.	99394		Exc. Lesion Malignant		Mono Test	86308
Well Exam 18–39 yrs.	99395		Benign		Pap Smear	88155
Well Exam 40–64 yrs.	99396		Location		Pregnancy Test	84703
Obstetrics			Exc. Skin Tags (1–15)	11200	Obstetric Panel	80055
Total OB Care	59400		Each Additional 10	11201	Pro Time	85610
Injections			Fracture Treatment		PSA	84153
Administration Sub. / IM	90772		Loc		RPR	86592
Drug			w/Reduc w/o Reduc		Sed. Rate	85651
Dosage			I & D Abscess Single/Simple	10060	Stool Culture	87045
Allergy	95115		Multiple or Comp	10061	Stool O & P	87177
Cocci Skin Test	86490		I & D Pilonidal Cyst Simple	10080	Strep Screen	87880
DPT	90701		Pilonidal Cyst Complex	10081	Theophylline	80198
Hemophilus	90646		IV Therapy—To One Hour	90760	Thyroid Uptake	84479
Influenza	90658		Each Additional Hour	90761	TSH	84443
MMR	90707		Laceration Repair		Urinalysis	81000
OPV	90712		Location Size Simp/Comp		Urine Culture	87088
Pneumovax	90732		Laryngoscopy	31505	Drawing Fee	36415
TB Skin Test	86580		Oximetry	94760	Specimen Collection	99000
TD	90718		Punch Biopsy		**Other:**	
Unlisted Immun	90749		Rhythm Strip	93040		
Tetanus Toxoid	90703		Treadmill	93015	**Pain Meds Rx**	
Vaccine/Toxoid Admin <8 Yr Old w/ Counseling	90465		Trigger Point or Tendon Sheath Inj.	20550	**Ultrasound/CT of Low Back**	
Vaccine/Toxoid Administration for Adult	90471		Tympanometry	92567	**R/O Kidney Stones**	

Diagnosis/ICD-9: **Low Back pain**

I acknowledge receipt of medical services and authorize the release of any medical information necessary to process this claim for healthcare payment only. I do authorize payment to the provider.

Patient Signature *Mark Lapooze*

Total Estimated Charges: _____

Payment Amount: _____

Next Appointment: _____

FIGURE 13-5 Encounter Form #3

Physician Note:

S: Established patient Mark Lapooze presents with lower back pain that comes and goes in "waves." Has worsened over past 24 hours. Not relieved by OTC pain medications or resting.

O: Mark's vital signs are WNL. Area that is sore is not consistent with muscular pain, not red, not inflamed, but patient in pain.

A: Unknown etiology of back pain.

P: Script for pain medications, referral to E.R. for ultrasound of back and/or CT scan. Spent 45 minutes with patient ruling out other diagnoses through history and physical.

Patient: Mark Lapooze   **Medical Record Number:** 201775

FIGURE 13-6   Physician Note #3

Final Claim Audit

Medicare audits are triggered by errors, the majority of which are claims that lack justification for medically necessity as required by Medicare guidelines. The claims must be reviewed for documentation to show the appropriateness and necessity of the treatment provided to the patient. When you are examining the claim for proper coding, review the E/M code for the accurate level of history obtained and the extent of examination performed. After it has been determined that the E/M code is correct, the claim is sent for processing.

> ▶ **CRITICAL THINKING QUESTION:** What should a medical biller or health claims examiner do when an encounter form indicates diagnoses and/or procedures that do not match the documentation in the medical record?

ACTIVITY #4

Extent of History and Examination

Directions: From the documentation provided, determine the E/M extent of history and extent of examination.

(See Figure 13-7 ●.)

1. Extent of History, #1: _____
2. Extent of Examination, #1: _____

(See Figure 13-8 ●.)

3. Extent of History, #2: _____
4. Extent of Examination, #2: _____

(See Figure 13-9 ●.)

5. Extent of History, #3: _____
6. Extent of Examination, #3: _____

History of Present Illness: This is a 41-year-old Caucasian man with no apparent past medical history who presented to the emergency room with the chief complaint of weakness, malaise and dyspnea on exertion for approximately one month. The patient also reports a 19-pound weight loss. He denies fever, chills and sweats. He denies cough and diarrhea.

Past Medical History: Essentially unremarkable except for chest wall cysts which apparently have been biopsied by a dermatologist in the past, and he was given a benign diagnosis. He had a recent PPD which was negative in August 1994.

Medications: None

Allergies: NKDA

Social History: He occasionally drinks and is a nonsmoker. The patient participated in homosexual activity in Haiti during the 1980's which he described as "very active". Denies IV drug use. The patient is currently employed full-time.

Family History: Unremarkable.

Physical Examination:

General: Thin, cachectic man speaking in full sentences with 2L oxygen.

Vital Signs: BP: 96/56; P: 120; Temp: 101.6; R: 30.

HEENT: All WNL except has oral thrush.

Lymph: He has marked adenopathy including right bilateral epitrochlear and posterior cervical nodes.

Neck: No goiter, no jugular venous distention.

Chest: Bilateral basilar crackles, and egophony at the right and left middle lung fields.

Heart: Regular rate and rhythm, no murmur, rub or gallop.

Abdomen: Soft and nontender.

Genitourinary: Normal.

Rectal: Unremarkable.

Skin: Multiple, subcutaneous mobile nodules on the chest wall that are non-tender.

Laboratory: Sodium 133, potassium 5.3, BUN 29, creatinine 1.8. Hemoglobin 14, white count 7100, platelet count 515. Total protein 10, albumin 3.1, AST 131, ALT 31. Urinalysis shows 1+ protein, trace blood. Total bilirubin 2.4, bilirubin 0.1. Arterial blood gases: pH 7.46, pCO_2 32, pO_2 46 on room air.

X-Ray Data: Electrocardiogram shows normal sinus rhythm. Chest x-ray shows bilateral alveolar and interstitial infiltrates.

Assessment:
1. Bilateral pneumonia; suspect atypical pneumonia, rule-out pneumocystis carinii pneumonia and tuberculosis.
2. Thrush.
3. Elevated unconjugated bilirubins.
4. Hepatitis.
5. Elevated globulin fraction.
6. Renal insufficiency.
7. Subcutaneous nodules.
8. Risky sexual behavior in 1982 in Haiti.

Plan:
1. Induced sputum, rule out pneumocystis carinii pneumonia nad tuberculosis.
2. Begin intravenous Bactrim and erythromycin.
3. Begin prednisone.
4. Oxygen.
5. Nystatin swish and swallow.
6. Dermatologic biopsy of lesions.
7. Check HIV and RPR.
8. Administer Pneumovax, tetanus shot and Heptavax if indicated.

FIGURE 13-7   History and Physical #1

Chief Complaint: This is the 3rd hospital admission for this 80 year old woman with a long history of hypertension who presented with the chief complaint of substernal "toothache like" chest pain of 12 hours duration.

History of Present Illness: Female is a retired nurse with a long history of hypertension that was previously well controlled on diuretic therapy. She was first admitted to the hospital in 2005 when she presented with a complaint of intermittent midsternal chest pain. Her electrocardiogram at that time showed first degree atrioventricular block, and a chest X-ray showed mild pulmonary congestion, with cardiomegaly. Myocardial infarction was ruled out by the lack of electrocardiographic and cardiac enzyme abnormalities. Patient was discharged after a brief stay on a regimen of enalapril, and lasix, and digoxin, for presumed congestive heart failure. Since then she has been followed closely by a cardiologist.

Aside from hypertension, the patient denies other coronary artery disease risk factors, such as diabetes, cigarette smoking, hypercholesterolemia or family history for heart disease. Since her previous admission, she describes a stable two pillow orthopnea, dyspnea on exertion after walking one block, and a mild ankle edema which is worse when she stands for a long period of time. She denies syncope, paroxysmal nocturnal dyspnea, or recent chest pains.

She was well until 11pm on the night prior to admission when she noted the onset of "aching pain under her breast bone" while sitting, watching television. The pain was described as "heavy" and "toothache" like. She denied nausea, vomiting, diaphoresis, palpitations, dizziness, or loss of consciousness. She took 2 tablespoon of antacid without relief, but did manage to fall sleep. In the morning she awoke free of pain, however upon walking to the bathroom, the pain returned with increased severity. At this time she called her son, who gave her an aspirin and brought her immediately to the emergency room. Her electrocardiogram on presentation showed sinus tachycardia at 110, with marked ST elevation in leads I, AVL, V4-V6 and occasional ventricular paroxysmal contractions. Patient immediately received thrombolytic therapy and cardiac medications, and was transferred to the intensive care unit.

Current Medications
Kcl 20mg once daily
Digoxin 0.125mg once daily
Enalapril 20mg twice daily
Tylenol 2 tabs twice daily PRN
Lasix 40mg once every other day

Medical History
General: Relatively good
Infectious Diseases: Usual childhood illnesses. No history of rheumatic fever.
Immunizations: Flu vaccine yearly. Pneumovax 2006
Allergic to Penicillin-developed a diffuse rash after an injection 20 years ago.
Hospitalizations, Operations, Injuries:
   1) Normal childbirth 48 years ago
   2) 1980 Gastrointestinal hemorrhage, see below
   3) 9/2005 chest pain- see history of present illlness

ROS
1. Constitutional: energy level generally good, weight is stable at 160 lbs, height 5'8"
2. HEENT:
   No headaches
   Eyes: wears reading glasses but thinks vision getting is worse, no diplopia or eye pain
   Ears: hearing loss for many years, wears hearing aid now
   Nose: no epistaxis or obstruction
   No history of tonsillitis or tonsillectomy
   Wears full set of dentures for more than 20 years, works well.
3. Respiratory: No history of pleurisy, cough, wheezing, asthma, hemoptysis, pulmonary emboli, pneumonia, TB or TB exposure
4. Cardiac: See HPI
5. Vascular: No history of claudication, gangrene, deep vein thrombosis, aneurysm. Has chronic venous stasis skin changes for many years

FIGURE 13-8   History and Physical #2

6. G.I.: Admitted to CPMC in 1980 after two days of melena and hematemesis.
   Upper G.I. series was negative but endoscopy showed evidence of gastritis, presumed to be caused by ibuprofen intake. Her hematocrit was 24% on admission and she received four units of packed cells. Colonoscopy revealed multiple diverticuli. Since then her stool has been brown and consistently hematest negative when checked in clinic. Several months after this admission she was noted to be mildly jaundiced and had elevated liver enzymes, at this time it was realized that she contracted hepatitis B from the transfusions. Since then she has not had any evidence of chronic hepatitis.
7. GU: History of several episodes of cystitis, most recently E Coli 3/1/90, treated with Bactrim. Reports dysuria in the 3 days prior to hospitalization. No fever, no hematuria. No history of sexually transmitted disease. Menarche was at 15, menstrual cycles were regular interval and duration, menopause occurred at 54. Seven pregnancies with 5 normal births and 2 miscarriages.
8. Neuromuscular: Osteoarthritis of the both knees, shoulder, and hips for more than 20 years. Took ibruprofen until 1980, has taken acetaminophen since her GI bleed, with good relief of intermittent arthritis pain. There is no history of seizures, stroke, syncope, memory changes.
9. Emotional: Denies history of depression, anxiety.
10. Hematological: no known blood or clotting disorders.
11. Rheumatic: no history of gout, rheumatic arthritis, or lupus.
12. Endocrine: no know diabetes or thyroid disease.
13. Dermatological: no new rashes or pruitis.

Personal History
1. Widowed and lives with one of her daughters.
2. Occupation: she worked as a nurse to age 69, is now retired.
3. Habits: No cigarettes or alcohol. Does not follow any special diet.
4. Born in South Carolina, came to New York in 1931. She has never been outside of the United States.
5. Present environment: lives in a one bedroom apartment on the third floor of a building with and elevator.
6. Financial: Receives social security and Medicare, and is supported by her children.
7. Psychosocial: The patient is generally an alert and active woman despite her arthritic symptoms. She understands that she is having a "heart attack" at the present time and she appears to be extremely anxious.

Family History
The patient was brought up by an aunt; her mother died at the age of 39 from kidney failure; her father died at the age of 47 in a car accident. Her husband died 9 years ago of pneumonia. She has 3 daughters (ages 65, 62, 48) who are all healthy, and one son (age 57) who has hypertension and type 2 diabetes. She has 12 grandchildren, 6 great grandchildren and 4 great, great grandchildren. There is no other known family history of hypertension, diabetes, or cancer.

Physical Exam
1. Vital Signs: temperature 100.2 Pulse 96 regular with occasional extra beat, respiration 24, blood pressure 180/100 lying down
2. Generally a well developed, slightly obese, elderly woman sitting up in bed, breathing with slight difficulty. She complains of resolving chest pain.
3. HEENT:
   a. Eyes: extraocular motions full, gross visual fields full to confrontation, conjunctiva clear. sclerae non-icteric, pulpils equal round and reactive to light and
   b. accomodation, fundi not well visualized due to possible presence of cataracts. Ears: Hearing very poor bilaterally. Tympanic membrane landmarks well
   c. visualized.
   d. Nose: No discharge, no obstruction, septum not deviated.
   e. Mouth: Complete set of upper and lower dentures. Pharynx not injected, no exudates. Uvula moves up in midline. Normal gag reflex.
4. Neck: jugular venous pressure 8cm, thyroid not palpable. No masses.
5. Nodes: No adenopathy

FIGURE 13-8   (*Continued*)

6. Chest: Breasts: atrophic and symmetric, non-tender, no masses or discharges. Lungs: bibasilar rales. No dullness to percussion. Diaphragm moves well with respiration. No rhonchi, wheezes or rubs.

7. Heart: PMI at the 6th ICS, 1 cm lateral to MCL. No heaves or thrills. Regular rhythm with occasional extra beat. Normal S1, S2 narrowly split; positive S4 gallop.
   a. A grade II/VI systolic ejection murmur is heard at the left upper sternal border without radiation.
   b. Pulses are notable for sharp carotid upstrokes.
   c.
Pulses:	Carotid	Brachial	Radial	Femoral	DP	PT
R	2+	2+	2+	2+	1+	0
L	2+	2+	2+	2+	1+	0

8. Spine: mild kyphosis, mobile, non-tender, no costovertebral tenderness

9. Abdomen: soft, flat, bowel sounds present, no bruits. Non-tender to palpation. Liver edge, spleen, kidney not felt. No masses. Liver span 10cm by percussion.

10. Extremities: skin warm and smooth except for chronic venous stasis changes in both legs. 1+ edema to the knees, non-pitting and very tender to palpation. No clubbing nor cyanosis.

11. Neurological: Awake, alert and fully oriented. Cranial nerves III-XII intact except for decreased hearing.

12. Motor: Strength not tested, patient moves all extremities. Sensory: Grossly normal to touch and pin prick.

13. Cerebellar: no tremor nor dysmetria. Reflexes symmetrical 1+ throughout, no Babinski sign.

14. Pelvic: deferred until patient more stable.

15. Rectal: Prominent external hemorrhoids. No masses felt. Stool brown, negative for blood

Labs

WBC: 12,400 Hgb 12.0 Hct 38.0 MCV 80.0 Plts 218,000 Retic 1.3 Diff Na 143 K4.1 C1 103 CO229 Glu 102 BUN 9 Creat 0.8; T bili 0.5 Dbili 0.1 Alk Phos 155 AST 55 ALT 26 LDH 274 CPK 480, MB fraction positive, Troponin 25

U/A   Sp Gr 1.008 pH 6.5 2+ Alb many WBC many RBC 3+ bact

ABG: pH 7.46 pCO234 PO284 O2Sat 98% (room air)

EKG: NSR 96, ST elevations I, AVL, V4-V6; rare unifocal VPC's

CXR: portable AP, probable cardiomegaly, mild PVC

Diagnostic

This 80 year old woman with a history of congestive heart failure, and coronary artery disease risk factors of hypertension and post-menopausal state presents with substernal chest pain. On exam she was found to be in sinus tachycardia, with no JVD, but there are bibasilar rales and pedal edema, suggestive of some degree of congestive heart failure. There were EKG changes indicate an acute anterolateral myocardial infarction, and the labs shows elevation of CPK and troponin.

Assessment

1. Acute anteloraeral myocardioal infarction, complicated by mild left ventricular dysfunction. Patient has received thrombolysis therapy.
2. Hypertension
3. Dysuria - 3+ bacteria in urine with pyuria

Plan

1. Continue aspirin, heparin, nitrates, beta blockers, nasal oxygen. Follow serial physical exams, EKGs, and labs.
2. Obtain echocardiogram to assess post MI heart function and murmurs heard on cardiac exam. If LV ejection fraction is preserved, to start early beta blocker therapy.
3. Continue ACE inhibitor therapy, and monitor blood pressure.
4. Dysuria and pyuria- probable recurrent cystitis, as she is afebrile and without costovertebral tenderness.
5. Start Bactrim treatment for presumed uncomplicated urinary tract infection and follow up on urine culture result.

FIGURE 13-8 (*Continued*)

Chief Complaint: This 65-year-old black male was seen in my office on Month DD, YYYY. Patient was recently discharged from the Hospital after he was treated for pneumonia. Patient continues to have severe orthopnea, paroxysmal nocturnal dyspnea, cough with greenish expectoration. His exercise tolerance is about two to three yards for shortness of breath. The patient stopped taking Coumadin for reasons not very clear to him. He was documented to have recent atrial fibrillation. Patient has longstanding history of ischemic heart disease, end-stage LV systolic dysfunction, and is status post ICD implantation. Fasting blood sugar this morning is 130.

Physical Examination:

VITAL SIGNS:	Blood pressure is 120/60. Respirations 18 per minute. Heart rate 75-85 beats per minute, irregular. Weight 207 pounds.
HEENT:	Head normocephalic. Eyes, no evidence of anemia or jaundice. Oral hygiene is good.
NECK:	Supple. JVP is flat. Carotid upstroke is good.
LUNGS:	Severe inspiratory and expiratory wheezing heard throughout the lung fields. Fine crepitations heard at the base of the lungs on both sides.
CARDIOVASCULAR:	PMI felt in fifth left intercostal space 0.5-inch lateral to midclavicular line. First and second heart sounds are normal in character. There is a II/VI systolic murmur best heard at the apex.
ABDOMEN:	Soft. There is no hepatosplenomegaly.
EXTREMITIES:	Patient has 1+ pedal edema.

Current Medications:
1. Ambien 10 mg at bedtime PRN
2. Coumadin 7.5 mg daily.
3. Diovan 320 mg daily.
4. Lantus insulin 50 units in the morning.
5. Lasix 80 mg daily.
6. Novolin R p.r.n.
7. Toprol XL 100 mg daily.
8. Flovent 100 mcg twice a day.

Assessment
1. Atherosclerotic coronary vascular disease with old myocardial infarction.
2. Moderate to severe LV systolic dysfunction.
3. Diabetes mellitus.
4. Diabetic nephropathy and renal failure.
5. Status post ICD implantation.
6. New onset of atrial fibrillation.
7. Chronic Coumadin therapy.

Plan
1. Continue present therapy.
2. Patient will be seen again in my office in four weeks.

FIGURE 13-9   History and Physical #3

Postaudit Review

After a Medicare audit, results are sent to the organization for review and acceptance or appeal. The audit can be a learning experience for those who are documenting and coding claims. Linking the error to its cause is the first step in creating a plan for better documentation. The second step is educating the documentation staff about the changes the need to be made to secure the appropriate reimbursement amount. Figure 13-10 ● shows a claim that was originally approved by Medicare, then denied by a Medicare audit. Medicare is seeking repayment for the claim. The reason for this Medicare audit finding can be seen in Figure 13-11 ●. In the history and description of the physical examination of this new patient, it is clear that although the multiple diagnoses justify a potential extensive Medical Decision Making, the amount of data reviewed and the risk of morbidity or morality did not justify it; thus, the E/M code should have been 99204 rather than 99205. The incorrect code caused Medicare to overpay the claim.

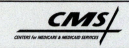

Medicare Summary Notice

July 1, 2012

BENEFICIARY NAME
STREET ADDRESS
CITY, STATE   ZIP CODE

CUSTOMER SERVICE INFORMATION

Your Medicare Number: 111-11-1111A

If you have questions, write or call:
Medicare (#12345)
555 Medicare Blvd., Suite 200
Medicare Building
Medicare, US XXXXX-XXXX

Call: 1-800-MEDICARE (1-800-633-4227)
Ask for Hospital Services
TTY for Hearing Impaired: 1-877-486-2048

BE INFORMED: Beware of "free" medical services or products. If it sounds too good to be true, it probably is.

This is a summary of claims processed from 05/10/2012 through 08/10/2012.

PART A HOSPITAL INSURANCE – INPATIENT CLAIMS

Dates of Service	Benefit Days Used	Non-Covered Charges	Deductible and Coinsurance	You May Be Billed	See Notes Section
	0	$0.00	$0.00	$0.00	
	0	$0.00	$0.00	$0.00	

PART B MEDICAL INSURANCE – OUTPATIENT FACILITY CLAIMS

Dates of Service	Services Provided	Amount Charged	Non-Covered Charges	Deductible and Coinsurance	You May Be Billed	See Notes Section
Claim Number: 12435-8956-8458						
Medicare Hospital, 123 Medicare Lane, Dallas, TX 75209						
Referred by: N/A						
05/10/CCYY						
	E/M 99205 New Patient	293.00	0.00	58.60	58.60	
	Claim Total	**$293.00**	**$0.00**	**$58.60**	**$58.60**	

(continued)

FIGURE 13-10   Medicare Summary Notice

July 1, 2012

Your Medicare Number: 111-11-1111A

Notes Section:

Deductible Information:

You have met the Part A deductible for this benefit period.

You have met the Part B deductible for 2012.

You have met the blood deductible for 2012.

General Information:

You have the right to make a request in writing for an itemized statement which details each Medicare item or service which you have received from your physician, hospital, or any other health supplier or health professional. Please contact them directly, in writing, if you would like an itemized statement.

Compare the services you receive with those that appear on your Medicare Summary Notice. If you have questions, call your doctor or provider. If you feel further investigation is needed due to possible fraud and abuse, call the phone number in the Customer Service Information Box.

Appeals Information – Part A (Inpatient) and Part B (Outpatient)

If you disagree with any claims decisions on either Part A or Part B of this notice, your appeal must be received by **November 1, 2006**. Follow the instructions below:

1) Circle the item(s) you disagree with and explain why you disagree.

2) Send this notice, or a copy, to the address in the "Customer Service Information" box on Page 1. (You may also send any additional information you may have about your appeal.)

3) Sign here _____   Phone number _____

Revised 08/06

FIGURE 13-10   *(Continued)*

Annette Adams
Address
Phone Number

Date: 00/00/CCYY

RE: MAC Audit due to out of proportion high level E/M codes.

Overpayment

Provider was overpaid in several instances due to upcoding E/M codes. Corrective action recommended includes: education of practitioners about documentation of decision making complexity and extent of examination; biller education of interpretation of documentation and use of E/M codes. A QA committee should be established to review claims prior to submission

Claim Findings

The findings for each claim in the sample, including a specific explanation of why any services were determined to be non-covered or incorrectly coded would be listed here. For the purpose of this example only one case is shown:

Claim number: 12435-8956-8458

In the history and physical of this new patient, it is clear that although the multiple diagnoses justify a potential extensive Medical Decision Making, the amount of data reviewed and the risk of morbidity or morality did not; thus, the E/M code should have been 99204 versus 99205 resulting in an overpayment by Medicare.

General Information:

You have the right to make a request in writing for an itemized statement which details each Medicare item or service which you have received from your physician, hospital, or any other health supplier or health professional. Please contact them directly, in writing, if you would like an itemized statement.

Compare the services you receive with those that appear on your Medicare Summary Notice. If you have questions, call your doctor or provider. If you feel further investigation is needed due to possible fraud and abuse, call the phone number in the Customer Service Information Box.

General Information:

If you have and questions, feel to contact us.

Center for Medicare and Medicaid Services

FIGURE 13-11 Medicare Audit Findings

PRACTICE **PITFALLS**

After a Medicare audit, the employees involved are likely to be anxious to correct claims and may undercode to avoid making the same mistakes as the ones that were found in the audit. Unfortunately, Medicare auditors will not upcode claims that are found to be undercoded. Therefore, it is important to maintain a standard of coding practices that allow for accuracy and best reimbursement on Medicare claims.

ACTIVITY #5

Learning from Postaudit Findings

Directions: Assume that the following report is a portion of an audit received from a Medicare audit. Determine five items that would need to be included in a training session on improving documentation to justify service provided.

Recommended Education Items. (See Figure 13-12 ●.)

1. _____
2. _____

3. _____
4. _____
5. _____

Recommended Education Items. (See Figure 13-13 ●.)

1. _____
2. _____
3. _____
4. _____
5. _____

Overpayment: Ventilator Support of 96+ hours—Ventilation hours begin with the intubation of the patient (or time of admittance if the patient is admitted while on mechanical ventilation) and continue until the endotracheal tube is removed, the patient is discharged/transferred, or the ventilation is discontinued after a weaning period. Provider is improperly adding the number of ventilator hours resulting in higher reimbursement. (Incorrect Coding).

Overpayment: Durable Medical Equipment, Prosthetics, Orthotics, and Supplies (DMEPOS) Provided During an Inpatient Stay- Medicare does not make separate payment for DMEPOS when a beneficiary is in a covered inpatient stay. Supplier is inappropriately receiving separate DMEPOS payment when the beneficiary is in a covered inpatient stay. (Billing for Bundled Services Separately).

FIGURE 13-12 Medicare Example Audit #1

Overpayment: Extensive Operating Room Procedure Unrelated to Principal Diagnosis—The principal diagnosis and principal procedure codes for an inpatient claim should be related. Errors occur when providers bill an incorrect principal and/or secondary diagnosis that results in an incorrect Medicare Severity Diagnosis-Related Group assignment. (Incorrect Coding)

Overpayment: Durable Medical Equipment, Prosthetics, Orthotics, and Supplies (DMEPOS) Provided During an Inpatient Stay- Medicare does not make separate payment for DMEPOS when a beneficiary is in a covered inpatient stay. Supplier is inappropriately billing for services performed after the date of death.

FIGURE 13-13 Medicare Example Audit #2

Electronic Billing Systems

For the most part, the billing and tracking of claims is done electronically. Different software programs have varying abilities to identify discrepancies in a claim, but a computer program is not able to review a chart note and determine whether it justifies the coding on the bill. This is why continual internal auditing is so important. Turnover in the medical staff who are doing the documenting presents a new challenge to the claims examiner, who must identify any gaps in the new employees' documentation to support appropriate billing. Already, there are electronic documentation programs that walk the documenter through each stage of documentation, requiring him or her to answer each question that leads to a determination of the E/M code. If a documenter is using this type of program and a Medicare audit shows disagreement with the automated coding, a more in-depth claims audit and training on use of the software will be required.

Requests for Supplemental Information

When the processor on the Medicare end receives a Medicare claim, he or she may determine that there is insufficient information on the claim to process it. In this situation, the claim is sent back to the provider with a request for more information. Prioritizing these requests will ensure timely payment. The supplemental information that is requested commonly includes the current history and physical, encounter note, extended information on the facts of an injury, and results of lab or other diagnostic reports. Keeping a log of issues from these requests is also a way to avoid making the same error in coding future claims. See Table 13-2 ● for an example log.

▶ CRITICAL THINKING QUESTION: If you find a pattern of documentation lacking sufficient information to accurately code a claim, as a medical biller what are your options?

TABLE 13-2 Log of Claim Errors

Date	Error	Education Provided	Comments/ Follow-up
2/15/CCYY	Lack of documentation to support medical necessity for Diabetic Labs	Physicians provided a checklist for documentation of medical necessity for labs	
3/5/CCYY	Denied preventative women's service, less than one year	Schedulers trained to check for last date of annual exam before scheduling routine annual exams	

ACTIVITY #6

Supplemental Information

Directions: Match the request with the probable document that would contain the requested information.

Request

1. Medicare is always last payer. Claim diagnosis is _____ (fracture of foot). Please provide explanation of how this injury occurred to rule out other insurance liability.
2. Payment for similar service was already made for this date. Please provide modifier and documentation of duplicate service.
3. This screening test is only covered if medically necessary. Please provide medical necessity documentation.
4. Plastic surgery is not covered as an elective procedure. Please provide indication for surgery for claim determination.

Document

a. Add modifier -55 to claim and physician notes for both visits.
b. Labs or other tests with history of symptoms showing need for this screening test.
c. History and physical showing indication for surgery and change diagnosis as appropriate.
d. History gathered from patient documenting injury.

CHAPTER REVIEW

Summary

- Determining the appropriate E/M procedural codes is essential to filing an accurate Medicare claim. Review the extent of history taken at the encounter, the examination time and technicality, and the level of medical decision making that was necessary to verify that the E/M code is correct.
- To identify why a Medicare audit downcoded a service, review the diagnosis and the procedure to ensure that they match. The most frequent audit reason for downcoding is lack of substantiation for the E/M code used.

- To prevent downcoding during an audit, choose key information from the medical record to complete a claim (rather than just using the codes indicated by the practitioner). Reviewing the Medicare claim for accuracy and medical necessity will also prevent declarations of overpayment due to an audit.
- When further information is requested from Medicare, produce the information from the medical record in a timely and thorough manner. This is the opportunity to justify the claim coding and avoid a reduction in payment.

- To ensure that a claim is ready for submission, conduct a team audit in which participants review a part of the claim that they did not initiate.

Review Questions

Directions: Answer the following questions without looking back at the material just covered. Write your answers in the space provided.

Multiple Choice

1. Which of the following criteria is least likely to affect the E/M code chosen by the medical biller?

   a. Extent of history taken at this encounter

   b. Examination time and technicality

   c. Level of medical decision making necessary

   d. Coordination of care conducted at this encounter

2. What medical decision-making criterion provides the highest reimbursement when you are coding E/M of a patient encounter?

   a. Straightforward

   b. Low complexity

   c. High complexity

   d. Problem focused

3. What is the first step in addressing postaudit findings?

   a. Review claims for audit findings validity.

   b. Review claims for underlying documentation issues.

   c. Create an education plan for practitioners and medical billers.

   d. Repay Medicare monies owed.

4. What key item(s) are important to pick out of a history and physical note written during an encounter?

   a. The extent of information gathered

   b. The time spent with the patient

   c. The level of complexity of decision making to reach the diagnosis

   d. The treatment plan

5. Which of the following diagnoses coded on a Medicare claim is likely to be returned with a request for supplemental information?

   a. Diabetes

   b. Hip fracture

   c. Influenza

   d. Face-lift

True/False

6. The information required on a Medicare claim is the same as any health insurance claim.

7. E/M codes are directly related to the time that the physician spends in the exam room with the patient.

8. If a patient is new, it does not affect the E/M coding.

9. A Medicare audit is required by law for every healthcare facility.

10. Internal audits to prepare for Medicare audits are necessary.

After completing this chapter, you will be able to:

- Identify potential workers' compensation (WC) claims from history and physical.

- Use the appropriate form to request information from a patient when there is a possible WC claim.

- Review physician notes to complete a Doctor's First Report of Injury.

- Review physician notes to complete progress reports and termination of treatment.

- List the steps to investigate WC claims for legitimacy.

- Recognize when previous diagnoses could have an effect on the validity of a WC claim.

- Determine appropriate diagnoses to submit a clean claim to a WC insurance agency.

Continuing our exploration of health claims examining, this chapter covers the duties of a medical biller working for a provider or as a workers' compensation (WC) claims examiner. The activities in the chapter will provide practice for a biller in screening claims for potential WC issues, gathering information for the Doctor's First Report of Injury or for Right to Work letters, and gathering progress report information to supplement claims. We also cover the steps of investigating a claim, which will be of interest to claims adjusters. Finally, this chapter reviews the clean claim criteria for a WC claim.

Workers' Compensation—The Billing Perspective

As previously discussed in this text, there are specific requirements for billing WC claims. If the provider is not an approved WC provider for that particular insurance company, payment could be delayed and/or denied. WC laws allow the patient to choose from a variety of approved WC physicians, but sometimes workers go to their primary care physician without considering the overall WC process. Therefore, it is important for medical billers to watch for common diagnoses that could be work related and thus denied by the patient's primary insurance.

These diagnoses involve injuries from slips, falls, lifting, chemical spills, inhalation of noxious fumes, or cuts. Occupations with the most dangerous WC injuries include construction, agriculture, forestry, fishing, and mining. The most common causes of injuries are falls, faulty equipment, or misuse of equipment. When you see that an injury is caused by one of these most common reasons, make sure you identify whether the injury potentially falls under WC.

ACTIVITY #1

Identifying Potential Workers' Compensation Claims

Directions: Indicate WC next to the diagnosis if it is a potential WC claim and an X next to the diagnoses that are unlikely to be potential WC claims.

1. 163 _____
2. 140-239 _____
3. 799.01 _____
4. 799.02 _____
5. 836.2 _____
6. 847.9 _____
7. 354. _____
8. 389.9 _____
9. 940.2 _____
10. 750.6 _____
11. 346.40 _____
12. 728.71 _____
13. 782.1 _____
14. 584.9 _____
15. 070.30 _____

Doctor's First Report

As discussed in Chapter 9, the first step in processing a WC claim is completing the Doctor's First Report of Injury report. This report includes the following information:

- Date, time, and location of the injury/illness
- Treatment provided
- Patient's subjective complaints
- Physician's objective findings
- Diagnosis
- Treatment plan
- Whether the worker can return to work and, if so, at what level

It is important for the biller to be able to identify these items in a physician note so that the report can be presented to the insurance company and/or employer in a timely manner. Some patients may make different decisions about medical treatment depending on who is paying for the care.

ACTIVITY #2

Preparing a Doctor's First Report

Directions: For the following three physician notes (shown in Figure 14-1 ●, Figure 14-2 ●, and Figure 14-3 ●), pick out the appropriate information and complete a Doctor's First Report using the forms in Appendix B.

Physician Note #1

Patient Name: _____   Date: _____

S: 33-year-old, female patient presents with lower back pain after sustaining a fall at work. Patient states, "I was mopping the floor when I slipped and fell backwards." The patient indicates shooting pain down her legs starting from the lower back area. She reports no tingling or numbness.

O: Upon examination, the patient is tender in the lower back area; there is no bruising or redness and no change in skin temperature. Movement is restricted when bending forward or side to side. No other issues with any system are reported.

A: Probable lower back sprain from fall at work today 10:30 a.m.

P: Ice, ibuprofen, and physical therapy referral. RTW on modified duty tomorrow.

Annette Adams, M.D.

FIGURE 14-1   Example Physician Note #1 (for Activity #2)

Physician Note #2

S: 21-year-old male presents at clinic with reported cut on his right index finger. Patient reports that he obtained the cut at work where he is a prep cook. He reports that the incident occurred at 1:00 p.m. today.

O: Upon examination, the right index finger has been cut 10 cm long and 3 cm wide with what appears to be tendon damage.

A: Tendon damage and laceration to right index finger consistent with knife cut. Will require surgery to fix the tendon and repair the damage from the cut. Surgery scheduled for two days from today. Patient will be unable to work until finger healed enough to get wet. Approximately 2 weeks.

P: Surgery scheduled, patient instructed to keep clean area and dry. Bandage provided.

Annette Adams, M.D.

FIGURE 14-2   Example Physician Note #2 (for Activity #2)

Physician Note #3

S: 62-year-old female arrived at Urgent Care complaining of hip pain. Patient states she fell at 2:00 a.m. walking to her car after work. She reports that there was ice on the parking lot and the lighting was poor.

O: Upon examination and X-ray, the left hip is broken and will require surgical reduction and subsequent immobilization and rehabilitation.

A: Left hip fracture from fall. Surgery pending, patient will be unable to work for approximately 6 weeks.

P: Surgery scheduled, patient will be admitted to the hospital for surgery and aftercare.

Annette Adams, M.D.

FIGURE 14-3   Example Physician Note #3 (for Activity #2)

Progress Reports and Termination of Treatment

Another important piece of WC claims is timely notification of the WC Agency of patient progress, missed appointments, and ending of treatment due to satiation in progress. The biller is often asked to prepare progress reports and termination of treatment information for the agency.

ACTIVITY #3

Progress Reports

Directions: Using the following physician notes (shown in Figure 14-4 ●, Figure 14-5 ●, and Figure 14-6 ●), complete a progress report for each of the three patients. Use the forms provided in Appendix B.

Workmans' Compensation Claim # 10000001

Patient:

S: Patient has been seen by PT for 3 visits. She has been working FT on modified duty. Patient states her back feels fine and she no longer wants to continue in PT.

O: Strength testing completed and patient appears back to base line.

A: Healed lower back sprain from fall at work.

P: Stop PT, return to work FT no restrictions.

Annette Adams, M.D.

FIGURE 14-4   Physician's Progress Note #1 (for Activity #3)

Physician's Progress Note

S: Patient reports difficulty in bending his finger. Has been attending PT 2 times a week and his surgeon tells him he needs to do the PT exercises so his finger will maintain joint movement.

O: Patient PT records show that he has not shown progress in movement of the affected joint in his finger. PT relates this to the lack of home exercises for the patient. Patient unable to bend finger joint. No other problems or concerns.

A: Patient needs to utilize the PT and homework assignments from PT for finger to heal properly. Suggest PT be increased to 3 times a week. Reevaluate 1 week. Continue PT and home exercises.

P: Postop therapy has been unsuccessful, need to increase frequency of PT for another week or so. May return to work full duty.

Annette Adams, M.D.

FIGURE 14-5   Physician's Progress Note #2 (for Activity #3)

Physician's Progress Note

S: Patient is postoperative from a hip fracture repair 2 weeks ago. Patient states that she has mild pain but is able to participate in her PT without difficulty.

O: Upon examination, patient is doing remarkably well for a S/P hip fracture. No signs and symptoms of infection or complication.

P: Patient requires at least 2 more weeks of PT before she can return to work. Must be able to tolerate sitting for 8 hours. Could return to work part-time if PT clears for sitting time of part-time work as receptionist.

Annette Adams, M.D.

FIGURE 14-6 Physician's Progress Note #3 (for Activity #3)

Investigating Workers' Compensation Claims

For medical providers, WC is a risk because the payer of record is unknown until the claim is reviewed and approved by the WC insurance company. This process can take time because the WC insurance agency wants to make sure the claim is legitimate. The insurance company's own claims investigators investigate the claim for evidence of fraud.

Interviews

One method of investigating an injury is interviewing the witnesses to the injury, including coworkers, the employer, and possibly police, family, and friends. They can provide information about what happened and how the claimant's life has been altered by the injury. The witnesses may have already submitted a statement that the investigator will clarify for validation of the claim.

Records Review

Part of investigating a WC claim is reviewing the claimant's medical records for previous injuries or conditions that could invalidate the WC claim. In some cases, the claims adjuster will require an evaluation from an independent physician to add an unbiased medical opinion to the file.

Writing Reports

After the investigation is complete, the claims investigator evaluates the information that he or she has found and writes a report summarizing the findings. This report will include the investigator's determination of the validity of the claim and whether the WC insurance company is responsible for paying the claim.

FINISHING THE CLAIM. If the claim is approved, the claim investigator works with the claimant to determine the settlement payment. If the claim is denied, the adjuster consults with the insurance company's attorney or legal department in the event that the case goes to court. A case manager (usually a registered nurse) may be assigned to supervise and coordinate all care in the case. If the case goes to court, the medical adjuster works with expert witnesses and the attorneys to defend the company's decision.

ACTIVITY #4

Preparing for a Claims Investigation

Directions: Take on the role of the claims investigator for the WC claim situations in the previous activities. Create a list of items to be reviewed and potential parties to be interviewed to determine the validity of each of the claims.

Patient #1: Lower back pain from fall
Records to Review: _____
_____
_____
People to Interview: _____
_____
_____

Patient #2: Cut tendon of index finger
Records to Review: _____
_____
People to Interview: _____
_____
_____

Patient #3: Hip pain from slipping on ice and falling
Records to Review: _____
_____
People to Interview: _____
_____
_____

ACTIVITY #5

Denial of Workers' Compensation Claim

Directions: Continuing the previous activity, what findings would cause suspicion of fraud or inappropriate assignment to WC in each of the cases?

Patient #1: Lower back pain from fall _____

_____

_____

Patient #2: Cut tendon on index finger _____

_____

_____

Patient #3: Hip pain after slipping on ice and falling

_____

_____

_____

Workers' Compensation Clean Claims Criteria

WC claims are filed in the same manner as regular health insurance or Medicare claims. The difference is that the workers' compensation claim will need to be reviewed for appropriate diagnosis and procedure coding to justify the treatment provided, and it must indicate where and how the injury occurred.

ACTIVITY #6

Verifying Workers' Compensation Claims

Directions: For each of the three WC claims used throughout this chapter, choose the appropriate diagnostic codes that show the correct coding to ensure the claim is clean.

Patient #1: Lower back pain from fall

Diagnosis Codes: _____

_____

_____

Patient #2: Cut tendon on index finger

Diagnosis Codes: _____

_____

_____

Patient #3: Hip pain after slipping on ice and falling

Diagnosis Codes: _____

_____

_____

ACTIVITY #7

Investigation Reporting

Directions: For each of the scenarios in Figure 14-7 ● and Figure 14-8 ●, write a summary report of your findings as if you are the WC claims examiner who has just concluded an investigation. You can extrapolate to fill in any gaps that you need to complete your report.

Julie is a United States Postal Worker. She sorts the mail and then delivers it on her assigned route. Julie noticed her wrist and elbow hurting while she was sorting the mail. When the pain continued to get worse for about two weeks, she went to her personal physician. She was diagnosed with carpal tunnel syndrome from repetitive movement at work while sorting mail. Julie asked her physician to submit the evaluation to her WC representative at work. The representative took the information and sent her to a WC physician for further evaluation. The WC doctor confirmed that Julie has probable carpal tunnel syndrome and prescribed rest, anti-inflammatory medication, and a wrist brace. The physician released her to go back to work full-time.

During an investigation of the injury, the investigator found that Julie is an avid computer gamer, playing and winning in tournaments. She plays with a game controller that could also be a cause of carpal tunnel syndrome. In addition, the investigator discovered that Julie played in a tournament a week before she went to the doctor for the wrist and elbow pain.

FIGURE 14-7   Case Scenario #1

Allen works in a care center for the elderly. The care center has a "no-lift" policy which dictates that the employees are not supposed to lift a patient alone. Instead, they must use one of the many mechanical lift options deemed right for the patient by the physical therapist. Employees are trained prior to working with patients and then annually are retrained on these procedures. Allen is a strong person who can carry patients or lift them on his own, and as he works the night shift he is able to do things "his way" (which is not using the mechanical lifts as directed in policy).

One night Allen was assisting an elderly woman to the bathroom from her bed. During this transfer, the elderly woman wet herself and a puddle developed on the floor. When Allen took his next step, he slipped and fell in the urine, causing a back injury.

He completed an incident report and went to the emergency room to have his back examined. He went to the WC-authorized emergency room because the office was closed during the night hours when the injury occurred. The X-ray on his back showed that Allen had an acute compression fracture in his back, most likely from the fall. The physician completed the Doctor's First Report of Injury and put Allen on "light duty," meaning he could not do any lifting, bending, or twisting for six weeks.

The care center appealed his WC claim due to findings in the incident report that Allen completed, where he indicated that he was "lifting Miss Jones out of the bed to help her to the bathroom." The employee handbook states that if employees are injured when they are not following policy and procedure, the injury will not be covered by WC.

FIGURE 14-8   Case Scenario #2

CHAPTER REVIEW

Summary

- The medical biller must be aware of the types of injuries that occur in workplace settings. By knowing the most common injuries, a medical biller can identify WC claims and bill the proper party. This information is found in the history and physical.
- If the medical biller determines that an illness or injury is potentially work related and therefore subject to WC insurance, the medical biller sends a letter with questions that will determine which party to bill for services. WC requires a Doctor's First Report of Injury to be submitted before a case can be approved to be pursued through workers' compensation insurance. Subsequent progress reports and a final termination of treatment are also required. The medical biller may be asked to review physician notes to complete these forms.
- Part of a claims examiner's job may be to investigate the validity of a WC claim. The steps in this process include record reviews, interviews, and writing of a report.
- To avoid paying for fraudulent claims, a WC claims examiner (and medical billers on the provider end) must be diagnostically fluent enough to recognize when previous diagnoses could have an effect on the validity of the WC claim.
- Medical billers and the WC claims examiner should know how to determine that the appropriate diagnosis is being used in a WC claim.

Review Questions

Directions: Using the information in this chapter, answer the following questions.

Multiple Choice

1. What is the most common WC injury?

   a. burns

   b. falls

   c. broken bones

   d. whiplash

2. Which of the following diagnoses is most difficult to determine whether it is a valid WC claim?

   a. lung cancer

   b. chemical burns

   c. sprains and strains

   d. cuts

3. Which of the following people would not likely be interviewed in a WC investigation?

   a. witnesses of the injury

   b. the spouse of the injured worker

c. the employer

d. the treating physician

4. Other than interviewing, what is the claims examiner's best investigative approach?

   a. examining record reviews

   b. replaying the incident

   c. conducting surveillance of the workplace

   d. videotaping the patient at his or her home

5. What should the coding on a WC claim include?

   a. all of the patient's medical history

   b. potential underlying illnesses of the patient

   c. the code for the activity and setting where the injury occurred

   d. rule-out diagnoses that would invalidate the WC claim

True/False

6. It is common for construction workers to be injured on the job.

7. The Doctor's First Report of Injury is the only form that is required to file a WC claim.

8. If WC insurance will not pay for a claim, the federal government can be billed for the charges.

9. A physician does not need to complete a history and physical on a patient who is being seen for a WC claim.

10. Misuse or malfunctioning equipment contributes to WC injuries.

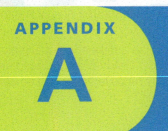

Contracts

Ball Insurance Company Contract

Winter Insurance Company Contract

Summer Insurance Company Contract

BALL INSURANCE CARRIERS

3895 Bubble BOULEVARD, SUITE 283, Boxwood, CO 85926 (970) 555-5432

INSURANCE CONTACT: BETTY BELL

PHONE NUMBER: (970) 555-5433

POLICY: **XYZ CORPORATION**

INSURANCE GROUP # AND SUFFIX: **62958/XYZ**

Basic/Major Medical Plan   **Effective 09/1/CCYY**

Eligibility

EMPLOYEE: Must work a minimum of 30 hours per week. Is eligible for coverage the first of the month following three consecutive months of continuous employment.

DEPENDENTS: Are eligible for coverage from birth to age 26. Not eligible as a dependent if eligible as an employee. Unmarried natural children, legally adopted children, and foster children are included (includes legal guardianship). If both parents are covered by the plan, children may be covered by one employee only.

Effective Date

EMPLOYEE: If written application is made prior to eligibility date, coverage becomes effective the first of the month following three months of continuous employment.

DEPENDENTS: The date acquired by the covered employee becomes the effective date if written application is made within 31 days of eligibility date. If confined in a hospital on date of eligibility, coverage will not start until the first of the month following the date the confinement ends. Newborns are automatically covered for the first 30 days following birth. Coverage will be terminated after 30 days unless written application for coverage is submitted by the employee within 31 days of birth.

Termination of Coverage

EMPLOYEE: Coverage terminates the last day of the month following termination of employment, when the employee ceases to qualify as an eligible employee, or following request for termination of coverage.

DEPENDENTS: Coverage terminates the date the employee's coverage terminates or the last day of the month during which the dependent no longer qualifies as an eligible dependent.

EXCLUSIONS

1. Expenses resulting from self-inflicted injuries.
2. Work-related injuries or illnesses.
3. Services for which there is no charge in the absence of insurance.
4. Charges or services in excess of UCR or not medically necessary.
5. Charges for completion of claim forms and failure to keep appointments.
6. Routine or preventative or experimental services.
7. Eye refractions, contacts or glasses, orthotics (eye exercises), radial keratotomy, or other procedures for surgical correction of refractive errors.
8. Custodial care.
9. Cosmetic surgery unless for repair of an injury or surgery incurred while covered or result of mastectomy.
10. Reversal of voluntary sterilization.
11. Diagnosis or treatment of infertility, including artificial insemination, in vitro fertilization, etc.

Questions: Call **1-800-XXX-XXXX** or visit us at www.insurancecompany.com.
If you do not understand any of the terms used in this form, see the Glossary at www.insuranceterms.gov.

BALL INSURANCE COMPANY

Policy Period: CCYY– CCNY

Plan Type: Basic / Major Medical

Summary of Coverage: What This Plan Covers

Important Questions	Answers	Why This Matters
What is the overall deductible?	$125 / Individual	You must pay this amount out of pocket before Ball Insurance Company will pay any healthcare costs. There is a three-month carryover provision: You can count the money spent on healthcare during the last three months of the year toward your deductible the following year.
	$250 / Family	Two members of the family must meet their deductible before Ball Insurance Company will pay any healthcare costs.
Deductibles for In-Patient Hospitalization services?	$50 / Per Admission	If you are hospitalized, you must pay a $50 deductible before Ball Insurance Company will pay any hospital expenses.
What is the coinsurance?	80% / Standard	After the deductible is paid, Ball Insurance Company will pay 80% of the usual, customary, and routine amount of expenses. This means you pay the other 20% of the bill.
What is the coinsurance for professional services in an inpatient setting?	40%	After the deductible is paid, Ball Insurance Company will pay 40% of the usual, customary, and routine amount of professional expenses incurred in the hospital. This means you pay the other 60% of the bill. Professional services do not include room and board charges (after the deductible, these are covered at 100%).
Is there an out-of-pocket limit on my expenses?	$400	After you have paid $400 toward deductibles and coinsurance, Ball Insurance Company pays 100% thereafter.
	$800 / Family	After a family has paid $800 toward deductibles and coinsurance, Ball Insurance Company pays 100% thereafter.
Does this plan use a network of providers?	No	You can visit any provider of your choosing.

Questions: Call 1-800-XXX-XXXX or visit us at www.insurancecompany.com.
If you do not understand any of the terms used in this form, see the Glossary at www.insuranceterms.gov.

WINTER INSURANCE COMPANY

9763 WESTERN WAY, WHITTIER, CO 82963, (970) 555-2963

POLICY: ABC CORPORATION   POLICY NAME: ABC   EFFECTIVE DATE: 06/01/CCYY

INSURANCE GROUP # and SUFFIX: <u>36928/ABC</u>

INSURANCE CONTACT: <u>Wilma Williams</u>   PHONE NUMBER: <u>(970) 555-2964</u>

Eligibility

EMPLOYEE: Must work a minimum of 35 hours per week. Is eligible for coverage the first of the month following 60 consecutive days of continuous employment.

DEPENDENTS: Are eligible for coverage from birth to age 26 if a full-time student or handicapped prior to age 26 (proof of disability must be furnished within 31 days after dependent reaches limiting age). Dependent is not eligible as a dependent if eligible as an employee. Unmarried natural children, legally adopted children, and foster children are included (also includes legal guardianship). If both parents are covered by the plan, children may be covered by one employee only.

Effective Date

EMPLOYEE: If written application is made prior to the eligibility date, coverage becomes effective the first of the month following 60 days of employment. Note: late applicants' coverage becomes effective on the first of the month following application.

DEPENDENTS: The date acquired by the covered employee becomes the effective date if written application is made within 31 days of the eligibility date. Newborns are automatically covered for the first seven days following birth; well-baby charges are excluded. Coverage will terminate after seven days unless written application for coverage is submitted by the employee within 31 days of birth.

Termination of Coverage

EMPLOYEE: Coverage terminates the last day of the month following termination of employment, when the employee ceases to qualify as an eligible employee, or following request for termination of coverage.

DEPENDENTS: Coverage terminates the date the employee's coverage terminates or the last day of the month during which the dependent no longer qualifies as an eligible dependent.

Extension of Benefits

If covered under the plan when disabled, employee may continue coverage for 12 months following the date of termination or until no longer disabled, whichever is less.

EXCLUSIONS

1. Work-related injuries or illnesses.
2. Services for which there is no charge in the absence of insurance.
3. Charges or services in excess of UCR or not medically necessary.
4. Charges for completion of claim forms and failure to keep appointments.
5. Routine or preventative or experimental services.
6. Eye refractions, contacts or glasses, orthotics (eye exercises), radial keratotomy, or other procedures for surgical correction of refractive errors.
7. Custodial care.
8. Cosmetic surgery
9. Reversal of voluntary sterilization.
11. Diagnosis or treatment of infertility, including artificial insemination, in vitro fertilization, etc.

Questions: Call **1-800-XXX-XXXX** or visit us at www.insurancecompany.com.
If you do not understand any of the terms used in this form, see the Glossary at www.insuranceterms.gov.

WINTER INSURANCE

Policy Period: CCYY– CCNY

Plan Type: Comprehensive Major Medical

Summary of Coverage: What This Plan Covers

Important Questions	Answers	Why This Matters
What is the overall deductible?	**$100 / Individual**	You must pay this amount out of pocket before Winter Insurance Company will pay any health care costs. There is a three-month carryover provision: You can count the money you spent on healthcare during the last three months of the year toward your deductible the following year.
	$200 / Family	Two members of the family must meet their deductible before Winter Insurance Company will pay any health care costs.
Deductibles for In-Patient Hospitalization services?	**$0 / Per Admission**	If you are hospitalized, you need not pay any deductible before Winter Insurance Company will pay for hospital expenses.
What is the coinsurance?	**90% / Standard** **40% / Lab** **90% / DME**	After the deductible is paid, Winter Insurance Company will pay 90% of the usual, customary, and routine amount of expenses. This means you pay the other 10% of the bill. The indicated percentages apply for Lab and DME.
What is the coinsurance for professional services in an inpatient setting?	**90%**	After the deductible is paid, Winter Insurance Company will pay 90% of the usual, customary, and routine amount of professional expenses incurred in the hospital. This means you pay the other 10% of the bill. Professional services do not include room and board charges (after the deductible, these are covered at 100%).
Is there an out-of-pocket limit on my expenses?	**$750**	After you have paid $750 toward deductibles and coinsurance, Winter Insurance Company pays 100% thereafter.
	$1500 / Family	After a family has paid $1500 toward deductibles and coinsurance, Winter Insurance Company pays 100% thereafter.
Does this plan use a network of providers?	**No**	You can visit any provider of your choosing.

Questions: Call 1-800-XXX-XXXX or visit us at www.insurancecompany.com.
If you do not understand any of the terms used in this form, see the Glossary at www.insuranceterms.gov.

SUMMER INSURANCE COMPANY
18932 SPRING ROAD, AUTUMN, CO 82974
(970) 555-9631
Policy Name: Ninja
INSURANCE CONTACT: Sammy Rock

Contract Holder: Rocky Corporation
1234 Ribbon Road, Rudolph, CO 81208
Effective Date of Contract: January 1, CCYY
Insurance Group # and Suffix: 67980/ROC
PHONE NUMBER: (970) 555-9632

Eligibility

EMPLOYEE: Actively at work for a minimum of 35 hours per week. Is eligible after 30 continuous work days.

Employees who enroll more than 30 days after their employment date are considered late enrollees and are subject to this Contract's Preexisting Conditions limitation. Coverage terminates the date an employee ceases to be an actively-at-work, full-time employee for any reason.

DEPENDENTS: Dependents include the employee's legal spouse and unmarried dependent children who are under age 26.

The Role of a Member's Primary Care Physician

A member's primary care physician (PCP) provides basic health maintenance services and coordinates a member's overall health care. Any time a member needs medical care, the member should contact his or her PCP. In a medical emergency, a member may go directly to the emergency room. If a member does so, then the member must call his or her PCP or the care manager and member services within 48 hours. If the member fails to make this call, we will provide services under this HMO plan only if we determine that notice was given as soon as was reasonably possible.

Referral Forms

A member can be referred for specialist services by his or her PCP. Except in the case of a medical emergency, a member will not be eligible for any services provided by anyone other than his or her PCP (including but not limited to specialist services) if a member has not been referred by his or her PCP. Referrals must be obtained prior to receiving services and supplies from any practitioner other than the member's PCP.

Medical Necessity

Members will receive designated benefits only when medically necessary and appropriate. We or the care manager may determine whether any benefit was medically necessary and appropriate, and we have the option to select the appropriate participating hospital to render services if hospitalization is necessary. Decisions as to what is medically necessary and appropriate are subject to review by our quality assessment committee or its physician designee.

Limitation on Services

Except in cases of medical emergency, services are available only from participating providers. We shall have no liability or obligation to cover any service or benefit sought or received by a member from any physician, hospital, or other provider unless we make prior arrangements.

Schedule of Services and Supplies

The services or supplies covered under the contract are subject to all copayments and are determined per calendar year per member, unless otherwise stated. Maximums apply only to the specific services provided. Note: No services or supplies will be provided if a member fails to obtain preauthorization of care through his or her PCP or health center or care manager. Read the member provisions carefully before obtaining medical care, services, or supplies.

EXCLUSIONS

1. Expenses resulting from self-inflicted injuries.
2. Work-related injuries or illnesses.
3. Services for which there is no charge in the absence of insurance.
4. Charges or services in excess of UCR or not medically necessary.
5. Charges for completion of claim forms and failure to keep appointments.
6. Routine or preventative or experimental services.
7. Custodial care.
8. Cosmetic surgery unless for repair of an injury or surgery incurred while covered or result of mastectomy.

Questions: Call 1-800-XXX-XXXX or visit us at www.insurancecompany.com.
If you do not understand any of the terms used in this form, see the Glossary at www.insuranceterms.gov.

SUMMER INSURANCE

Policy Period: CCYY– CCNY

Plan Type: HMO

Summary of Coverage: What This Plan Covers

Important Questions	Answers	Why This Matters
What is the overall copayment for services?	**$15 / Visit** **$25 / Prenatal care**	You must pay this amount out of pocket before Summer Insurance Company will pay any health care costs. Visits include outpatient surgery, office visits, diagnostic imaging, chiropractic, podiatry, and preadmission testing. For prenatal care, the copayment is a one-time copay of $25.
What is the overall copayment for supplies?	**$0**	Two members of the family must meet their deductible before Summer Insurance Company will pay any health care costs.
copayment for In-Patient Hospitalization services?	**$50 / Per ER** **$150 / Per Day Admission**	If you are admitted to the ER, you must pay a $50 copay. If you are admitted to the hospital that same day, the copay transfers to the hospital copayment of $150 per day for the first five days.
What is the coinsurance for prescriptions?	**50% / Pharmacy** **$15 / Carrier**	Summer Insurance Company will pay 50% of the usual customary and routine amount of prescription expenses. This means you pay the other 50% of the bill. If the prescription is filled through Summer Insurance Carrier, the copayment is $15.
Is there an out-of-pocket limit on my expenses?	**$1500.00**	The limit of out-of-pocket costs for hospitalization is $1500 a year.
Does this plan use a network of providers?	**Yes**	No services or supplies will be provided if a member fails to obtain preauthorization of care through his or her PCP or health center or care manager. Read the Member provisions carefully before obtaining medical care, services, or supplies.

Questions: Call 1-800-XXX-XXXX or visit us at www.insurancecompany.com.
If you do not understand any of the terms used in this form, see the Glossary at www.insuranceterms.gov.

CMS-1500

UB-04

COB Calculations Worksheet

Patient Bill (also called "Supplemental Bill")

Family Deductible Tracking

Request for Copy of Denial of Claim

Request for More Information

Doctor's First Report of Injury

Workers' Compensation Progress Notes

CMS-1500

1500

HEALTH INSURANCE CLAIM FORM

APPROVED BY NATIONAL UNIFORM CLAIM COMMITTEE 08/05

☐☐PICA

CARRIER

PICA☐☐

1. MEDICARE MEDICAID TRICARE CHAMPVA GROUP FECA OTHER	1a. INSURED'S I.D. NUMBER (For Program in Item 1)
CHAMPUS HEALTH PLAN BLK LUNG ☐(Medicare #) ☐(Medicaid #) ☐(Sponsor's SSN) ☐(Member ID#) ☐(SSN or ID) ☐(SSN) ☐(ID)	

2. PATIENT'S NAME (Last Name, First Name, Middle Initial)	3. PATIENT'S BIRTH DATE SEX MM ⎪ DD ⎪ YY M☐ F☐	4. INSURED'S NAME (Last Name, First Name, Middle Initial)

5. PATIENT'S ADDRESS (No, Street)	6. PATIENT RELATIONSHIP TO INSURED Self☐ Spouse☐ Child☐ Other☐	7. INSURED'S ADDRESS (No, Street)

CITY	STATE	8. PATIENT STATUS Single☐ Married☐ Other☐	CITY	STATE

ZIP CODE	TELEPHONE (Include Area Code)	Full-Time Part-Time Employed☐ Student☐ Student☐	ZIP CODE	TELEPHONE (Include Area Code)

9. OTHER INSURED'S NAME (Last Name, First Name, Middle Initial)	10. IS PATIENT'S CONDITION RELATED TO:	11. INSURED'S POLICY GROUP OR FECA NUMBER
a. OTHER INSURED'S POLICY OR GROUP NUMBER	a. EMPLOYMENT? (Current or Previous) ☐YES ☐NO	a. INSURED'S DATE OF BIRTH SEX MM ⎪ DD ⎪ YY M☐ F☐
b. OTHER INSURED'S DATE OF BIRTH SEX MM ⎪ DD ⎪ YY M☐ F☐	b. AUTO ACCIDENT? PLACE (State) ☐YES ☐NO └___┘	b. EMPLOYER'S NAME OR SCHOOL NAME
c. EMPLOYER'S NAME OR SCHOOL NAME	c. OTHER ACCIDENT? ☐YES ☐NO	c. INSURANCE PLAN NAME OR PROGRAM NAME
d. INSURANCE PLAN NAME OR PROGRAM NAME	10d. RESERVED FOR LOCAL USE	d. IS THERE ANOTHER HEALTH BENEFIT PLAN? ☐YES ☐NO **If yes**, return to and complete item 9 a-d

READ BACK OF FORM BEFORE COMPLETING & SIGNING THIS FORM.

12. PATIENT'S OR AUTHORIZED PERSON'S SIGNATURE I authorize the release of any medical or other information necessary to process this claim. I also request payment of government benefits either to myself or to the party who accepts assignment below. SIGNED _____ DATE_____	13. INSURED'S OR AUTHORIZED PERSON'S SIGNATURE I authorize payment of medical benefits to the undersigned physician or supplier for services described below. SIGNED _____

PATIENT AND INSURED INFORMATION

14. DATE OF CURRENT MM ⎪ DD ⎪ YY ◄ ILLNESS (First symptom) OR INJURY (Accident) OR PREGNANCY (LMP)	15. IF PATIENT HAS HAD SAME OR SIMILAR ILLNESS, GIVE FIRST DATE MM ⎪ DD ⎪ YY	16. DATES PATIENT UNABLE TO WORK IN CURRENT OCCUPATION FROM MM ⎪ DD ⎪ YY TO MM ⎪ DD ⎪ YY

17. NAME OF REFERRING PHYSICIAN OR OTHER SOURCE	17a. 17b. NPI	18. HOSPITALIZATION DATES RELATED TO CURRENT SERVICES FROM MM ⎪ DD ⎪ YY TO MM ⎪ DD ⎪ YY

19. RESERVED FOR LOCAL USE	20. OUTSIDE LAB? $ CHARGES ☐YES ☐NO

21. DIAGNOSIS OR NATURE OF ILLNESS OR INJURY (Relate Items 1,2,3 or 4 to Item 24E by Line) 1. └___ ___┘ 3. └___ ___┘ 2. └___ ___┘ 4. └___ ___┘	22. MEDICAID RESUBMISSION CODE ⎪ ORIGINAL REF. NO. 23. PRIOR AUTHORIZATION NUMBER

	24. A. DATE(S) OF SERVICE From To MM DD YY MM DD YY	B. PLACE OF SERVICE	C. EMG	D. PROCEDURES, SERVICES, OR SUPPLIES (Explain Unusual Circumstances) CPT/HCPCS ⎪ MODIFIER	E. DIAGNOSIS POINTER	F. $ CHARGES	G. DAYS OR UNITS	H. EPSDT Family Plan	I. ID. QUAL.	J. RENDERING PROVIDER ID. #
1									NPI	
2									NPI	
3									NPI	
4									NPI	
5									NPI	
6									NPI	

25. FEDERAL TAX ID NUMBER SSN EIN ☐☐	26. PATIENT'S ACCOUNT NO.	27. ACCEPT ASSIGNMENT? (For govt. claims, see back) ☐YES ☐NO	28. TOTAL CHARGE $	29. AMOUNT PAID $	30. BALANCE DUE $

31. SIGNATURE OF PHYSICIAN OR SUPPLIER INCLUDING DEGREES OR CREDENTIALS (I certify that the statements on the reverse apply to this bill and are made a part thereof) SIGNED _____ DATE _____	32. SERVICE FACILITY LOCATION INFORMATION a. b.	33. BILLING PROVIDER INFO & PH. # a. b.

PHYSICIAN OR SUPPLIER INFORMATION

NUCC Instruction Manual available at: www.nucc.org   *PLEASE PRINT **OR** TYPE*   APPROVED OMB 0938-0999 FORM CMS-1500 (08/05)

UB-04

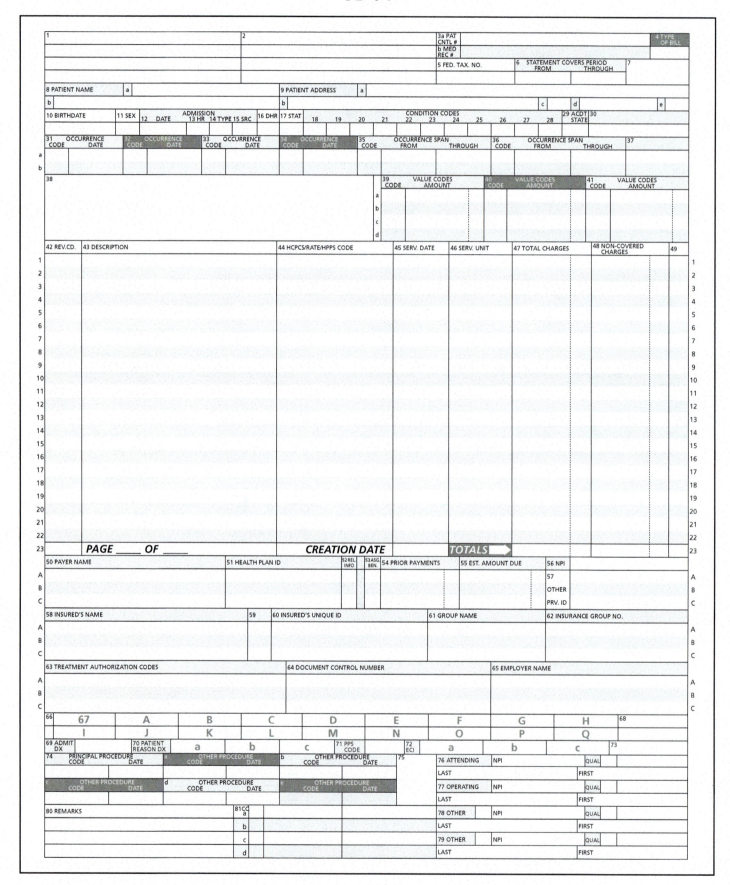

Coordination of Benefits
Calculation Worksheet

Patient's Name: _____   Year: _____

Payment Calculation:

1. Total allowable amount for this claim is the greater of either the primary plan's allowable amount or the secondary plan's allowable amount.   _____

2. Total primary insurance carrier payment for this claim   _____

3. Difference between Line 1 and Line 2   _____

4. Secondary insurance carrier's normal liability for this claim   _____

5. The lesser of Line 3 or Line 4   _____

   This is the amount of the secondary insurance carrier's actual payment on this claim.

Credit Reserve:

6. Normal liability for this claim (Line 4)   _____

7. Actual payment for this claim (Line 5)   _____

8. Subtract Line 7 from Line 6.   _____

9. Credit reserve on all previous claims for this patient   _____

10. Total credit reserve (sum of Line 8 and Line 9)   _____

Instructions:

Enter the patient's name and the year that services were rendered at the top of the calculation sheet.
1. Enter the total allowable amount on this claim. The total allowable amount is the greater of either the primary plan's allowable amount or the secondary plan's allowable amount.
2. Enter the total amount that other insurance companies have paid on this claim.
3. Subtract Line 2 from Line 1.
4. Enter the normal liability amount for this insurance company for this claim.
5. Enter the lesser of either Line 3 or Line 4. This is the actual amount paid by the secondary insurance on this claim.

To Calculate Credit Reserve:

6. Enter the normal liability amount for the secondary insurance carrier for this claim.
7. Enter the actual payment for the secondary insurance carrier for this claim.
8. Subtract Line 7 from Line 6. This is the amount of money the secondary carrier has saved by paying secondary on this claim. This amount becomes part of the credit reserve.
9. Enter the credit reserve amount for all previous claims for this patient.
10. Add Line 8 and Line 9. This is the total credit reserve for this patient.

Annette Adams, MD
5858 Peppermint Place
Anytown, USA 12345
(765) 555-6768

Patient Bill

Patient:	Date of Birth:	Account Number:

Date of Service	Service Provided	Insurance Payment	Patient's Responsibility

Family Tracking Form

Family Name: _____

Insurance: _____

Date of Service	Name of Patient	Total Charge	Family Deductible _____	Coinsurance _____	Out-of-Pocket Expenses (Family) _____

REQUEST FOR COPY OF DENIAL OF CLAIM

Date: _____

Dear Provider:

We are unable to process your Medicare claim at this time. Please provide proof that _____ insurance has denied the claim in order for us to reconsider this claim.

Attached is a copy of your original claim.

Sincerely,

MAC Administration

REQUEST FOR MORE INFORMATION

Date:_____

Dear Provider:

We are unable to process the attached claim due to missing information. Please fill in the requested information and return this form to our office.

This claim is made for an injury. Please indicate which of the following is true about the cause of the injury:

_____ Injured while participating in a recreational activity

Describe activity, place, and equipment being used: _____

_____

_____

_____ Injured while working for an employer

Name of employer: _____

Activity when injured: _____

Did the patient seek Workers' Compensation Evaluation?_____

If so, which provider: _____

_____ Injured in a car accident or pedestrian/car accident

Name of car insurance: _____

Describe incident: _____

Has a claim been filed with the automobile insurance? _____

If not, explain why not: _____

_____

Thank you,

Ball Insurance Company

STATE OF CONFUSION

DOCTOR'S FIRST REPORT OF OCCUPATIONAL INJURY OR ILLNESS

Within five days of your initial examination, for every occupational injury or illness, send two copies of this report to the employer's workers' compensation insurance carrier or the insured employer. Failure to file a timely doctor's report may result in assessment of a civil penalty. In the case of diagnosed or suspected pesticide poisoning, send a copy of the report to Division of Labor Statistics and Research, P.O. Box 555555, Anytown, USA 12345-6789, and notify your local health officer by telephone within 24 hours.

	PLEASE DO NOT USE THIS COLUMN
1. INSURER NAME AND ADDRESS	
2. EMPLOYER NAME	Case No.
3. Address: No. and Street City Zip	Industry
4. Nature of business (e.g., food manufacturing, building construction, retailer of women's clothes.)	County
5. PATIENT NAME (first name, middle initial, last name) 6. Sex ☐Male ☐ Female 7. Date of Birth: Mo. Day Yr.	Age
8. Address: No. and Street City Zip 9. Telephone number ( )	Hazard
10. Occupation (Specific job title) 11. Social Security Number - -	Disease
12. Injured at: No. and Street City County	Hospitalization
13. Date and hour of injury or onset of illness Mo. Day Yr. Hour _____ a.m. _____ p.m. 14. Date last worked Mo. Day Yr.	Occupation
15. Date and hour of first examination or treatment Mo. Day Yr. Hour _____ a.m. _____ p.m. 16. Have you (or your office) previously treated patient? ☐Yes ☐No	Return Date/Code

Patient please complete this portion, if able to do so. Otherwise, doctor please complete immediately, inability or failure of a patient to complete this portion shall not affect his/her rights to workers' compensation under the California Labor Code.

17. **DESCRIBE HOW THE ACCIDENT OR EXPOSURE HAPPENED.** (Give specific object, machinery or chemical. Use reverse side if more space is required.)

18. **SUBJECTIVE COMPLAINTS** (Describe fully. Use reverse side if more space is required.)

19. **OBJECTIVE FINDINGS** (Use reverse side if more space is required.)
A. Physical examination

B. X-ray and laboratory results (State if none or pending.)

20. **DIAGNOSIS** (if occupational illness specify etiologic agent and duration of exposure.) Chemical or toxic compounds involved? ☐Yes ☐ No
ICD-9cm Code ___ ___ ___ - ___ ___

21. Are your findings and diagnosis consistent with patient's account of injury or onset of illness?   ☐Yes ☐No   If "no", please explain.

22. Is there any other current condition that will impede or delay patient's recovery?   ☐Yes ☐No   If "yes", please explain.

23. **TREATMENT RENDERED** (Use reverse side if more space is required.)

24. If further treatment required, specify treatment plan/estimated duration.

25. If hospitalized as inpatient, give hospital name and location   Date   Mo.   Day   Yr. Estimated stay
admitted

26. WORK STATUS -- Is patient able to perform usual work?   ☐Yes ☐No
If "no", date when patient can return to: Regular work ____/____/____
Modified work ____/____/____   Specify restrictions _____

Doctor's Signature _____   License Number _____
Doctor Name and Degree (please type) _____   IRS Number _____
Address _____   Telephone Number _____

FORM 5021 (Rev. 4)

Workers' Compensation Progress Report

Patient Name: Claim Number:

Status Update:

S:

O:

A:

P:

Work Status:

☐ Return to work full-time with no restrictions

☐ Return to work part-time with no restrictions

☐ Return to work full-time with the following modifications in duty:

_____

_____

_____

☐ Do not return to work. Anticipated date of return: _____

Physician Signature   Date

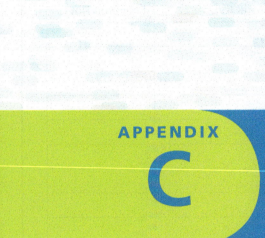

Tables

RVS Schedule

UCR Conversion Report

Denial Reasons

List of Remarks

Durable Medical Equipment Guidelines

Potential Medical Case Management Claims

Assistant Surgeon Procedures

Relative Value Study

CPT®/HCPCS	Description	Total RVUs	Followup Days
00215	ANESTHESIA FOR CRANIOPLASTY	9.0	--
00400	ANESTHESIA, INTEGUMENTARY SYSTEM, EXTREMITIES	3.0	--
00520	ANESTHESIA FOR CLOSED CHEST PROCEDURES	6.0	--
00534	ANESTHESIA FOR TRANSVENOUS INSERTION	7.0	--
00868	ANESTHESIA FOR RENAL TRANSPLANT	10.0	--
01230	ANESTHESIA FOR UPPER 2/3 OF FEMUR, OPEN	6.0	--
01480	ANESTHESIA ON BONES OF LOWER LEG, OPEN	30	--
01990	PHYSIOLOGICAL SUPPORT, BRAIN-DEAD PATIENT	7.0	--
15570	FORMATION OF DIRECT OR TUBED PEDICLE	10.0	90
15952	EXCISION TROCHANTERIC PRESSURE ULCER	8.0	90
19125	EXCISION OF BREAST LESION	7.0	30
19126	EXCISION OF BREAST LESION, EACH ADDITIONAL	3.5	30
20205	BIOPSY, MUSCLE, DEEP	2.4	15
21800	CLOSED TREATMENT OF RIB FRACTURE, EACH	18.0	90
24102	ARTHROTOMY, ELBOW WITH SYNOVECTOMY	14.5	90
25622	CLOSED TREATMENT OF CARPAL SCAPHOID FRACTURE	3.5	60
27350	PATELLECTOMY OR HEMIPATELLECTOMY	12.0	60
27372	REMOVAL OF FOREIGN BODY, DEEP, THIGH REGION	5.2	30
27758	OPEN TREATMENT OF TIBIAL SHAFT FRACTURE	12.7	30
27784	OPEN TREATMENT OF PROXIMAL FIBULA SHAFT FX	12.7	90
28456	PERCUTANEOUS SKELETAL FIXATION OF TARSAL BONE FX	3.9	90
30125	EXCISION DERMOID CYST NOSE, UNDER BONE	8.5	30
31200	ETHMOIDECTOMY	7.0	90
31225	MAXILLECTOMY WITHOUT ORBITAL EXENTERATION	22.5	120
32800	REPAIR LUNG HERNIA THROUGH CHEST WALL	12.0	30
33217	INSERTION OF A TRANSVENOUS ELECTRODE	9.5	15
33225	INSERTION OF PACING ELECTRODE	BR	--
33240	INSERTION OF SINGLE OR DUAL CHAMBER PACING	0.7	15
36430	TRANSFUSION, BLOOD	0.4	00
38100	SPLENECTOMY, TOTAL	16.0	45
39520	REPAIR, DIAPHRAGMATIC HERNIA	17.0	90
39545	IMBRICATION OF DIAPHRAGM FOR EVENTRATION	12.0	90

(continued)

40808	BIOPSY, VESTIBULE OF MOUTH	0.7	00
43840	GASTRORRHAPHY, SUTURE PERFORATED ULCER	14.0	45
47630	BILIARY DUCT STONE EXTRACTION	7.0	45
49560	REPAIR INITIAL INCISIONAL OR VENTRAL HERNIA	11.5	45
52500	TRANSURETHRAL RESECTION OF BLADDER NECK	10.0	90
58700	SALPINGECTOMY, COMPLETE OR PARTIAL	11.4	90
59400	ROUTINE OBSTETRIC CARE	20.0	45
59820	TREATMENT OF MISSED ABORTION	4.5	30
61703	SURGERY OF INTRACRANIAL ANEURYSM	13.0	90
62000	ELEVATION OF DEPRESSED SKULL FRACTURE	8.3	90
65800	PARACENTESIS OF ANTERIOR CHAMBER OF EYE	3.0	00
69400	EUSTACHIAN TUBE INFLATION	0.3	00
70250	RADIOLOGIC EXAM, SKULL	3.1	--
70260	RADIOLOGIC EXAM, SKULL, COMPLETE	5.0	--
70450	CAT SCAN, SKULL	21.7	--
71020	RADIOLOGIC EXAM, CHEST	3.2	--
73100	RADIOLOGIC EXAM, WRIST	2.5	--
73130	RADIOLOGIC EXAM, HAND, MINIMUM 3 VIEWS	2.8	--
73550	RADIOLOGIC EXAM, FEMUR	2.8	--
73590	RADIOLOGIC EXAM, TIBIA AND FIBULA	2.5	--
73718	MRI LEG	55.0	--
74250	RADIOLOGIC EXAM, SMALL INTESTINE	6.6	--
76090	MAMMOGRAPHY, UNILATERAL	4.5	--
76092	SCREENING MAMMOGRAPHY, BILATERAL	4.5	--
76870	ECHOGRAPHY, SCROTUM AND CONTENTS	8.0	--
76872	ECHOGRAPHY, TRANSRECTAL	13.8	--
78810	TUMOR IMAGING	100.0	--
80048	BASIC METABOLIC PANEL	1.3	--
80053	COMPREHENSIVE METABOLIC PANEL	1.6	--
81000	URINALYSIS	0.7	--
82310	CALCIUM, TOTAL	1.0	--
83540	IRON	1.6	--
85025	BLOOD COUNT, COMPLETE, AUTOMATED	0.8	--
85610	PROTHROMBIN TIME	0.6	--
86901	BLOODTYPING, RH (D)	1.1	--

(continued)

87040	CULTURE, BACTERIAL; BLOOD	1.2	--
87070	CULTURE, BACTERIAL OTHER SOURCE	1.3	--
88150	CYTOPATHOLOGY, SLIDES, CERVICAL OR VAGINAL	0.9	--
90782	THERAPEUTIC, INJECTION	2.5	--
93000	EKG	7.8	--
93545	INJECTION DURING ANGIOGRAPHY	22.0	--
94060	BRONCHOSPASM EVALUATION	20.0	--
97116	GAIT TRAINING	7.0	--
99201	OFFICE OR OTHER OUTPATIENT VISIT, NEW	6.5	--
99213	OV ESTABLISHED PATIENT, EXPANDED	9.0	--
99284	EMERGENCY VISIT, DETAILED	25.0	--
99285	EMERGENCY VISIT, COMPREHENSIVE	37.0	--

UCR Conversion Factor Report

The following list of UCR Conversion Factors is intended to be used for training and reference purposes only.

Zip	Area	Including Zip Codes	Surgery	Medicine	X-Ray & Lab (DXL)	Anesthesia
006	Puerto Rico	006-009	35.58	31.13	26.68	22.14
039	Maine	039-049	31.01	27.13	23.26	31.34
100	New York City	100-102	66.02	57.77	49.51	30.30
125	Poughkeepsie, Monticello, NE NY	125, 127-129, 136	40.71	35.62	30.53	32.71
153	Southwestern PA	153-158	36.76	32.16	27.57	25.25
210	Baltimore Area	210, 211, 214	48.00	42.00	36.00	35.35
255	Huntington, Wheeling, Parkesburg, Morgantown	255, 257, 260, 261, 265	32.94	28.82	24.70	31.14
302	Atlanta	302, 303	38.86	34.00	29.14	47.43
354	Alabama-Miscellaneous	354-357, 359-360, 363-365, 368, 324	30.90	27.04	23.18	32.06
441	Cleveland, Youngstown Area	441, 444	37.10	32.46	27.83	38.69
480	Detroit	480-482, 485	36.63	32.05	27.47	31.41
550	Minneapolis-St. Paul Area	550, 551, 553	26.42	23.12	19.81	29.46
580	North Dakota	580-588	28.00	24.50	21.00	23.12
606	Chicago	606	45.64	39.94	34.23	49.57
640	Kansas City Area	640-641, 661-662	33.48	29.29	25.11	40.30
770	Houston	770,772,775	40.60	35.52	30.45	42.66

(continued)

777	Austin & Beaumont	777,779,787,788	33.10	28.96	24.82	50.31
801	Denver, CO Springs, Alamosa, Glenwood Springs Area	801-803,806,808, 811,816	32.32	28.28	24.24	41.69
890	Reno & Area	890, 895, 897	34.38	30.08	25.78	49.11
904	Santa Monica, Long Beach, Glendale	904, 908, 912	45.18	39.53	33.89	47.94
970	Portland & Western OR	970, 971, 974, 975	30.87	27.01	23.15	34.20

Denial Reasons

Charge exceeds amount covered under your plan.
This procedure does not require the attendance of an assistant surgeon.
Personal convenience items are not covered under your plan.
"item" – Duplicate Charge.
"item(s)" is/are not covered under your plan.
Services not covered. Patient is over the age limit.
Services were denied as not medically necessary.
Non-prescription medication not covered under your plan.
"patient" is not covered under this plan.
Test performed is not related to the diagnosis indicated.
Pended. Additional Information Needed.
Pended. Please verify if charges are for professional services or facility fees.
Pended. Need anesthesia time.
Pended. Please submit narrative explaining use of Polaroid camera.
Charge exceeds Medicare's approved amount.
Group responsibility, covered under capitation.
Charges included in global maternity fee.
Charges incidental to above procedure.
"procedure" is not covered under your plan.
Charge exceeds amount covered under your plan. All x-rays combined under full mouth x-ray w/ bitewings.
Fluoride treatment only covered for children under 14.
No additional base units allowed for secondary procedures.
Monitoring blood gasses is an integral part of anesthesia. No extra units allowed.
Room and Board covered up to $"amount" per day.
Charge exceeds average semiprivate room rate.
Charges due to preexisting conditions which are excluded under your plan.
Exceeds purchase price of rental item.
Not covered, exceeds maximum amount covered for this service.

Remarks List

No Deductible Taken Due To Common Accident Provision.
Accident Benefit, First $500 Payable At 100%.
Accident Benefit Has Already Been Applied For On This Accident.
Lifetime Maximum Has Been Reached. $"amount" Exceeds Your Lifetime Maximum.
Charges Have Been Applied To Your CCYY Deductible.
20YY Individual Deductible Limit Has Previously Been Met.
20YY Individual Deductible Has Been Met On This Claim.
CCPY Carryover Deductible Does Not Apply To CCYY Family Deductible Limit.
CCYY Family Deductible Limit Has Previously Been Met.
CCYY Family Deductible Has Been Met On This Claim.
CCYY Individual and Family Deductibles Have Been Met On This Claim.
CCYY Individual and Family Deductible Limits Have Previously Been Met.
CCYY Individual Out-Of-Pocket Limit Has Previously Been Met.
CCYY Individual Out-Of-Pocket Limit Has Been Met On This Claim.
CCYY Family Aggregate Out-Of-Pocket Limit Has Been Met On This Claim.
CCYY Family Aggregate Out-Of-Pocket Limit Has Previously Been Met.
CCYY Family Coinsurance Limit Has Been Met On This Claim.
CCYY Family Coinsurance Limit Has Previously Been Met.
CCYY Individual And Family Coinsurance Limits Have Previously Been Met.
CCYY Individual And Family Coinsurance Limits Have Been Met On This Claim.
CCYY Individual Coinsurance Limit Has Previously Been Met.
CCYY Individual Coinsurance Limit Has Been Met On This Claim.
Benefits Reduced To #%.
Benefits Payable At #%.
Non-Network Provider Benefits Payable At #%.
Benefits Have Been Adjusted Due To Medicare's Payment.
Credit Reserve = $"amount"
Medicare's Payment Exceeds Your Plan Normal Liability, Therefore, No Benefit Is Payable.
Provider Does Not Accept Medicare Assignment.
Provider Accepts Medicare Assignment.
Lab Professional Charges Paid at #% of UCR.

(continued)

Deductible Waived For Network Facilities.
Network Provider. Benefits Paid At #%.
Network Facility. Benefits paid at #%.
Maximum Dental Benefit Payable is $1,000. Per Calendar year.
Maximum Payable For Ambulance Is $150. Each Way.
Hospital Inpatient Deductible $200.
Benefits Have Been Adjusted Due To COB With Primary Carrier.
Benefits Are Adjusted Due To Payment By Primary Payer.

Durable Medical Equipment Coverage Guidelines

The following is a list of commonly billed DME items and coverage guidelines. This list is intended to be used for training and reference purposes only, as the particular company or plan guidelines may differ from the guidelines stated.

Item	Description	Coverage Guidelines
Action bath hydro massage	(See Whirlpool.)	Rx required. Refer for medical review.
Adjust-a-bed	(Lounger.)	Not covered. Comfort item.
Aero-massage	(See Whirlpool.)	See Whirlpool.
Aero-pulse Surgical Leggings	(Non-reusable support leggings.)	Rx required following surgery.
Air Conditioner	(Circulates and cools the air in a home.)	Not covered. Environmental control equipment.
Air-fluidized Bed	(Institutional equipment.)	Not covered. Not for home use.
Air Purifier	(Electronically cleans house environment.)	Not covered. Environmental control equipment.
Allergy-free Items	(Not primarily medical.)	Not covered. Preventive in nature. nondurable
Alternating Pressure Pads	(Prevents pressure sores in patient confined to bed or wheelchair)	Rx required when ordered for treatment of decubitus ulcers or when a person is susceptible to ulcers.
Ankle Weights	(As exercise equipment for postoperative care.)	Not a covered medical expense. Covered only when prescribed in a post-op situation to return function (e.g., knee surgery).
Apnea Monitor	(Monitors apnea, cessation of breathing, episodes in infants.)	Medical documentation of condition necessary. Rx required.
Aqua-matic K-pad	(Heating pad.)	Not covered. Comfort item, nondurable medical equipment.
Aqua-matic K-thermia	(Warm water system.)	Used only in institutions or acute care facility. Not covered.
Aqua Massage Pump	(See Whirlpool.)	See Whirlpool.
Aqua-whirl	(See Whirlpool.)	See Whirlpool.
Arch Supports	(Removable in-shoe support. See Orthotics.)	Not covered. Nondurable medical equipment.
Arterio Sonde	(Automatic blood pressure monitor.)	Covered as home blood pressure monitoring device.
Artificial Kidney	(Home hemodialysis unit.)	Covered for chronic renal disease; ancillary supplies essential to medical use may also be covered. Refer to medical review.
Astromatic Bed, Astropedic Bed, Comfort-a-bed	(Comfort bed. Not medical equipment.)	Not covered. Comfort item.
Autolift, Bathtub	(Bathtub lift.)	Possible convenience item. Rx required, patient's weight and statement of medical necessity; refer for medical review.
Backtrak, Cotrell	(Home back traction unit.)	Not covered.
Barbells	(As exercise equipment. For post-op rehabilitation.)	Not a covered medical expense. Covered only if prescribed in a post-op situation to return function.
Bathtub Rail and Seat	(Attached to bathtub for patient assistance.)	Rx required or statement of medical necessity. Covered for

(continued)

		paraplegics, quadriplegics, or stroke patients.
Beautyrest Adjustable Bed	(Not a hospital bed, not primary medical.)	Not covered. Convenience item. See Hospital bed (standard).
Bed Bath	(Hygienic equipment.)	Convenience item. Not for treating disease or injury.
Bedboard	(Provides firm support under mattress.)	Not covered. Not for treatment of disease or injury.
Bed Lift	(Sling, either manual or electronic; lifts person to and from bed.)	See Bathtub rail and seat. Rx required, patient's weight and statement of medical necessity.
Bed Lounge, Power or Manual	(Not a hospital bed.)	Convenience item (power or manual). Not covered. See Hospital bed, standard.
Bed Mattress	(Standard mattress for adjustable hospital bed.)	Covered when hospital bed is allowed.
Bedpan	(Hospital type.)	Covered for bed-confined or immobilized patients.
Bed Siderail	(Attached to hospital bed, protective device, often standard bed equipment.)	Covered if person is confined to bed, or if condition of vertigo, seizure, or neurologic disorder is present; also covered for small children.
Bed, Oscillating Type	(Swings back and forth.)	Not covered for home use. Institutional equipment.
Bell & Howell Master	(Speech teaching machine, training aid.)	Not covered.
Bendix-type Oxygen Concentrator	(Concentrates room air oxygen to a therapeutic level.)	Rx required. Covered for person with severe breathing impairment.
Bennett IPPB Machine	(Intermittent positive-pressure breathing.)	Rx required. Covered for person with severe breathing impairment.
Bicycle, Standard	Not covered.	Not covered.
Bicycle, Stationary	(For cardiac medical exercise program only.)	Refer for medical review.
Bidet	(Hygienic toilet item.)	Not primarily for treatment of disease or medical condition. Not covered.
Bimler Appliance	(Orthodontic dental appliance, corrects tongue thrust.)	Not covered.
Bi-osteogenic Electromagnetic Treatment System	(Electrical currents used to treat nonunion fracture.)	Covered to treat fractures. Medical documentation required.
Bird Respirator	(IPPB Machine for respiratory therapy.)	Rx required. Covered for person with severe breathing problem.
Blood Pressure Cuff	(Measures blood pressure; necessary for home management.)	Covered with documented diagnosis of hypertension; also used with home hemodialysis units.
Body Braces, Back, Foot, Leg, Arm	(Supportive devices.)	Rx required. Covered if durable and necessary.
Bra, Jobst Surgical	(Support item following surgery.)	Initial bra only following post-surgical reconstruction and mastectomy.
Braille Teaching Aid	(Training and vocational equipment.)	Not covered.
Breast Pump	(Assists mother in breastfeeding; may be either manual or electric.)	Not covered. Elective device for patient comfort.

(continued)

Canes	(Straight, quad, ambulatory aids.)	Covered for ambulatory impairments.
Cardiac Phone Monitor	(Telephone-relayed EKG reporting devices.)	Charges covered within physician's office fee.
Cast Guards	(A waterproof [usually plastic] coverlet for casts.)	Covered for all covered casting procedures.
Cast Shoes (fracture boot)	(A wood or rubber-based shoe with canvas sides to support casts in ambulation.)	Covered with documentation by diagnosis.
Catheter	(Medical supply item, not reusable.)	For bed-confined or similarly disabled persons; for urinary retention problems.
Centrifuge Readocrit	(Blood testing equipment.)	Rx required. Covered for person on home dialysis.
Cervical Collar	(Neck support item.)	Covered for appropriate diagnosis, such as cervical sprain.
Cervical Pillow	(Neck support item.)	Covered for appropriate diagnosis, such as cervical sprain.
Colostomy Supplies, Bags and Accessories	(Used after ostomy procedures.)	Covered for colostomy patients, post-rectal surgery.
Commode	(Bedside toilet chair.)	Covered for bed or wheelchair-confined person.
Computerized Equipment for Mobility and Speech	(For paraplegics.)	Not covered.
Contact Lens, Bandage	(Protects cornea following surgery or injury.)	Rx required.
Contact Lens, Orthokeratology	(Myopia or refractive.)	Refer for medical review.
Corset	(Supportive item.)	Covered with appropriate diagnosis, such as thoracic sprain.
Crutches	(Ambulatory aids.)	Covered for ambulatory impairments.
Cushion-lift Power Seat	(Assist person in/out of seat.)	Covered for person with hip, knee arthritis, or other neuromuscular conditions.
Dehumidifier	(Room or central system type.)	Not covered. Environmental control equipment.
Deluxe Padding	(Comfort item, special order for wheelchairs, other seating.)	Not covered.
Denis Browne Splint or Bar	(Metal support to maintain and correct adduction.)	Covered for child with clubfoot or metatarsus deformity (includes one pair of shoes).
Dextrometer/Glucometer/Diabetic Supplies	(Measures blood sugar levels.)	Rx required. For diabetic treatment.
Dialysis Equipment and Supplies	(Artificial kidney.)	Covered for chronic renal disease. See hemodialysis.
Diapulse Machine	(Diathermy machine.)	Not covered for home use.
Diathermy Equipment	(Heat treatment.)	Not covered for home use.
Disposable Sheets and Bags	(Supplies.)	Not covered. Nondurable medical equipment.
Ear Molds	(Prevents water from entering inner ear canal.)	Refer for medical review.
Ease-o-matic Bed Spring	(Comfort item, not adaptable to hospital bed.)	Not covered. See Hospital bed (standard).
Eaton E-Z Bath	(Bathtub seat.)	See Bathtub rail and seat.
Egg-crate Pad, Mattress	(Portable pad for preventing	Rx required. For treatment of

	bedsores.)	decubitus ulcers.
Elastic stocking, Jobst type	(Supportive, medical item following surgery.)	Rx required. Covered post-surgical expense or for diagnosis of circulatory problems.
Electra-Rest Bed	(Not a hospital bed)	Not covered.
Electrocardiocorder	(Diagnostic equipment.)	Covered only as part of a physician's diagnostic charge.
Electrostatic Air Purifier Machines	(Air cleanser, environment control apparatus.)	Not covered. Environmental control equipment.
Elevators	(Convenience item.)	Not covered.
Emesis Basin	(Basin for vomitus fluids.)	Covered expense for home bed-confined patients.
Enema Supplies	(For stimulating lower colon activity.)	Rx required.
Enuresis Equipment	(Monitoring and training devices for involuntary urination.)	Not covered.
Enurtone	(Training device for enuresis.)	Not covered.
Ergometer	(Tension measuring device for stationary bicycle.)	See bicycle (stationary).
Esophageal Dilator	(To open esophagus.)	Used only by physician. Not covered for home use.
Exercise Equipment	(Not primarily medical.)	Not covered.
Exercise Pad	(Flat soft surface.)	Not covered.
Exercycle	(Stationary bicycle.)	Rx required. For cardiac patients in active program. See Bicycle (stationary).
Face mask, Oxygen	(Necessity for oxygen therapy.)	Covered when oxygen therapy is required.
Face mask, Surgical	(For contagious diseases, isolation care.)	Rx required.
Flowmeter, Oxygen	(Oxygen regulator.)	Covered when oxygen therapy is required.
Fluidic Breathing Assistor	(Positive-pressure machine.)	Covered when IPPB care is necessary.
Foundation Garment	(Padding, bras, etc.)	Not covered. Check under specific items such as Corset.
Freika Pillow Splint	(Maintains adduction.)	Covered for small child with hip disorder.
Gatchboard	(Bedboard.)	Not covered.
Gel Flotation Pad and Mattress	(Treats and prevents pressure sores.)	Covered for treatment of decubitus ulcers.
Glideabout Chair	(Chair with small wheels.)	Rx required. Covered in lieu of wheelchair.
Glucometers	(Measures blood sugar levels.)	Rx required. For medical management of covered conditions.
Gravitronics Gravity Device	(Antigravity treatment for back condition.)	Not generally accepted medical practice.
Hand-E-Jet	(Portable whirlpool machine.)	See Whirlpool.
Hand-D-Vent	(Similar to IPPB machine; manual respiratory therapy.)	Rx required. Covered for severe respiratory impairment.
Hearing Aid	(To assist hearing.)	No coverage when specifically excluded by policy.
Heating Lamp	(External thermal applicator.)	Not covered outside hospital setting.

(continued)

Heating Pad	(Applies external heat.)	Not covered. Nondurable medical equipment.
Hemodialysis Equipment	(Artificial kidney device for blood filtering.)	Rx required. For chronic renal disease.
Holter Monitor	(24-hour cardiac measurement.)	Used only in physician's office. Charges payable within office fee as billed by physician.
Hospital bed, Electric	(Power multipurpose Bed.)	Rx required. May be necessary when person is required to self-change bed position. Refer for medical review.
Hospital bed, Standard	(Multilevel positioning Bed.)	Rx required. For bed-confined person who requires frequent position changes.
Hot Tub	(Thermal home spa system.)	Not covered.
Hoyer lift, Hydraulic	(Hydraulic patient Lift.)	Rx required. Generally a convenience for lifting person from bed to wheelchair, etc. Patient's weight and statement of medical condition necessary. Refer for medical review.
Humidifier, Component of Oxygen Equipment	(Adds moisture to oxygen.)	Covered when oxygen therapy unit is covered.
Humidifier, Room or Central	(Environmental control.)	Not covered. Environmental control equipment.
Hydrocollator Heating Unit	(Applies local external heat.)	Rx required. Expense should be incurred through physician's office.
Hydro-jet Whirlpool Bath	(Comfort whirlpool.)	See Whirlpool.
Hypodermic Needles and Supplies, Hypospray	(Administration of intramuscular, intradermal injections.)	Rx required. For medical management of covered condition.
Incontinence Pads	(Nondurable, disposable supply.)	Covered only for post-surgical urinary conditions for one month.
Infusion Pump	(Stimulates constant infusions of medication subcutaneously or intra-arterially.)	Rx required. Refer for medical review.
Insulin Pump	(Artificial pancreas function surgically implanted.)	Procedures still investigational. Submit records for medical review.
Inhalator	(Respiratory assistance.)	Rx required.
IPPB Machines	(For respiratory therapy.)	Rx required.
Irrigation Kit	(For hygienic use.)	Covered for respiratory paralysis, wound drainage, etc. 60 days rental.
Jacuzzi Portable Pump	(For use in bathtubs.)	Rx required. Refer for whirlpool medical review.
Jobst Hydro Float	(Special Flotation cushion.)	Covered for prevention or treatment of decubitus ulcers.
Jobst Pneumatic Appliance and Compressor, Pump	(Pneumatic full-limb appliance that maintains surface pressure.)	Rx required. Covered for intractable edema, post-radical mastectomy, etc. Refer for medical review.
Jobst Fabric Support, Houses, Sleeves, Stockings	(Nonreusable items, anti-embolism hose.)	Rx required. For circulatory conditions, pre- and post-op situations.
Lambs' Wool Pad	(Soft padding, deluxe item,	Covered for bed sores, etc.

(continued)

	nondurable.)	
Laser Equipment, any kind	(High-intensity light source.)	Covered service only in physician's office.
Lattoflex Spring Base	(Not a hospital-type bed.)	Not covered. Comfort item.
Lenox Hill Knee Brace	(Supportive orthopedic device.)	Rx required. Charges based on individual custom-ordered appliance.
Leotards	(Tight body apparel.)	Not covered.
Life-O-Gen Tank	(Portable oxygen.)	Rx required. Covered for persons with respiratory impairment.
Limb-O-Cycle	(Exercise equipment.)	Not covered.
Linde Oxygen Walker	(Portable oxygen system.)	Rx required. Covered for persons with respiratory impairment.
Lumex Chair Table	(Like a rollabout chair.)	Covered in lieu of regular wheelchair.
Lymphedema Pump	(Appliance that maintains surface pressure.)	Rx required. Covered for intractable edema of extremity.
Mask Devices	(To mask ringing in ears.)	Refer for medical review.
Mask, Oxygen	(Used to deliver oxygen.)	Covered for persons who require oxygen.
Massage Devices	(Comfort item.)	Not covered.
Massage Pillow	(Comfort item.)	Not covered.
Mattress, Medical	(For use with hospital bed.)	Covered when hospital bed is allowed.
Maxi-Mist Machine	(Delivers medicines as mist to be inhaled.)	Rx required.
Medasphere Portable Oxygen Unit	(Portable oxygen system.)	Covered when oxygen is necessary with exercise or walking.
Medcolator	(Physical therapy equipment.)	Not covered.
Medi-Cool Refrigerator	(For cooling medication.)	Not covered.
Medi-Jector, Injection Gun	(Delivers insulin without use of needles, convenience item.)	Not covered.
Micronaire Environmental Control	(Equipment to control environment; air purifier.)	Not covered. Environmental control equipment.
Milwaukee Back Brace	(Supportive orthopedic brace.)	Rx required.
Mobile Geriatric Chair	(Wheelchair with smaller than normal wheels.)	Covered in lieu of regular wheelchair.
Nebulizer	(Delivers medicine in mist form for inhalation.)	Covered for respiratory impairment.
Neck Halter	(Supportive device.)	Rx not required.
Nolan Bath Chair	(For assistance in bathtub.)	Rx required. Possible convenience item. Statement of medical necessity. See Bathtub rail and seat.
Nonvocal Communication System	(Daily living assistance system, electronic.)	Not covered.
Obturator	(Oral prosthesis.)	Rx required. Cleft palate prosthesis.
Orthopedic Shoes	(Custom shoes.)	Not covered.
Orthosis	(Adjustable back brace.)	Rx required.
Orthotics, Foot Stabilizers	(Acrylic arch supports.)	Covered only when dispensed by physician and when not excluded by policy provisions.
Osci Lite	(Heat lamp.)	Not covered.

(continued)

Oscillating Bed	(Alternating motion bed.)	Not covered for home use.
Ostomy Bags	(Used after ostomy procedures.)	Covered post-surgically.
Ottobock Cosmetic Stockings	(Covers existing prosthesis.)	Not covered. Nondurable medical equipment.
Overbed Tables	(For use with hospital bed, comfort item.)	Not covered.
Oxygen	(Compressed gas or liquid in tank.)	Rx required.
Oxygen Concentrator	(Condenses oxygen from room air.)	Rx required. Covered for persons with severe respiratory impairment.
Oxygen Humidifier	(Adds moisture to oxygen before inhalation.)	Rx required. Used in conjunction with oxygen tank system.
Oxygen Regulator	(Measures oxygen flow.)	Covered when oxygen unit is allowable.
Oxygen Tent	(Plastic overbed cover.)	Rx required.
Oxygen Tank, Spare	(Precautionary supply.)	Not covered.
Pace Trac	(Pacemaker monitor.)	Rx required. Refer for medical review.
Poli-Axial Knee Cage Brace System	(Lightweight supportive athletic knee cage and brace; very costly.)	Not covered. Athletic support device.
Paraffin bath Unit, Portable and Standard	(Wax immersion of affected joints.)	Covered for home use for arthritis patients.
Parallel Bars	(Exercise equipment.)	Not covered.
Penile Implant	(Inflatable penile prosthesis.)	Covered for those with diabetes, spinal cord injury, vascular disease, hypertension, post-surgical impotence.
Penile Monitor	(Electronic measuring device.)	Covered only in hospital under medical supervision.
Percusser	(Striking instrument used to perform percussion.)	Refer for medical review.
Phonic Mirror, Handi-Voice	(Electronic device that produces words by pressing buttons.)	Not covered.
Pogon Buggy, Stroller Type	(Adaptive wheelchair for child.)	Covered for nonambulatory child who requires more support than standard wheelchair provides.
Pollen Extractor	(For home environment use air purifier.)	Not covered. Environmental control equipment.
Portable Oxygen System	(Transportable.)	Regulated, adj. flow. Rate – Rx required. – Preset, one flow rate – (For general use.) – Not covered.
Portable Room Heater	(Environmental control.)	Not covered.
Posture Support Chairs	(Comfort item.)	Not covered.
Posturpedic Mattress	(Special mattress.)	Covered only when a hospital bed is allowable.
Pressure-Eze Pad	(Alternating pressure pad.)	Covered for treatment of decubitus ulcer.
Pressure Leotard	(Form-fitting apparel.)	Not covered.
Pulmo-Aide	(Medicated nebulizer system.)	Covered for upper respiratory disease.
Pulse Tachometer	(Electronic pulse reader.)	Not covered.
Reading Lamp	(For home use.)	Not covered.
Rib Belt	(Supportive elastic item.)	Rx not required. Covered for appropriate diagnosis such as rib injury.

(continued)

Sacro-Ease Car Seat	(For auto use.)	Not covered.
Sanitation Equipment	(For environmental use.)	Not covered.
Sauna Bath	(Comfort item.)	Not covered.
Scolitron Stimulator	(For curvature of the back, similar to TENS unit.)	Refer for medical review.
Seat Lift	(Seat that raises and lowers person in and out of chair.)	Rx required. For arthritis or other degenerative type diseases when the person is ambulatory.
Selectron Air Purifier	(Air cleaner for environmental control.)	Not covered. Environmental control equipment.
Shoe Wedging	(Sole modification.)	Rx required.
Shoes	(Wearing apparel item.)	Not covered. See Orthopedic shoes.
Sitz Bath	(Moist heat application.)	Not covered for home use.
Sleek Seat	(Supportive chair for atonic child.)	Rx required. For children with atonic muscle condition.
Spectrowave Machine	(Diathermy machine.)	Not covered for home use.
Speech Teaching Aids	(Education devices.)	Not covered.
Sphygmomanometer	(Blood pressure equipment.)	Covered with documented diagnosis of hypertension; also used with home hemodialysis units.
Spircare Incentive Breathing Device	(Usually shows pulmonary function.)	Not covered.
Stairglide	(Home elevator system.)	Not covered.
Stand Alone	(Device that allows a paraplegic to stand without assistance. Comfort item.)	Not covered.
Standing Table	(Special table for use in standing position.)	Not covered.
Stethoscope	(Blood pressure monitoring equipment.)	Covered only with home blood pressure monitoring system.
Stimulators, TENS	(Electronic pulse.)	Rx required. Refer for medical review.
Stryker Flotation Pad and Mattress	(Gel flotation pad treats and prevents pressure sores.)	Rx required.
Suction Machine	(Removes secretions from airway, etc.)	Rx required. Must have qualified person in home to handle machine.
Sun Lamp	(Thermal application to skin.)	Not covered.
Superpulse Machine	(Diathermy machine.)	Not covered for home use.
Surgical Stockings and Leggings	(Support apparel, anti-embolism hose.)	Rx required. See Jobst fabric.
Telemedic II	(Telephone cardiac monitor.)	Covered only when done in physician's office.
Telephone Arm	(Attaches to receiver, comfort item.)	Not covered.
Thermo-Jet	(Whirlpool pump.)	See Whirlpool.
Thermometer, Clinical	(Measures temperature.)	Not covered.
Thermophore Fomentation Device	(Heat applicator, external heat source moist heating pad.)	Not covered. Nondurable medical equipment.
Tilt Table	(Adjustable exercise table.)	Not covered.
Toilet Seat, Raised	------------------------	Rx required. Hip replacement surgeries. See seat lift for other conditions.

(continued)

Traction Device	(Weighted device for physical therapy.)	Rx required.
Trapeze Bar	(Supportive device used for lifting self in hospital bed.)	Rx required. For use with a standard hospital bed only.
Travel Type	Covered in lieu of regular wheelchair.	
Treadmill Devices	(Home walking exercise unit.)	Rental covered with Rx and appropriate cardiac diagnosis.
Truss	(Hernia support.)	Rx not required. Covered with appropriate diagnosis.
Tub Chair	(Bathtub use. Comfort item.)	Not covered.
Twister Cable Medical Device	(Pediatric orthopedic.)	Rx required. Refer for medical review.
Ultrasound Machine	(Sound waves applied to muscles, tendons, etc.)	Covered only in physician's office. Not for home use.
Ultraviolet Equipment	(Directs ultraviolet light to body areas.)	Covered for persons with psoriasis when medical necessity is documented and home use approved by physician.
Urinal, Autoclaveable Hospital Type	(Not a comfort item.)	Rx not required. Covered for bed-confined able person.
Vaporizer	(Delivers water mist to limited area in home.)	Not covered. Does not dispense medication as a nebulizer does.
Vasculating Bed	(Special hospital bed providing movement.)	Not covered for home use.
Vision Therapy Training Aids	(For adjunctive home use with vision therapy program.)	Not covered.
Walker	(Ambulatory aid.)	Rx not required.
Water Bed	(Comfort item.)	Not covered. See standard adjustable hospital bed.
Water Pressure Pad and Mattress	(Treats and prevents pressure sores, hospital bed type.)	Rx required.
Weighted Quad Boot	(Physical fitness equipment.)	Not covered. See ankle weights.
Wheel-O-Vater	(Home elevator.)	Not covered.
Wheelchair	Regular manual standard model.	Rx not required if documented by diagnosis.
Wheelchair	Electric type.	Rx required. Person must require independent mobility.
Wheelchair	Accessories and repair to function.	
Wheelchair	(Rubber wheel linings, ball appropriate and bearings, batteries, seat pad.)	Rx required. Covered only when policy provisions do not exclude. Convenience items or modifications not functional in nature such, as color coordination, deluxe padding, and trays, are not covered expenses.
Wheelchair Insert	(For small child, when chair seat does not fit.)	Rx not required.
Whirlpool Pumps	(Portable units for home use in baths.)	Rx required. Refer for medical review.
Wigs and Toupees	(Cosmetic appliance for conditions of alopecia, hair loss.)	Refer for medical review.

Potential Medical Case Management Claims

The following list consists of diagnoses that are potentially medical case management claims. This list is intended to be used for training and reference purposes only, since the particular company or plan guidelines may differ from those stated.

Section 1: Potential medical case management claims listing by condition are as follows:

Neurologic Patients	Neonatal Patients	Malignancy Patients
Brain tumors	Premature birth	Multiple surgeries
TIA (transient ischemic attack)	Hydrocephalus	Radiation treatments
Closed head injury	Respiratory distress and in ICU over one week	Cancer in children
Unconsciousness (any cause)	Meningomyelocele	Chemotherapy
Cerebral aneurysm or AV malformation	Bronchopulmonary dysplasia	Acute leukemia
Meningitis or encephalitis	Major or multiple congenital anomaly	Aplastic anemia
Reye's syndrome		Kaposi's sarcoma
Anoxic encephalopathy	TRANSPLANT/DIALYSIS PATIENTS	OBSTETRIC PATIENTS
Guillain-Barre	Heart, liver, or bone marrow transplant	Expected multiple birth of three or more infants
Quadriplegia	Organ rejection	Previous history of neonatal ICU confined infant
Paraplegia	Cardiomyopathy	Bleeding during pregnancy
Chronic stroke	Biliary atresia	
Multiple sclerosis (MS)	Renal failure	
Amyotrophic lateral sclerosis (ALS)		
Alzheimer's disease		

Psychiatric Conditions	Traumatically Injured Patients	Cardiovascular Conditions
Anorexia nervosa	Thermal burns or frostbite	Ruptured abdominal aortic aneurysm
Adolescent adjustment reaction	Child over 10% or adult over 20%	Myocardial Interaction (heart attack)
Manic depression; bipolar disorder	Crash injuries	Intractable angina
Schizophrenia	Amputations	Peripheral vascular disease, w/ pending amputation
Sexual abuse	Multiple trauma or fractures	
Chemical dependency	Spinal cord injury	
Depression with or without suicide attempt		

Respiratory Conditions	Other Diagnoses
Respirator dependency (any cause)	AIDS
Emphysema	Lupus
Chronic bronchitis or asthma	Any condition causing paralysis

(continued)

Section II: Potential medical case management claims by ICD–9–CM® codes are as follows:

Cases ICD-9-CM	Description	Cases ICD-9-CM	Description
High-risk mothers		**Other**	
640.x – 644.0	Complications of pregnancy	344.x	Other paralytic syndromes
646.x – 648.x		045.x	Poliomyelitis
760 – 779	Perinatal conditions		
Highly suggestive of AIDS		**Traumatic brain injury**	
031.0	Pulmonary infection by *Mycobacterium*	850.x—854.x	Various types of head injury
		800.x—804.x	Skull fracture
112.0*	Candidiasis of mouth (thrush)	780.0x	Coma and stupor
112.4	Candidiasis pneumonia	**Non-traumatic brain injury**	
112.5	Systematic candidiasis		
112.81 – 112.89*	Candidiasis of other sites	191.x	Brain tumors
114	Coccidioidal meningitis	293.x	Transient organic psychotic conditions
114.0	Pulmonary coccidioidomycocis		
114.9	Coccidioidomycocis, unspecified	294.x	Other organic psychotic conditions
115.0 – 115.9	Histoplasmosis		
130.0	Toxoplasmosis encephalitis	310.x	Mental disorders due to organic brain damage
130.3 – 130.9	Toxoplasmosis of other sites		
136.3	*Pneumocystis carinii* pneumonia	348.x	Brain conditions
176.x	Kaposi's sarcoma	349.x	Other and unspecified diseases of CNS
279.3	Deficiency of cell-mediated immunity		
279.3	Unspecified immunity deficiency	**Stroke**	
279.9	Unspecified disorder of immune system	342.x	Hemiplegia
		430	Subarachnoid hemorrhage
279.10	Immunodeficiency with predominant T-cell defect, unspecified	431	Intercerebral hemorrhage
		432	Other unspecified intracranial hemorrhage
279.19	Other immune disorders		
780.6*	Fever of unknown origin	433.x	Occlusion and stenosis of cerebral arteries
785.6*	Lymphadenopathy		
790.8*	Viremia, unspecified		
Spinal cord injury		**High-risk infants**	
952.x	Spinal cord injury without evidence of spinal bone injury	343.x	Infantile cerebral palsy
		741.x	Spina bifida
805.x – 806.x	Fracture of neck and trunk	742.x	Other congenital anomalies of the nervous system
336.x	Diseases of spinal cord		
		644.2	Early onset of delivery
Multiple fractures		**Burns**	
733.81	Malunion (fx)	940.x—949.x	Burns
733.82	Nonunion (fx)		

Assistant Surgeon Procedures

Following is a list of surgical procedures by CPT® code for which an assistant surgeon is considered NOT necessary. This list and is intended to be used for training and reference purposes only, as the particular company or plan guidelines may differ from those guidelines stated.

17108	19125	19126	19328	21616
23020	24101	24105	24110	24351
25295	25909	26037	26358	26516
27358	27619	27831	28290	30130
30140	30520	30620	31502	33470
36469	37700	42220	46700	52510
54110	54430	55040	55680	56304
58660	59821	61556	62142	63308
63746	64862	65155	66605	67101
67311	67875	68505	69631	69670

Glossary

Abortion—Abortion is a premature expulsion of an embryo or nonviable fetus.

Accident—An accident is an unintentional injury that has a specific time, date, and place.

Accidental injury—An accidental injury is a sudden and unforeseen event that has a specific time and place.

Accumulation period—The accumulation period is the period each year between the time that an insurance policy starts and the time that it renews (normally January 1 through December 31).

Active work—Active work refers to actively working in a position for a full day.

Actively-at-work—An "actively-at-work" stipulation states that a person must be at work (or actively engaged in his or her normal activities if the person is a dependent) on the date that insurance coverage becomes effective.

Acts of Third Parties (ATP)—Acts of Third Parties (ATP) and subrogation are provisions that are included in many benefit plans to allow the insurance company to recover money paid on claims that were incurred as a result of a third party's act or acts for which that party is financially responsible.

Actuarial statistics—Actuarial statistics are studies that an insurance company uses. For a carrier which covers health insurance, these can include statistics on average lifespan, number of days spent in the hospital per year for each age group, number of doctor visits, costs of all medical services, and so on.

Acupuncture—Acupuncture is the ancient Chinese practice of inserting fine needles into various points in the body to relieve pain, induce anesthesia, and regulate and improve body functions.

Adjudicated—When a patient is released to work, all benefits have been paid, and the case is closed, the claim is said to have been adjudicated.

Adjustment—An adjustment in the medical billing world is really a write-off. In the claims examiner world, it is the reprocessing of a claim to correct prior errors.

Affordable Care Act of 2010—The Affordable Care Act of 2010 is the healthcare reform started by President Obama in 2009, which sets forth several mandates, including the removal of preexisting conditions clauses by 2014, coverage for preexisting conditions by the federal government until 2014, and 100% coverage of preventative services and women's services.

Aggregate—Aggregate means that any amounts paid toward the deductible by any member of the family will be added up until the deductible is reached.

Air ambulance—An air ambulance is a helicopter or other flight vehicle that is used to transport severely injured or ill persons to a hospital.

Allowable expense—An allowable expense is any necessary, reasonable, and customary item of a medical or dental expense that is at least partly covered under at least one of the plans covering the person for whom a claim is made.

Allowed amount—The allowed amount is what the insurance company considers to be a reasonable charge for the procedure performed, often less than the amount that the doctor bills.

Alternative Birthing Centers (ABCs)—Alternative birthing centers (ABCs) are outpatient care centers that provide special rooms for routine deliveries. As a rule, these centers provide quiet, nontraditional, homelike rooms which are designed to allow the parents to be together and participate in the birthing experience.

Alternative medicine treatments—Alternative medicine treatment includes chiropractic care, acupuncture, massage therapy, and other nontraditional medical services.

Ambulance expenses—Ambulance expenses are charges billed for transporting an injured or ill person to a medical facility. Ambulance services are not considered professional or hospital services.

Ambulatory Surgical Centers (ASCs)—Ambulatory surgical centers (also called surgi-centers) are equipped for the performance of surgery on an outpatient basis. These centers may be freestanding or attached to a major acute care facility.

Ancillary expenses—Ancillary expenses are miscellaneous services or supplies that are provided by the hospital on an inpatient or outpatient basis, which are necessary for the medical care or treatment of an individual.

Anesthesia—Anesthesia is the artificially induced loss of feeling and sensation, with or without loss of consciousness.

Arthroplasty—An arthroplasty is a procedure in which a portion of the joint is surgically removed and the toe is straightened.

Assignment of benefits—A statement, usually included on the claim form, that permits the member to authorize the administrator to pay benefits directly to the person or institution that provided the service.

Assistant surgeon—The assistant surgeon assists the primary surgeon, as required.

Audit—An audit is a formal examination or systematic check of a program. Medicare and Medicaid conduct audits on claims.

Audit analysis report—After the audit, the audit information is analyzed and put into an audit analysis report that includes recommendations for corrective action and a compliance plan.

Audit of findings—A process for validating audit results.

Audit scope—The audit scope details what is being investigated, who will conduct the audit, and when the process will occur.

Automatic Annual Reinstatement (AAR)—An automatic renewal of a policy occurs each year as long as the payment is being made.

Balance billing—Balance billing is the practice of charging patients for more than the Medicare allowance. Participating physicians in a plan agree not to engage in this practice.

Basic benefit—A Basic benefit provides a specified allowance for a certain type of service (e.g., preventative tests), is usually paid at 100% of covered expenses, and is paid before major medical benefits are paid.

Batch files—Batch files are groups of claims that are categorized for the convenience of the biller or examiner, whichever is the case.

Beneficiary—The beneficiary is the person who would receive payment on a claim if he or she has not signed an assignment of benefits to the provider.

Benefit—Benefits are outlined in an insurance contract and may include payment of healthcare expenses, the replacement or repair of personal property, or payment for the expenses of others who have been injured by you or on your property.

Benefit period—A benefit period for Medicare begins with the first day of admission to the hospital. A benefit period ends after the patient has been discharged from the hospital or skilled nursing facility for a period of 60 consecutive days (including the day of discharge).

Bilateral procedure—A bilateral procedure is a surgery that involves a pair of similar body parts (e.g., breasts, eyes).

Biofeedback—Biofeedback is training an individual to consciously control automatic, internal bodily functions.

Block procedures—Block procedures are multiple surgical procedures that are performed during the same operative session, in the same operative area.

Bone spur—A bone spur is a bony overgrowth on the bone. Bone spurs have a variety of causes and usually result in pain, interfere with the use of the foot, and detract from its appearance.

Bunion—A bunion is an enlargement of a bone in a joint at the base of the big toe.

By Report (BR)—Some procedures are so unusual or variable that it is impossible to determine a standard UCR or unit value allowance for them. These procedures are called By Report (BR) procedures.

Capitation—Capitation is the practice of paying a provider a set amount per month to provide treatment to MCP members and for providing other administrative duties.

Capsulotomy—A tenotomy and capsulotomy are performed to release the buckling of a toe by cutting the top and bottom tendons. The joint capsules may also have to be cut.

Carriers—Private insurance companies, called carriers or Part B MACs, process Part B claims.

Carryover (C/O) deductible—A carryover deductible means that any amounts which the patient pays toward his or her deductible in the last three months of the year will carry over and will be applied toward the next year's deductible.

Certificate of Compliance Agreement (CCA)—After the compliance plan is complete, the organization receives a certificate of compliance agreement. This certificate is only applicable as long as the organization continues to follow the compliance plan.

Chromosomal analysis—Amniocentesis is the transabdominal perforation of the uterus and withdrawal of a sample of the amniotic fluid surrounding the fetus. Chromosomal analysis is the diagnostic study performed on the fluid to study the number and structure of the chromosomes to determine whether any abnormalities are present.

Claim—By filing a claim, the insured individual is notifying the insurance company, via the provider, of the member's loss or entitlement to reimbursement for any losses incurred.

Claim determination period—A claim determination period is usually a calendar year. It does not include any part of a year before the effective date of duplicate coverage under the secondary plan. It does not include any remaining amount during a calendar year that occurs after the termination date of the primary plan.

Claim files—Claim files or batches in the provider office contain the information for which claims have been submitted, returned to insurance companies with supplemental information, and denied.

Claim investigation—When a provider investigates a claim, the provider is inquiring about the status of a claim, such as a lost or denied claim, and seeking to obtain payment on the claim.

Claim processing—Claim processing is a process of determining benefit amounts and paying, pending, or denying a claim.

CMS-1500—The CMS-1500 claim form is a standardized form that has been approved by the American Medical Association for use as a "universal" form for billing outpatient professional services.

Coinsurance—Coinsurance is similar to a copayment; however, it is a percentage and usually is limited as an out-of-pocket expense for the insured.

Coinsurance limit—Many insurance carriers have a coinsurance limit which stipulates that if the coinsurance portion of a patient's bill reaches a certain amount, all subsequent claims will be paid at 100% of the allowed amount.

Common accident provision—A common accident provision states that only one deductible, under Major Medical, will be taken for all members of a family involved in the same accident.

Company activities—Company activities are activities sponsored by an employer for the purpose of obtaining some business gain, are activities in which employees participate and for which the company provides remuneration, or refer to normal workplace environments. An employee might file a claim for an injury sustained while attending a company activity.

Compensatory damages—Compensatory damages are designed to compensate an insured for all of the actual losses or damages to make that person whole again. For example, a person might be unable to pay his or her home mortgage or car payment because he or she did not receive a monthly disability check. If the person's home and car are therefore repossessed, he or she may be able to recover equity for the home and car, attorney fees, and damages for emotional stress.

Computed tomography (CT) scan—Computed tomography (CT) scans use multiple X-ray images to create three-dimensional images of body structures.

Concurrent review—Concurrent reviews determine whether the estimated length of time and scope of the inpatient stay is justified by the diagnosis and symptoms.

Consideration—Consideration is anything that is given, done, promised, forbidden, or suffered by one party as an inducement for the agreement. The most common form of consideration is the payment of money in exchange for a promise. For insurance, consideration is the premium paid by the group policyholder.

Consolidated Omnibus Budget Reconciliation Act of 1985 (COBRA)—In 1986, President Ronald Reagan signed into law HR3128, the Consolidated Omnibus Budget Reconciliation Act of 1985 (COBRA), also referred to as continuation of coverage, which allowed employees to retain health insurance coverage in between jobs by paying for it.

Consultation—A consultation is provided by a specialist who has been requested to provide an opinion only, not treatment.

Contract—A contract is any agreement between two or more persons that is enforceable by law.

Contributory plan—In a contributory plan, the employees contribute to the cost of the coverage, usually through payroll deductions.

Convalescent facilities—Convalescent facilities are usually considered to be midrange facilities that provide non-acute care for persons who are recovering from an acute illness or injury.

Conversion—Most states have legislatively mandated that insurance policies contain a continuation of coverage provision known as conversion. Conversion permits employees and dependents to continue their insurance protection on an individual basis when their coverage under a group plan ceases.

Coordination of Benefits (COB)—Coordination of benefits (COB) is the process used to ensure that an insured person who has more than one insurance plan is reimbursed for all costs, but no more.

Copayment—Copayments allow the insured party to share in the cost of the service, depending on the service but at a set amount each time the person obtains that service.

Corrective action—Corrective action is taken to correct lapses in regulations that are found during an audit.

Cosmetic procedure—Cosmetic procedures are performed solely to improve the appearance of a body part and are not usually covered by benefit plans.

Cosmetic surgery—Cosmetic surgery is a surgical procedure that is performed solely to improve appearance and that is usually not covered by benefit plans.

Cosurgeons—Under some circumstances, two surgeons, usually with similar skills, may operate simultaneously as primary surgeons performing distinct, separate parts of a total surgical service. They are referred to as cosurgeons.

Covered expense—An expense that is allowable under the insurance plan is a covered service or allowed amount.

Credit Reserve (CR)—The Credit Reserve (CR) is a cumulative amount within a claim determination period that is derived from the amount of funds that a plan has saved by being the secondary carrier.

Cumulative benefit—Many types of medical while hospitalized (MWH) benefits are available. One of the more common types is called a cumulative benefit. To calculate benefits under this provision, multiply the number of days hospitalized by the benefit amount.

Current Dental Terminology (CDT)—*Current Dental Terminology (CDT)* is a reference book that provides language for dental healthcare claims.

Current Procedural Terminology (CPT)—*Current Procedural Terminology (CPT)* is a systematic listing of all the procedures or services performed by a physician, with the appropriate codes.

Custodial care—Custodial care is primarily done in order to meet the personal daily needs of the patient and can be provided by personnel without medical care skills or training.

Day care centers—Day care centers provide treatment during the daylight hours and release the patient at night.

Death benefits—Death benefits compensate the family of a deceased employee for the loss of income which the employee would have provided to the family.

Deductible—A deductible is the amount which the member must pay before the insurance pays any benefits.

Deficit Reduction Act of 1984 (DEFRA)—The Deficit Reduction Act of 1984—and its amendments—have redirected the financial responsibility for medical coverage of active employees aged 65 years and older and their spouses aged 65 years and older.

Diagnosis-related group (DRG)—In the early 1980s, Medicare instituted diagnosis-related group (DRG) payments for inpatient hospital claims. Under DRG, a flat-rate payment is made on the basis of the patient's diagnosis, rather than using the hospital's itemized billing.

Diagnostic charges—Diagnostic charges are charges for initial testing to confirm a diagnosis or to rule out other diagnoses.

Diagnostic procedures—Diagnostic procedures are performed to determine the presence of disease or the cause of the patient's symptoms.

Diagnostic X-rays—Diagnostic X-rays are flat or two-dimensional pictures of a particular body part or organ.

Dialysis—Dialysis is a treatment given to patients who have suffered acute kidney failure and must have their kidney functions taken over artificially.

Disclaimer—A disclaimer is a denial or renunciation of responsibility. In the health claims examiner's world, it means to use words and phrases that refuse to promise an outcome.

Doctor's First Report of Occupational Injury or Illness (First Report)—On an injured employee's first visit to a physician, the physician completes a "Doctor's First Report of Occupational Injury or Illness" or "First Report" to submit to workers' compensation.

Documentation—Documentation is the substance of a claim.

Dorsal osteotomy—A dorsal osteotomy is performed by removing a small wedge of bone from the top (dorsal) side of the base of the fifth metatarsal bone.

Durable medical equipment (DME)—Durable medical equipment (DME) includes any item that can be used for an extended period of time without significant deterioration (i.e., it can stand repeated use).

Dwyer procedure—The Dwyer procedure is the treatment for a deformity of the calcaneus or large heel bone. It consists of a wedge resection of a portion of the calcaneus bone, closed with a staple, pin, or screw fixation.

Effective date—The effective date is the date on which the contract begins to be in force.

Electronic claims—All healthcare claims are submitted electronically to insurance carriers. These claims are called electronic claims.

Electronic claims submission—Electronic claims submission is a process whereby insurance claims are submitted via an EDI directly from the provider to the insurance company.

Electronic Data Interchange (EDI)—The Electronic Data Interchange (EDI) is the system that claims examiners and medical billers use to send and receive information from regarding claims.

Electronic Health Records (EHR)—Electronic Health Records (EHR) are collections of all the information about a patient, kept in an electronic record rather than in a traditional medical chart/record.

Electronic Remittance Notice (ERN)—The Electronic Remittance Notice (ERN) is the electronic version of the Medicare Remittance Advice (MRA) form.

Eligibility—Eligibility refers to having the qualifications which make the person eligible for coverage.

Eligibility requirements—Eligibility requirements are the baseline standards that the insured must meet in order to receive coverage.

Eligibility roster—Check the eligibility roster to determine the effective dates of the patient's coverage, the contract under which he or she is covered, and the patient's PCP (the Group/IPA responsible for his or her primary care).

Eligible—Qualifying for coverage.

Embezzlement—When an employee illegally takes funds from the company for which he or she works, it is embezzlement.

Emergency medical technicians (EMTs)—Emergency medical technicians (EMTs) are personnel who are trained in basic life support.

End-Stage Renal Disease (ESRD)—End-stage renal disease (ESRD) is the condition in which a person's kidneys fail to function.

Endogenous obesity—Endogenous obesity is obesity that is caused by an internal malfunction, usually hormonal (e.g., thyroid disorder).

Epidural anesthesia—Epidural anesthesia is a procedure that blocks the nerves in the epidural space.

Evidence of insurability—The prospective member of an insurance plan and all eligible dependents sometimes have to provide proof of good health, also known as evidence of insurability, by filling out health questionnaire.

Exclusions—Every contract has a list of exclusions, conditions or expenses for which no coverage is provided.

Exclusive Provider Organization (EPO)—In an Exclusive Provider Organization (EPO), the patient must select a primary care provider and can only visit physicians who are part of the network or who are referred by the primary care physician.

Exogenous obesity—Exogenous obesity is caused by overeating.

Explanation of Benefits (EOB)—An explanation of benefits (EOB) is a letter from a payer indicating how a member's benefits have been applied in response to the submission of a claim for services. The EOB indicates deductibles, coinsurance amounts, nonallowable amounts, UCR limitations, and other pertinent information. An EOB is required by law to be generated on each claim submission showing the disposition of the claim.

Extended benefits—Extended benefits are the continued entitlement of a member, under certain circumstances, to receive benefits after the coverage has terminated.

Facility services—Facility services are those services provided at a "place," for example, a hospital or clinic.

False nail—The treatment for an ingrown toenail is usually a total matrixectomy, in which the nail and growth plate are removed either surgically or chemically. The body then produces a "false nail,": tough skin that mimics a real nail. This false nail usually grows in within a few months after surgery.

Fee schedule—Some plans have established their own calculations of the amount payable for particular services. These amounts are listed on what is commonly called a fee schedule.

Flat feet—Flat feet (pes planus) are hereditary and are caused by a muscle imbalance.

Followup days—Followup days are the days immediately following a surgical procedure in which a doctor must monitor a patient's condition related to that particular procedure.

Fraud—Fraud is the use of deception to cause a person to give up property or something to which the person has a lawful right.

Full-credit adjustment—A Full-Credit Adjustment is an adjustment that completely reverses a claim payment because the original submission should not have been paid at all.

Ganglions—Ganglions are fluid-filled sacs that may grow on a joint capsule or tendon.

Gatekeeper PPO—In the Gatekeeper PPO scenario, the member chooses a family provider or physician and must see him or her before being referred to a specialist.

General anesthesia—General anesthesia produces a state of unconsciousness. It may be brought about by inhalation of gases such as ether, nitrous oxide, and ethylene or by drugs administered intravenously, such as sodium pentothal.

Global approach—Nearly all multiple surgery claims are calculated using a global approach. In a global approach, the total billed amount should be compared with the total UCR amount.

Global COB—A Global COB is a COB that is applied to both medical and dental charges combined. All savings are kept intermingled.

Group contract—The group contract offers an instrument through which an insurance company can meet the financial security needs of a group of persons. In essence, it is an agreement between the insurance company and the policyholder to insure the lives and/or health of the members of a defined group of persons and to pay the insurance benefits to the insured persons or their beneficiaries.

Group insurance—Group insurance provides coverage for several people under one contract, called a master contract.

Group model—In a Group model HMO, a medical facility or Group bands together to provide services for HMO patients at their own facilities.

Group Plan—A form of coverage where several individuals are covered under one insurance plan.

Hammertoes—Hammertoes are inherited muscle imbalances or abnormal bone lengths that can make the toes buckle under, causing their joints to contract.

Health Maintenance Organization (HMO)—A Health Maintenance Organization (HMO) is a type of prepayment policy in which the organization bears the responsibility and financial risk of providing agreed-on healthcare services to the members enrolled in its plan, in exchange for a fixed monthly membership fee.

The Healthcare Common Procedure Coding System (HCPCS)—The Healthcare Common Procedure Coding System (HCPCS), Commonly referred to as "hicpics" in the medical community, was created to correct the limitations in the *CPT* and *RVS* for billing services such as injections, medication, supplies, durable medical equipment, and chiropractic and dental services.

Heel spur—A heel spur is an overgrowth on the heel bone.

High-arched feet—High-arched feet (pes cavus) are caused by an imbalance of muscles and nerves and are often inherited.

Hospice care—A palliative care program offered at the end of life to support the family and patient through the end of life process.

Hospital services—Hospital services are performed in a hospital setting. The term is used generically to refer to charges billed by a hospital, urgent care center, surgi-center, alternative birthing center, or similar institution.

Hospital staff anesthesiologist—A hospital staff anesthesiologist is an anesthesiologist who is employed by the hospital.

Hypnosis—Hypnosis is a state in which the subconscious mind is allowed to take over and the conscious mind is more or less inactive. Some patients choose hypnosis over conventional forms of anesthesia.

***In utero* fetal surgery**—*In utero* fetal surgery is surgery performed on a fetus while it is in the mother's womb. It also refers to the removal of the fetus from the womb, surgery on the fetus, and return of the fetus back to the womb, with the pregnancy continuing to term.

***In vitro* fertilization**—*In vitro* fertilization is the fertilization of the ovum outside the body (i.e., within a test tube or a petri dish).

In-network—An in-network provider is a physician or other service provider who is contracted with a managed care plan.

Incidental procedure—An incidental procedure is one that does not add significant time or complexity to the operative session.

Independent anesthesiologist—An independent anesthesiologist is self-employed or not employed by the hospital.

Independent Physician Associations (IPAs)—Independent Physician Associations (IPAs) are groups of providers who have banded together for the sole purpose of signing a contract with a Managed Care Plan.

Individual deductible—If an individual deductible is assigned, the individual expenses must be paid by the individual family member before the plan pays for any benefits.

Individual insurance—Individual insurance is issued to insure the life or health of a named person or persons, rather than the life or health of the members of a group.

Individual Practice Organizations (IPOs)—Individual Practice Organizations or IPOs (sometimes called Independent Practice Associations) are legal entities composed of a network of private physicians who have organized to negotiate contracts with insurance companies and HMOs.

Infusion pump—A machine that administers fluids and/or medications at regular intervals usually through an IV.

Ingrown toenail—An ingrown toenail is a nail in which one or both corners or sides of the nail grow into the skin of the toe.

Inpatient care—Inpatient care describes care that is provided when the patient has been admitted into the hospital and stays for a period of time, usually a minimum of 24 hours.

Insurance—Insurance is an agreement between insurance companies, who collect fees or premiums, and individuals, who pay the premiums in return for specific benefits.

Insurance carrier—The insurance carrier is a corporation or association whose business is to develop insurance contracts.

Insurance company—An insurance company sells policies offered by insurance carriers.

Insurance policy—An insurance policy outlines the benefits that the insured receives for payment of premiums and the requirements that he or she must meet in order to receive these benefits.

Insurance premium—An insurance premium is the amount of money that is required for coverage under a specific insurance policy for a given length of time.

Insurance speculation—Insurance speculation occurs when someone buys insurance coverage for the purpose of making a profit. It may include staging a fake death or an accident in order to file claims under more than one policy.

Insured—An insured person (also called member or guarantor) obtains or is otherwise covered by insurance on his or her health, life, or property.

Intermediaries—Medicare Part A claims are processed by third party claims administrators called intermediaries or Part A MAC's.

International Classification of Diseases – 9th Revision Clinical Modification (ICD-9-CM)—The *International Classification of Diseases—9th Revision—Clinical Modification (ICD-9-CM)* is the reference book used for coding healthcare claims with diagnostic information.

International Classification of Diseases – 10th Revision Clinical Modification Manual (ICD-10-CM) or Procedure Coding System (ICD-10-CM)—The *International Classification of Diseases—10th Revision—Clinical Modification and Procedure Coding System (ICD-10-CM/PCS)* is the reference book that is used for coding healthcare claims with diagnostic and procedural information. The 10th version takes effect on October 1, 2014.

Intractable pain—Intractable pain is pain that is difficult to manage and is often severe enough to limit a patient's movement or abilities.

Intravenous (IV) sedation—Intravenous (IV) sedation is the intravenous administration of a medication composed of a sedative and a painkiller to produce a semiconscious state.

Investigation—Investigation is an organized effort to discover the facts or truth of a matter.

Job-related injuries—Job-related injuries happen during the performance of work-related duties, whether they occur in or out of the office.

Joints—Joints are where two bones meet.

Laboratory examinations—Laboratory examinations involve the analysis of body substances to determine their chemical or tissue make-up.

Lapse in coverage—If the insured does not renew his or her insurance, the individual may have a lapse in coverage, which is defined as time without insurance coverage.

Legal damages—Generally, the law of bad faith allows an insured to attempt to recover various types of legal damages above and beyond the benefits that are provided by the plan.

Lien—A lien is a legal document that expresses claim on the property of another for payment of a debt.

Ligaments—Ligaments are flexible bands of fiber that join one bone to another.

Limiting charge (LC)—A limiting charge (LC) is the maximum amount that the federal government allows nonparticipating physicians to charge Medicare patients for a given service.

Local anesthesia—Local anesthesia affects only a localized area.

Loss date—The loss date is the date of the accident or injury.

Maintenance of benefits—Maintenance of benefits refers to a provision in many group health plans that allows a person who has Medicare to "maintain" the same group benefits as members who do not have Medicare.

Major Medical benefits—Major Medical benefits are benefits that are paid after Basic benefits, and which are usually subject to a deductible and/or coinsurance.

Malice—Malice is an intention to cause injury or conduct that is carried on with the conscious disregard of the rights of others.

Managed care—Managed care is a strategy for reducing or controlling healthcare costs by closely monitoring and restricting the use and cost of services. Under this type of system, the insurer manages the delivery of healthcare and controls costs by emphasizing primary and preventive care services. Managed care plans use quality assurance and utilization review to ensure the appropriate delivery of care.

Management Service Organization (MSO)—A Management Service Organization (MSO) is a separate corporation that is set up to provide management services to a medical group for a fee.

Mandates—Mandates are laws enacted by states that require insurance carriers to cover certain services, dependents, or services provided by certain providers.

Mandatory program—A mandatory program requires the patient to obtain an second surgical opinion for specific procedures. If the patient does not do so, there is an automatic reduction or denial of benefits.

Matrixectomy—A matrixectomy is a procedure in which the nail and growth plate are removed, either surgically or chemically.

Maximum—The maximum amount payable by the plan applies only to agreed-on fees between the insurance company and the provider (e.g., managed care programs). As of 2014, annual and/or lifetime maximums are no longer written into insurance policies.

Medicaid—Medicaid is a jointly funded federal–state entitlement program that is designed to provide healthcare services to certain low-income and medically needy people.

Medicaid Fraud Control Unit (MFCU)—Medicaid Fraud Control Units (MFCUs) investigate and prosecute Medicaid fraud, as well as patient abuse and neglect in healthcare facilities.

Medical Case Management (MCM)—Medical Case Management (MCM) is the process of evaluating the effectiveness and frequency of medical treatments by reviewing services to determine whether the care that is being rendered or that is going to be rendered is appropriate.

Medical dictionary—Medical dictionaries list medical terms and their definitions, synonyms, illustrations, and supplemental information.

Medical groups—Medical groups are groups of physicians who are signed under or work for the same company.

Medical management—Medical management X-ray/lab charges are incurred to control or manage a diagnosis (e.g., monitoring blood glucose levels on a patient with diabetes).

Medically oriented equipment—Medically oriented equipment is primarily and customarily used for medical purposes (i.e., it is designed to fulfill a medical need).

Medicare—Medicare is the Federal Health Insurance Benefit Plan for the Aged and Disabled, Title XVIII of Public Law 89-97 of the Social Security Act of 1965. This program is for people 65 years of age or older and certain persons who are totally disabled or have a diagnosis of ESRD.

Medicare allowance—The total fee that a physician may receive from Medicare and from beneficiaries for an assigned bill is limited by the Medicare allowance, the amount that Medicare deems to be an appropriate fee for the particular service or procedure.

Medicare Part A—Medicare Part A is considered the basic plan, or hospital insurance. This part covers facility charges for acute inpatient hospital care, skilled nursing, home healthcare, and hospice care.

Medicare Part B—Medicare Part B is the medical (supplementary, voluntary) insurance that covers physician services, outpatient hospital services, home healthcare, outpatient speech and physical therapy, and durable medical equipment.

Medicare Part C—Part C is the Medicare advantage portion and includes coverage in an HMO, PPO, or other insurance.

Medicare Part D—Part D is the prescription drug component, which was introduced by the Medicare Prescription Drug, Improvement, and Modernization Act of 2003 and became effective in 2006.

Medicare Remittance Advice—The Medicare Remittance Advice is used to convey payments to providers who accept assignment for Medicare claims.

Medicare Summary Notice (MSN)—The Medicare Summary Notice (MSN) is an explanation of benefits sent to the Medicare beneficiary, detailing the processing of claims submitted for payment.

Medicare supplements—Medicare supplements (also called Medigap) are private insurance separate plans that are written exclusively for Medicare participants.

Member file—The member file is an electronic file for an individual patient stored at the provider's office or facility. The insurance company also keeps member files for its members.

Mental Health and Substance Abuse Treatment Expenses—Mental Health and Substance Abuse Treatment Expenses include claims submitted for psychiatric services, marriage and family counseling services, and drug and alcohol treatment.

Merck Manual—Medical professionals rely on the *Merck Manual* to identify symptoms, prognosis, treatment protocols, etiology, and other miscellaneous information regarding diagnoses.

Metatarsal plantar callus—A metatarsal plantar callus occurs when the metatarsal bone is longer or lower than the others so that it hits the ground first at every step with more force than it is equipped to handle. As a result, the skin under this bone thickens and becomes hardened into a callus.

Miscellaneous services—Miscellaneous services are all types of services that are not included in another category. For example, prescriptions, medical equipment (e.g., wheelchairs, crutches), and ambulance charges are all considered miscellaneous types of expenses.

Mobile intensive care unit—A mobile intensive care unit is a life support vehicle that is equipped to provide care to critically ill patients who require transportation to a hospital or from one hospital to another. It is designed to serve as an extension of an intensive care unit at a hospital.

Modifier codes—Modifier codes are two-digit numerical codes or alphanumeric codes that are attached to a *CPT* code to indicate special circumstances that affect reimbursement for that particular service.

Monitored anesthesia care (MAC)—Monitored anesthesia care (MAC) is the monitoring of a patient's vital signs during an operation in anticipation of the need for general anesthesia.

Multiple procedures—Multiple procedures are more than one surgical procedure performed during the same operative session.

Necessity—A treatment or item of equipment is a necessity when it is expected to make a meaningful contribution to the treatment of the patient's illness or injury or to the improvement of the functioning of a malformed body part.

Nerve block anesthesia—For a nerve block anesthesia, a drug is injected close to the nerve so that the nerve impulses are interrupted, producing a loss of sensation.

Network model—In a network model, the HMO contracts with several providers in a locale, allowing some overlap of geographic area.

Neuroma—A neuroma is a tumor that arises from the connective tissue of the nerves.

Night care centers—Night care centers allow a patient to pursue a normal routine during the day, such as working, and be treated at the center and cared for overnight.

Nonaggregate—In a nonaggregate policy, a specified number of individual deductibles must be satisfied before the family limit is met.

Noncontributory plan—In a noncontributory plan, the employer bears the complete cost of the coverage and the employee does not contribute.

Nondisability claims—Nondisability claims are for minor injuries that do not prevent a patient from continuing to work.

Nonparticipating physicians—Nonparticipating physicians treat Medicare-eligible patients but decide whether to accept assignment on a case-by-case basis.

Normal Liability (NL)—Normal Liability (NL) is the amount payable under a secondary plan's provisions without regard to any other coverage (what the plan normally would have paid if there were no other insurance).

Nuclear medicine—Nuclear medicine combines the use of radioactive elements and X-rays to image an organ or body part.

Nursing homes—Also called long-term care facilities. Nursing homes specialize in custodial care, that is, care that is primarily for the purpose of meeting the activities of daily living for the patient.

Occupational illnesses—Occupational illnesses are any disorders, illnesses, or conditions that arise at work or from exposure to factors at work.

Offer—When making an offer, an individual is proposing to undertake or to do or give something in exchange for a return promise from the person to whom the act or gift is being offered.

Office of Inspector General (OIG)—The Office of Inspector General (OIG) was created under the Inspector General Act of 1978. The responsibilities have changed to include oversight over programs funded through the American Recovery and Reinvestment Act of 2009. The OIG assesses whether the Department of Health and Human Services is using funds from the Recovery and Reinvestment Act in accordance with legal and administrative requirements. The OIG is involved with the CMS in conducting audits of the Medicare and Medicaid programs.

Office or other outpatient visits—Office or other outpatient visits are encounters between a physician and patient that occur outside a hospital setting.

Open enrollment—Open enrollment is a process that allows all applicants to enroll in an insurance plan or change their current insurance coverage.

Open letters—Open letters notify the industry of changes or OIG initiatives to prevent fraud and abuse in the Medicare and Medicaid system.

Ophthalmology care—Ophthalmology care is eye care provided either by an optometrist (O.D.) or an ophthalmologist (M.D.).

Oppression—Oppression is putting a person through cruel and unjust hardships and consciously disregarding the person's rights.

Optional modifiers—Optional modifiers denote special conditions for anesthesia services.

Order of Benefit Determination (OBD)—Order of Benefit Determination (OBD) rules were established to provide standardized rules for coordination among health plans.

Orthoptics—Orthoptics is the retraining of the muscles that control vision.

Orthosis—An orthosis is an orthopedic appliance that in many cases is as effective as surgery for restoring functionality to the patient.

Orthotic devices—Orthotic devices are prescribed custom-made arch supports that fit inside most shoes and "bring the floor up to your feet."

Osteopathic treatment—Osteopathic treatment is based on the idea that the body can cure itself if it is in a normal state and provided with the proper environmental conditions.

Out-of-network—An out-of-network provider is a healthcare provider with whom the relevant managed care organization does not have a contract to provide healthcare services.

Out-of-pocket (OOP) costs—A member's "out-of-pocket" (OOP) costs include the deductible, cost sharing arising from the operation of the coinsurance clause, and medical expenditures that are deemed by the plan to exceed reasonable and customary charges. To calculate the OOP expense, use the reverse of the coinsurance amount.

Out-of-pocket (OOP) maximum—The out-of-pocket (OOP) maximum is a yearly limit on the OOP that the insured is responsible for paying.

Outliers—Outliers are cases that are atypically expensive (for on the diagnosis) because of complications or an abnormally long confinement. These cases are reimbursed on an itemized or cost percentage basis rather than using the DRG system.

Outpatient provider—The outpatient provider of service is a hospital facility (the title may be Hospital, Medical Center, Surgi-center, or Birthing Center) in which there are no room and board charges.

Overinsurance—Overinsurance occurs when a person is covered under two or more policies and is eligible to collect an accumulation of benefits that actually exceeds the amount charged by the provider.

Panel tests—Panel tests are composed of multiple tests that are combined and run from one specimen.

Papanicolaou or "Pap" smear—A Papanicolaou or "Pap" smear is a diagnostic laboratory test for detecting the absence or presence of infection, viruses, trauma, or cancer in a specimen of cervical cells.

Paramedics—Paramedics are specially trained emergency medical personnel who render emergency treatment at the scene of the injury or illness.

Partial-credit adjustment—A partial-credit adjustment is an adjustment that partially reverses a claim payment when the original claim was overpaid.

Participating physician—To encourage physicians to accept assignment for bills, the Medicare allowance is higher for physicians who agree to accept assignment for all bills for Medicare-eligible persons. These physicians are called participating physicians.

Patient Protection and Affordable Care Act of 2010—The Patient Protection and Affordable Care Act of 2010 prohibits lifetime limits on most benefits in any health plan or insurance policy that was issued or renewed on or after September 23, 2010.

Pended claim—A pended claim is on hold awaiting further information.

Per period of disability—Basic benefit waiting periods and deductibles are referred to as per period disability; these may apply on a per illness basis or on a waiting period basis.

Permanent and stationary—Permanent and stationary means that the patient will have the disability for the rest of his or her life.

Permanent disability—Permanent disability usually commences after temporary disability when it is determined that the patient will not be able to return to work.

Personal items—Personal items are items that are primarily for the comfort of the patient and are not medically necessary.

Physical medicine—Physical medicine is the manipulation and physical therapy associated with the nonsurgical care and treatment of the patient.

Physical status modifiers—Physical status modifiers are used for anesthesia services and are represented by the initial P, followed by a single digit from 1 to 6.

Physician Hospital Organization (PHO)—A Physician Hospital Organization (PHO) is an organization of physicians and hospitals that band together for the purpose of obtaining contracts from payer organizations.

Physicians' Desk Reference (PDR)—The *Physicians' Desk Reference (PDR)* is a manual that provides information on prescription drugs, including usage, dosage, appearance, prescription status, makeup, and other details.

Podiatry—Podiatry is the medical treatment of the feet.

Policy—Every health benefit plan, whether it is insured or not, is required by law to have a written document describing the plan benefits, which is called a contract or policy.

Positional bunion—A positional bunion develops when a bony growth on the side of the metatarsal bone enlarges the joint, forcing the joint capsule to stretch over it.

Preadmission testing—Preadmission testing consists of routine laboratory and X-ray tests performed on an outpatient basis before a scheduled inpatient admission.

Preauthorization—Preauthorization is gaining approval for services that are to be performed, as well as finding out whether the insurance carrier will provide coverage for these services.

Precertification—Precertification means preapproval for admission on an elective, nonemergency hospitalization.

Predetermination—Predetermination is an estimate of maximum benefits that may be paid under the plan for the services. It is not, however, a guarantee that benefits will be paid.

Preexisting condition—A preexisting condition is a medical condition that an individual had before he or she purchased a particular insurance policy.

Preferred Provider Organization (PPO)—A Preferred Provider Organization (PPO) is a group of healthcare providers who agree to provide services to a specific pool of patients for an agreed fee (contractual).

Premium—A premium is the fee that members pay in order to receive insurance.

Preventive coverage—Preventive coverage includes coverage of services such as an annual physical, cancer screening (Pap smears, mammograms, etc.), flu shots, immunizations, and well-baby care.

Primary care provider (PCP)—Members of an HMO choose a specific provider for their care called a primary care provider or a primary care physician (PCP).

Primary plan—The primary plan is the benefit plan that determines and pays its benefits first, whether or not there is any other coverage.

Procedure code—A procedure code is a five-digit numerical code used to designate medical services according to standardized, industry-accepted methods, usually reflected in the *CPT* manual.

Products—Products are any items that are packaged to be sold to a consumer. In the case of insurance, products include health plans, life insurance, and policies covering the various properties belonging to a consumer.

Professional component (PC)—The professional component (PC) is the interpretation or the reading of the results of the test and is denoted by adding modifier -26 to the *CPT* code.

Professional services—Professional services are performed by a licensed individual, such as a medical doctor, physician's assistant, advanced nurse practitioner, or chiropractor.

Prosthetic devices—Prosthetic devices are designed to replace a missing body part or to restore some function to a paralyzed body part.

Provider of service (Provider)—The provider of service is the medical professional or facility that provides service to the insured patient.

Punitive damages—Punitive damages are intended primarily to punish wrongdoing by the defendant and to make an example of the individual to help deter others from committing such actions in the future.

Qualified beneficiary—A qualified beneficiary is anyone who, on the day before the qualifying event, is covered under the health coverage plan as an employee, a dependent spouse, or a dependent child.

Qualifying event—A qualifying event is an event that results in the loss of eligibility or becoming eligible under the employer-sponsored health plan.

Radiation oncology—Radiation oncology is the use of radiation to treat a medical condition.

Reasonable charges—Medicare payments are based on "reasonable charges," which are the amounts approved by the Medicare carrier according to what is considered reasonable for the geographic area in which the doctor practices.

Reasonableness—Reasonableness is an evaluation of the need for Durable Medical Equipment in the rehabilitation process.

Rebundling—If unbundling of a charge has occurred, the claims examiner should perform rebundling by denying the component parts of the procedure as already included within the allowable charge for the single procedure.

Reconstruction—Reconstruction is performed to rebuild or aesthetically restore a part of the body that was damaged or defective as a result of an illness or injury.

Recovery Audit Contractors (RACs)—Recovery Audit Contractors (RACs) are government-contracted auditors whose task is to find and stop Medicare fraud.

Red Book and Blue Book—The *Red Book* is primarily used by pharmacists for drug information and wholesale pricing, and the *Blue Book* is used normally by providers and patients to compare pricing for their geographical area.

Reexamination Report—If the patient's condition changes significantly, after a claim has been filed, a Reexamination Report, or a detailed progress report, should be filed with the insurance carrier.

Referral—The term referral is different for the medical biller and the claims examiner. A medical biller checks that a patient obtained required referrals from his or her primary care provider before visiting a specialist. In the same manner, a claims examiner verifies that such a referral was made (if required), but the term is also used when the claim is referred to a technical specialist for review.

Regional anesthesia—Regional anesthesia is the loss of sensation of a part of the body due to the interruption of nerve conduction.

Rehabilitation benefit—If an employee is found to have a permanent disability, some states allow for a rehabilitation benefit. This benefit gives the employee training in a physical ability that will help him or her to seek future employment.

Rehabilitation facilities—Rehabilitation facilities specialize in long-term, postsickness, or postinjury care.

Reinstatement—After a member's insurance policy has lapsed due to nonpayment of premiums, the member can pay his or her old premiums to get coverage reinstated.

Reinsurance—Reinsurance is a program that reimburses the employer when losses exceed a specific amount agreed on by the employer and the reinsurance carrier.

Relative Value Scale (RVS)—The Relative Value Scale (RVS) is a payment methodology devised by Harvard University and adapted by CMS to be used in the American Medicare system. It assigns a value to procedures performed by a physician. The relative value differs by geographic region and is adjusted annually.

Relative Value Units (RVUs)—Relative Value Units (RVUs) represent the total RVS for components of the schedule, which is revised every five years.

Renewal—A renewal is the payment of a premium in order to continue an individual's coverage after the initial or subsequent policy periods have expired.

Retrospective review—A retrospective review, conducted after discharge, is used to determine whether the hospitalization and treatment were medically necessary and covered by the terms of the benefit program.

Saddle block—A saddle block is a type of spinal anesthetic, named because the injection produces a loss of feeling in the region of the body that corresponds to the area which makes contact with a riding saddle (buttocks, perineum, and thighs).

Second Surgical Opinion (SSO) Consultation—A Second Surgical Opinion (SSO) or confirmatory consultation allows the insurance company to verify that another physician recommends surgery for the patient. Patients often are required to get a second opinion for surgeries that have a reputation for being done needlessly.

Secondary plan—A secondary plan pays after the primary plan has paid its benefits. The benefits of the secondary plan take into consideration the benefits of the primary plan, and the secondary plan may reduce its payment so that only 100% of allowable expenses are paid.

Self-disclosure protocol (SDP)—A part of any compliance plan is the education of employees on self-disclosure protocol (SDP), essentially letting them know that it is important to report fraudulent or abusive practices.

Self-funded plan—In a self-funded plan, the total and ultimate responsibility for providing all plan benefit payments rests solely with the employer, group, or association.

Serial surgery—Serial surgery is surgery on several individual toes or joints, with one surgical procedure being performed in each operative visit (i.e., surgery on one toe, followed by surgery on another toe one week later, followed by still other surgeries after that). Alternatively, it is surgery on one joint, followed by surgery on a different joint of the same toe at a later date.

Speech therapy—Speech therapy is usually provided to correct speech that has been impaired because of sickness or injury, but it can also be used to correct speech impediments or to help a deaf person to speak.

Spinal anesthesia—In spinal anesthesia, nerves in the subarachnoid space are blocked.

Staff model—The staff model is the original concept of HMO services. A physician or provider is hired to work at the HMO's own facility, is usually paid a salary, and may receive additional bonuses. The provider works only for the HMO and sees no outside patients.

Stat fees—Stat fees are a charge for DXL services that are performed on an expedited priority basis.

State insurance regulatory department—The insurance industry is overseen in each state by an insurance regulatory department. These departments for each state hold the primary legal authority over the operations of all insurance companies within that state.

Statistical adjustment—A statistical adjustment changes the claim data (e.g., procedure coding, type of benefit paid, diagnosis) but does not increase or decrease the original claim payment.

Statistical sampling—Statistical sampling is a method that selects and analyzes enough claims to form a statistically valid sample but not all the claims in the group.

Stop-loss insurance—Stop-loss insurance, or reinsurance, is a program that reimburses the employer when losses exceed a specific amount agreed on by the employer and the reinsurance carrier.

Stop-loss protection—Stop-loss protection means that if the costs to the provider exceed a specified amount, the provider will be reimbursed by the group or IPA for at least 90% of expenditures over that amount.

Structural bunion—A mild structural bunion occurs when the angle between the first and second metatarsal bones exceeds the normal angle.

Subjective findings—Subjective findings are feelings that cannot be discerned by anyone other than the patient.

Subpoena duces tecum—A subpoena duces tecum is a demand for a witness or a document to appear.

Subrogation—Subrogation, like ATPs, is a provision that is included in many benefit plans to allow the insurance company to recover money it has paid on claims incurred as a result of a third party's act or acts for which that party is financially responsible.

Supplemental adjustment—A supplemental adjustment increases the original claim payment. A statistical adjustment is often but not always involved as well, as the original claim coding may have caused the incorrect payment.

Surgery—Surgery is the branch of medicine that treats diseases, injuries, and deformities through operative or invasive methods. Surgery is anything that involves removing, altering, repairing, entering, or carrying out any other invasion of the body.

Take-home prescriptions—Take-home prescriptions are medications to be taken after the patient is released from the hospital.

Tax Equity and Fiscal Responsibility Act of 1982 (TEFRA)—The Tax Equity and Fiscal Responsibility Act of 1982 (TEFRA)—and the Deficit Reduction Act of 1984 (DEFRA) and amendments—have redirected the financial responsibility for medical coverage of active employees aged 65 years and older and their spouses aged 65 years and older.

Technical component (TC)—The taking of the specimen or X-ray is called the technical component (TC). It includes the expenses for the personnel performing the test and the cost of the necessary equipment.

Telemetry charges—Telemetry charges are charges for specialized observation equipment.

Temporary disability—Temporary disability claims are filed when the patient is not able to perform his or her job requirements until he or she recovers from the injury involved.

Tenotomy—A tenotomy and capsulotomy are performed to release the buckling of a toe by cutting the top and bottom tendons.

Termination date—The termination date of an insurance policy is the date on which coverage ceases.

Termination of coverage—Termination of coverage is a cessation of eligibility under the plan, however, coverage will often continue until the end of the month in which an employee terminates.

Therapeutic procedures—Therapeutic procedures are performed to remove or correct the functioning of a body part that is diseased or injured.

Third-party administrator (TPA)—A third-party administrator (TPA) is a professional firm that is under contract by the insurance company to deal solely with administering the eligibility and claim payment services, including all of the paperwork (and various other administrative services) for self-funded benefit plans.

Third-party liability (TPL)—Under third-party liability (TPL), the plan advances money to the injured person with the understanding that, if the claimant is successful in obtaining reimbursement from a third party, the claimant will reimburse the plan for its losses.

Topical anesthesia—Topical anesthesia is applied directly to the surface of the area to be anesthetized.

Treatment Authorization Request (TAR)—Most MCPs require that the provider or member obtain preauthorization for services which are the financial responsibility of the MCP. This is often done using a Treatment Authorization Request (TAR) form. The provider lists the diagnosis and proposed treatment plan along with any needed followup care, on the form.

TRICARE—TRICARE (formerly CHAMPUS) provides a comprehensive program of healthcare benefits for active duty and retired services personnel, their dependents, and the dependents of deceased military personnel.

Ultrasonography—Ultrasonography provides a more definitive type of picture than X-rays. Instead of using radiation, ultrasounds bounce sound waves off the desired structure to form a picture of the organ.

Unbundling—Unbundling (also called fragmentation or code splitting) refers to the practice of billing multiple procedure codes for a group of procedures that are covered by a single comprehensive code.

Uniform Bill-2004 (UB-04)—The Uniform Bill-2004 (UB-04) is a form that hospitals or hospital-type facilities use for inpatient and outpatient billing.

Unit value—The unit value is a numerical value assigned by a relative value study to a procedure code.

Unnecessary surgery—Unnecessary surgery is recommended as an elective procedure when an alternative method of treatment may be preferable for a number of reasons.

Unusual services—Unusual services are services that are rarely provided, unusual, or variable and that may warrant an additional anesthesia fee.

Urgent care center—An urgent care center is a facility that follows professionally recognized standards to provide urgent or emergency treatment.

Usual, customary, and reasonable (UCR) calculation—The unit value is multiplied by the conversion factor to determine the usual, customary, and reasonable (UCR) allowance or a basic allowance for medical services.

Van transportation units—Van transportation units are specially equipped to handle wheelchairs and patients who are unable to get in and out of a regular vehicle.

Version 4010/4010A—The 4010/4010A forms were the previous versions of the CMS-1500 form for outpatient services and the UB-04 for hospital or inpatient services.

Version 5010—The 5010 form is the current version of the CMS-1500 form and the UB-04 form.

Vocational rehabilitation—Many states provide employees with vocational rehabilitation or retraining in a different job field when the employees are unable to return to their former positions.

Voluntary program—A voluntary program encourages participants to obtain an SSO Consultation, but there is no automatic reduction of benefits if the patient does not comply.

Waiting period—If the insurance is a provision from an employer, there may be a waiting period before coverage begins (e.g., 30 days after date of hire).

Warts—Warts are skin growths caused by a virus and are contagious.

Withhold—The MCP may retain a withhold, a portion of the monthly capitation amount, to protect the HMO from inadequate patient care or financial management by the PCP.

Work hardening—Some states participate in a "work hardening" program, wherein an employee is assigned therapy similar to their work in an attempt to strengthen him or her and build up the individual's endurance toward a full day's work.

Workers' compensation (WC)—Workers' compensation (WC) is a separate medical and disability reimbursement program which provides 100% coverage for job-related injuries, illnesses, or conditions arising out of and in the course of employment.

X-rays—X-rays are created by sending low-level radiation through the body and capturing the resulting image on a sheet of film.

Zone Program Integrity Contractor (ZPIC)—Zone Program Integrity Contractor (ZPIC) is the latest auditing program paid by CMS and designed to look at billing trends and patterns of Medicare billing. The purpose of the ZPICs is to prevent waste, fraud, and abuse in the Medicare system.

Index

A

Abortion, 193
Accidental death and dismemberment insurance, 5
Accidental injury, 101
Accident benefits, 66, 101
Accumulation period, 95
Actively-at-work (active work), 65, 72
Acts of Third Parties (ATP), 78
Actuarial statistics, 6
Acupuncture, 166, 206
Adjudicated, 239
Adjustments, 152
Administrative sanctions, 17
Administrative Simplification and Compliance Act (ASCA) (2001), 129
Affordable Care Act. *See* Patient Protection and Affordable Care Act (2010)
Aggregate deductibles, 67, 97
Air ambulance, 177–178
Allergy and clinical immunology, 164
Allowed amount, 107
Alternative birthing centers (ABCs), 175
Alternative medicine treatment expenses, 67
Ambulance services, 177–178
Ambulatory/surgical centers, 175
American Recovery and Reinvestment Act (ARRA) (2009), 11, 267
Amniocentesis, 193
Anatomic pathology, 170
Ancillary expenses, 173
Anesthesia, 104, 166
    acupuncture, 166, 206
    allowance calculation, 208
    coding, 206
    general, 205, 211
    handling procedures, 206–207
    intravenous sedation, 166, 205–206
    medical direction of, 210
    monitored, 209–210
    pain control, 210
    qualifying circumstances, 209
    regional, 205
Anesthesiologist, hospital versus independent, 206
Anti-Kickback Statute, 17
Appendectomies, 188
Arthroplasty, 202
Artificial insemination, 193
Assignment of Benefits form, 130, 141, 219–220
Assistant surgery/surgeons, 104, 199–200, 204, 358
Attorneys, communicating with, 127
Auditory system, 188
Audits
    certificate of compliance agreement, 270–272
    of findings, 270
    Medicaid Fraud Control Units, 269
    Medicare final, 294–299
    Medicare postaudit review, 299–303
    phases, 269–270
    Recovery Audit Contractors, 269
    role of, 269
    scope, 269–270
    self-disclosure protocol, 273
    Zone Program Integrity Contractor, 269
Authorization to Release Information form, 130
Automatic Annual Reinstatement, 96

B

Bad faith awards, 20
Balance billing, 219
Basic benefits
    calculating, 100–104
    description of, 66–67, 101–104
    order of payments, 104
Batch files, 126
Beneficiary, 71
Benefit calculations
    automatic annual reinstatement, 96
    basic, 100–104
    coinsurance, 96
    copayments, 97
    major medical, 104–106
    out-of-pocket costs, 97
    worksheets, 330–332
Benefit period, 217
Benefits, 3
    accumulation period, 95
    basic, 66–67, 100–104
    coordination of, 145–149
    covered expenses, 95
    extension of, 73–74, 96
    loss date, 96
    major medical, 67–68, 104–106
    maximums, 96
    out-of-pocket costs, 67, 96
    per period of disability, 96
    unit value, 96
Bilateral procedures, 190
Billing for services rendered, 276
Biofeedback, 163
Blepharoplasty, 194–195
Block procedures, 191–192
Blue Book, 25, 30, 142
Bone marrow transplants, 187–188
Bone spurs, 202–203
Breast surgical procedures, 195, 196–197
Bunions, 201–202
By report (NR) procedures, 190

C

Capitation payments, 252
Capsulotomy, 202
Cardiovascular services, 164, 187
Care plan oversight services, 161
Carryover deductibles, 67, 98
Case management services, 161
Cataract surgery, 188
Category II and III codes, 167
Central nervous system assessments/tests, 164
Certificate of compliance agreement, 270–272
Cheiloplasty, 195
Chemical peels/abrasion, 195
Chemistry, 170
Chemotherapy administration, 165
Chiropractic treatment, 166
Chromosomal analysis, 193
Civil monetary penalties (CMPs), 17–18
Claim files
    batch, 126
    defined, 126
    family financial, 126
    member, 126
Claims, 4
    See also Auditing; Coordination of benefits (COB);
        Electronic claims; Medicare claims; Prescription drug
        claims; Workers' compensation claims
    adjustments, 152
    Assignment of Benefits form, 130, 141
    committee review of, 277
    coordination of benefits, 145–149
    denial, common reasons for, 92, 344
    denials, ERISA and, 141
    denials, request for copy of, 335
    documentation to substantiate, 126–127
    dual coverage, recognizing, 150
    examining, 281
    Explanation of Benefits (EOB) form, 147
    Family Benefits Tracking Sheet, 142, 144
    files, maintenance of, 125–126
    Inventory/Production Sheet, 142, 143
    investigations, 128
    mutually exclusive code pairs, 133
    overpayments, collecting, 152–154
    payees, determining, 141
    payment history, updating, 141–142
    payment worksheet, 134, 135–136, 138–141, 142
    pending, 128–129
    processing, 129–133, 275–285
    remarks list, 345–346
    request for more information, 335
    Right of Reimbursement Claims Log, 82–84
    tracking, 126
    unbundling of services, 133
Claims auditing. *See* Auditing
Claims examiners
    duties of, 7–8, 128
    referrals, 128, 129
Cleft lip/palate, 196, 197
Clinton, B., 11, 87
CMS-1500 form, 8
    claim processing using, 134
    example of, 31, 137, 138, 323–328
    illness information, 32–33
    insured information, 32
    patient information, 32
    place of service codes, 34–36
    procedures performed information, 33
    provider of services information, 33
    secondary insurance information, 32
    signatures, authorized, 32
    third-party liability information, 32
    Version 5010, 37
COBRA (Consolidated Omnibus Budget Reconciliation Act) (1985), 73
    applicability, 75
    duration of coverage, 75
    eligibility notification, 75–77
    premium payments, 77
    qualified beneficiaries, 75
    qualifying event, 75
    termination of coverage, 77
    Title X, 74
Coding. *See* Current Procedural Terminology (CPT)
Coinsurance
    calculating, 96
    defined, 67
    limits, 67
Collagen injections, 196
Committee review of claims, 277
Common accident provision, 98
Company activities, 234
Compensatory damages, 20
Compliance education, 270–272
Compliance plan, 270
Component charges, 171
Computed tomography (CT) scans, 168
Concurrent review, 117
Confirmatory consultations, 160
Congenital abnormalities, 196
Conscious sedation, 166
Consideration, 64
Consultations, 159–160, 170
Continuation of coverage, 73–77
Contracts
    basic benefits, 66–67
    benefits of written, 63
    continuation of coverage, 73–77
    effective date, 65
    eligibility, 65, 69–72
    enrollment, 71–72, 73
    examples of, 316–321
    exclusions, 68
    group, 64
    major medical benefits, 67–68
    provisions, 65, 78
    termination of coverage, 65, 73
    validity of, 63–64
Contributory plan, 71
Convalescent facilities, 176
Conventional insurance, 6
Conversion factor, 96
Conversion policies, 74
Coordination of benefits (COB)
    calculation worksheet, 151
    definitions and example of, 146–147
    Medicare, 220–226
    order of benefit determination rules, 148
    reason for, 145–146
    right of recovery, 148–149
    right to receive and release information, 148
Copayments
    calculating, 97
    defined, 67
Corporate Integrity Agreements (CIAs), 267
Corrective actions, 270
Cosmetic surgery, 186–187, 194–198

Cost containment programs, 115
    preadmission testing, 116
    preauthorization, 116
    precertification, 117
    predetermination, 116
    second surgical opinion consultations, 117–118
    utilization review, 117
Cosurgeons, 199
Covered expenses, 95
Critical care services, 160
Cumulative benefits, 103
Current Dental Terminology (CDT), 25
Current Procedural Terminology (CPT), 25, 26–27
    anesthesia, 206
    care plan oversight services, 161
    case management services, 161
    consultations, 159–160, 170
    critical care services, 160
    custodial care services, 161
    dialysis, 163
    disability services, 162
    emergency department services, 160
    home services, 161
    hospital inpatient services, 159
    hospital observation services, 159
    newborn care services, 162
    non-face-to-face physician services, 162
    nursing facility services, 161
    office/outpatient services, 159
    pathology, 169–171
    preventive medicine services, 161–162
    prolonged services, 161
    second surgical opinions, 160
Current Procedural Terminology, Medicine section
    acupuncture, 166
    allergy and clinical immunology, 164
    anesthesia, 166
    biofeedback, 163
    cardiovascular services, 164
    Category II and III codes, 167
    central nervous system assessments/tests, 164
    chemotherapy administration, 165
    chiropractic treatment, 166
    conscious sedation, 166
    dermatological procedures, 165
    education and training, 166
    endocrinology services, 164
    gastroenterology, 163
    health/behavior assessments/interventions, 165
    home health services, 166
    home infusion services, 166
    immune globulins, immunizations, vaccines/toxoids,
        162–163
    list of, 162
    medication management services, 166
    neurology and neuromuscular procedures, 164
    non-face-to-face nonphysician services, 166
    nutrition therapy, 165
    ophthalmological services, 163–164
    osteopathic treatment, 166
    otorhinolaryngologic services, 164
    photodynamic therapy, 165
    physical medicine and rehabilitation services, 165
    psychiatry, 163
    pulmonary services, 164
    radiology services, 168–169
    X-ray and laboratory services, 168–169
Current Procedural Terminology, surgery
    auditory system, 188
    cardiovascular system, 187
    digestive system, 188
    endocrine system, 188
    eye and ocular adnexa, 188
    female genital system, 188
    gender designated, 191
    hemic and lymphatic systems, 187–188
    integumentary system, 187
    intersex surgery, 188
    list of, 187
    male genital system, 188
    maternity care and delivery, 188, 192–194
    mediastinum and diaphragm, 188
    musculoskeletal system, 187
    nervous system, 188
    operating microscope, 188
    podiatry, 200–204

    respiratory system, 187
    urinary system, 188
Custodial care services, 161
Cytogenetic services, 170
Cytopathology, 170

D

Day care centers, 174
Death benefit, 236
Deductibles
    calculating, 97–98
    carryover, 98
    common accident provision, 98
    types of, 67
Deficit Reduction Act (DEFRA) (1984), 216
Dental insurance, 7
Dependent eligibility, 70–71, 72
Dermabrasion, 196
Dermatological procedures, 165
Diagnosis-related group (DRG) billing, 226–227
Diagnostic X-rays and laboratory (DXL) services,
    102, 168
Dialysis, 163, 216
Digestive system, 188
Disability claims, workers' compensation, 235–236
Disability insurance, 5
Disability services, 162
Disclaimers, legal issues and, 10–11
Doctor's First Report, 235, 237, 238, 307–308
Documentation to substantiate claims, 126–127
Dorsal osteotomy, 202
Drug assays, therapeutic, 170
Drug testing, 170
Dual coverage, recognizing, 150
Durable Medical Equipment (DME)
    billing procedures, 178–180
    coverage guidelines, 347–355
Dwyer procedure, 202

E

Education and training, 166
Effective date of coverage, 3, 65, 72
Electrolysis epilation, 196
Electronic claims
    See also Claims
    Assignment of Benefits form, 130, 141
    Authorization to Release Information form, 130
    processing, 129–133
    submission, 129
Electronic Data Interchange (EDI), 8, 14, 129
Electronic health records (EHRs), privacy issues, 11
Electronic Remittance Notice (ERN), 215
Electronic transmission of health information, 14
Eligibility requirements, 3, 65, 69–72
Eligibility roster, 258
Email, use of, 14
Embezzlement, 19
Emergency department services, 160, 178
Emergency Medical Technicians (EMTs), 178
Employee benefits, 6
Employee eligibility, 69
Employment Retirement Income Security Act (ERISA)
    (1974), 141
Encounter forms, use of, 288–294
Endocrinology services, 164, 188
Endoscopies, 188
End-stage renal disease (ESRD), 216
Enrollment, 71–72, 73
Epidural anesthesia, 205, 211
Evidence of insurability, 71–72
Exclusions, 68
Exclusive provider organizations (EPOs), 119
Explanation of Benefits (EOB) form, 147
Extension of benefits, 73–74, 96
Eye and ocular adnexa, 188

F

Facelift, 197
Facility services, 158
False Claims Act (2009), 17
Family Benefits Tracking Sheet, 142, 144
Family deductibles, 67
Family financial file, 126
Family tracking form, 334
Faxing, 14

Fees
    physician fees, formulas for determining, 114–115
    physician fee schedules, RVUs for, 107–112
    professional, 174
    schedules, 115, 116
Female genital system, 188
Fertilization, 193
Fetal surgery, 193
First Report, 235, 237, 238, 307–308
Flat feet, 203
Followup days, 189–190
Fraud
    case, establishing a, 15, 18
    defined, 14
    forms of, 15
    indicators of, 15–17
    investigating, 18–19
    legal issues and, 14–19
    Medicaid, 269
    Medicare, 269
    workers' compensation, 239–240
Fraud Enforcement and Recovery Act (FERA)
    (2009), 17
Full-credit adjustments, 152

G

Ganglions, 203
Gastroenterology, 163
Gatekeeper PPO, 119
Gender designated surgery, 191
Geographical Process Cost Index (GPCI),
    112–114
Global approach, 191
Grievance systems, 91–92
Group contracts, 64
Group insurance, 5–6

H

Hair transplantation, 196
Hammertoes, 202
Health/behavior assessments/interventions, 165
Health Care Common Procedure Coding System
    (HCPCS), 25, 27–28
Healthcare costs, rising, 4–5
Health Care Reform, 78
Health information, electronic transmission of, 14
Health Information Technology for Economic and Clinical
    Health Act (HITECH), 11, 13, 14, 129
Health insurance
    defined, 5
    types of plans, 6–7
Health Insurance Portability and Accountability Act
    (HIPAA) (1996)
    credible coverage, 88
    development of, 11, 87
    fraud issues, 17
    maximum periods, 89
    preexisting conditions, 87–89
    pregnancies, newborns, adopted children, 89
    prior coverage credit, 88
    prior notification, 88
    privacy issues, 11, 13, 14
Health maintenance organizations (HMOs)
    closed panel, 7
    coordination of benefits, 149
    coverage, 249–250
    fees, 118–119
    group model, 247, 248
    individual practice organizations, 248–249
    network model, 249
    open access, 7
    staff model, 247–248
Heel spurs, 202
Hematology and coagulation, 170
Hemic and lymphatic systems, 187–188
Hernia repair, 188
High-arched feet, 203
HIPAA. *See* Health Insurance Portability and
    Accountability Act
HITECH. *See* Health Information Technology for
    Economic and Clinical Health Act
Home health services, 166
Home infusion services, 166
Home services, 161
Hospice care, 176

Hospital benefits, 102–103
Hospital services/charges
  inpatient charges, 173–174
  inpatient services, 159
  observation services, 159
  outpatient charges, 174
  typical, 172
Hypnosis, 206
Hysteroscopy, 188

I

ICD-9-CM (International Classification of Diseases-9th Revision-Clinical Modification), 25–26
ICD-10-CM/PCS (International Classification of Diseases-10th Revision-Clinical Modification/Procedure Coding System), 25, 26
Immune globulins, 162–163
Immunizations, 162–163
Immunology, 170
Indemnity plans, 6–7
Independent physician associations (IPAs), 250–252
Individual deductibles, 67, 97
Individual insurance, 5–6
Individual practice organizations (IPOs), 248–249
Infusion pump, 210
Ingrown toenails, 203
Injuries
  accidental, 101
  nonaccidental, 102
In-network providers, 118
Inpatient hospital charges, 173–174
Inspector General Act (1978), 267
Insurance
  conventional, 6
  defined, 3
  individual versus group, 5–6
  self-funded plans, 6
  terms, 3
  types of, 5–6
Insurance carrier, 64
Insurance company, 64
Insurance identification card, 3, 4
Insurance policies
  See also Contracts
  conversion, 74
  defined, 3, 19
Insurance speculation indicators, 16
Insured, 64
Integumentary system, 187
Intermediaries, 217
International Classification of Diseases-9th Revision-Clinical Modification. *See* ICD-9-CM
International Classification of Diseases-10th Revision-Clinical Modification/Procedure Coding System. *See* ICD-10-CM/PCS
Intersex surgery, 188
Intravenous (IV) sedation, 166, 205–206
Inventory/Production Sheet, 142, 143
Investigating fraud, 18–19
In vitro fertilization, 193
In vivo services, 170

J

Job-related injuries, 233

K

Keloid removal, 196

L

Laboratory services, 168
Laparoscopy, 188
Lapse in coverage, 3
Laws
  mandates, 90–91
  prompt-pay laws, 91
Legal damages, 19–20
Legal issues
  disclaimers and, 10–11
  fraud and, 14–19
  privacy guidelines, 11–14
  subpoenas duces tecum and notification, 21
Lesions, 187
Liens, 240–243
Life insurance, 5
Lifetime maximum, 67
Limiting charges, 220

Lipectomy, 196, 198
Look-back time, 88
Loss date, 96
Lymphatic system, 187–188

M

Maintenance of benefits, 222
Major medical benefits
  calculating, 104–106
  comprehensive, 105
  description of, 67–68
Male genital system, 188
Malice, 20
Mammoplasty, 196
Managed care
  appeals, 262
  billing for services, 253
  capitation payments, 252
  claim payments, 258–259
  claim processing, 259–261
  defined, 118
  denial of service/claim, 257, 261–262
  exclusive provider organizations, 119
  gatekeeper PPO, 119
  health maintenance organizations, 118–119, 247–250
  management service organizations, 119
  medical groups/independent physician associations, 250–252
  outpatient surgery, 257
  physician hospital organizations, 119
  preauthorization, 253, 255–256
  preferred provider organizations, 118, 250
  prescription coverage, 257–258
  referrals, 256
  second opinions, 256–257
  stop-loss, 262
  utilization review, 256
Management service organizations (MSOs), 119
Mandates, 90–91
Mastectomy, 196–197
Master contract, 5
Maternity care and delivery, 188, 192–194
Maximums, 96
Mediastinum and diaphragm, 188
Medicaid, 5, 227
Medicaid Fraud Control Units (MFCUs), 269
Medical billers, duties of, 8, 128
Medical Case Management (MCM), 119
  claims, 356–357
Medical dictionaries, 29
Medical groups, 250–252
Medically oriented equipment, 178
Medical plan provisions. *See* Contracts
Medical record release form, 12
Medical while hospitalized (MWH), 102–103
Medicare
  allowance, 219
  Assignment of Benefits form, 219–220
  coordination of benefits, 220–226
  diagnosis-related group billing, 226–227
  eligibility, 216
  formation of, 5, 215
  fraud, 269
  limiting charges, 220
  Part A, 217–218
  Part B, 217, 218
  Part C, 217, 218–219
  Part D, 217, 219
  participating physicians, 219–220
  payments, calculating, 226
  payments based on reasonable charges, 219
  providers of service, 216–217
  secondary payer rules, 223
  supplements, 226
Medicare claims
  electronic billing and tracking, 303
  encounter forms, use of, 288–294
  evaluation and management coding, 287–288
  final audit, 294–299
  postaudit review, 299–303
  supplemental information requests, 304
Medicare Prescription Drug, Improvement, and Modernization Act (2003), 217, 219
Medicare Remittance Advice, 215
Medicare Remittance Notice (MRN), 215
Medicare Summary Notice (MSN), 215

Medication management services, 166
Medigap, 226
Member, 64
Member files, 126
Mental health and substance abuse treatment expenses, 67
Mentoplasty/genioplasty, 197
Merck Manual, 25, 29, 87
Microbiology, 170
Miscellaneous services, 159
Mobile intensive care unit, 178
Modifiers, 27
  evaluation/management with medicine codes, 167–168, 169
  optional, 208
  pathology, 172
  physical status, 208
  radiology, 169
  surgery, 205
Moles, 198
Monitored anesthesia care (MAC), 209–210
Multiple procedures, 190
Musculoskeletal system, 187
Mutually exclusive code pairs, 133

N

National Council for Prescription Drug Program (NCPDP), 37
National Uniform Billing Committee (NUBC), 37
Nerve block anesthesia, 205
Nervous system, 188
Neurology and neuromuscular procedures, 164
Neuromas, 203
Newborn care services, 162
Night care centers, 174
Nonaccidental injuries, 102
Nonaggregate deductibles, 67, 97
Noncontributory plan, 71
Nondisability claims, 235
Nonparticipating physicians, 220
Nuclear medicine, 169
Nursing facility/home services, 161, 176
Nutrition therapy, 165

O

Obama, B., 78, 90
Obesity, surgery, 198–199
Occupational illnesses, 233, 234–235
Office of the Inspector General (OIG), 17–18, 267–268
Office visits, 104, 159
Open enrollment, 73
Open letters, 267, 268
Operating microscope, 188
Ophthalmological services, 163–164
Oppression, 20
Order of Benefit Determination (OBD) rules, 148
Orthoptics, 164
Orthotic devices, 203
Osteopathic treatment, 166
Osteotomy procedures, 202
Otoplasty, 197
Otorhinolaryngologic services, 164
Outliers, 226–227
Out-of-network providers, 118
Out-of-pocket costs (OOP)
  calculating, 97
  defined, 67
  maximum, 96
Outpatient facility charges, 66–67, 174
Outpatient services, 159
Overinsurance, 145–146
Overpayments, collecting, 152–154
Oxygen use, 180

P

Pain control, 210
Panel tests, 169
Pap (papanicolaou) smear, 171
Paramedics, 178
Partial-credit adjustments, 152
Participating physicians, 219–220
Pathology codes/modifiers, 169–172
Patient bill example, 333
Patient Protection and Affordable Care Act (2010), 66, 67, 68, 78, 90, 101, 132
Payment history, updating, 141–142

Payment worksheet
  description and steps for, 134, 135–136, 138–141
  quick reference formulas, 142
Pelvic examinations, 188
Pended, 8
Pending claims, 128–129
Permanent disability claims, 236
Per period of disability, 96
Personal Health Information (PHI), electronic
    transmission of, 14
Personal items, 174
Per-visit benefits, 103
Photodynamic therapy, 165
Physical medicine and rehabilitation services, 165
Physician fees, formulas for determining, 114–115
Physician fee schedules, RVUs for, 107–112
Physician hospital organizations (PHOs), 119
Physicians' Desk Reference (PDR), 25, 28–29, 142
Physician's Final Report, 237, 239
Physician's first report of occupational injury or illness, 336
Plantar calluses, 202
Podiatry, surgery codes, 200–204
Point-of-service (POS) plans, 7
Policies. *See* Contracts
Postaudit review, 299–303
Preadmission testing (PAT), 66, 116
Preauthorization, 116, 253, 255–256
Precertification, 117
Predetermination, 116
Preexisting conditions
  defined, 68, 85
  handling, 85–87
  HIPAA and, 87–89
  workers' compensation and, 243
Preferred provider organizations (PPOs), 7, 118, 250
  coordination of benefits, 149
  Explanation of Benefits, 149
Premiums, 3
Prescription drug claims
  Blue Book, 25, 30, 142
  criteria drugs must meet, 142
  determining payment, 145
  outpatient guidelines, 145
  Red Book, 25, 30, 142
  take-home, 173–174
Prescription drug insurance 7
Preventative care services, 91, 101, 161–162, 249
Primary care provider/physician (PCP), 247
Privacy guidelines, 11–14
  workers' compensation and, 236–239
Procedure codes, 26–27
Professional services, 158
Prolonged services, 161
Prompt-pay laws, 91
Prosthetic devices, 180
Providers
  in-network, 118
  out-of-network, 118
Psychiatry, 163
Public Health Service Act (PHSA), 74, 75
Pulmonary services, 164
Punitive damages, 20

Q
Qualified beneficiaries, 75
Qualifying event, 75

R
Radiation oncology, 169
Radiology services, 168–169
Railroad Retirement benefits, 216
RAT-STATS, 270
Reagan, R., 74
Reasonable charges, 219

Rebundling, 133
Record keeping, 20–21
Recovery Audit Contractors (RACs), 269
Red Book, 25, 30, 142
Reexamination report, 237
Referrals, 128, 129, 256
Rehabilitation benefit, 236
Rehabilitation facilities, 176
Reimbursement
  payment worksheet, 134, 135–136, 138–141
  Right of Reimbursement Claims Log, 82–84
Reinstated, 3
Reinsurance, 6, 262
Relative Value Scale (RVS), 25, 27, 104, 206, 339–341
Relative Value Units (RVUs)
  for physician fee schedules, 107–112
Renewal, 3
Reproductive procedures, 171
Respiratory system, 187
Retrospective review, 117
Rhinoplasty, 197
Rhytidoplasty, 197
Right of Reimbursement Claims Log, 82–84

S
Saddle block, 205
Second opinions, 66, 117–118, 160, 256–257
Self-disclosure protocol (SDP), 273
Self-funded plans, 6
Separate procedures, 134
Septoplasty, 197–198
Signatures, authorized, 32, 130
Skin grafts, 187
Social Security Disability, 216
Speech therapy, 164
Spinal anesthesia, 205
State insurance regulatory department, 9–10
State mandates, 90–91
Stat fees, 160
Statistical adjustments, 152
Statistical sampling, 270
Stem cell transplants, 187–188
Sterilization, 193–194
Stop-loss insurance, 6, 105–106, 262
Subjective findings, 237
Subpoena notification, 21
Subpoenas duces tecum, 21
Subrogation, 78, 84–85
Suicides, attempted, 102
Supplemental adjustments, 152
Surgeons
  assistant, 199–200, 204, 358
  co-, 199
Surgery
  See also Current Procedural Terminology, surgery
  ambulatory/surgi centers, 175
  cosmetic, 186–187, 194–198
  diagnostic procedures, 186
  followup days, 189–190
  modifiers, 205
  multiple/bilateral procedures, 190
  obesity, 198–199
  pathology codes, 170
  in physician's office, 189
  preoperative care, 189
  reconstructive, 186
  therapeutic procedures, 186
  unnecessary, 118
  while hospitalized, 103–104

T
Take-home prescriptions, 173–174
Tax Equity and Fiscal Responsibility Act (TEFRA)
    (1982), 216

Taylor's procedure, 202
Telemetry charges, 173
Telephone information sheet, 127
Temporary disability claims, 236
Temporomandibular joint surgery, 198
Tenotomy, 202
Termination date, 3
Termination of coverage, 65, 73
Third-Party Administrators (TPAs), 6
Third-Party Liability (TPL), 78–82
Three-month carryover, 98
Toxoids, 162–163
Transfusions, 170
Transplants, bone marrow/stem cell, 187–188
Treatment Authorization Request (TAR),
    253, 255
TRICARE, 5
  Explanation of Benefits, 149–150
Tubal ligation, 193–194

U
UB-04 (Uniform Billing Form 2004), 37
  example of, 38, 329
  form locator number, name and description,
    37, 51, 55–57
  hospital form locator codes, 51–55
  hospital revenue codes, 39–50
  reviewing, 172–177
Ultrasound, 168–169
Unbundling of services, 133, 192
Unit value, 96
Unnecessary surgery, 118
Unusual circumstances, 208–209
Urgent care centers, 175
Urinalysis, 170
Urinary system, 188
Usual, customary, and reasonable (UCR) charges, 67
  calculating, 106–107
  conversion factor report, 342–343
  global, 191
Utilization review (UR), 117, 256

V
Vaccines, 162–163
Van transportation units, 178
Version 5010, 37
Vision insurance, 7

W
Waiting period, 3
Warts/moles removal, 198, 203
Women's services, 91
Workers' compensation, 5, 233
  employee activities, 234–235
  fraud and abuse, 239–240
  liens, 240–243
  privacy in processing, 236–239
  reversals, 243–244
  types of claims, 235–236
Workers' compensation claims
  billing requirements, 307
  clean claims criteria, 311–312
  doctor's First Report, 235, 237, 238, 307–308
  investigating, 310–311
  progress reports and termination of treatment,
    309–310, 337
Work hardening, 236

X
X-ray services, 168–169

Z
Zone Program Integrity Contractor (ZPIC), 269